CRC Handbook of Management of Radiation Protection Programs

Editors

Kenneth L. Miller
Health Physics Office
Milton S. Hershey Medical Center
Hershey, Pennsylvania

William A. Weidner
Department of Radiology
Pennsylvania State University
Hershey Medical Center
Hershey, Pennsylvania

CRC Series in Radiation Measurement and Protection
Editor-in-Chief

Allen Brodsky
Certified American Board of Health Physics
American Board of Radiology
American Board of Industrial Hygiene

CRC Press, Inc.
Boca Raton, Florida

Library of Congress Cataloging in Publication Data
Main entry under title:

CRC handbook of management of radiation protection programs.

(CRC series in radiation measurement and protection)
Bibliography: p.
Includes index.
1. Radiation—Safety measures—Handbooks, manuals, etc. I. Miller, Kenneth L. II. Weidner, William A. III. Title: C.R.C. handbook of management of radiation protection programs. IV. Title: Handbook of management of radiation protection. V. Series.
RA569.C86 1986 363.1′79 84-21461
ISBN 0-8493-3769-0

Direct all inquiries to CRC Press, Inc., 2000 Corporate Blvd., N.W., Boca Raton, Florida, 33431.

International Standard Book Number 0-8493-3769-0

Library of Congress Card Number 84-21461

Printed in the United States

SERIES PREFACE

The purpose of this handbook series is to provide data and methods for dealing with the design and evaluation of radiation measurement instruments; monitoring and survey methods; selection of protective facilities, equipment and procedures for handling radioactive materials; effluent control and monitoring; radioactive waste diposal; transportation of radioactive materials; and many other related subjects. Aspects of these subjects involve not only all of the sciences but also management, legal, insurance, and public information considerations. The sciences themselves include the entire range of basic scientific and engineering methods, as broad a range as in the entire field of public health itself. This series of volumes will be divided as far as possible into logical groupings that hopefully will tend to maximize the usefulness of each volume, as well as the series of volumes, to its users.

The primary aim of the handbook series will be to include as much useful data as possible for the specialist needing ready access for the solution of problems most likely to arise in the radiation protection professions. However, some selected review of fundamental concepts is also included to enable persons with a basic science or engineering background to acquire the necessary knowledge to solve a majority of problems in especially important aspects of radiation protection. Also, since the profession is broad in discipline, an attempt has been made to fulfill the frequent need of professionals for a refresher course in some of the more important fundamentals needed to utilize data included in the handbook. Principles of management, organization, and procedures related to radiation safety are also summarized in this and later volumes, with attention to presentation of methods for establishing new radiation safety programs based on the accumulated experience of others.

This series of volumes should, therefore, be useful in industrial, academic, medical, and governmental institutions and to scientists carrying out both applied and basic research in subjects related to radiation protection, to engineers designing protective facilities and equipment, to applied health physicists establishing radiation safety programs, to physicians involved with caring for patients exposed to radiation or radioactive materials, to public health and other government officials concerned with regulating radiation safety and developing national standards, to professors and students studying and synthesizing a broad base of knowledge in radiation protection, and to practically every other type of professional involved in radiation protection problems. The editor and publisher hope that the many users will offer continued suggestions for improving these volumes and for including data that will make them more useful.

A general acknowledgement of gratitude must be made to the advisory board, to the contributors, and to the authors and publishers who have granted permission to include material in this series. Contributors of the sections in this series have been selected for their professional knowledge in the respective subject areas, and in most cases have generously devoted their own personal time to this effort without monetary compensation. Material included in this handbook series was selected according to the professional opinions of authors, compilers, and editors and does not necessarily reflect any official sanction of the agencies or companies with which the contributors are employed. Addresses indicated for the contributors are for identification and correspondence purposes only. The collective responsibility for the total content lies, of course, with the editor, who is solely responsible for any omissions either from inadvertence or necessity.

On the other hand, the editor has purposely built in some redundancy of certain important types of data, since it is advisable to cross-check values obtained from different literature sources or approaches. The editor has also, to some degree, allowed repetition of similar data in different sections of the handbook where it was deemed advisable for the continuity of individual sections or for the convenience of the user due to the need for frequent cross reference between text and data. In cases where the users intend to rely on a tabulated or calculated value for the protection of humans, it is, of course, necessary to arrive at values in different ways in order to not only avoid inadvertent mistakes but also to ensure better understanding of the degree of reliability or range of uncertainty of the end result. Frequently, in radiation protection design as in general engineering practice, factors of safety must be included that are based on knowledge of the ranges of uncertainty in estimated risks. A further purpose of the redundance of sources is also to include older as well as newer approaches in cases where the changes themselves may be of interest in evaluating the need for protective actions or changes in regulations or policies.

The editor is grateful to CRC Press for generally providing an outstanding facility and staff for the publication of data and reference sources currently needed in science and technology. The publishers, Bernard, Florence, and Earl Starkoff have also given invaluable guidance in determing the philosophy, scope, and organization of this handbook series. Their continued enthusiam and encouragement has been an inspiration to the editor. Gerald A. Becker, Editorial Director when the project began, also provided early inspirational leadership in developing the concepts and format of this series. Kay Harter was helpful in the initial administration of this series. The editor would also like to acknowledge the invitation of Professors Niel Wald and Yen Wang to contribute to the CRC Handbook of Radioactive Nuclides; reprinting of some of the editor's sections from the above handbook ultimately inspired the development of this handbook series. Special mention should be made of the continued interest and able assistance with this series given over the years by Paul Gottehrer, Senior Editor, and Sandy Pearlman, Managing Editor.

Allen Brodsky
Editor-in-Chief
Derwood, Maryland
May 1984

PREFACE

This volume provides a continuation of the *CRC Handbook of Radiation Measurement and Protection* series. Its emphasis is on various aspects of radiation safety from the regulatory or management standpoint. A great deal of the material included in this volume could come under the category of "lessons learned"; either lessons learned through early mistakes, radiation litigations, or in the aftermath of the Three Mile Accident.

In this volume, Vincent Collins provides a unique historical evaluation of radiation litigations from both the scientific and legalistic view point. His section provides a comprehensive documentation that ranges from the first case to more recent cases, including some in which the final outcome is still pending. His section should be of interest to everyone, and especially those who may have occasion to appear as a professional witness. Ron Kathren and Barbara Matthews have reviewed the public relations responsibilities in Health Physics and offer unique insights into the public perception of radiation risk. They also review the correct procedures for dealing with and responding to the news media. Ken Miller has documented a number of uniquely different perspectives on public information from the Health Physicists' and the journalists' point of view.

Ed Durkosh and Ken Miller's section on the organization and management of a radiation safety office provides a checklist of basic considerations and requirements for establishment of, or evaluation of a radiation safety program. Bill Allen has done the same with special emphasis on the management of radioactive waste. His section also reviews the changes in regulations governing low level radioactive waste disposal.

Bob Gallagher has called upon his many years of experience in responding to various radiation emergencies to develop his section on radiation emergency control procedures for minimizing damage. His checklists of appropriate actions are an invaluable resource for anyone responding to a radiation emergency situation. The accidents at Three Mile Island and elsewhere have taught us about the need for approriate preparation for and response to such accidents when the need arises. Syd Porter reviews these lessons learned and gives us guidance for improved response to future emergencies. Ideally, one would be able to predetermine every conceivable situation that could arise in a nuclear power plant accident and preplan appropriately for each situation. Jim Martins' section on predetermined actions for predetermined conditions does just that while his section on release characteristics and consequences covers the entire spectrum of possible releases following an accident at a light water nuclear power plant.

Frank Bradley has done a thorough review of the cumbersome regulations and requirements relating to transportation of radioactive materials. He has analyzed these requirements and presents them in a manageable format. His treatise of the subject should be refreshing for anyone who has ever been entangled in the jungle of regulations governing the subject.

We hope this volume will add usefully to this Handbook series.

The Editors are indebted to the contributors for their willingness to share this wealth of information.

Kenneth L. Miller
William A. Weidner

THE-EDITOR-IN-CHIEF

Dr. Allen Brodsky has a broad professional background and interest in the scientific, engineering, and management aspects of radiation protection. After graduation with a B.E. in Chemical Engineering (Johns Hopkins University) and 1 year of postgraduate study in Radiological Physics at the Oak Ridge National Laboratory, his broad career in health physics and radiation measurements pinpointed the need for further study, which led to the degrees of M.A. in Physics (Johns Hopkins University) and Sc.D. in Biostatistics and Radiation Health (University of Pittsburgh). He is also certified by the American Board of Health Physics, The American Board of Industrial Hygiene, and the American Board of Radiology.

In addition to his education, positions as Physicist and Health Physicist, Naval Research Laboratory; Radiological Defense Officer, Federal Civil Defense Administration: Health Physicist, U. S. Atomic Energy Commision: Associate Professor of Health Physics, University of Pittsburgh: Radiation Therapy Physicist and Radiation Safety Officer, Mercy Hospital; and Adjunct Research Professor, School of Pharmacy, Duquesne University stimulated his interest in the need for readily available data to solve radiation measurement and protection problems, and to design facilities, equipment, and procedures for the safe handling of radiation sources and radioactive materials.

The Editor's research interests include the development of radiation measurement and dosimetry methods, hazard evaluation, facility design, methodology for health and mortality follow-up of radiation workers, and the theory of cancer induction by environmental agents. His present position at the U.S. Nuclear Regulatory Commision involves the development of guides for radiation protection in medical institutions, industry, and universities.

The editor welcomes suggestions or offers of further contributions of data for the handbook series at the following address:

Dr. Allen Brodsky
P.O. Box 34471
West Bethesda, MD 20817

THE EDITORS

Kenneth L. Miller received his B.S. degree in Education, with majors in mathematics, physics and general science, in 1965 from the Lock Haven State College in Lock Haven, Pennsylvania. After a year of teaching high school he accepted a position as Health Physics Assistant at the Pennsylvania State University. In 1969, he was awarded a Public Health Service Fellowship from the University of Pittsburgh's Graduate School of Public Health. Upon receiving his M.S. degree in 1970, he returned to Penn State as Associate Health Physicist. In 1971, he accepted appointment as Director of Health Physics and Research Associate at The Milton S. Hershey Medical Center of The Pennsylvania State University.

Mr. Miller developed the radiation safety program at the Hershey Medical Center and has been very active in the development of education and research programs dealing with various aspects of radiation protection. His research endeavors are practical in nature and deal primarily with applied health physics. His interests and research have led to presentation of over 100 papers and scientific exhibits at national and international meetings and publication of nearly half that many papers, chapters for books, and booklets. Ken now serves as Director, Division of Health Physics and Associate Professor of Radiology. He is certified in Health Physics by the American Board of Health Physics. He is active in numerous professional societies, and received the 1982 Elda E. Anderson Award from the Health Physics Society.

William A. Weidner has a broad professional background in Radiology and the administration and management of Radiology departments. His undergraduate and graduate training were received at the University of Wisconsin where he was awarded an M.D. degree in 1952. He served a rotating internship at the Medical College of Virginia and was a flight surgeon in the U. S. Navy from 1953 to 1956.

After a year of general surgery, he began his residency in Radiology at the Los Angeles County-USC Medical Center in Los Angeles in 1958 and after completion of his residency, was the first NIH Fellow in neuroradiology at UCLA in 1963. He was appointed Chief Radiologist at Harbor General Hospital in 1965 and through his contact with Dr. George Taplin, and an appointment in the Laboratory of Nuclear Medicine and Radiation Biology at UCLA, developed an interest in radiation protection programs. He was Chairman of Diagnostic Radiology at the Medical College of Virginia in 1968 and in 1971 was appointed the first Professor and Chairman of the Department of Radiology of The Milton S. Hershey Medical Center of The Pennsylvania State University College of Medicine. Shortly after his appointment as Chairman, he recruited Kenneth L. Miller to be Director of Health Physics at Hershey. Their programs for radiation protection and emergency response were tested during the nuclear power plant accident at Three Mile Island on March 28, 1979. Some of their experiences during that accident were presented in a paper entitled. "The Impact of a Nuclear Crisis on a Radiology Department" at the 65th Scientific Assembly and Annual Meeting of the Radiological Society of North America in November, 1979. This paper was also subsequently published in RADIOLOGY. Dr. Weidner is interested in radiation protection, medical radiation emergencies and public health consequences of nuclear attack. He has presented his views on the role of non-governmental organizations in the event of nuclear attack at the 1981 annual meeting of the NCRP and participated in the development of The American Medical Associations' *Guide to the Hospital Management of Injuries Arising from Exposure to or Involving Ionizing Radiation.*

ADVISORY BOARD MEMBERS

Dr. J. Newell Stannard
Professor Emeritus
Department of Radiation Biology and Biophysics
The University of Rochester
17441 Plaza Animado
Apt. 132
San Diego, California 92128

Dr. Conrad P. Straub
2330 Chalet Drive
Minneapolis, Minnesota 55421

Dr. Niel Wald
Chairman
Department of Radiation Health
Graduate School of Public Health
University of Pittsburgh
130 DeSoto Street
Pittsburgh, Pennsylvania 15261

CONTRIBUTORS

William D. Allen
Health Physics Consultant
Allen Nuclear Associates
San Clemente, California

Dr. F. J. Bradley
Principal Radiophysicist
Radiological Health Unit
N.Y.S. Department of Labor
Division of Safety and Health
New York, New York 10047

Vincent P. Collins
Clinical Professor
Department of Radiation Therapy
University of Texas Medical Branch
Galveston, Texas

E. D. Durkosh
Radiation Safety Officer
Radiation Safety Office
University of Pittsburgh
Pittsburgh, Pennsylvania

Mr. Robert G. Gallaghar
President
Applied Health Physics, Inc.
Venture, Inc.
17 Park Avenue
East Greenbush, New York 12061

Ronald L. Kathren
Staff Scientist
Battelle, Pacific Northwest Laboratories
Affiliate Associate Professor of Radiological Science
University of Washington
Richland, Washington

James A. Martin, Jr.
U.S. Nuclear Regulatory Commission
Washington, D. C.

Barbara L. Matthews
Manager
Public Relations
Battelle, Pacific Northwest Laboratories
Richland, Washington

Kenneth L. Miller
Assistant Professor of Radiology
Department of Radiology
The Milton S. Hershey Medical Center of the Pennsylvania State University College of Medicine
Hershey, Pennsylvania

Sydney W. Porter, Jr.
President
Porter Consultants, Inc.
Head
TMI Effluent & Dose Assessment Branch
Ardmore, Pennsylvania

TABLE OF CONTENTS

SUMMARY OF EXPERIENCE IN RADIATION LITIGATION

Vincent P. Collins

This is a review of courtroom encounters between law and science in the field of radiation injuries since the discovery of the X-ray. Over the years that radiation has been in court, the voice of science has been faintly heard and poorly understood. Perhaps if science had a better appreciation of the purpose and mechanisms of law, it might yet make a more effective contribution.

When differences of opinion, disputes, or claims arise that require present resolution and are not satisfied by personal debate or barter, then the courtroom is the arena where all our knowledge, called evidence, is displayed in an adversary system. Each view is presented as strongly as possible to sway the mind of judge and jury. This route to truth and proof is apt to be in conflict with the precision science seeks, but the scientist is the guest in court and he has rules to learn. The court's purpose and function is decision-making on the basis of conflicting evidence. While this is also the nature of scientific enquiry, science can wait for answers. In law, the parties have their day in court and at its end a decision is due. The law, with centuries of experience in dealing with conflicts and uncertainty, has developed rules and devices to accomplish its purpose of decision. These may be rigidly followed, sometimes to the exasperation of an informed observer, or they may be molded or overturned to the amazement or applause of the parties involved. As an aid to understanding it is necessary to see all participants as individuals, the product of their heritage, their training and their environment. It is particularly necessary to see a judge as a person, the product of all the forces that brought him to his position, with reactions and responses elicited by preferences and biases, rather than the impersonal, faceless force referred to as "the Court". His decision will be a result of the evidence, the manner of its presentation, precedents to restrain, and social forces to evolve, all acting upon a complex personality to respond with a solution bound to be seen by one party as correct, but by the other as in error. Oliver Wendell Holmes defined truth as "what I can't help believing". Josh Billings' definition is even more appropriate to the needs of the legal decision-maker, "The truth is anything that has got itself believed by me". For a party at interest who feels his just cause has been denied, he must see this as his failure to present the facts and theory of his case in such a fashion as judge and jury "can't help believing". Science must come to court prepared to teach, clearly and convincingly.

When Roentgen's publication caught the attention of the world in January 1896, the equipment to produce the "invisible light" was present and available around the world. X-ray photography exploded into clinical use and into the courtroom within weeks, in London, in Montreal, in Wichita, and in Denver, to mention only those that vie for first to court. In the case of Smith vs. Grant that came to court in Denver in December of 1896, Mr. Smith attempted to introduce as evidence an X-ray photograph of his hip to prove that Dr. Grant had failed to diagnose a fracture. Judge Owen E. LeFevre admitted the plaintiff's X-ray photograph into evidence with a welcoming fanfare. "We have been presented with a photograph taken by means of a new scientific discovery, the same being acknowledged in the arts and sciences. It knocks for admission at the temple of learning; what are we to do or say? Close fast the doors or open wide the portals?... The law is the acme of learning throughout all ages. It is the essence of wisdom, reason, and experience. Learned priests have interpreted the law. They classified reasons for certain opinions which, in time, have become precedents, and these ordinarily guide and control, especially trial courts. We must not, however, hedge ourselves round about with rule, precept, and precedent until we can advance no further. Our field must ever grow as trade, the arts and science seek to enter it. It must not be said of the law that it is wedded to precedent, and will not lend a helping hand. Rather let the courts throw open the doors to all well-considered scientific discoveries. Modern science has made it possible to look beneath the tissues of the human body and has aided surgery in telling of the hidden mysteries. We believe it to be our duty in this case to be the first if you please to so consider it, in admitting in evidence the process known and acknowledged as a determinate science. The exhibits will be admitted in evidence.''

The doctors of Denver were being harassed by a rash of damage suits at the time and the appearance of the X-ray in court was seen more as a prop for plaintiffs' lawyers than a scientific advance. But this case dealt with X-ray as a diagnostic tool and neither law not medicine had recognized that a dangerous agent had been unleashed. Enthusiasm for X-ray photography was sweeping the world and the aftermath of injuries was quick to appear.

Actually, the first recorded injury occurred before Roentgen's announcement. Emil Grubbe had been producing and testing vacuum tubes for scientific studies and consulted his family physician about a rash on his hands sometime in 1895. When Roentgen's publication reached the public in January of 1896, Grubbe and his physician recognized the association. They promptly applied this biologic effect and are credited with treating a breast cancer on February 22, 1896, but the effect is not recorded. Grubbe went on to become a physician and practiced radiology for many years in Chicago. At the time of his death in 1958, he had lost several fingers, part of his nose and upper lip from surgery for skin cancer and he combatted an anemia with his own prescription of port wine and fresh beef blood from the abattoirs.

This account must be more a sampling than a summary of experience in radiation litigation. The series of cases is presented in chronologic order to illustrate the evolution of the problems of radiation injury and the legal solutions over a span of more than 80 years. Where facts in a given case are scanty and decisions seem based on inadequate information it is justifiable conjecture to consider that another outcome might have resulted if science had supplied, and law had understood, the missing knowledge of radiation physics and biology.

THE ORME MURDER CASE (NY, 1897)[1]

The Ormes, man and wife, maintained a boarding house in Horseheads, N. Y. Returning home unexpectedly on July 8, 1897, Mr. Orme found his wife in the embrace of an Italian boarder, James Punzo. In the melee that ensued, Mr. Orme was battered about the head and retaliated by firing two shots, one striking Mrs. Orme in the mouth, removing a portion of her tongue, and the other lodging in the brain of the boarder, Punzo. Punzo was taken to Arnot-Ogden Hospital in nearby Elmira where he made a surprising recovery. By July 31st, Punzo was walking about the hospital, his wound had healed and on this date ''an unsuccessful attempt was made to locate the bullet in Punzo's brain with Roentgen Rays''.

The X-ray examination was carried out under ether anesthesia. A Crookes tube was placed $1^1/_2$ in. from the head and attached to a Holtz Static Generator with a capacity of producing 500,000 V. A 35-min exposure was made but no picture of the bullet was obtained, only a dark outline of the skull appeared upon the sensitive plate. From that day on, the patient remained in a semi-comatose condition until his death 12 days later. An autopsy was performed. ''In my opinion'', said pathologist E. H. Davis, ''James Punzo came to his death from injuries to the brain caused by a gunshot wound, anesthetics, and the X-ray.''

Defendant Orme was acquitted.

Comment

This appears to be a contest between expert witnesses, Dr. John T. Pitkin of Buffalo for the defendant Orme, and Dr. Frank Ward Ross of Elmira, N. Y. for the prosecution. The tables were turned on the prosecution who attempted to establish a first in crime detection by identifying a bullet in the brain by X-ray photography but instead, provided a contributing factor in Punzo's death that absolved Orme of the charge of murder. Dr. Ross, in a later address at the Medico-Legal Society in New York indicated some chagrin in stating, ''My greatest consolation, in this case, was the same argument would have been used had I failed to use the X-ray to locate the bullet. Had the case died, then the omission would have been claimed as neglect''. He raises a current concern of physicians involved in malpractice suits, ''Evidence which to our trained surgical senses or deductive logic may be sufficient for us to use as a guide for treatment which holds a human life, may count for naught in a court of law; and our efforts to save life and best intentions are often looked upon with suspicion by the court and jury. Especially is this true in regard to new discoveries, which are viewed rather in the light of experiments.''

THE FRANK BALLING CASE (ILL., 1897) [2]

On September 2, 1895, in Chicago, Frank Balling was thrown from his buggy and fractured his right ankle. Frank Balling's accident occurred within a few days of Roentgen's observation of fluorescence in his laboratory that led to the deduction of the presence of an invisible light he called the ''X-ray''. During the ensuing year, while Balling continued to complain of pain and stiffness in his ankle, X-ray photography became available throughout the country and on September 19, 1896 he was referred for this new examination. There were 3 exposures of 35 to 40 min with the tube placed 5 to 6 in. from the skin surface. An erythema developed which progressed to blistering and extensive ulceration that required amputation on November 28, 1896, and further amputation of the stump on August 27, 1897.

''Professor H. P. Pratt, M. D., was called as an X-ray and electrical expert for the purpose of establishing the fact that the X-ray or electrical discharge produced while the X-ray was in operation, was competent to produce injurious results, and that such injuries results were more apt to occur in an exposure where the tube was placed as close as from 5 to 6 in., than a farther distance. There were four or five X-ray and electrical experts called by the defense, who disagreed widely one from another, with reference to the effects of the X-ray and the distance of the tube from the part exposed which could produce those effects, yet, taking the testimony of each one as a whole, there was no substantial difference, so far as to the fact that injurious results might follow an exposure to the X-ray. The jury awarded $10,000 damages.''

Comment

This is the first encountered case of radiation brought to court. The number of expert witnesses available is evidence of the experience with radiation injuries gained in the first year of X-ray photography. The record has a familiar ring in the disagreement between experts on the physical factors and biologic effects but the jury ''could see no substantial difference'' in the testimony and, as still happens when science cannot make itself clear, it is easier for the judge and jury to see what happened, rather than why it happened, and award damages accordingly. An award of $10,000 in 1897 might be the equivalent of at least $1 million in today's market.

HENSLIN VS. WHEATON (MINN., 1904)[3]

This is an action for negligence and unskillfulness in the use of ''the device known as Roentgen's X-rays''. Mr. Henslin thought he had inhaled the gold crown of one of his teeth. Dr. Wheaton attempted, unsuccessfully, to locate the crown by X-ray photography and about 2 weeks later his patient developed an ''X-ray burn'' on his back. The only details recorded are that there were several exposures of 30 to 40 min with the tube placed within 2 in. of the patient.

The patient's allegation was that the exposure was too long and the tube placed too close to his body. His expert witness was Professor Freeman who testified that he was familiar with electricity and had been since childhood — that he knew the X-ray and its properties and had used the X-ray more or less since its discovery by Roentgen. The testimony of this witness, if received, would tend to show unskillfulness and negligence on the part of the defendant. The defendants objected that in an action against a physician for malpractice — unskillfulness in treatment being charged — the physician was entitled to have the propriety of his treatment tested by a physician of the same school. Judge Brown ruled that this might be so if the application of the X-ray to the plaintiff was for the purpose of treating a disease or ailment, but here the purpose of the examination was that of locating a foreign substance thought to be in the lungs.

In a Minnesota Supreme Court decision Judge Brown writes, ''This is the first case to come before us involving alleged negligence on the part of physicians in applying the recently discovered X-rays, and no rule of care in such cases has been laid down. But there can be no doubt that the rule applicable to the care and skill required of physicians toward their patients in other cases applies. . . .The legal obligation of the physician to his patient, where his conduct is questioned in an action of this character, demands of him no more than the exercise of such reasonable care and skill as is usually given by physicians and surgeons in good standing. . . .The so called X-rays discovered by Roentgen, have been recognized as known to scientists both in and out of the medical profession for some eight years. . . It may be applied by anyone possessing the requisite scientific knowlege. . . .The rule (a physician is entitled to have the propriety of his treatment tested by a physician of the same school) might apply did it appear that the application. . . .was for medical purposes and not for the scientific purpose of discovering the presence of a foreign substance in his lungs''.

Judge Brown held that Professor Freeman's testimony should have been admitted.

Comment

The plaintiff has been injured and the cause is clear. It is also clear that the injury might have been prevented if the skill and knowledge of Professor Freeman were brought to bear.

Judge Brown's decision must be to choose between the standard represented by Dr. Freeman, a professor of physical sciences, or the standard of physicians and surgeons in good standing. If the standard is that of physicians and surgeons in good standing, Professor Freeman's testimony must be rejected, Dr. Wheaton's treatment is proper and the plaintiff cannot recover for his injury. But if Dr. Wheaton was not actually treating the patient, then ''propriety of treatment'' would not be in question. Judge Brown rules that the taking of X-ray photographs was not for treatment but a search for a gold crown. Anyone familiar with X-ray equipment could do this. Professor Freeman is such an expert and his testimony may be admitted to pass on the use of X-ray not for treatment purposes. This is a good example of innovative judicial reasoning to avoid a rule that would prevent a recovery that must seem well deserved.

SAUERS vs. SMITS (Washington, 1908)[4]

Early in 1906, in Aberdeen, Washington, Dr. Smits treated Mrs. Sauers for an ''ailment of the foot'' not otherwise described. Treatment consisted of ''the daily exposure of the affected member or part to the light rays of an X-ray machine for a period of about a month, each exposure lasting about 15—30 minutes. ...at the close of the ... treatment there was an X-ray burn of the fourth degree on the foot which is generally considered incurable. ...by reason of the treatment, the foot is permanently injured, the patient has been rendered a cripple for life and the injury will probably necessitate amputation of the foot''.

There was conflicting testimony on many essential points. The charge was negligence. No shield was used. The affected part was about the size of a nickel. The tube or bulk of the X-ray machine was placed not to exceed 2 or 3 in. from the foot. The condition gradually grew worse from day to day but treatment was continued. The defense was contributory negligence, that the patient disobeyed instructions, discontinued treatment, that there was no X-ray burn of any kind, and that at the time of trial the foot was entirely cured and in a healthy condition.

Judge Rudkin notes that "the X-ray is comparatively a new discovery and was not well understood by physicians and surgeons practicing in such communities as Aberdeen at the time the treatment was given .... If it should appear that the physicians and surgeons in such communities as Aberdeen were ignorant of the effect of X-ray exposure, ... jury might well conclude that the use of such a dangerous agent by one who had little or no knowledge as to the possible consequences was negligence per se".

All seven members of the Supreme Court of Washington heard the case on appeal, reversed a judgment for the physician, and ordered a new trial.

Comment

That the Supreme Court of the state of Washington would hear this personal injury case has some implication for the novelty of X-ray injury and a less crowded docket in 1908. That "physicians and surgeons in such communities as Aberdeen" might be "ignorant of the effects of X-ray exposure" suggests that the judge felt no inhibiting incompetence in dealing with the evidence presented. Established rules of law were readily applicable. No estimate has been encountered of the number of X-ray machines in use but such accounts suggest that within 10 years of Roentgen's discovery there was a large, widely distributed number of these machines, and that the incidence of acute and late effects in patients and personnel must have exceeded by far the isolated cases that came to attention in litigation.

COOMBS vs. KING (Maine, 1910)[5]

Lillian Coombs was first treated by Dr. King in 1901 for "scrofulous glands of the neck". These were "cut out" but in 1903 "bunches again appeared". A diagnosis of Hodgkin's Disease was made and X-ray treatment advised. This was administered 2 or 3 times a week for 25 treatments, the first 3 or 4 by Dr. King, the rest by his office girl. During treatments, lasting 10 to 15 min, the patient was seated in a chair with head thrown back and face protected down to the lips with a sheet of lead. As a result the patient developed a "very severe and greatly disfiguring X-ray burn on the left side of the neck and lower part of the face." The charge was negligence and in the trial court Mrs. Coombs was awarded damages in the amount of $3500. Dr. King appealed.

Judge Savage sets forth the accepted basis for a physician's legal responsibility, "to possess the ordinary skill of members of his profession in like situation, and exercise reasonable care and diligence, to use his best judgment; he is not an insurer, he is not liable even for mistakes in judgment; the burden is on the plaintiff to show malpractice." Dr. King's defense is that his responsibility must be considered with reference to the science of X-ray treatment in 1903. In reviewing the basis of the patient's claim of failure to use reasonable care and exercise his best judgment, Judge Savage discusses treatment technic, distance, strength of current, frequency and length of treatment, soft and hard vacuum tubes, and personal sensitivity of the patient. "There is testimony that great advances have been made in X-ray knowledge since 1903, but it does not appear what they are". However, even in 1903, he knew that X-rays could burn and that watchfulness was necessary to detect the signs of burning in order that it might be prevented.

In confirming the jury verdict of negligence, Judge Savage also confirms recovery for "mental chagrin, mortification and discomfort at her disfigurement", a "question that has never been before the law court" (in Maine). He holds that mental suffering is a real injury and the plaintiff may have damages awarded for it.

Comment

If early X-ray photography produced numerous radiation injuries, the early applications of X-ray therapy represented an even greater hazard. The problem for Judge Savage's decision is to recognize negligence in the use of radiation within 8 years of Roentgen's discovery. He carefully puts forth the basis for physician's liability which is unchanged over the years. If his concept of the physical and biologic effects of radiation is necessarily primitive, the law's grasp of these subjects is not greatly improved in modern cases nor does this seem to handicap the decision-making process. This 1910 opinion awarding damages for mental suffering, preceeded by nearly 50 years the opinion in Ferrara vs. Galluchio that seemed to believe it was introducing mental anguish as a compensible injury.

SWEENEY vs. ERVING (U.S. Supreme Court, 1913)[6]

Anne Sweeney claimed she had suffered a fractured rib due to the negligence of a railroad company. The company requested an X-ray examination. Seen first by one specialist in X-ray diagnosis who failed to find a fracture, her physician referred her to Dr. Erving, another specialist in the use of X-ray for diagnostic purposes. There was evident apprehension, since her employer had warned her that the X-ray was dangerous but Dr. Erving assured her he had never had an accident in over 1000 exposures. She went to his office on four occasions and on each visit several exposures were made. About 2 weeks after her fourth visit she returned to Dr. Erving and informed him of the burn on her back. Despite treatment by Dr. Erving, other physicians, and in hospitals, the burn did not heal. Mrs. Sweeney sued to recover damages for injury sustained through negligence in making the X-ray tests. There was a judgment for the defendant in the lower courts and plaintiff's appeal reached the U. S. Supreme Court.

The plaintiff contended that the doctrine of res ipse loquitur applied — 'that the thing speaks for itself' — that from the evident injury there is an inference of negligence that must stand unless the defendant can explain or rebut the inference.

The opinion provides an excellent example of the use of precedent in reaching back to an 1839 case, Stokes vs. Saltonstall, a case in which a stage coach owner was absolved from liability for injury sustained by a passenger when the coach overturned. Although the overturning was evidence of negligence, it was not necessary for the defendant to show some other cause for the accident, but only that the driver was a person of competent skill and that the equipment was properly made and maintained.

Applying this principle to the X-ray injury, although there might be an inference of negligence, it would not be necessary for Dr. Erving to prove some other cause or factor, but only that he exercised the skill and competence required of him and that the equipment was in good working order. Expert witnesses did testify to Dr. Erving's competence and to the adequacy of his X-ray apparatus.

Dr. Justice Pitney found no error in the record and affirmed the judgement for the defendant doctor.

Comment

Information is lacking to explain how this case reached the U.S. Supreme Court. The patient and her attorney must have felt strongly that her claim had merit and the Supreme Court would recognize it. That the Supreme Court accepted the case may indicate a curiosity about the mysterious X-ray and its strange effects.

The essential question before the court is, whether the patient-plaintiff bears the burden of her injury or whether it should be shifted to the defendant by monetary damages. The decision rests on a finding as to negligence on the part of Dr. Erving. Mr. Justice Pitney does not strain to weigh the details of the X-ray examination that resulted in the injury. His decision-making process is to accept expert testimony that the examination is in accordance with careful and prudent X-ray operators and to turn to the precedent of an ancient case to establish whether the patient must prove negligence or physician must prove care. As the stage coach owner was required only to prove that his driver was competent and his equipment properly made, so Dr. Erving did not need to prove how the radiation injury was caused, but only that he was a person of competent skill and his machine was a good one of its kind.

It is evident that Mr. Justice Pitney relies on a strictly legalistic analysis as compared to later cases that admittedly seek to "find some basis for redress in a proper case" .

COOVER vs. PAINLESS PARKER, DENTIST (California, 1930)[7]

Rowena Coover was a 45-year-old patient of Painless Parker, Dentist, a corporation. She sustained severe radiation burns of the facial area "as a result of over-exposure in taking of dental X-ray photographs". The plaintiff was awarded a judgement of $10,250 and the defendant appealed on the basis that the amount was "grossly excessive and suggests passion or prejudice on the part of the jury".

The report details the "terrible suffering lasting three months", the residual atrophy, scarring, telangiectasis, and impaired vision. Weighing her plight the judge notes "while.. ..advancing years bring a change in....the appearance....even a person of middle age has a substantial right not to have this change hastened or aggravated by the wrongful act of another". The possibility of cancer is raised and a physician testified, "Our medical literature is full of cases of cancer-carcinoma (sic) that have developed upon a senile skin following an X-ray burn, ...a cancer may develop in this region....it is common". To the objection that this is "wholly conjectural and uncertain", Judge Finch holds that "this predisposition in itself is some damage .... which must be held to be a real and not a fanciful element of damage".

Comment

The early instances of radiation injury were prompt responses to heavy exposure. There was no new problem for the courts in identifying cause and effect, and traditional rules of law were readily applicable. Delayed and nonspecific effects raised problems of proof; conjecture and speculation are not supportive.

In this decision, Judge Finch sees the possibility of developing a future cancer as a 'predisposition' and an injury in itself. A similar result in later cases is obtained by seeing the injury as an anxiety neurosis or simply allowing recovery for "future injury". When a delayed effect has the threat of cancer, judge and jury are likely to see a possibility raised to a probability.

The testimony indicates again the vast experience in radiation injuries that had accumulated in the first 30 years of X-ray usage and refers particularly to skin cancer as a sequela of radiation burns. Judge Finch finds nothing in the amount of the verdict "to shock the sense of justice" or that it was "the result of passion or prejudice". The development of cancer may be conjectural and uncertain but that there is a threat of cancer inherent in the visible injury was presented clearly enough that Judge Finch "can't help believing" that it is a real element of damage. The inclusion of this case is to record that 50 years ago the possibility of cancer as a delayed effect was interpreted as a predisposition which is itself recognized as a compensable injury.

VALLAT vs. RADIUM DIAL CO. (Illinois, 1935)[8]
LA PORTE vs. U. S. RADIUM CORP. (New Jersey, 1935)[9]

Inez Vallat was employed by the defendant company in 1929, painting dials with luminous paint containing radium, and in the course of her employment 'inhaled, swallowed or otherwise took into her system' dust containing particles of radium. The complaint charged that the defendant employer failed to provide methods of prevention of occupational diseases and the plaintiff contracted "anemia, rarefaction of the bones, alveoli of the jaws and other bone complications and disorders".

Miss Valet asks $50,000 damages for her illness resulting from a violation of the Occupational Diseases Act of 1911, requiring provision of "reasonable and approved devices....for the prevention of....occupational diseases....incident to such work or process". The requirement is found "unconstitutional because uncertain, vague and indefinite". Further, the plaintiff failed to show that she had suffered any disablement during her employment, she was not an employee when the disease affected her, and the suit was not filed within 2 years after her illness was discovered.

Justice Farthing affirmed the lower courts judgement dismissing the plaintiff's claim.

Mrs. La Porte was employed by the defendant company from May 1917 to December 1918, and for a period of about 6 weeks in 1920, painting watch dials with luminous paint containing radium. There were 80 girls working in a large room, described in detail as to working conditions and the technic of painting with a camel's hair brush pointed with the tip of the tongue. The plaintiff married in 1921 and was in good health until 1927 when she began to have a fear of radium poisoning. She told her dentist and her physician about her fear but they reassured her. The diagnosis of radium necrosis was made in October 1930 by Dr. Harrison Maitland, who reviewed X-rays of her jaws taken in 1925 and recognized typical areas of radiation osteitis. She presented a claim for damages on May 4, 1931 and died on June 16, 1931. An autopsy established the diagnosis of osteogenic sarcoma of the pelvis.

The question is whether an action for damages should be barred by the 2 year statute of limitations. The last exposure and time when her action could have accrued was in 1920 and the 2 year statute of limitations would have barred her recovery in 1922, 2 years before radium necrosis was recognized as a diagnosis, and 7 years before she was diagnosed.

"Today (1935), industrial methods which the defendant then employed would be not merely negligent but criminal. But....this case must be decided on the facts as they existed in the light of the knowledge of 1917 to 1920.... This is a case where both the plaintiff and defendant were ignorant of the facts". The defendant company did not know of the danger in the period when the plaintiff was exposed so there could be no fraudulent concealment. Even with the plaintiff's expressed concern her physicians could not diagnose the injury until 1930. ".... can her employer be charged with responsibility of anticipating such dangers in the light of the learning of the years 1917 to 1920?"

Judge Forman holds the bill must be dismissed.

Comment

In both cases the decision illustrates adherence to the letter of the law. A new type of injury has come to light that was unrecognized by either party at the time of occurrence. Without knowledge of its existence or effect, no preventive measures could be invoked, and the latent period far exceeded the statute of limitations. If the decision must be "decided on facts as they existed in the light of knowledge of 1917 to 1920", then the decision itself must be considered in the light of science and society of 50 years ago.

In the Vallat case, Judge Farthing finds a 20-year-old statute invalid as uncertain, vague and indefinite. It seems likely that this deficit is related to a newly recognized dangerous agent for which existing standards might give no guidance as to protective methods or devices. "....courts have no power to supply the omissions of this statute". Making no attempt to utilize, or cope with science in the court, Judge Farthing holds the statute unconstitutional and the claim invalid under workers compensation because the 2-year statute of limitations is exceeded.

In the La Porte decision by Judge Forman, the documented details give evidence of the depth of his inquiry into every aspect. He describes the workplace for 80 girls who worked,

$5^1/_2$ days a week, the materials, tools, and the technic of painting luminous numerals, the estimation of ingested radium sulfate (43 μg/working day), background information on Madame Curie and Lord Rutherford, the decay scheme of radium, the medical prescription of radium, the mounting literature of harmful effects, and the ultimate acknowledgement that she died of cancer resulting from radium ingested in the course of her employment years before. Weighed against the law, science cannot stay the running of the statute of limitations. A party wronged by fraud may be relieved of the bar to recovery, but no fraud or fault can be found. Time alone settles the rights of the parties. "The statute of limitations and its exceptions were not conceived for this extraordinary situation.... Only forward looking legislation can protect future situations such as the one here presented".

In dismissing the plaintiff's case Judge Forman recognizes the dilemma of an injury without a wrong and without a remedy. "But a court has no power to adjust the law which has been enacted to meet the needs of a time when no such case as this could be forseen".

The concern of Judge Forman for the conflict of the unfolding truths of science, and established man-made rules of law, presages a shifting balance and the change in legal thinking that will occur over the next 4 decades.

FERRARA vs. GALLUCHIO (New York, 1958)[10]

As a result of a series of X-ray treatments for bursitis of her right shoulder, Eleanor Ferrara developed a severe local reaction that healed with residual atrophy, irregular pigmentation, and telangiectasis. In the course of an action for malpractice, her attorney referred her to a dermatologist for examination. Based on his diagnosis of radio-dermatitis, the dermatologist advised her that "the area of the burn might become cancerous". The record indicates that the treatment consisted of 1400 R in seven treatments, elapsed time not stated. One expert witness for Mrs. Ferrara supported her claim of excessive radiation, four expert witnesses testified that Dr. Galluchio's dosage was not excessive under any view of the facts. A neuropsychiatrist testified that she was suffering from a severe cancerophobia and that she might have permanent symptoms of anxiety. The jury rendered a verdict in favor of Mrs. Ferrara for $25,000; $10,000 for the radiation injury itself and $15,000 for mental anguish flowing from the cancerophobia.

In this Appellate decision, Chief Judge Conway, writing the majority opinion, affirmed the judgment for Mrs. Ferrara. He bases his opinion on "common knowledge....that wounds which do not heal over long periods of time frequently become cancerous. Physical culture lectures..., radio advice...newspaper daily articles — all give the same advice". A very revealing statement is made, "The very clear tendency of the recent cases is to refuse to admit incompetence to deal with such a problem, and to find some basis for redress in a proper case".

Judge Froessel entered a strong dissent. His objection is, "...recovery would depend upon the subjective mind of the litigating plaintiff, and speculation by the physician, without even an opinion by the latter based on reasonable certainty.... The decision of the majority introduces into the law a new field of damages for cultivation by plaintiffs and affording countless opportunities for fraudulent unverifiable claims".

Comment

By Judge Oliver Wendell Holmes' definition of truth, the majority of Judge Conway's court "can't help believing" that Mrs. Ferrara received an excessive dose of radiation and that her cancerophobia is a compensable injury. The defense has failed to disturb this belief despite the conservative dose recorded. No question of error was raised. The cancerophobia may be real but the probability of cancer could be shown to be remote on the basis of clinical experience with thousands of patients treated to higher doses and equivalent reactions in the course of cancer therapy.

The kindest appraisal of this decision is that a decision must be had, the judges favoring the decision acknowledge conflicting testimony and views but accept available 'common knowledge' and assume competency to decide. Medicine and science have failed to present this information in the community and in the courts for lack of preparation, invitation or assumption of a responsibility to teach.

This opinion is sometimes credited with introducing anxiety neurosis and cancerophobia as a compensable injury although there has always been a tort termed 'interference with peace of mind' compensable when accompanied by physical injury, as indeed there is here. It is particularly cautionary to note that the anxiety neurosis was precipitated by a consulting physician's thoughtless remark that cancer might develop. Judge Conway finds support in 'common knowledge' that he 'can't help believing'. Science might have offered a better opinion but apparently did not come to court, was not heard, or was not believed.

The opinion demonstrates the gradual evolution of decisions toward a more ready relief for the injured party and provides a sharp contrast to the decisions in the radium dial painters cases.

NATANSON vs. KLINE (Kansas, 1960)[11]

Mrs. Natanson underwent radical mastectomy for breast cancer and a course of postoperative radiotherapy by Dr. Kline, which resulted in an injury that is vividly described, "the skin, flesh and muscles beneath her left arm sloughed away and the ribs of her left chest were so burned that they became necrotic, or dead". Despite this dramatic description of the injury, all issues of fact were resolved in favor of the defendants and the jury found Dr. Kline not guilty of any act or acts of negligence. The appeal is based on the contention that the defendants are negligent as a matter of law. The argument is developed in this fashion.

The opinion written by Judge Schroeder sets forth his understanding of 'irradiation therapy', dosimetry, radiobiology and testimony of physicists, "Radioactive cobalt is so powerful that the Atomic Energy Commission specified the contruction of the room... The walls are forty inches thick... The room is sunken down in a courtyard outside the hospital....the operator in the outer room looks through a specially designed thick lead quartz glass which gives a telescopic view.... These facts are not commonly known and a patient cannot be expected to know the hazards or danger of radiation unless the patient is informed by the radiologist".

In denying the allegation of negligence and carelessness, Dr. Kline counters with the pleading that Mrs. Natanson "assumed the risk as hazard of treatment". This is a long established defense termed 'assumption of risk' but Judge Schroeder writes that this is only applicable where a plaintiff and defendant are equally competent to judge the hazards and the risks. Raising this defense implies that Dr. Kline was aware that Mrs. Natanson would have to be so informed to consent to assume this risk as hazard of treatment. "Dr. Kline gave the appellant no explanation whatever. He made no disclosures. He was silent on the state of the record. Dr. Kline failed in his legal duty to make a reasonable disclosure to the appellant who was his patient, as a matter of law.... Whether or not a physician has advised his patient of the inherent risks and hazards...is a question of fact concerning which lay witnesses are competent to testify.... we think the evidence is sufficient and would authorize a jury to infer that had she been properly informed the appellant would not have taken the cobalt irradiation treatments".

This decision by Judge Schroeder reverses the trial court judgment for Dr. Kline and the hospital, and renders judgment for Mrs. Natanson.

Comment

This landmark case in the development of the doctrine of informed consent is clear legal logic and provides a route to recovery for the injured plaintiff where negligence in the treatment itself could not be shown. It conforms to the reasoning in the case of Ferrara vs. Galluchio in avoiding the need to admit incompetence to deal with the intricacies of radiation treatment and finds a basis for redress that does not require a showing of negligence or carelessness. In Judge Schroeder's opinion, Mrs. Natanson would not have consented had she been ''properly informed'', and the jury could decide on what might be necessary to meet this requirement. That such a result could not be forseen by Dr. Kline and he would not, in wild speculation, have warned of such an injury as is luridly described, is not weighed as a consideration. How a jury of laymen could know probable or possible effects and how they should be presented to a patient, is not asked. What is required is a basis for redress and by the device of 'fiction of law' this serves its purpose.

The report contains a hidden clue as to the reason for the unexpected complication. It records that at the time the patient was referred for treatment, there was persistent drainage from the operative wound. This indicates a seroma or collection of serum in the operative site. This acts as a sterile foreign substance and causes a local increase in vascularity. It is a basic rule of radiobiology that an increase in vascularity or oxygenation increases sensitivity to radiation. Under these circumstances a reaction may appear in the first week of treatment that would not be expected for 3 or 4 weeks. This particular effect is little known, has apparently not appeared in medical literature, and there is no way that Dr. Kline could have known or warned the patient.

Had medical science been aware and been in court to explain the mechanism of injury, it might still have been beyond the comprehension of a judge or jury that obtains its basic understanding from physical culture lectures, radio advice, and newspaper daily articles.

Informed consent as a legal concept should not be confused with the understanding that is required in the view of science.

KUHNE vs. UNITED STATES OF AMERICA & U.S. FIDELITY & GUARANTY CO. (Tenn., 1965)[12]

Kuhne was an electrical engineer who worked in Oak Ridge during the years of 1943 to 1945 for the Tennessee Eastman Company. During this period he alleged that he was repeatedly exposed to radiation (not further described or documented) but none since that time. Gradually developing incapacitation led to a diagnosis of ''myelofibrosis-myeloid metaplasia''. He now brings suit against U.S.F & G Co. for workmen's compensation benefits for total disability caused by exposure to radiation at Oak Ridge, and against the United States under Federal Torts Act for negligence in connection with his radiation exposure. The Tort Claims Act specifically states, ''An occupational disease which an employee had on March 12, 1947, shall not be covered hereunder''. Since Kuhn's employment at Oak Ridge terminated nearly 2 years earlier the case is dismissed as to the insurance company. As to the government, although there is a 2-year statute of limitation on tort claims, there is precedent to toll the statute of limitations if there has been concealment or negligence and ''in view of the mischievous nature of radioactive materials the government had a responsibility to see that care was taken by the independent contractor''.

Comment

For the purpose of decision-making, ''mischievous'' is as good a term as any for Judge Taylor's concept of radiation. It implies an unpredictable, harmful nature rendering credibility to the late appearance of a strange and polysyllabic diagnosis. The essential warning here is that when delayed effects are ascribed to radiation exposure, any evidence of negligence or concealment are likely to void the protection of the statute of limitations.

Quite apart from instruction and monitoring of activities of public, personnel and patients, this places a heavy burden of recordkeeping on the radiation safety officer.

BESNER vs. KIDDE NUCLEAR LABORATORY (N.Y. 1965)[13]

Besner was a physicist who had been employed by Kidde for 1 year when he developed acute myeloblastic leukemia and died 1 year later. He handled no radioactive materials although there was a shielded ion exchange column, a 201-mCi Cobalt 60 source and a 1-mCi Cobalt 60 source in the laboratory. His exposure was said to be 2250 mR during the year.

Workmen's Compensation death benefits were granted to his widow and an appeal was taken. Expert testimony stated there was no threshold or safe dose. New York Workman's Compensation Law requires proof of an exposure that could cause the injury in question. A presumption then exists that the exposure did cause the injury unless disproven, as, for example, another nonwork-related cause could be shown. Here expert witnesses testified that there was no threshold dose for radiation injury, no other cause of leukemia could be shown, and the judgement for the plaintiff was affirmed.

Comment

Workmen's Compensation laws are intended to place the burden of work-related injury on the employer who may pass this on as a cost of doing business. The only decision required is whether or not an injury is work-related. Medicine and science cannot establish the etiology of leukemia in a given case, but given the question the court must produce an answer. "The presumptions" provide a decision-making device. The workman must prove his exposure. Expert witnesses advanced the 'no threshold' concept as to causation. This raises the presumption that the radiation did not cause the leukemia. If the presumption is not disproven, as by showing another cause, then the presumption stands.

Science's contribution to law's decision here is attesting to the no-threshold concept for radiation effect. Law accepts this at face value and accomplishes its purpose of decision-making by means of legal presumptions. Science would have to consider alternate or contributory causes, weigh medical or other exposures, and then might stall in indecision. For its purposes, law is superior to science in its decision-making power.

EMPLOYERS MUTUAL vs. PARKER (Texas, 1967)[14]

Alton Parker was first employed in 1961 in a government installation involved in assembling and storing nuclear weapons. His job was described as "material handler". Over the next 4 years he had some contact with radioactive materials and was issued a film badge on four occasions. The recorded exposure totalled 36 mrem but some parts of the body may have received a higher dose estimated at 540 rem. In 1965 a biopsy of the swelling in the neck yielded a diagnosis of metastatic cancer, probably seminoma, although in this record the primary site is not established. In the trial court there was a jury verdict to the effect that the plaintiff was totally and permanently disabled due to cancer resulting from his exposure in the course of his employment to radiation from radioactive materials.

The insurance company appeals on the grounds that there was no evidence that the cancer was the result of work-incurred radiation. Expert testimony was to the effect that exposure to radiation was a "possibility" and that under some circumstances it "could" or "can" cause cancer. Judge Cadena's assessment of the entire testimony is that "an inference of causal connection can be no more than speculation and conjecture....testimony to the effect that radiation may have, could have, or possibly caused plaintiff's tumor is, standing alone, no evidence of a causal connection between such exposure and the subsequent development of cancer." The judgment of the trial court was reversed and judgment entered that the plaintiff take nothing.

Comment

When a cancer arising on a basis of chance cannot be distinguished from a cancer caused by radiation, science may postpone an opinion indefinitely, but the parties in court must have a decision. Devices for decision distinguish between "reasonable medical probability" or they may place the burden of proof on the plaintiff to prove that radiation caused his cancer ("a Sisyphian task") or on the defendant to prove it did not. Texas requires expert testimony to be based only on reasonable medical probability. The expert witnesses could go no further than a possibility, and this does not support the plaintiff's claim to the level of reasonable medical probability. Here the court finds no need to delve into radiation biology and carcinogenesis but, staying within its area of special competence, utilizes its expert witnesses to assess the probability of work-related injury and finds that conjecture and speculation are an inadequate basis for believing.

WILKINSON vs. VESEY (Rhode Island, 1972)[15]

In 1951, Winifred Wilkinson, then aged 33, was found to have a mediastinal tumor. Lymphoma or substernal thyroid were considered. A 5-day course of external radiotherapy was undertaken and when shrinkage of the shadow occurred within 10 days, a clinical diagnosis of malignant tumor was made. A series of X-ray treatments was concluded in January of 1952. In 1955, breakdown of skin began and in 1960, the first plastic surgery was undertaken. "At trial time, Winifred's medical-surgical box score listed eight operations, numerous skin grafts, the removal of seven ribs, the clavicle and the sternum. Her heart has been moved and is cushioned and supported by muscle taken from the left arm. She has had innumerable and lengthy hospitalizations. Testimony was adduced which showed that the condition which caused Winifred to seek the assistance of the plastic surgery was radiation burns which were attributable to the 1951—52 treatments."

Mrs. Wilkinson brought suit against Dr. Vesey and Dr. Hunt on three grounds. She charged the defendant doctors with negligence in that (1) they incorrectly diagnosed her ailment; (2) the X-ray therapy was improperly administered; and (3) they failed to obtain her knowing consent to the treatment given her. At the conclusion of testimony, the trial justice granted directed verdict in favor of the defendant doctors. The plaintiff and her husband appealed. This appellate opinion sustains the appeal and overrules the trial court on all three grounds.

As to the correctness of diagnosis, Judge Kelleher reasons: "Either the X-ray beams had destroyed the cancer or Winifred never had cancer. The posit of the case being what it is, the reasonable inference to be chosen is the latter."

Judge Kelleher's concept of the treatment technic is described at length if not in detail. "There were three areas which were exposed to X-ray beams...the tube of the X-ray machine would be lowered so that the X-ray filter which had been attached to the tube would rest on the plaintiff's body..." "Dr. Hunt was somewhat imprecise as he described (the) technique of centering the filter — about five to eight centimeters to the right of the mid-line, — to radiate the hilar (sic) of the left lung, the filter was centered a "little below" the left nipple and approximately six to seven centimeters to the left of the mid-line. It is obvious (from) the use of such imprecise terms...that the goal of preciseness...was rarely if ever attained."

In the matter of informed consent, Judge Kelleher writes, ..."There is no necessity for expert testimony (as to) what the medical fraternity in the community tells its patients ...The jury can decide if the doctor has disclosed enough information to enable the patient to make an intelligent decision ... It is obvious from the record that Winifred...would have refused to undergo the proposed therapy had she been properly informed."

Lastly this opinion overules the trial court and holds that the doctrine of res ipsa loquitur (the thing speaks for itself) is applicable based on the three "traditional" conditions, (1) the event is one which ordinarily does not occur in the absence of negligence, (2) it must be caused by an agency controlled exclusively by the defendant, and (3) it must have no voluntary act or contribution by the plaintiff.

Comment

The decision in this case is written some 20 years after the treatment that resulted in the injury. This injects the difficulty, not only of fact-finding after a lapse of 20 years, but also of weighing knowledge, custom, and technique involving cancer and radiation therapy, two subjects where opinions as to diagnosis and treatment are in constant evolution and development.

The matter for consideration is not whether the plaintiff should have been allowed or denied relief but whether science and medicine could or should have influenced the outcome. More is required than offering science's truths to the court, there must be convincing presentation. Justice Kelleher is left with the impression that treatment without an histologic diagnosis is negligent. Circumstances govern, but a clinical opinion could be strongly presented to justify such treatment in the face of unacceptable surgical risk. In the matter of technique, it is clear that Justice Kelleher has not profited greatly by whatever testimony science brought to court, whether this was deficient in content or in force of presentation. Nevertheless the judge decides boldly on the basis of the information as he perceives it. In dealing with the concepts of informed consent and res ipsa loquitur he demonstrates the evolution of legal thought. He sees no necessity for expert testimony by the medical fraternity of the community. It is beyond question that if Mrs. Wilkinson had known the outcome in 1971, she would not have consented in 1951. It is equally certain that if Dr. Vesey had known, he would not have treated and, if he did not know, he could not have informed. It is evident that Judge Kelleher was more impressed by the vivid description of the injury than by testimony present on diagnosis and technic of treatment.

The decision awards compensation for injury to an innocent victim, an outcome in keeping with the now well-established trend that society can share the burden when this is passed on as a 'cost of doing business' through insurance mechanisms. The lingering need of law is to require fault or wrongdoing to justify the award. The injury is clear, but the element of negligence in diagnosis, treatment, and the matter of informed consent after a lapse of 20 years seems a belief based more on conviction than expert testimony.

STATE COMPENSATION FUND vs. CORA MAE JOE AND FANNIE DICK (Arizona, 1975)[16]

The plaintiffs are widows of David Joe and Clark Dick, American Indians and uranium miners. David Joe had worked for 15 years and Clark Dick for 20 years in the mines before developing anaplastic lung cancers. Joe survived 31 months and Dick 9 months beyond the time of diagnosis. During their working years both had moved "from one mine to another as is typical among uranium miners", both had moved from Arizona to Colorado 2 years before their lung cancers were diagnosed. The widows have applied for workmen's compensation benefits in Arizona and death benefits under the Occupational Disease Disability Act of Colorado.

There are two issues to be decided. The first is whether a widow may recover compensation under a Workmen's Compensation Act, when the workman died of disease defined under the Occupational Disability Act. The second issue is assignment of liability when exposure has occurred with multiple employers in different workplaces.

Dr. Victor E. Archer, expert witness specializing in lung cancer among uranium miners, testified that exposure to radiation in uranium mines was the probable cause of lung cancer in both men. Mr. Joe had accumulated a total exposure of 1450 work level months of which approximately 834 were in Arizona and 60 to 100 in Colorado. Mr. Dick had a cumulative exposure of 1280 work level months of which 777 were in Arizona and approximately 20 were in Colorado. Dr. Archer testified that the Colorado exposure represented the last injurious exposure for both men in that it would probably increase their chances of developing lung cancer.

Although there is no question that the accumulative exposure in Arizona increased the risk of lung cancer, more radiation was accumulated in Colorado. The legal principle is stated, "When a disability develops gradually, or when it comes as a result of a succession of accidents, the insurance carrier covering the risk at the time of the most recent injury or exposure bearing a causal relation to the disability is usually liable for the entire compensation". The Colorado employer hired these men knowing that they had worked in the Arizona mines for years. The last working environment that injuriously exposed these men to the hazards of radiation was in Colorado and the widows may not recover under the Arizona Workmen's Compensation Act.

Comment

The nonspecific nature of cancer as to etiology, the delayed appearance, and the assignment of liability among multiple exposures are recurrent decisional problems for radiation and cancer. The years of radiation exposure in uranium mines is not challenged as the cause of cancer. The essential problem is to assign liability among multiple employers. The solution here is arbitrary and simple, "the last injurious exposure", this is acceptable legal logic based on a principle that it may be better to be consistent than right particularly if right is not readily recognizable.

Science's contribution here is to confirm the work related causation of lung cancer in uranium miners. If this were a law suit in civil court, science could present a convincing case that the duration of cancer before diagnosis is such that inception of these cancers could only have occurred in Arizona before the miners moved to Colorado. But statutory law is not to be altered in the courts, the result is consistent and the families of the injured miners are compensated.

DAYTON vs. BOEING (Montana, 1975)[17]

Dayton sought damages against his employer, Boeing, for injuries due to exposure to "electromagnetic pulses and laser radiations". His wife sought damages in the same suit, for loss of consortium. Dayton and his wife are bringing action under common law and attempt to avoid compensation law that would limit recovery.

An employee suffering from an occupational disease has no common law remedy because the Occupational Disease Act binds both employer and employee. The Act defines radiation injury but Dayton urged that "electromagnetic impulse is (sic) neither radioactive, nor X-ray, nor is it ionizing radiation". Judge Smith ruled that there was no purpose in the Act to cover one kind of radiation and not another. The Act distinguishes radiation disability from other disabilities to provide that liability falls on the last employer if the employee had been employed by him for a period of 90 days or more.

Comment

The employee proposes a basis in physics, and perhaps biology, to distinguish his injury from radiation injuries covered by the Occupational Disease Act and allow him to bring a personal injury suit for a unique type of injury directly against his employer. This might require lengthy and possibly conflicting expert testimony to establish. Judge Smith's decision does not require an enquiry into a physical or biologic basis. He sees this as a matter of law, and, taking account of the purpose of the legislation, disposes of the question succinctly and simply. One may see Dayton's position as correct, this is not ionizing radiation and not specifically covered by the Act, and disagree with the decision; or one may see the legal logic and agree. The matter is settled and becomes precedent for some future case unless, of course, a cogent argument can be conceived to overturn.

Note also in this case, a useful if arbitrary rule to identify the responsible employer. Here again the answer is a device to aid decision-making in the face of uncertainty. In which period of employment did the cancer arise? What is the duration of cancer before diagnosis? Less than 90 days by law.

PEGRAM vs. SISCO (Arkansas, 1976)[18]

Mrs. Pegram had an early carcinoma of the cervix and was advised by her gynecologist, Dr. Applegate, to have a ''radium implant''. Arrangements were made with Dr. Sisco by telephone, and she was admitted to the hospital on September 14, 1970. The procedure was carried out on the following morning but she did not meet or see Dr. Sisco until that evening. She testified she did not know the radium was in her uterus until it was removed by Dr. Sisco 3 days later. Following release from the hospital she had burning, fatigue, and diarrhea with pain and discomfort. In January 1971, a fecal fistula developed, requiring hysterectomy and bowel resection in March 1971.

Her recovery of $13,700 was compensatory damages for malpractice based on failure to obtain informed consent and on negligent treatment.

Judge Williams accepted expert testimony, that it was standard medical practice to inform a potential patient of alternative procedures and of the possibility of radium burns and fistulae. He found that Dr. Sisco's defense, 'that he was only a consultant and assumed that Dr. Applegate had obtained consent', did not adhere to the medical community standards. On the theory of negligent treatment Judge Williams quoted, ''... a specialist should be held to the standard of care and skill of the average member of the profession practicing the specialty, taking into account the advances in the profession.'' Dr. Sisco was held negligent for failure to take X-rays which were necessary for two reasons, first to determine the shape and location of the uterus to guide the insertion of the radium, and second ''to determine how much radiation the surrounding organs are receiving''.

Comment

The fundamental problem is a failure of patient-physician communication not only in the matter of discussion of alternatives and complications but in personal contact to offset fear and apprehension. Although in this case lack of informed consent is adequate basis for recovery, Judge Williams has heard expert testimony on technique for use of intracavitary radiation. It has not been necessary to detail the anatomy of the pelvis or the steps in determining the dosimetry of the radium application. It has been enough that he recognizes negligence in failing to obtain X-rays of the pelvis before and after placement of the radium. The physician can expect to have the adequacy of his technique evaluated in court, and this case illustrates that pertinent expert testimony can be offered and understood. The points of chief significance here are the phrases ''taking into account the advances in the profession'', and ''...it is permissable to consider the medical resources available to him''. As expressed, these are legal considerations rather than scientific but they have a message for radiotherapists, physicists, and hospital administration.

MARTINEZ vs. UNIVERSITY OF CALIFORNIA (New Mexico, 1978)[19]

Ramon Martinez was employed as a foundry technician by the University of California at the Los Alamos Scientific Laboratories for some 30 years. His exposure to radioactive materials is not detailed but he was required to wear a film badge. No mention is made of his exposure record. The report describes that during his years of employment, some of his fellow employees developed cancers, fatal illness of unknown origin, and blindness, with the implication that these were work-related. In February 1976, a 'growth' diagnosed as "Bowen's lesion" was removed from his right eye. His physicians did not attribute this to radiation exposure but Martinez believed otherwise. Worried this might be a cancer that would spread, he developed symptoms of extreme anxiety and terminated his employment in July 1976.

On a diagnosis of 'anxiety neurosis' he was classified as "a total physical disability by reason of an occupational disease... unable to perform any work for remuneration or profit". He was awarded compensation under the Occupational Disease Disablement Act in the amount of $124.97 per week for 600 weeks plus medical and legal expenses. First reversed by the Court of Appeals, the Supreme Court of New Mexico now reverses the Court of Appeals and affirms the judgment for the workman.

Comment

Again we see that different judges "can't help believing" quite different conclusions from the same evidence. This may be due to ambiguous presentation of the evidence or to what the mind of the decision-maker is prepared to receive. The decision to compensate for work-related anxiety neurosis has precedent in an acrophobia following a scaffold accident (Bailey vs. American General Insurance (Texas, 1955), but the possibilities for the extrapolation and exploitation of this ruling are tremendous in the present atmosphere of fear and apprehension for even minimal exposures that occur in the public, patients, and radiation workers in medicine and industry.

CROCKER vs. STATE OF TEXAS (Tex 1978) [20]

Kerry Andrus Crocker was convicted on May 2, 1974 of castrating his 13 year old son, Kirk, by exposure to radiation, and sentenced to 10 years in prison and a fine of $5000.

Kerry Andrus Crocker, a petroleum engineer, had two sons, Kirk, age 13, and Patrick, age 9, at the time of his divorce in February, 1971. By agreement he had custody of the boys 2 weekends a month and 1 month a year. In November 1971, he obtained a license to possess a 1 Ci source of Cesium 137, amended in March of 1972, to 2 sources of 2-Ci each, for oil well logging purposes. There is no record that the sources were ever used for this purpose. Beginning in April, 1972 and continuing until January 1973, a series of episodes occurred in which Kirk was apparently deliberately exposed by his father to the Cesium 137 sources. In the recalled events the boy was given orange juice with a pill at bedtime. On several occasions he awakened to find small cylinders in his bed and at least twice there was nausea and vomiting the next day. He developed a rash that progressed to an ulcer of his thighs, thumb, and ankle. He was hospitalized and seen by multiple consultants including a psychiatrist, but it was not until December, 1973 that Dr. Cronin, a plastic surgeon, consulted because of the ulcers, recognized radiation necrosis. A radiotherapist concurred and a urologist reported one testis "sloughed out" and the other damaged beyond recovery. Some 16 surgical procedures were necessary to repair the damage, but the boy was castrated. At trial, expert witnesses were in agreement as to causation and Kerry Andrus Crocker was convicted on May 10, 1978. An appeal was based on ten separate errors in the trial court but Judge Douglas affirmed the conviction and Judge Odom concurred.

On January 14, 1981, Kerry Andrus Crocker was arrested by FBI agents in Wyoming where he was working under a false name as a petroleum consultant. He was returned to Houston to begin serving his sentence with an additional 5 years for bond jumping when his appeal was denied.

Comment

This is the only discovered instance of felonious as opposed to tortious radiation exposure. The outstanding feature is that from the first exposure on April, 1972 until ultimate recognition by Dr. Cronin in December 1973, 20 months elapsed. With increasing disability, the boy dropped out of school, was hospitalized and seen by 16 physicians, none of whom recognized or considered the possibility of radiation exposure. This may not be surprising, since only a radiotherapist or a surgeon experienced with this injury could be expected to recognize radiation necrosis. It is alarming, because with increasing use and availability of radiation sources, it is likely that such injuries have occurred, and will occur again, unrecognized.

NEUBERG vs. MICHAEL REESE HOSPITAL (D.C. Illinois, 1978) [21]
DUBIN vs. MICHAEL REESE HOSPITAL (App. Illinois, 1979) [22]

At one time radiotherapy for tonsillitis was favored over the risks of tonsillectomy and in the period from 1947 to 1951 a number of patients were so treated at Michael Reese Hospital. When instances of carcinoma of the thyroid were reported, follow up enquiries on Michael Reese patients were made. These two cases represent patients who have brought suit against the hospital some 30 years later. The suits are against the hospital rather than the physicians involved and, lacking a basis for a charge of negligence, the doctrine of product liability or strict liability is invoked for the first time in the matter of injury related to radiotherapy. The principle of product liability is that if the product is made and sold for profit, then the cost of injury resulting from its use should be borne by those who market such products, to be passed on as a cost of doing business, rather than by the injured persons who are powerless to protect themselves.

In the Neuberg case, the principle of product liability was held not applicable, since radiotherapy was offered as a service rather than a product for sale.

In the Dubin case, the trial court dismissed the charge on the same basis but on appeal the judgment is reversed and the case remanded for a new trial. Justice Downing writes, "We do not agree with the Neuberg court in its refusal to extend the doctrine of product liability to the defendant's supply of X-radiation because it was incidental to the rendering of a service". His concept is that an X-ray is derived from and composed of electricity, prepared, manufactured, distributed, and sold and injected into the bodies of the patients for profit, and that the defendant has the ability to distribute the risk of injury by passing the loss on to the public. "Therefore X-radiation, a form of electricity, should also be held to be a product for the purpose of stating a cause of action based on strict liability in tort".

Comment

These two cases offer a classic illustration of two decision-makers arriving at frankly contradictory opinions on the same evidence. The different result must be differing background and sensitivity of the judicial mind or the effectiveness of the testimony presented. But science must take the credit or the blame, for the truth achieved is what each judge "cannot help believing".

Of landmark importance is this introduction of the principle of strict or product liability into the field of radiation injury in the course of radiotherapy. At this time it applies to the hospital operating the radiotherapy equipment for a fee and would be readily extended to the manufacturer. The ultimate extension to the prescribing physician must be considered when the distinction between product and service is eroded by a convincing argument for a prepared mind.

Overlooking Justice Downing's novel concepts of radiation and radiotherapy, this is a development to overcome the objection to the opinion in the Wilkinson vs. Vesey case where it was necessary to establish negligence on the part of the physician if compensation was to be awarded to the innocent victim. Under strict liability in tort, or product liability, only injury and causation need be proven and society will share the burden of the injury without the need to brand the defendant as a 'wrong-doer'.

Addendum

Dubin vs. Michael Reese Hospital reached the Supreme Court of Illinois and in a decision handed down on December 1, 1980, the Appellate Court was reversed and the Circuit Court affirmed. Justice Moran held that X-radiation is not "unreasonably dangerous" per se and that the danger is the medical decision as to when it may be used, the manner of administration, and the amount applied. He ruled that strict liability does not come into play in determining the negligence of professional conduct and the Appellate Court decision by Justice Downing erred in finding X-radiation a product subject to the doctrine of strict liability in tort.

SILKWOOD vs. KERR MCGEE CORP. (Oklahoma, 1979)[23]

Karen Silkwood was an employee at the Cimmarron nuclear fuel reprocessing facility operated by the Kerr McGee Corporation. Plutonium found in the Silkwood apartment constituted the basis for an action in product liability and an award to the plaintiff of $505,000 for actual damage and $10,000,000 for punitive damages. The injury was contamination in the plaintiff's apartment where plutonium was found, and the related anxiety caused by such contamination. There is no showing or claim of a biological effect of radiation. In fact, it is indicated that "Silkwood's burden was within the regulation limits for a lifetime exposure" although there is "some evidence that the level of plutonium in Silkwood's apartment may potentially have exceeded that permitted in an unrestricted area such as a residence" .

This appeal from the trial court's verdict is based on a motion for a judgement, not withstanding the verdict, or a new trial.

The essential points are these:

1. Plutonium from the defendant's processing facility was found in the Silkwood apartment.
2. Responsibility for escape of the plutonium from the facility must fall on the defendant company. It does not matter how it reached Silkwood's apartment even if she herself brought it there; there could be no injury if it had not escaped.
3. The presence of the plutonium in the plaintiff's apartment is the injury. This is outside the workplace.
4. Even if the exposure in the apartment is less than the permissible occupational exposure, the plaintiff is not a worker outside of her place of employment and the lower level of permissible exposure to the public applies.
5. Compliance with all standards and regulations is not a defense to a charge of negligence, this in only evidence of care to be weighed by the jury.
6. The principle of ALARA (as low as reasonably achievable) overrides the maximum permissible dose, and will be weighed by the jury.
7. The principle of product liability applies.

Plutonium is a dangerous substance being manufactured and processed for profit. The defendant company is liable in damages in the allowing of plutonium to escape from the plant, without a requirement to show fault or carelessness. It would not matter if another party, or Silkwood herself, had carried it out, only that a dangerous product for profit caused an injury. The company also argued that a recovery of $10,505,000 was excessive, but Judge Theis finds it reasonable. Thus the decision sweeps away all arguments of the defense and concurs in the original decision.

Comment

The significance of this case lies in the reasoning rather than the result. The dessicated and lengthy opinion in the law report gives no recognition to the lurid accounts of Karen Silkwood's troubled personal life, involvement in union and company conflict, allegations of defective products and safety violations and rallying of anti-nuclear personalities of screen and television to her cause after her death in a one-car accident. These accounts in such diverse sources as *Saturday Evening Post* and *Science* are background to understanding the legal decision.

Anxiety as a compensable injury is well-established in this series of radiation cases that have been presented and product liability is an accepted legal device for redress where a product for profit is involved. The denial of observation of safety standards and regulations as a defense is an alarming development that must have some cautionary effect on participation of private enterprise in the nuclear energy program. This is a forseeable outcome of the application of the principle of ALARA where 'reasonable' is to be determined by a jury of average citizens.

A succinct appraisal of Judge Theis' opinion is that it presents Karen Silkwood's injury and the need for redress as a reflection of the public's concern for any radiation exposure, rather than science's weighing of danger vs. risk, or possibility vs. probability. It is likely that further appeal will be taken, but if the decision is not modified it may be precedent for a proliferation of suits involving low level radiation exposures that will be sustained despite all reasonable precautions short of prohibition of radiation.

Addendum

In December 1981 the 10th Circuit Court of appeals reversed the judgement of the lower court as to the damages of $505,000 awarded for personal injuries and punitive damages of $10,000,000. In a decision by Circuit Judge Logan it was held that the contamination of Karen Silkwood's person was job related. Worker's compensation legislation provides the remedy to the employee for accidental injury in the course of employment and at the same time protects the employer from other liability to the employee. Punitive damages were overruled because federal regulation of atomic energy precludes states from exercising regulatory authority over the handling of nuclear material. Judgement in the sum of $5000 was affirmed as to damages due to contamination of personal property in Silkwood's apartment. (667 Fed 2nd 908, 10th C.A., 1981)

Silkwood appealed this ruling to the U.S. Supreme Court which reversed and remanded back to the Appellate Court for reconsideration. (104 S. Ct. 615, 1984) This Supreme Court decision should be read in its entirety as an illustration of how a body of evidence can induce opposing interpretations and opinions in the minds of justices of our highest court.

Justice White rendered the majority opinion rejecting Kerr-McGee's submission that the punitive damages award conflicts with Congress' expressed intent to preclude dual regulation of radiation hazards. It finds ample evidence that Congress had no intention of forbidding state remedies for radiation injuries in a nuclear plant since it had provided no federal remedy for persons injured by such conduct.

Separate dissents were written by Justice Blackmun and Justice Powell, joined by Chief Justice Burger and Justice Marshall. They present that the majority opinion "wreaks havoc with the regulatory structure that Congress carefully constructed."

The dissent states that "The Nuclear Regulatory Commission (NRC) found no relevant violation of its stringent regulatory requirements worthy of punishment," and "There is no evidence that Silkwood suffered any specific injury, temporary or permanent, other than mental distress for a short period." They note that the jury was instructed that "compliance with federal standards was not a complete defense" and that "Your duty is to determine what constitutes the exercise of reasonable care in handling plutonium." The dissent continues, "The Court defends — judgements by lay juries with no competency to understand highly sophisticated technology of nuclear facilities." "Today the Court opens a wide and inviting door to indirect regulation by juries authorized to impose damages to punish and deter on the basis of inferences even when a plant has taken the utmost precautions provided by law."

At this time reconsideration by the 10th Circuit Court is awaited.

SINDELL vs. ABBOTT LABORATORIES (California, 1980)[24]

The plaintiffs are daughters of women who were given DES to prevent abortion and are representative of those who developed pelvic cancer apparently due to an effect of the drug upon the fetus. The obstructions to recovery are the uncertain etiology, the long latent period, the nonspecific injury, the uncertainty of causation particularly with regard as to what manufacturer produced the drug actually dispensed and ingested. The judgment was entered in favor of the defendant drug companies. Plaintiffs appealed. The appellate court and the Supreme Court of California reversed the lower court and entered judgment for the plaintiffs.

The basis for recovery is in previously established legal doctrines of product liability or strict liability in tort, the manufacturers had produced a dangerous product for profit, that the manufacturers could better sustain the burden of injury than the plaintiffs, and damages could be charged as a cost of doing business. The new element is a theory of liability based on market share. When multiple manufacturers produced the drug, and the producer of the specific drug ingested by the patient could not be identified, all manufacturers may be held liable for the proportion of the judgment represented by its share of the market.

Comment

The possible extension of this "market share" theory of liability to defendants in actions involving other hazardous agents and occupations is evident. Radiation is one agent among many too numerous to list. Where an individual has been employed by a number of firms involved in such activities as industrial radiography, a formula for assigning liability has not been established but the possibility of shared liability may evolve on a similar basis. Should the substance of this decision be confirmed on further appeal, which may well go to the U. S. Supreme Court, it will clearly affect all concerned with any aspect of radiation production or utilization.

As a device to protect the consumer, product liability, or strict liability has its justification in compensating the innocent victim, as any damage to equipment might be passed along to the public as a cost of doing business, without requirement of proof of fault or negligence.

DISCUSSION

Historical Background

The explosion of information in our time, and the reciprocal explosion of ignorance,[25] leaves little time for history, and means that immense amounts of information may be lost forever or must await costly rediscovery. This sampling of radiation injuries that were severe enough to come to court, can only hint at the much larger number of injuries that are not in the available legal reports or were sustained in silence, and an immense number of individuals exposed to levels of irradiation that would make population exposures due to the Utah fallout or the Three Mile Island incident seem insignificant. In a text, *Roentgen Rays and Phenomena of the Anode and Cathode,* published in 1896,[26] there is a photograph of the Edison X-ray exhibit at the New York Electrical Exposition of the Electric Light Association in June of that year. It shows a line of visitors awaiting their turn to see their hands shown on a fluoroscopic screen (Figure 1). The text describes, "Thousands of people, through the beneficence of Dr. Edison were permitted to see the shadows of their bones surrounded by living flesh. The screen was made of calcic tungstate. The hand and arm were placed behind and viewed from the front". The geometry and factors can only be surmised, but visitors and exhibitors would receive a substantial or even alarming dose in

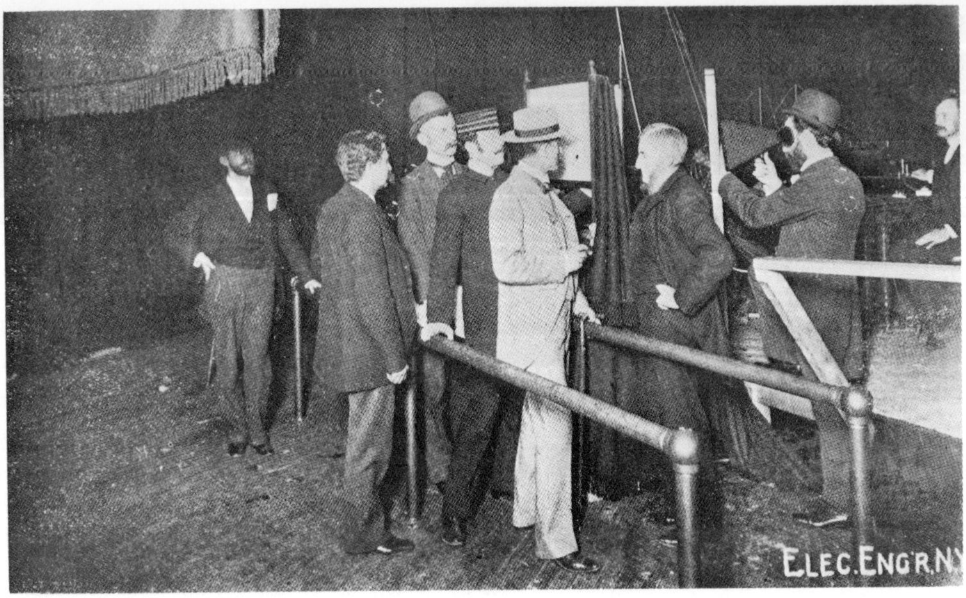

FIGURE 1. Visitors to the New York Electrical Exposition of the Electric Light Association on June 3, 1896 see their bones on a calcic tungstate screen (left) and a sciascope (near right) with no evident protection for the attendant. (From Thompson, Edward, P., *Roentgen Rays and Phenomena of the Anode and Cathode*, D. Van Nostrand Co., New York, 1896. With permission.)

this demonstration within 6 months of Roentgen's publication, when biologic effects were barely considered and the need for protection was not a concern. The same book contains advertisments of five manufacturers offering X-ray "outfits", apparatus, and tubes for sale (Figure 2). Manufacturers, physicists, physicians, patients, the public, and press were enthusiastic. The *Scientific American* for February 22, 1896, carried a progress note, "During the last week innumerable reports of work in X-ray photography have appeared in the columns of various journals, scientific and otherwise, but with comparatively little new matter in them. It still appears that Prof. Roentgen gave the matter so thorough a treatment before publishing his results that it has taken the rest of the scientific world a month to catch up with him".

The American record is only a reflection of a world-wide application of this new tool of science, medicine, and industry. Clearly there were martyrs and victims who paid the price of introducing a modality with benefits we would not choose to lose. The story points to a lesson learned and the need for caution in the introduction of new technologies. Still, a publication on "The Hazards to Man of Nuclear & Allied Radiation" by the Medical Research Council of Great Britain speaks of the 'appurtenances of civilization', "Since the discovery of X-rays and radioactive materials man has adapted them increasingly for certain of his needs. In medicine they now prove invaluable, and often irreplaceable, aids to diagnosis and treatment. They are also used extensively in industry and in the amenities of modern civilized life". If the introduction of the X-ray usage levied a toll of acute injuries that may be seen as the price of this amenity of civilization, we have had some 80 years and 3 or 4 generations to reap and recognize chronic and delayed effects. However these may be assessed they have been overwhelmed by improved health and longevity and the race is not in jeopardy on this account.

THE COURT

An essential difference to consider when law and science confront each other over problems

X-RAY OUTFITS.

The Edison Manufacturing Company

ARE PREPARED TO SUPPLY

MR. THOMAS A. EDISON'S ORIGINAL APPARATUS

As exhibited at the recent Electrical Exhibition in New York.

OUTFITS FOR TRAVELLING EXHIBITORS.
OUTFITS FOR SCIENTIFIC INSTITUTIONS.
OUTFITS FOR PHYSICIANS.
EDISON X-RAY TUBES.
EDISON-LALANDE BATTERIES FOR X-RAY APPARATUS.

WRITE FOR PARTICULARS.

EDISON MANUFACTURING COMPANY,
110 East 23d St., New York City.

X Ray Apparatus

OF ALL KINDS.

(1) **RUHMKORFF COILS.** (Immersed in oil;—the highest insurance of insulation.)

(2) **HOLTZ MACHINES.** (Latest type. Efficient, portable.)

(3) **HIGH FREQUENCY SETS.** (For alternating currents. Designed by Prof. Elihu Thomson.)

(4) **CROOKES TUBES.**

(*a*) Double-focussing (Thomson Universal).
(*b*) Single-focussing.
(*c*) Globular.
(*d*) Elongated pear-shape.

Our Thomson Universal Tube is the only one in the market that is provided with simple means of adjusting the vacuum.

(5) **FLUOROSCOPES.** (Approved patterns, various sizes.)

(6) **FLUORESCENCE SCREENS.** (Even distribution, various sizes.)

(7) **CALCIUM TUNGSTATE.** (Fine crystals, chemically pure.)

EDISON DECORATIVE & MINIATURE LAMP DEPT.,
Sussex and Fifth Streets,
HARRISON, N. J.

FIGURE 2. Advertisment(s) for X-ray apparatus appearing within a year of Roentgen's discovery. (From Thompson, Edward P., *Roentgen Rays and Phenomena of the Anode and Cathode,* D. Van Nostrand Co ., New York, 1896. With permission.)

such as the cases presented here, is that while both seek to establish truth and reach a conclusion, law is deliberative but science is investigative. The court, made up of judge and jury as individuals, weighs only testimony and evidence presented. They need not, and may not, inquire beyond what the parties in contest offer in support of their positions. There is no requirement to establish the court's credentials to deal with the specific matter in dispute. A comparison of classroom and courtroom may serve to illustrate. In class, the burden is on the student audience to absorb information and be tested by their teacher. In court, the burden is on the parties to the suit to present their information with credibility and be accepted or rejected by the audience of judge and jury. Viewed in this fashion any dissatisfaction or criticism of the reasoning or outcome must be looked upon as a failure to provide a believable account. The verdict or opinion is what the court "can't help believing" after the parties have had their day in court.

Society generally has shown an increasing willingness to share the burden of illness or injury that befalls the individual, by the mechanisms of insurance premiums, increased cost of products and services, or tax-supported welfare systems. There has been a similar evolution in legal thinking, in the area of litigation involving liability and damages for injury. That this is particularly evident in matters of radiation and cancer over the past 50 years, from the radium dial painters cases to the Silkwood case, only illustrates that the personnel of the courts share public apprehension on these subjects. From the mounting urgency of problems to be solved it must be expected that a body of law on radiation and cancer will grow. Science has a stake in this development that calls for vigorous and thoughtful participation.

THE EXPERT WITNESS

Science, in the role of expert witness, clearly has knowledge in the area of radiation litigation that is beyond the knowledge of the courts. But in many cases there is no need for science's expertise. Radiation is only another dangerous agent and in acute injury, where cause and effect are not in doubt, established legal rules determine liability. Beginning with the radium dial painters cases, and with increasing frequency as current problems of medical and industrial use and disposal of radioactive materials are fanned by inflammatory rather than informational reports, a more urgent need for the expert witness arises. Appraisal of dose from low level exposure, greatly delayed effects, intervening or contributing factors and nonspecific or spontaneously occurring conditions, cloud the issues of injury and causation. The court can and will decide, with or without the advice of science, but the testimony of the expert witness may have an effect that goes far beyond the case at hand.

As an ordinary witness, any individual may be subpoenaed to court to give testimony as to facts within his personal knowledge, any object, act, or happening that he personally perceived, or action that he himself has taken. He may not offer inferences or conclusions, nor hearsay, i.e. what someone else has said about a fact, as proof of that fact. There are fixed exceptions to the rule, e.g. a dying declaration, declaration as to bodily condition or state of mind, such as a patient may relate to a physician in the course of a medical history, but these do not bear specifically on our purpose.

Expert opinion is called upon when the information and facts are beyond the experience and knowledge of laymen on the jury. The expert witness has special status. Because of his special knowledge, his opinion based on such knowledge may be helpful to the court. First he will be called upon to recite his qualifications. If accepted by the court he may be asked to present his opinion and conclusions. These are not binding, the jury decides upon his credibility. In the adversary atmosphere of the courtroom, the expert witness will be subject to cross-examination. At the end of the cross-examination the expert witness is entitled to rehabilitation, which is the term for defense to impeachment. The witness must be given the opportunity to explain, mitigate, or deny.

In examining the role of the expert witness, in our sampling of radiation litigation, the first observation is on contradictory opinions that may be expressed. The legal presentation is deliberately and necessarily adversary between plaintiff's and defendant's attorneys. But it is a little startling to find that the facts of science, at least when presented in the opinions and conclusions of expert witnesses lend themselves so well to the support of adversary opinions from radiation's earliest appearance in court in 1896 to our most recent example in 1979. This raises the matter of credibility in the eyes of the jury. We must assume that expert witnesses of different convictions are themselves convinced of the validity of their views; they need only offer a presentation that judge and jury "can't help believing", and this in the face of cross-examination aimed at discrediting. Preparation must include careful briefing of attorneys for all too often consultation may be a hurried meeting at the courtroom door.

The areas for opinion of expert witnesses are likely to be the nature of radiation exposure, the nature of the radiation effect or injury, the relation between the two called causation, and customary conduct under the circumstances of the case which may indicate care or lack of it. The physical basis for exposure and the biological basis for injury are clear to the expert witness perhaps, but although his opinions and conclusions are admissible, it is his communication with the jury, his credibility, that renders his testimony effective. The expert witness must come to court to convince as well as instruct.

RECOMMENDATIONS

1. The professional societies that deal with radiation research, biology, physics, diag-

nostic, and therapeutic radiology and nuclear medicine should have committees on law and legislation.

2. These committees should maintain a surveillance of litigation involving radiation and publish lists and abstracts of such cases.
3. The committees should have an ongoing instructional program dealing with radiation and the law.
4. They should encourage interested members to consider law as one area for graduate study and make full use, in an advisory capacity, of any member who does proceed to a degree in law. Radiation law is a burgeoning area and there is need for individuals who can speak the languages of both law and science.

GLOSSARY OF LEGAL TERMS

INJURY — Any wrong or damage done to another, either in his person, rights, reputation, or property.

DANGER — The *possibility* of injury. This is inherent to a given situation and there is no liability for danger as such. Dangerous procedures are made feasible by the careful conduct of a physician.

RISK — The *probability* of injury. It is in the power of the physician to decrease or increase this probability by care, or lack of it, in a given circumstance. This is the basis for liability.

LIABLE — To be bound or obligated to make satisfaction, compensation or restitution for an injury to another as determined by rules of law or equity.

TORTS — This is the study of a continuously evolving area of law which has to do with the rights, wants, and desires of the individual. When these are recognized in law (and this is a state of mind, restrained by the past, and urged by the future), one who interferes with their realization will be liable.

TORT — This is the offense. It has four essential components. A legal injury must be proven. There must be a duty which one party owes another. There must be a violation of this duty. The injury must result from such violation.

INTENTIONAL TORT — The types are assault, battery, interference with peace of mind, and false imprisonment.

UNINTENTIONAL TORT — This is negligence.

NEGLIGENCE — An unintentional tort that arises when a duty of care between two parties is breached by act or omission that is at odds with what a reasonable and prudent person would do. It is necessary to prove the injury, the act, and that the act caused the injury. The act was not intended to cause the injury, but the injury was forseeable, and the act entailed an unreasonable risk.

FAULT — Any deviation from prudence, duty or rectitude; any shortcoming or neglect of care, of performance resulting from inattention, incapacity, or perversity.

MALPRACTICE — Bad, wrong, or injudicious treatment of a patient, professionally, or in respect to a particular disease or injury, resulting in injury, unnecessary suffering, or death to the patient, proceeding from ignorance, carelessness, want of proper professional skill, disregard of established rules or principles, neglect, or malicious or criminal intent.

EVIDENCE — The content of legal presentation in court—records, documents, objects or verbal accounts — for the purpose of inducing judge and jury to believe the contentions of the parties to the trial of an issue.

TESTIMONY — Information presented orally by a competent witness under oath, sometimes used synonymously with the broader term evidence which includes all testimony.

EXPERT WITNESS — An individual competent to give expert testimony because of special knowledge, skill, or experience not likely to be possessed by the ordinary layman. Where an ordinary witness may give testimony only to what he has experienced by his five senses, the expert is entitled to give an opinion or an inference. The jury determines his credibility.

ARGUMENT — An effort to establish belief by a course of reasoning.

PROOF — The conviction or persuasion of the mind of a judge or jury by the exhibition of evidence and the presentation of argument, of the reality of a fact alleged. (Anything you can get judge or jury to believe).

CORRELATIVE — Having a mutual or reciprocal relation, in such sense that the existence of one necessarily implies the existence of the other. (Left and right, up and down, duty and right).

RIGHT — That which a man is entitled to have, or to do, or to receive from others, by custom, by law, or by agreement. There is no right unless there is an identifiable person with a duty to satisfy the desire.

DUTY — The obligation to meet the expectations of another as to his person, his possessions and his actions, such as are recognized by custom, by law, or by agreement. There is no duty unless there is an identifiable person with a right to receive the obligation.

CRIME — An offense prosecuted by the state for conduct prohibited by law or failure to comply with a requirement of law. The essential feature is the existence of legislation or regulation requiring or prohibiting a specific act or conduct.

PRODUCT LIABILITY or STRICT TORT LIABILITY — The elements are (1) a product marketed for profit, (2) a defect in the product which may be in its manufacturing, its design or its marketing including packaging or warning, (3) an injury due to such defect. It is not necessary to prove negligence on the part of the manufacturer. Liability may exist even if the product has passed through several hands to an ultimate user.

FICTION OF LAW — Something known to be false is assumed to be true. A rule of law which assumes as true, and will not allow to be disproved, something which is false but not impossible. The assumption is of a beneficial nature as a device to aid decision-making by extending a procedure from cases where it is applicable, to others where it is not strictly applicable, e.g. it is a rule of law that consent, to be valid, must be informed, but it is a fiction of law that assumes that a patient can be fully informed about radiation and cancer in order to consent to radiotherapy.

REFERENCES

1. **Pitkin, John T.,** The Orme Murder Case, The roentgen ray in the Orme murder trial, *Am. X-Ray J.*, 4, 531—534, 1899; **Ross, Frank Ward,** *The X-ray in forensic medicine, Medico-Legal J.*, 16, 142—149, 1898.
2. The Frank Balling Case, *Am. X-Ray J.*, 4, 566, 1899.
3. Henslin vs. Wheaton, 97 N.W., 882, 1904.
4. Sauers vs. Smits, 95 P. 1097, 1908.
5. Coombs vs. King, 78 A. 468, 1910.
6. Sweeney vs. Erving, 233 U.S. Sup. Ct., 815, 1913.
7. Coover vs. Painless Parker, 286 P. 1048, 1930.
8. Vallat vs. Radium Dial Co., 196 N.E. 485, 1935
9. LaPorte vs. U.S. Radium Corp., 13 F. Supp., 263, 1935.
10. Ferrara vs. Galluchio, 152 N.E. 2d 249, 71 ALR 2d 331, 1958.
11. Natanson vs. Kline, 354 P. 2d 670, 1960.
12. Kuhne vs. U. S. A./U. S. Fidelity & Guaranty Co., 250 F. Supp. 523, 1965.
13. Besner vs. Kidde, 24 A.D. 2d 1045, 1965.
14. Employers Mutual vs. Parker , 418 S.W. 2d 570, 1967.
15. Wilkinson vs. Vesey, 295 A.2d 676, 1972.
16. State Compensation Fund vs. Cora Mae Joe & Fannie Dick, 543 P. 2d 790, 1976.
17. Dayton vs. Boeing, 389 F. Supp. 433, 1975.
18. Pegram vs. Sisco, 426 F. Supp. 776, 1976.

19. Martinez vs. Univ. of Calif. D. C., 1st Judicial District County of Rio Arriba, N.M. 5 April, 1978; 601 P.2d 425, 1979.
20. Crocker vs. State of Texas, 573 S.W. 2d 190, 1978.
21. Neuberg vs. Michael Reese Hospital, 377 N.E. 2d 215, 1978.
22. Dubin vs. Michael Reese Hospital, 393 N.E. 2d 588, 1979.
23. Silkwood vs. Kerr McGee Corp., 485 F. Supp. 566, 1979.
24. Sindell vs. Abbott Laboratories, App. 149 Cal. Rptr 138 (1978); Cal., 607 P. 2d 924, 1980.
25. **Lukasiewicz, J.** The ignorance explosion, *Trans. N. Y. Acad. Sci.* 34, 373—391, 972.
26. **Thompson, Edward, P.,** *Roentgen Rays and Phenomena of the Anode and Cathode*, D. Van Nostrand Co., New York, 1896.

PUBLIC RELATIONS RESPONSIBILITIES IN HEALTH PHYSICS

Ronald L. Kathren and Barbara L. Matthews

RESPONSIBILITIES AND OBLIGATIONS

Public relations is a term with many meanings. Frequently it is taken to be synonymous with publicity, promotion, and propaganda, as practiced by press agents, politicians, and advertising personnel. Thus, for many scientists engaged in radiation protection, public relations has little or no relevance to their workaday world. Only in the event of a radiological accident may practitioners of radiation protection perceive themselves as involved in public relations, and then perhaps only to the extent of supplying the news media with a terse factual statement of the event, usually via the company public information officer.

Public relations, however, is much broader in scope and considerably more important than creating a favorable public image or providing an after-the-fact accounting of an accidental occurrence. Rather, it includes the sum total of communication between the practitioners of radiation protection and the public. From these communications, the public will gain a perception of radiation and radiation protection. The accuracy of this perception will, of course, depend on many factors, not the least of which are the accuracy of the information presented to the public, and the means of presentation. Also, the particular sector of the public will play an important role in the perception; other scientists will perceive radiation protection activities far differently than politicians, or students, or any other group of individuals.

The health physicist or other radiation protection specialist has certain basic responsibilities and obligations in the broad area of public relations. These include legal and contractual obligations as well as ethical responsibilities. In the latter regard, the single most important obligation is the need to communicate openly, honestly, and completely about radiation protection matters. Such communications must be straightforward and unbiased, and must present an accurate portrayal of the topic or situation. Note that the obligation of openness, completeness, and honesty is paramount but in some instances may be tempered by the responsibility to maintain certain information private. Thus, trade secrets or processes, personal information, and the right of the individual to privacy must be respected. Similarly, information, however newsworthy, must not be released prematurely.

Certain obligations of employment must also be fulfilled, assuming these do not conflict with laws, regulations, or professional ethics. Thus, it is incumbent upon the health physicist to use established management and other communication channels, and to avoid initiating direct communication with the news media unless this is in consonance with the policies of the employer. Ordinarily, employers will have a designated person who functions as public information officer, with responsibility for contact and liaison with the media. It is this person through whom the health physicist will ordinarily contact the press and other media.

In addition, an employee or consultant has a basic obligation to an employer not to reveal information classified for reasons of security, whether national or industrial. To do so would constitute a severe breach of ethics, and may well be in violation of a contract, a law, or a regulation. Also, the health physicist must refrain from revealing decisions or facts that could place his or her employer in an inferior competetive position, or that, if taken out of context, may give rise to erroneous conclusions on the part of the public, for the health physicist has an important and deep responsibility to try to ensure that the public receives an accurate, factual account of whatever event is being reported. Thus, the health physicist should avoid opinions and conjecture, particularly as these may relate to the aftermath of an accident, unless such opinion can be well supported by fact and is in consonance with generally accepted scientific data.

In addition to his employer, the health physicist also has certain obligations to his professional peers, other professionals with whom he may interface, and the public as a whole. In general, these responsibilities are met by the simple method of honesty and openness. However, in relationships with other professionals, reasoned opinion and conjecture as well as statements not fully supported by data may be necessary. When such statements are made, it is incumbent upon the health physicist to advise the other professionals of the most probable situation, and to assist by interpreting the available health physics data in a meaningful and understandable way. This is particularly important when dealing with physicians and other medical personnel, who may be charged with the care of a contaminated or overexposed individual, but who do not fully comprehend the biological or dosimetric implications of the case.

Perhaps the overriding responsibility in the public relations area is that owed the public. In addition to honesty, the public has a right to be informed on radiological safety matters, without being unduly alarmed or made complacent of the potential hazards. Rather the public should be given a fair and complete discussion of radiological safety and protection, and the health physicist should be accessible to those members of the public who may wish to ask questions relating to health physicists. To discharge this important responsibility adequately, the health physicist must answer in the *lingua franca* or common language; use of technical terminology, mathematical or statistical hedging, or exceptions should not be used when a simple yes or no or similarly simple answer will suffice. And, finally, the health physicist must not become polarized or present a biased or distorted point of view; rather he or she must strive for an honest and balanced point of view.

PUBLIC PERCEPTION AND PUBLIC OPINION

The perception of radiation, radioactivity, and nuclear power has undergone radical changes over the years. In the early years after the discovery of X-rays and radioactivity, these were imbued with phenomenal, almost magical, properties by the news media, who were prone to great exaggeration of beneficial effects of radiation, as well as of the physical aspects of these phenomena. A similar positive image was initially created about nuclear power and radionuclide applications in the first decade or so following World War II. Unlike the situation with radium and X-rays, this positive perception did not persist; by the late 1960s, organized opposition to nuclear power reactors began to appear, and what appeared to be a rather abrupt change in public perception became evident.

Public opinion is, of course, based in large measure on public perception. In the late 1960s and throughout the 1970s, a large body of data began to be collected by pollsters interested in public opinions of nuclear power as well as the underlying perceptions held by various respondents. The initial studies conducted about 1970 showed that while a majority or a significant plurality of those surveyed favored nuclear power, there was also a large segment of the population — as many as a third — who had no opinion. In general, men tended to favor nuclear power more than women; women also had a greater percentage of respondents in the no opinion or undecided category.

Opposition to nuclear power was generally based on nuclear or radiological safety concerns, with radioactive waste management and disposal being the primary area of concern. Thus, at least among the roughly one-fourth of the population opposed to nuclear power, there is a perception of danger — perhaps the fear of the control of technology not well understood. Many of those in favor of nuclear power share this type of perception. It is important to recognize that these perceptions are not based on calculations or objective risk estimates as are so-called expert perceptions or hazards evaluations. And, it should also be noted that as yet, the factors that control public perception of risk are as yet largely unknown.

For the health physicist, some clearly helpful information can be obtained from the polls which is directly applicable to public relations situations. First, the public in general has a great deal of confidence in what scientists say on matters relating to nuclear power and technology. In a large poll conducted in the mid-1970s, nearly three-fifths (58%) of the general public expressed confidence in the words of scientists. By contrast, no other group even approached 50%; for example, only about a third of public (34%) had a great deal of confidence in what was said by leading ''environmentalists'', a fourth (24%) in the President of the U. S., and about a fifth in the heads of electric utilities (i.e., business leaders) and news media personnel. The obvious interpretation of this result is one of credibility for the health physicist or other scientist involved in radiation protection activities.

Public opinion and quite possibly public perception of nuclear power appears to have remarkable stability over the years. Following the major accident at the Three Mile Island Nuclear Power Station on March 28, 1979, public sentiment in favor of nuclear power dropped. Similarly, the fraction opposed to nuclear power increased. However, within a few months, the percentages had ''rebounded'' to what they were prior to the accident. This suggests that the accident had no significant permanent effect on the basic public perception of nuclear power.

PUBLIC AFFAIRS

Public affairs is a newly emerging specialized area largely concerned with relationships between a company and governmental bodies and elected officials. Thus, it includes lobbying within its purview, although in general, public affairs is not synonymous with lobbying but rather includes many other activities relating to corporate citizenship. Thus, the public affairs role of a corporation may include political education of employees (and the public), support of various political causes and candidates (including formation of political action committees of PAC's), and participation in various activities (such as hearings) of public agencies, in addition to the more traditional lobbying role.

RELATIONSHIPS WITH THE NEWS MEDIA

Good communication skills are important in winning success for organizations, ideas, and programs. The fastest, most efficient way to reach a large number of people is through the mass media — newspapers, radio-television, and magazines. Newspapers and magazines are sometimes known as the ''print media'' and radio and television as the ''electronic media''. The latter are faster in response, and generally allow relatively little time for each story. However, the basic principles of working with reporters from each sector are the same.

People who understand the needs and operations of the mass media are in the best position to secure the media exposure their organizations want and need. The following are a few basic ideas for working with and through the news media .

1. *Understand the news media representatives* — They are people whose work constantly exposes them to differing points of view in America's open marketplace of ideas. That does not mean they are inherently biased or against your point of view. It does mean they are skeptical and will ask tough questions. Accept this as part of the mutual give and take in dealing with reporters.
2. *Remember that public relations is a long-term proposition* — Good public relations with the news media means establishing your credibility as a reliable source of news over a period of months. It involves getting to know individual reporters, understanding media needs, and being helpful to them.
3. *Know the media you are dealing with* — Begin by making or obtaining a list of local papers, radio-TV stations and magazines. Visit or call each one to learn their deadlines and how they prefer to receive information. For example, some newspapers like to

get a written news announcement of an upcoming meeting. Others prefer that you telephone in the information which their reporters can use to write a story. Get the name of contact people you should deal with and investigate news options that may be open to you: TV talk show interviews; public service announcements, or coverage of major meetings, conventions or speeches.

4. *When appropriate, offer personal service to the news media as an information source* — Most reporters have minimal background in radiation protection, and many are not sure where to get answers to basic questions. You can help build long-term good relationships by offering to explain technical information. Be modest in your approach. Do not try to educate everyone on all facets of your specialty. Be a source of information — one who can help others break through complex concepts and the technical jargon. This may well require practice and will be most effective if each local organization identifies members who are skilled at translating technical information to lay terms.
5. *Prepare carefully for interviews with reporters* — If you know the topic in advance, make a careful outline of the key points you want to make. Keep it simple and stick to the main points. Try out your explanations on a lay person to make sure you are communicating clearly. Avoid technical jargon and acronyms. When their use is unavoidable, provide written definitions /explanations which the reporter can refer to later in writing the story. For oral interviews, short, simple answers are best.
6. *Be prepared to respond to the news media* — Some of your dealings with the media may be in delicate or crisis situations. You can deal with these situations most effectively when you are prepared. Identify your organizational spokespersons and make sure they have copies of position statements on sensitive issues. Take time to prepare a response. It is perfectly fair to tell a reporter you will call him back after you have collected your thoughts. But, be timely! Good, longterm relationships are enhanced by observing news deadlines.

PREPARATION OF PUBLIC ANNOUNCEMENTS FOR THE MEDIA

The health physicist may occasionally find it necessary to prepare public announcements on meetings, new facilities, routine operations and accident and emergency situations, particularly if there are only limited public relations services available within his company. The media are deluged daily with news releases from hundreds of organizations. Paying some attention to journalistic style will increase (though not guarantee) the chances of getting your story published or used on the air.

There is no need to be uncomfortable with journalism. The need for good grammar and clarity of expression are guidelines for any writing. The change is in style, with emphasis placed on objectivity, accuracy, and brevity. Some important points to remember in writing are:

1. Use short sentences and paragraphs.
2. Use active verbs.
3. Be objective. Be fair and impartial in selecting facts and attribute statements of opinion to an authority.
4. Do not color your story with prejudicial words and labels, or with emotional statements or buzz words.
5. Be accurate; be specific. Pay attention to using exact days and dates. Avoid using "yesterday" or "Friday".
6. Keep it uncluttered. Try to stick to the important details.
7. Use attribution. Every story must have a source. Identify your source by name and title in the body of the story. Expressions of judgment or viewpoint should be directly attributed to the source throughout the story.

8. Avoid jargon and highly technical terms and discussions.

The oldest and most useful news structure is the inverted pyramid. It is essentially a mold that separates facts in diminishing order of importance. The most important points are covered in the beginning or ''lead''. The lesser ones are left to the end where they can be eliminated to fit the demands of time, space, and editorial decisions.

The most important element of the story is the lead, which introduces the story and, hopefully, will catch the interest of the reader. The lead may be one or two sentences or several paragraphs. The most common lead is the summary lead, which tells the reader the important facts: Who, What, When, Where, Why, and sometimes How. Reader interest is attracted by picking the most important of those elements and putting the primary focus on it.

The remainder of the story should be used to provide any necessary elaboration on the major points. The order may be based on chronology (such as in an account of an accident), priority (such as a meeting notice), or sequence (such as a cause-and-effect situation). However the body of the story is shaped, the important facts should come first.

MECHANICS OF NEWS RELEASE PREPARATION

1. Type news releases, double spaced, on 8 $^1/_2 \times 11$ in. white paper. Use only one side of the paper.
2. Start the text $^1/_3$ of the way down the first page.
3. In upper left hand corner of page 1, put your name and home and office telephone numbers. Just beneath your name, put a few words about the subject of the story.
4. Below the subject matter, type: ''For Immediate Release: (insert date).''
5. If there is more than one page, center the word ''more'' at the bottom of page 1. Continue the story about 2 in. down on page 2. Identify page 2 in the upper left hand corner with ''page 2'' and a couple of words about the subject matter. At the end of the story type ''end'' or ''30''.
6. Limit your information to those two pages, at a maximum.

REFERENCES

1. **Cutlip, Scott, M. and Center, Allen, H.,** *Effective Public Relations,* 4th Ed., Prentice-Hall, New York, 1971.
2. Louis Harris and Associates,Inc., A Second Survey of Public and Leadership Attitudes Toward Nuclear Power Development in the United States, Ebasco Services (privately printed), November 1976.
3. **Hébert, John, A. and Kathren, Ronald, L.,** Radiation and the Perception of Risk in the U.S.A., Book of Papers of the Fifth Int. Congr. International Radiation Protection Association, Jerusalem, Vol. I, March 9—14, 1980, 323—327.
4. **Lesley, Philip, Ed.,** *Lesly's Public Relations Handbook,* Prentice-Hall, Englewood, N.J., 1971.
5. **Marston, John,** *The Nature of Public Relations,* McGraw-Hill, New York, 1963.
6. **Nielander, William, A.,** *Public Relations,* University of Texas, Austin, 1967.

TECHNIQUES AND METHODS OF DISSEMINATING INFORMATION TO THE PUBLIC ABOUT RADIATION AND NUCLEAR POWER

Kenneth L. Miller

In its investigation of the March 28, 1979 accident at Three Mile Island, the Kemeny Commission discovered that the public and the news media had been poorly instructed in the aspects of radiation and nuclear power. In trying to correct this deficiency and improve upon past performances, various professional societies such as the American Nuclear Society and the Health Physics Society have expended considerable effort to develop improved programs. Additionally, there have been numerous conferences and symposia conducted in an attempt to determine the best methods for informing the public and to provide an opportunity for inter-change of ideas between representatives of news media and the professional societies. The following perspectives on the best approach have been abstracted with permission from the proceedings of a symposium held on May 30, 1981: INFORMING THE PUBLIC ABOUT RADIATION AND NUCLEAR POWER. This symposium was cosponsored by the Baltimore-Washington Chapter of the Health Physics Society and the Radiation Safety Section of the National Institutes of Health.

RADIATION PROFESSIONALS PERSPECTIVES

1. There is doubt as to whether or not the public wants to know more about radiation and nuclear power.
2. Industry should have well-trained spokespersons who will discuss emergencies in a truthful and forthright manner.
3. The reasons why nuclear plants are not atomic bombs should be carefully, simply, and thoroughly explained.
4. Hazards of exposure to radiation and radioactivity should be put into recognizable terms by comparison to everyday associations such as normal background levels.
5. Beneficial and positive uses of radiation and by-products of nuclear power such as beneficial uses of thermal discharges should be emphasized.
6. The nuclear industry should establish press centers.
7. Tours of nuclear power plants are encouraged.
8. Informational booklets should be prepared.
9. Attend antinuclear meetings to answer questions and insure accuracy of disseminated information.
10. The public wants reassurance rather than a plethora of facts, figures, and information which they do not understand.
11. Remember that most of the press consists of competent journalists who are incompetent in the radiation and nuclear field.
12. Never speak down to your audience.
13. Professional groups should view public information as a responsibility of the profession.
14. Professional organizations should insure their speakers are abreast of current controversies.
15. Education of the public on nuclear and radiation matters has to begin at the lower high school grade level or even in the elementary schools.
16. Candor is the first responsibility in reaching the public and disseminating the truth.
17. Tell the public what the benefits are and what the risks are and give them credit for being able to understand.
18. Polls have indicated that (a) the most significant group against nuclear power is woman, (b) the next closest group is young people, and (c) the group most in favor of nuclear power is highly educated people.

19. Attempting to inform the public about radiation is the same as embarking on a fools mission. The public does not want to and does not need to learn about radiation and atomic energy.
20. Most things that you talk to the public about tend to convince them that there is something to be afraid of.
21. Journalists deceive.
22. The news media lies.
23. When being interviewed by the media be prepared to give them background information.
24. If you do not have final approval over what is shown, do not let the news media tape you.
25. Speak on the level of the audience.

NEWS MEDIA PERSPECTIVES

1. The scientific community has to develop a way of effectively explaining to the public why a nuclear reactor cannot blow up like an atom bomb.
2. The public needs to know that the problems of waste disposal are not technical but political problems.
3. All malignant energy sources, whether fossil or nuclear, have to be opposed.
4. Broad data on nuclear issues should be given to the public.
5. If activities cannot be justified they should not be done.
6. All information should be shared with the public as it becomes available unless there are very strong reasons for keeping it secret, such as national security.
7. There are both good and bad reporters.
8. When public relations presents only the good side, it does a disservice to the organization which it represents.
9. The professional has got to talk to reporters and make them understand what the technology is.
10. During a crisis professionals need to be accessible.
11. The public needs to be in on the scientific decision-making process before it can understand the scientific process.
12. Have written information available for distribution when interviews are requested.
13. Honesty is the best policy, always tell the truth.
14. Handle interviews through your public relations office.
15. You should not answer all questions asked by reporters, only those to which you know the answers.
16. Do not assume a reporter has heard or understood all that you have said.
17. Handle media inquiries as quickly as possible.
18. Do not answer questions with ''no comment'', explain why you are not commenting.
19. Remember that reporters are exposed to a number of views on controversial subjects.
20. Remember, the judgement on continuing the nuclear power program will be made by the general public.
21. People tune out when they cannot judge technical issues for themselves, and they tend to go with the ones who give them the worst news.
22. Do not try to communicate too much, but communicate clearly on key points.
23. Technical people must overcome their distrust of the press if they are going to be effective.

In the words of Daniel J. Boorstin: ''As a nation we should cure ourselves of the contagious cliché that what we need is an ''informed citizenry''. What we really need is a knowledgeable citizenry''.*

* From Boorstin, D. J., Homo Up-to-Datum Is a Dunce, *Reader's Digest,* September 1982, 54—56. With permission.

MANAGEMENT OF RADIOACTIVE WASTE

William D. Allen

INTRODUCTION

A comprehensive radiation safety[1-6] program must encompass all aspects of the receipt, use, and disposal of radioactive material for protection of personnel and the environment. The management of waste produced during nuclear operations presents a challenge that must receive a health physicist's thorough attention. In this chapter the general concepts of managing various wastes will be discussed. It should be noted that a waste management program is facility specific and in some instances program specific. Detailed plans and procedures must be developed to assure adequate waste control measures are considered prior to the receipt and use of radioactive material.

WASTE CATEGORIES

Many previous attempts[7-10] have been made to categorize waste in groups such as "High", "Intermediate", and "Low". These arbitrary terms were often misleading due to the fact that the two lower hazard categories were defined with respect to the high level waste generated at fuel reprocessing plants.

More recently a new classification system was adopted[11] for radioactive wastes for near surface disposal: This system provides three classifications of waste:

- **Class A** — Waste which has the least radioactivity but may require segregation at the burial site if stability requirements of 10 CFR 61.56 (b) are not met.
- **Class B** — Waste which may be more radioactive than Class A and has more rigid requirements on structural stability.
- **Class C** — Waste with the maximum allowed radioactivity, requires structural stability and may require burial at greater depths or barriers to protect against inadvertent intrusion.

The classification, in general, is determined by the half life and type of radionuclide. For radioactive waste containing only those radionuclides listed in Table 1, classification is as follows:

- If the concentration does not exceed 0.1 times the value in Table 1, the waste is Class A.
- If the concentration exceeds 0.1 times the value in Table 1, but does not exceed the value in Table 1, the waste is Class C.
- If the waste exceeds the concentration values of Table 1, it is generally not acceptable for near-surface disposal.
- For wastes containing mixtures of the radionuclides in Table 1 if the sum of fractions exceeds unity, the waste is considered to be in the next higher classification.

If the radioactive waste does not contain any of the radioisotopes listed in Table 1, classification is determined based on the concentrations in Table 2.

If the waste contains radionuclides contained in Table 2 but not Table 1, classification is as follows:

- If the concentration does not exceed the value in Column 1, the waste is Class A.

Table 1

Radionuclide	Concentration (Ci/m³)
C-14	8
C-14 in activated metal	80
Ni-59 in activated metal	220
Nb-94 in activated metal	0.2
Tc-99	3
I-129	0.08

Radionuclide	Concentration (nCi/g)
Alpha emitting transuranic nuclides with half-life greater than 5 years	100
Pu-241	3,500
Cm-242	20,000

Table 2

Radionuclide	Concentration (Ci/m³)		
	Column 1	Column 2	Column 3
Total of all nuclides with less than 5 year half life	700	[a]	[a]
H-3	40	[a]	[a]
Co-60	700	[a]	[a]
Ni-63	3.5	70	700
Ni-63 in activated metal	35	700	7000
Sr-90	0.4	150	7000
Cs-137	1	44	4600

[a] There are no limits established for these radionuclides in Class B or C wastes. Practical considerations such as the effects of external radiation and internal heat generation on transportation, handling, and disposal will limit the concentrations for these wastes. These wastes shall be Class B unless the concentrations of other nuclides in Table 2 determine the waste to the Class C independent of these nuclides.

- If the concentration exceeds the value in Column 1, but does not exceed the value in Column 2, the waste is Class B.
- If the concentration exceeds the value in Column 2 but does not exceed the value in Column 3, the waste is Class C.
- If the concentration exceeds the value in Column 3, the waste is not generally acceptable for near-surface disposal.
- For wastes containing mixtures of the radionuclides listed in Table 2, if the sum of fractions exceeds unity, the waste is considered to be in the next higher classification.
- For mixtures of radionuclides from both Tables, the most restrictive classification applies.
- If the radioactive waste does not contain any nuclides listed in either Table 1 or 2, it is Class A.

Packaging requirements have been designed to facilitate handling at the disposal site and provide protection of disposal site personnel. Included in the restrictions are that disposal in cardboard or fiberboard boxes is unacceptable; liquid waste must be solidified or packaged in sufficient absorbent material to absorb twice the volume of the liquid; for solid wastes containing liquid, the liquid shall not exceed more than 1% of the volume; wastes must not be capable of explosion under normal temperatures or pressures or upon exposure to water; wastes must not contain or generate toxic gases, vapors or fumes; wastes must not be pyrophoric; wastes in gaseous form must not be packaged at pressures greater than 1.5 atm at 20°C and cannot exceed 100 Ci/container; biological pathogenic or infectious materials must be treated to minimize these hazards.

Waste Types

As the maximum permissible concentrations decrease, waste management controls should increase. Three types of radioactive waste,[12] regardless of concentrations, need to be addressed — solid, liquid, and gaseous. In addition, it should be emphasized that over-reaction in the control of one type of waste may adversely affect another. For example, an overzealous attempt at decontaminating a piece of equipment may generate an excessive volume of liquid waste containing perhaps chemical wastes as well as radioactive materials. If the equipment is prone to recurrent contamination, evaluation of the necessity for decontamination as well as the residual levels that may be safely permitted should be performed prior to the decontamination effort.

WASTE MANAGEMENT FACILITIES

When selecting or preparing facilities and space requirements to support a radiation safety program, the health physicist should consider, in detail, the waste management program necessary to support anticipated activities. This evaluation should include an estimate of solid, liquid, and gaseous waste production so that proper facilities may be dedicated.

Gaseous radwaste systems must be evaluated to review the production rate of filters and assure that adequate space is available for changeout, storage and preparation for disposal. In addition, if short lived radionuclides will be present on air handling equipment, consideration of storage space for decay may be required. Facilities should be reviewed during air handling system operation to assure that air movement is from areas of expected lower to higher concentrations. Modifications to or administrative control of doors or openings may be required to assure proper movement and balance. In addition, facilities surrounding air handling equipment should be reviewed to assure adequate space is available to support routine and special maintenance activities. Depending on types and quantities of materials to be handled, consideration of isolation or recirculation and treatment capability to minimize releases during an accident condition may require facility modifications.

Liquid waste collection and treatment systems should be reviewed to assure that facilities provide adequate space for operation, repair, or modification. Any anticipated decay of collected liquids will impact storage space requirements. Users of radioactive material should be consulted to determine the approximate volumes of liquid that will be generated to assure that proper facilities are available to house the proposed collection and treatment equipment. In addition, this review will assist in the selection of the best mode of treatment and disposal.

Solid waste facilities should be provided to facilitate and accomodate the receipt of waste from various points of use with due consideration of minimizing handling time. Ideally, a waste receiving storage and shipment area should be selected as close to work areas as practicable. The area should be provided with appropriate shielding so as to minimize exposure in any potentially occupied adjacent areas. Storage areas for unprepared and prepared packages should be appropriately shielded so as to minimize exposures to personnel preparing solid waste for shipment. The facility should be provided with adequate ventilation as as to minimize the buildup of airborne concentrations or noxious fumes. Following the selection of solid waste treatment equipment, the handling facility should be properly sized to accommodate empty shipment containers, input waste storage, treatment equipment, decontamination areas, and a holding area for necessary radiation and contamination surveys prior to shipment or storage. The layout should be properly designed to minimize handling time and provide for ease of decontamination.

COLLECTION AND HANDLING EQUIPMENT

A waste management program should include appropriate equipment for the safe collection and handling of waste. Types of equipment will vary widely and are dependent on the type, form and quantity of waste anticipated to be generated.

Solid waste containers should be provided as close to work areas as practicable, with consideration of anticipated exposure rates and occupancy, to minimize movement of wastes. Materials such as plastic bags or tubing should be available at work areas to provide for early isolation of contaminated materials and thus minimize the potential for contamination spread. Wherever practicable, waste containers with self-closing lids should be utilized to minimize the potential for generating airborne concentrations as well as to control contamination spread. Waste containers should be provided with heavy gauge plastic liners so that a full container may be sealed prior to movement to storage or solid waste treatment area. A specific written instruction or procedure should be developed that specifies proper use, handling, and limitations of solid waste containers.

Equipment necessary to manage liquid waste will vary from facility to facility. The ideal minimum would provide a dedicated drainage and collection system. This system should include a collection tank with level indication and alarm. To assure a representative sample is taken, a recirculation system should be utilized and at least three tank volumes should be circulated prior to sampling. Following appropriate analyses, controlled release rate may be calculated to assure compliance with regulatory requirements. Every reasonable effort should be made to minimize concentrations released by methods such as routing radioactive liquid releases to nonradioactive effluent streams to maximize dilution. If liquid waste input and storage capability permit, and short-lived isotopes exist, every reasonable effort should be made to allow maximum decay time prior to sampling and release. Equipment placement procedures should minimize the possibility of inadvertent injection of clean water to reduce the volume to be handled if liquid treatment is required. If separate drains and collection tanks are not feasible, existing drains may be modified and routed to a collection container. However, these should have positive indication of level and alarm to prevent overflow. A drip pan, curbing, or sumps should be provided as a second defense to contain overflow and thus control contamination spread. If practicable, short-lived isotopes should be restricted to one drain/collection system so that filled containers may be stored for decay prior to sampling and release.

Use of materials that are potentially volatile or operations potentially causing airborne concentrations should always be limited to well-ventilated areas, with air movement away from the user as well as from areas of lower to higher concentrations. Air movement patterns should be determined by the use of velometers, smoke tubes, or differential pressure indicators prior to radioactive material handling. Records of these studies should be maintained and reverified periodically and after modifications to ventilation systems. Ideally, any operation potentially generating airborne wastes should be performed within a confined and exhausted enclosure such as a fume hood. These enclosures should have a means of indicating proper air movements to the user. If airborne concentrations or materials handled warrant, an indication or alarm in the event of loss of flow should be provided. Exhaust flow should assure a linear velocity of 120 to 150 ft/min at openings. These flows should be routinely verified by velometer measurements. When activities are required to be performed away from fixed equipment such as fume hoods, the use of temporary local exhaust systems capable of routing any airborne concentrations from the local work area to other exhaust or treatment systems should be considered. When work areas are too large for local exhaust, temporary tents or enclosures may be erected and exhausted with portable devices to manage airborne concentrations. The exhaust point(s) from such enclosures should be selected to assure air movement is away from normally occupied areas. Air handling equipment should be provided with appropriate filters to minimize concentrations released whenever practicable. In addition, commercially available temporary plastic containments that may be placed on specific equipment to manage contamination and airborne spread during work activities may be utilized.

TREATMENT EQUIPMENT AND METHODS

Airborne radioactive wastes are generally treated by filtration and dilution. Equipment styles range from small filtered enclosures or hoods to complex ventilation systems with multiple filters. Certain facilities handling short-lived isotopes may also utilize a long off gas delay pipe to provide sufficient decay prior to release. Containers of gaseous radioactive material may be stored for decay or released in a controlled manner so as to assure minimal concentration at the release point. Filters should be placed upstream of exhaust fans or blowers, and an indication of differential pressure should be utilized as an indicator of proper filter function. Appropriate sampling and calculational techniques should be utilized to assure and document that releases of radioactive material are as far below regulatory limits as practicable. Filtered ventilation systems should provide adequate flow for areas of radioactive material use and be properly sized to minimize the production of spent filters which must then be processed as radioactive waste.

Liquid waste treatment equipment varies from facility to facility and is dependent on material and form. Waste liquid should be sampled and analyzed to assure proper methods to minimize releases are evaluated. For example, samples showing filterable solids would indicate that filtration to remove particulates may be appropriate. Other treatment methods could include ion exchange with organic or inorganic materials or evaporation. These treatment methods complicate the liquid waste problem by generating a more concentrated waste by-product for subsequent handling and disposal. The additional personnel exposure, increased equipment and processing costs, and the types, volumes, and concentrations of influent waste must be carefully evaluated to assure every practicable effort is applied to minimize liquid releases. Those facilities generating low volume and/or handling short-lived isotopes may utilize delay and controlled release as the only practicable treatment method to maintain releases below regulatory requirements. Solidification of liquid or solids suspended in liquids (such as ion exchange resin or evaporator bottoms) is usually utilized by only the largest of facilities as a practicable treatment method.

Solid radioactive waste treatment equipment usually consists of commercially available compaction devices to minimize the volume of waste for shipment. The most practicable method for treatment of short-lived containment solids is storage for decay and release as normal trash. However, this method requires careful planning, thorough surveys, and adequate records Waste collection recepticles should be identified for those short-lived isotopes and, if practicable, areas of use isolated from those areas using longer-lived materials. This method reduces cost to the facility and helps reduce burial ground impact. However, the importance of segregation must be emphasized during training to assure minimal handling during survey work prior to release.

Certain facilities are licensed to treat solid combustible waste by incinerator techniques. Licensing difficulties, extensive preparations, planning capital expense, and strict treatment and sampling requirements make incineration economically infeasible for the majority of facilities. It, however, is a viable alternative to filling shallow land burial sites with large volumes of material with small concentrations and hazard.

Solid noncompactible waste may be packaged and shipped in DOT-approved containers, or decontaminated for reuse or release. The necessity for decontamination as well as the impact on liquid waste production should be evaluated prior to implementing such measures as scrubbing, ultrasonic cleaning, high pressure water or steam, chemical cleaning, or electropolishing.

ADMINISTRATIVE CONTROLS

Plans and Procedures

Prior to use of radioactive material, adequate instructions or procedures should be developed by the user. These documents should be thoroughly reviewed not only from a radiation safety perspective, but from a waste estimation and control point of view. Considerations may include items such as:

- Availability of equipment to control leaks and spills
- Proper tools to safely handle material
- Adequate instructions for emergency response
- Precautionary measures to minimize time handling storage or open containers of radioactive material
- Assurance that only that amount of material necessary to complete a specific task utilized.

In addition to operational procedures, specific documents that define waste handling, collection, preparation, and shipment methods should be developed. The key elements of such waste management documents should be emphasized during training sessions so all users of radioactive material are familiar with program requirements.

Training

Users of radioactive material must receive training commensurate with activities to be performed. In addition to the minimal radiation safety training required by 10CFR19.[13] instruction in the waste control measures employed should be emphasized. Instructions should emphasize the importance of preplanned activities and the measures utilized to minimize waste production. A training program should also include mechanisms for re-instruction on a routine basis and special instruction on changes in waste handling techniques or requirements. A training program should address subjects such as:

- Waste storage containers and their use and limitations
- The packaging and containment of wastes
- Waste inventory mechanisms
- Good housekeeping practices
- Decontamination methods and limitations
- Waste minimization techniques.

The individual(s) responsible for radioactive waste preparation and shipment should receive specific instructions on applicable USNRC and USDOT regulations as well as burial ground requirements and restrictions.

Records

Liquid and airborne waste released from a facility must be thoroughly documented in order to justify compliance with applicable regulatory limits. In USNRC regulated states the applicable limits imposed by 10CFR 20.106[14] are contained in Appendix B, Table II, Columns 1 and 2. In addition, records must be evaluated to assure that releases are as far below these limits as practicable.

Solid waste records are required to assure that isotopic and curie content estimates for shipment purposes are accurate. An inventory log sheet on or near waste receptacles is a practicable way to account for contents by isotope. If the solid material is unknown, sampling or smear testing and analysis may be required to estimate the total curie content. Records of these analyses and calculations should be maintained to justify entries on shipping papers.

For most facilities, the balance of records related to the waste management program are an integral part of the health physics program and records system. Typical records in support of a waste management program include:

- Radiation and contamination surveys in preparation and storage areas
- Airborne surveys during waste handling and preparation
- Incident reports
- Decontamination projects
- Receipt, use, and disposal documents
- Personnel exposure
- Radiation surveys at restricted area perimeter
- Transport vehicle and waste shipping package surveys.

Personnel exposure records should include direct or indirect dosimeter results. If properly recorded, dosimeter results can be related to work function. This activity will permit analysis of functions which are causing the highest man-rem expenditures so that procedural or equipment changes may be evaluated to assure exposures are ALARA. Examples of such work functions for waste activities are:

- Waste collection
- Waste processing
- Packaging and preparation
- Survey work
- Decontamination
- Labeling and handling

Audits

As in radiation safety programs, a routine audit activity should be implemented to evaluate the effectiveness of waste management controls. This function can best be performed by an individual not intimately involved in day to day waste management. The findings from the audit should be formally documented and responsible individuals should develop a plan of action to evaluate and/or implement changes that respond to recommendations or deficiencies. Typical audit items that should be included are:

- Waste handling exposures
- Waste volumes and concentrations
- Volume reduction efforts
- Incident reports
- Waste management program training
- Shipment and disposal records

Of particular importance is the quantity of material used. The rate of usage should be compared to the amount of waste generated over the same time period so that trends may be established for future comparisons. Significant differences could indicate a breakdown in procedural control, failure of volume reduction efforts, or a need for training/retraining.

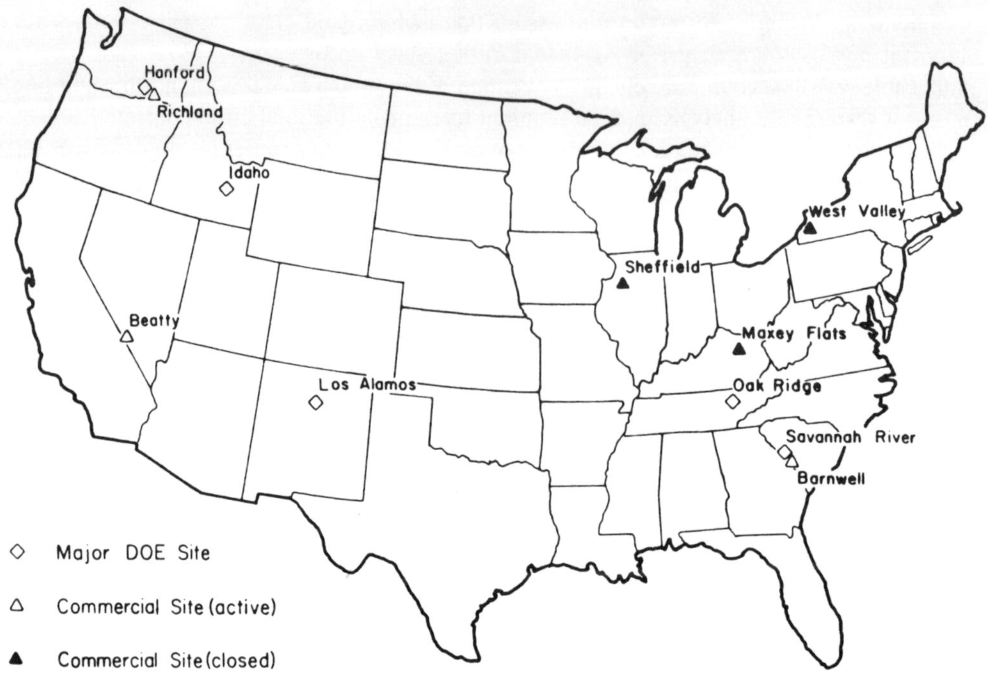

FIGURE 1. Commercial low-level radioactive waste disposal sites in the U.S.

REGIONAL RADIOACTIVE WASTE COMPACTS

Today it is necessary for disposal site users to be aware of the atmosphere surrounding the Low-Level Radioactive Waste (LLW) disposal industry. The larger users of disposal sites are somewhat insulated from the inelastic pricing and marketing policies of the disposal site operators. Nonetheless, all of us are affected to some degree by the policies and politics that have recently developed.

In 1970 the U.S. had access to six disposal sites located in reasonable proximity to the users. These sites were located (See Figure 1) in New York, Kentucky, South Carolina, Illinois, Washington, and Nevada. Trouble began in the early 1970's with the closing of West Valley and Maxey Flats followed by licensing and other delays at Sheffield in 1979. Closure was primarily due to continuing problems with material control at these sites. The associated costs of the closures has largely been borne by taxpayers. The problems which led to closure of these sites has led many to question the industry's ability to deal with problems and programs responsibly.

The closing of the three disposal sites in the 1970's led to an increase in the number of shipments at the three remaining sites with the biggest bulge occurring in South Carolina. Accordingly, the disposal prices soared. In addition, the governments of the three host states of Nevada, Washington, and South Carolina imposed unusual, but popular, restrictions on the continued use of these sites by out-of-state users. South Carolina was probably the most effective in using this power by initiating and winning from Congress a new law known as the Low-Level Waste Policy Act of 1980. This law gave legitimacy to the previous acts of the three states and stated that low level waste was no longer a national issue, but a state or regional issue and must be solved by the states. Concurrently, the Washington Environmental Council formed a coalition with environmental groups in the state of Washington to sponsor an initiative for the fall, 1980 ballot in Washington, to prohibit all out-of-state wastes from coming into the state of Washington including so-called defense wastes. That ballot item was approved overwhelmingly by the voters in Washington, but was subsequently overturned by the U.S. District Court. However, the practical effect of the initiative has been embodied in the LLW Policy Act of 1980.

While all of these other events were occurring, South Carolina was making efforts to impose a limit on the volume of waste permitted to be received at the Barnwell Site. In late 1979, a volume reduction program which required the site operator to cut site receipts by 50% by October, 1981, arriving at a ceiling of 1.2 million ft^3/year was proposed. The intent was to force the site users in the northeast to ship their LLW west to Nevada and Washington. Because of this ceiling, a Volume Allocation Plan, approved by the court and subsequently by the state of South Carolina, was imposed in January, 1980.

Through all of this, Nevada was making efforts to close the Beatty Disposal Site. The many turns of this effort seem to be politically motivated, particularly, for anyone who has visited the Beatty Site and seen the vast amount of unused space available for disposal. Suffice it to say that the Nevada Site remains open for now and the prospects for continued operation are unknown.

The LLW Policy Act of 1980, authorized states to form regional compacts and to exclude out of region wastes after 1986. However, the Congress of the U.S., must ratify all regional compacts and ratification may be unlikely in view of the fact that a majority of the Congress will be voting to exclude their own state from access to existing disposal sites. Table 3 compares and summarizes the status of compact activities in the nation.

Where the immediate future will lead no one can predict, except to say that the LLW Policy Act has produced a new constituency for maintaining the status quo. Prior to the Act waste generators had only to deal with the policies of the site operators. Now they must also deal with the Compact Committees who will overview disposal site activities in each region. These committees are formed by appointment of the Governor of each compact member state.

Low-level waste generators must remain informed about and involved with the issue of LLW Disposal even if as only a casual user of disposal space. All are going to be affected by almost every action taken by the site operators and the host state agencies responsible for oversight. Their actions could directly impact any waste management program by:

1. Introducing financial variables affecting waste budgets
2. Causing consideration of increased storage space contingencies
3. Instituting regulatory variables causing increased man hours in shipment preparation
4. Potentially requiring special processing, increased segregation and, therefore, handling.

Table 3
A COMPARISON OF PROPOSED REGIONAL LOW-LEVEL RADIOACTIVE WASTE COMPACTS[a]

Compact/Region	Midwest interstate low-level radioactive waste compact	Northwest interstate low-level radioactive waste compact	Central interstate low-level radioactive waste compact	Rocky Mountain low-level radioactive waste compact	Northeast interstate low-level radioactive waste compact●	Mid-Atlantic interstate low-level radioactive waste compact	Southeast interstate low-level radioactive waste compact
Initially eligible states plus those participating in discussions. (R) denotes ratified by legislature (*) denotes talking with other groups	Delaware(*), Illinois, Indiana, Iowa(*) Kansas, Kentucky(*), Maryland(*), Michigan, Minnesota(*), Missouri(*), Nebraska(*), North Dakota, Ohio, South Dakota, Virginia(*), Wisconsin	Alaska, Hawaii, Idaho, Montana, Oregon, Utah, Washington, Wyoming	Arkansas, Iowa(*), Kansas(R), Louisiana(R), Minnesota(*), Missouri(*), Nebraska(*), North Dakota, Oklahoma	Arizona, Colorado, Nevada, New Mexico, Utah, Wyoming	Connecticut, Delaware(*) Maine, Maryland(*), Massachusetts, New Hampshire, New Jersey, New York, Pennsylvania, Rhode Island, Vermont	Delaware(*), Kentucky(*), Maryland(*), North Carolina(*), Puerto Rico, District of Columbia, Virgin Islands, Virginia(*), West Virginia	Alabama(R), Florida(R), Georgia(R), Mississippi(R), North Carolina(*), South Carolina(R), Tennessee(R), Virginia(R)
General provisions							
Policy/purpose/objectives	All compacts either directly state or infer that the agreement is intended to provide for regional management of low-level radioactive waste as well as for providing for regional disposal facilities. Except for the Northwest Compact, all agreements include explicit language giving the Compact authority to limit the number of facilities in a region.						
Definitions	Care, commission, decommissioning disposal, eligible state, facility generator, host state, management plan, party state, person, region, regional facility site state, storage treatment, waste management. LLW definition is compatible with LLW Policy Act.	Facility, generator, host state LLW is defined as primarily beta/gamma-emitting radioisotopes. Excludes material containing more than 10 nCi of transuranics. Does not exclude milling tailings.	Commission, disposal, extended care, facility, generator, host state, management of waste, notification of each party state, person, region, regional facility, site, state, storage, treatment. LLW definition is compatible with LLW Policy Act.	Board, carrier, disposal, facility, generate, host state, management, operator, person, region, regional facility. Beatty, Nevada site is defined as a regional facility. LLW definition is not compatible with LLW Policy Act. Transuranic contaminants are limited to 10 nCl/g wastes from mining process not related to radium production are excluded (e.g., uranium mill tailings are excluded).	Commission, disposal, facility, generator, high-level waste, host state, party state, person, region, state, waste management, waste, postclosure maintenance and care, storage treatment. LLW definition is compatible with LLW Policy Act.	Commission, decommissioning, disposal, eligible state, facility, generator, host state, management plan, part state, person, post closure maintenance and care, region, regional facility, site, state, storage, treatment, waste management. LLW definition is compatible with LLW Policy Act.	Commission, facility, generator, high-level waste, host state, party state, person, region, regional facility, waste management. LLW definition is compatible with LLW Policy Act. The South Carolina Barnwell disposal facility is included in the definition of a regional facility, up to 12/31/92. Transuranic wastes are defined as materials containing transuranic elements with contamination levels with determined by NRC or *any host state that is an Agreement State.*

Exclusionary provisions	No waste may be imported into or exported from the region after 11/1/86 unless authorized by a vote of a majority of the Commission; import into the region also requires the affirmative vote of the host state.	As of 7/1/83, only party states may use the disposal site, unless approval is given by a 2/3 vote of the Compact Committee and the host state. Until 7/1/83, LLW from a nonparty state may be accepted only with a certificate of compliance issued by officials in the originating state No export restrictions.	No waste may be imported into or exported from the region, or transported from a generating site to anywhere but a regional facility after 1/1/86, unless authorized by the Commission and the affirmative vote of the host state.	No waste may be exported from or imported into the region after 1/1/86 without the approval of the Board; import requires the approval of the host state. Sets civil penalties for violation. No waste other than low-level waste may be managed at a regional facility, unless approved by the Board and the host state; sets civil penalties for violation.	No waste may be imported into the region after 1/1/86, unless authorized by the Commission and host state(s); no waste may be exported without Commission and host state approval after Compact goes into effect.	No waste may be exported from or imported into region without approval of Commission.	As of 1/1/86, no waste may be imported into the region unless authorized by the Commission. After 1/1/86, the Commission may prohibit exporting of waste by a majority vote.
Treatment of federal LLW	Compatible with LLW Policy Act.	Not compatible with Act. Does not exclude any federal generator waste from compact. Does exclude federal waste facilities.	Not compatible with Act; excludes all federal waste from Compact, not just DOE defense and federal RD waste.	Not compatible with Act: excludes all federal defense wastes, not just DOE defense waste.		Not compatible with Act. Excludes all defense wastes, not just DOE defense wastes.	Not completely compatible with Act. Excludes all defense wastes, not just DOE defense wastes.
Formal establishment of compact	Except for the import and export provisions which do not go into effect until 11/1/86, the agreement is effective on 7/1/83 or any date following, upon enactment by three eligible states.	Effective when two eligible states have enacted a statute to become party states.	Effective upon enactment of the legislation by three states.	Effective when two states have enacted legislation, except for import and export restrictions which would go into effect 1/1/86.	Effective in a party state upon enactment; as a regional compact upon enactment of legislation by three states and consent of Congress.	Effective upon enactment of legislation by three states.	Constituted upon enactment of legislation by three states.

[a] As of November 29, 1982.

[b] Still in draft form.

From Establishing Regional Compacts for Low-Level Waste Management — A National Conference. Sponsored by the Northwest Interstate Compact Committee on Low-Level Waste Management and the State of Washington, Seattle, November 30—December 1, 1982.

REFERENCES

1. Operational Radiation Safety Program, NCRP Report No. 59, National Council on Radiation Protection and Measurements, Washington, D.C., 1978.
2. **Cember, H.,** *Introduction to Health Physics,* Pergamon Press, New York, 1969.
3. **Overcamp, T. J.,** Low level radioactive waste disposal by shallow land burial, *Handbook of Environmental Radiation,* Klement, A. W., Ed., CRC Press, Boca Raton, 1982.
4. **Eliassen, R. and Lauderdale, R.,** Liquid and Solid Waste Disposal, in *Radiation Hygiene Handbook,* Blatz, H., Ed., McGraw-Hill, New York, 1959.
5. **Brodsky, A.,** Basic units of radiation measurement, in *Handbook of Laboratory* Safety, 2nd ed., Steere, N.V., Ed., CRC Press, Boca Raton, 1971.
6. **Bradley, F. J.,** Radioactive waste disposal, in *Handbook of Radioactive Nuclides,* Wang, Y., Ed., CRC Press, Boca Raton, 1969.
7. **Gera, F.,** The Classification of radioactive waste, *Health Phys.,* 27, 113—121, 1974.
8. Standardization of Radioactive Waste Categories, Technical Report Series No. 101, International Atomic Energy Agency, Vienna, 1970.
9. U.S. Nuclear Regulatory Commission, Code of Federal Regulations, Title 49, Part 173 subpart I, Radioactive Materials; Definitions, Office of the Federal Register, National Archives and Records Service, General Services Administration, Washington, D.C., 1983.
10. U.S. Nuclear Regulatory Commission, Code of Federal Regulations, Title 10, Part 71, Appendix C, Packaging of Radioactive Material for and Transportation of Radioactive Material Under Certain Conditions, Office of the Federal Register, National Archives and Records Services, General Services Administration, Washington, D.C., 1979.
11. U.S. Nuclear Regulatory Commission, Code of Federal Regulations, Title 10, Part 61, Management and Disposal of Low-Level Wastes by Shallow Land Burial and Alternative Disposal Methods, Office of the Federal Register, National Archives and Records Service, General Services Administration, Washington, D.C., 1982.
12. Safe Handling of Radioactive Materials, National Bureau of Standards Handbook 92, Superintendent of Documents, U.S. Government Printing Office, Washington, D.C. 1964.
13. U.S. Nuclear Regulatory Commission, Code of Federal Regulations, Title 10, Part 19, Notices, Instructions and Reports to Workers; Inspections, Office of the Federal Register, National Archives and Records Service, General Services Administration, Washington, D.C., 1980.
14. U.S. Nuclear Regulatory Commission, Code of Federal REgulations, Title 10, Part 20, Standards For Protection Against Radiation, Office of the Federal Register, National Archives and Records Service, General Services Administration, Washington, D.C., 1979.

ORGANIZATION AND MANAGEMENT OF A RADIATION SAFETY OFFICE

Edward D. Durkosh and Kenneth L. Miller

INTRODUCTION

Generally speaking the purpose and function of a radiation safety office are directly related to employer needs and regulatory requirements.

Any institution that possesses ionizing radiation sources that are stored, used, or processed has the responsibility of providing an assessment of the exposure potential to and protecting anyone who is or could be exposed to the radiation from such sources. This responsibility extends not only to potential occupational exposures but to nonoccupational exposures, to the population in the general area of the facility, and to the population at large who may be affected inadvertently to exposure from ionizing radiation sources due to transportation accidents or other unlikely circumstances. The radiation safety program thus includes the evaluation of exposure potentials, to prevent, minimize, or eliminate the associated hazards. This is best implemented by the professional; however, some aspects of the responsibilities may be carried out by semiprofessional or other individuals who receive adequate and proper supervision. In most cases knowledge and implementation of applicable standards requires the background of a radiation safety expert.

There exists a vast body of regulatory requirements and guidance governing the possession and use of sources of ionizing radiation. The regulatory groups exist at the Federal, State, and in some cases, at the local level (county, city, borough, etc.). Knowledge of and access to an understanding of the applicable regulatory requirements is best and often more efficiently handled by persons who work at radiation safety as a specialty occupation on a full, part-time, or consultation basis. A listing of various organizations involved in developing and publishing radiation protection recommendations is contained in Appendix A.

At the heart of the radiation safety program is the radiation safety office,[1-6] the size of which will depend on many factors ranging from the magnitude of source inventory, the hazard potential of sources, the organization's size, and to a large extent, on management's evaluation or emphasis on radiation safety. No magic formula exists to equate some defined ratio of radiation safety personnel per number of radiation workers and/or number of radiation sources. This ratio will vary with the particular circumstances and can best be established by an in-depth assessment made jointly by management and the professional radiation safety specialist. An indirect participant in determining the appropriate size of the radiation safety program appears in the form of one of the many regulatory agency representatives (program compliance auditors) who are trained to recognize understaffing deficiencies and suggest corrective action.

SOURCES OF RADIATION

Management is obligated to insure a safe working environment and compliance with applicable regulatory requirements. An audit of activities is necessary in order to determine if radiation sources are in use at one's installation. The following subsections present by general categories, the type of radiation sources that would require occupational exposure evaluation and control.

By-Product Material

The regulatory definition of by-product material is anything that (except source or special nuclear material) is yielded in or made radioactive by exposure to the radiation incident to the process of producing or utilizing special nuclear material. Therefore, radioactive material that results from nuclear fission or is made radioactive through bombardment of neutrons during a nuclear fissioning process is considered by-product material. This definition excludes anything made radioactive through bombardment in any of the various accelerator machines or materials that are found to be radioactive in nature. By-product material represents the type of radiation source that one is most likely to encounter in the occupational setting. Such sources are common in hospitals, universities, teaching and research settings, radiographic operations, and industrial applications. Relatively small amounts of certain by-product materials can produce significant exposure potentials.

Source Material

Source material is uranium or thorium (or any combination thereof in any physical or chemical form, or ores, that contained by weight 1/20 of 1% (0.05%) or more of uranium, thorium, or any combination thereof). Source material does not include special nuclear material.

Generally speaking, source material is low in specific radioactivity and small or exempt quantities may be found in most research laboratories, hospitals, etc. Large amounts of source material, requiring radiation control efforts, are usually associated with the nuclear fuel cycle and include mining, milling, processing, fuel element manufacture, and usage in nuclear reactor operations or subsequent reprocessing. Natural uranium and/or thorium in quantities less than several pounds have only a slight radiation safety control need which should be recognized and addressed.

Special Nuclear Material

Special nuclear material means plutonium-239, uranium-233, uranium-235, uranium enriched in the isotopes 233 or 235. This could also mean any other material that the Nuclear Regulatory Commission determines to be special nuclear material, but it does not include source material. The difference between fuel cycle usage and research laboratory usage of special nuclear material generally involves the quantity possessed. In general, the fuel cycle involves large quantities of special nuclear material, whereas the requirements of the research laboratory are usually satisfied by quantities not exceeding several grams.

Accelerator-Produced Radioactive Material

Accelerator-produced radioactive material is any material made radioactive through electronic acceleration of atomic or subatomic particles and subsequent bombardment of target atoms (for example, Van de Graaff generators, cyclotrons, synchro-cyclotrons, etc.). Aside from high energy physics programs, the most common presence of accelerator-produced material is in the health care field and support industries such as research labs or radiopharmaceutical suppliers. Nearly all nuclear medicine departments use some accelerator produced radiopharmaceuticals.

Naturally Occurring Radioactive Materials

Naturally occurring radioactive materials are those radioactive materials found in nature that are not "man-made" radioactive materials. The most widely used natural radioactive materials has probably been radium, but there are others that can and do present the potential for radiation exposure.

Electronically-Produced Ionizing Radiation

This classification of radiation is produced by machines or devices that are electronically activated. The most common type are the X-ray machines. X-ray machines have been in widespread use since 1896 for the purpose of diagnosis and treatment of human illness or diseases. Additionally, there are analytical devices and industrial-type X-ray units that are generally designed to be used on inanimate objects and materials. The operating voltages of these machines range from low kilovolts to megavolts, and each X-ray machine has unique characteristics and operational features that require separate exposure evaluations. X-rays can also be an unwanted by-product of the operation of certain electronic devices such as vacuum switches or other devices containing unshielded high voltage rectifier tubes, as well as other electronic devices that produce both X-rays and nonionizing types of radiation.

In addition to X-ray machines there are electronic-powered devices that produce radiations other than X-rays, such as particle accelerators and neutron generators. Generally the evaluation and quantitation of radiation hazards associated with this class of machine requires more than the casual radiation monitoring experience.

The types and sources of ionizing radiation vary from the very simple to the extremely complex. The specific characteristics of the ionizing radiation source must be taken into consideration when organizing the radiation safety program.

PURPOSES AND FUNCTIONS OF A RADIATION SAFETY OFFICE

As a radiation safety program is established it quickly becomes apparent that the responsibilities encompass more than the readily obvious. Quite frequently the radiation safety officer finds himself involved in more than the technical aspects of radiation monitoring and evaluation. These additional functions may quickly expand to any of the following.

Satisfying of Regulatory Requirements

In order to possess and use radiation sources in more than innocuous levels some form of licensing or registration is usually required by Federal, State, or local regulations. The licensing procedure[7-11] can be lengthy depending upon the complexity of the program and the hazard potential presented by the radiation sources to be licensed. In order to obtain the license it is necessary to explain in sufficient detail the radiation safety program that will permit safe usage of the sources. Paramount to granting of the license is a firm commitment on the part of management[12-13] to the establishment of the program and the continued execution of its functions to ensure adequate safety. Once the license is granted, the licensee can expect periodic inspections by the regulatory agency. Such inspections not only audit those procedures indicated in the license application, but also check to ensure that regulatory requirements and accepted safety practices are being adhered to. The preparation of license applications, registration forms, and renewal applications may occupy a sufficient amount of the radiation safety officers time. Appreciable time may also be spent in preparation for inspections and the correction of deficiencies found during the inspection.

Ensuring a Safe and Healthful Working Environment

At one time this could be interpreted as meaning that sufficient steps should be taken to keep radiation exposure below the regulatory specified maximum permissible doses. However, the current concept of ALARA[14-15] (As Low As Reasonably Achievable) mandates that, wherever reasonably and economically possible, exposures should be kept as far below the maximum permissible dose as possible. Therefore, there is significant diversity about what should now be considered acceptable maximum permissible doses. That which is readily achievable for one type of facility may be economically or practically impossible for another. It is the joint responsibility of administration and the radiation safety office and the regulatory agencies to determine those levels of radiation exposure that are reasonably achievable.

Control and Minimization of Deleterious Impact Beyond the Site Location

Regulations permit certain small concentrations of radioactive materials to pass beyond the site boundaries as effluent[15] (air or water). It is the responsibility of the user to provide adequate controls and monitoring to ensure that limits are not exceeded. In addition to controlled releases of material, the program must provide adequate assurances against uncontrolled releases that might exceed the limits. Where the potential exists for excessive releases, as the result of accidents or malfunctions, specific emergency criteria must be developed. In the case of nuclear reactors and fuel reprocessing, such preparations are extensive. Incorporated in any such plans should be adequate medical attention for anyone who might develop injuries from radiation exposure or who might have traumatic injuries also involving possible radioactive contamination. The user of radioactive materials is responsible for ensuring the safety of any radiation sources sent from or used away from the site boundaries, e.g., shipment of radioisotopes or radioactive waste or usage of sources in such procedures as industrial radiography.

Minimizing Damage to the Facility and Loss of Equipment

Facility damage, removal of the facility from service, or the loss of equipment through radiation exposure or contamination, can be hazardous and costly. It is therefore necessary to ensure that all radiation sources are used in a controlled and confined manner. Accidents that cause widespread radioactive contamination can result in curtailment of activities (research, manufacture, productions, etc.) and can lead to very costly decontamination efforts. Equipment and supplies (e.g. radiographic or photographic film) that may be sensitive to radiation exposure can be very costly to replace. Equipment that cannot be decontaminated may have to be discarded as radioactive waste. Certain situations require reporting to regulatory authorities and are discussed in Appendix B.

Training and Educating Radiation Workers

Those individuals who work with radiation sources must be adequately trained.[16] Although regulatory agencies usually require adequate training, it is generally left up to the licensee to justify the adequacy of his training program. For certain industries such as the nuclear industry there are national standards (e.g. ANSI standards) that outline training programs considered to be adequate. The radiation safety officer is relied upon to establish radiation safety training programs and to identify the appropriate individuals or groups in need of such training. At times the training requirements extend beyond the radiation workers, and include appropriate training or briefings for individuals who enter areas where radiation sources are used. Some examples would include maintenance personnel, housekeeping personnel, emergency personnel, sales representatives, consultants, members of the general public, and family or friends of the radiation worker.

Providing Assurance to Nonradiation Workers

For those individuals not specifically trained in radiation characteristics and radiation safety, the thought of possible exposure to a hazard that is undetectable by human senses can be very frightening. Accidents that have occurred have cast an aura of suspicion over the ability of radiation workers to effectively control the hazards with which they are working. Quite frequently the radiation safety officer is the only person with sufficient credibility to answer questions and alleviate the fears of the nonradiation worker.

Providing Public Relations

The complexity of understanding the relative magnitude of radiation risks, inappropriate headlines and continued controversies amplified in the media have generated public fear and distrust of radiation and its usages. The radiation safety expert must bear the brunt of responsibility for educating the public about measures taken to ensure the safe and controlled uses of radiation sources.

Participating in Administrative Responsibilities and Budgetary Requirements

Since radiation safety specialists generally have multifaceted backgrounds they are often called upon to lend their expertise in other areas. This may require involvement in nonradiation-related safety aspects such as safety inspections or participation on various safety committees. A good administrator will be increasingly pulled toward other areas of management and operations. The complexities and expense of operating a radiation safety program generally involve budgets of appreciable size. The radiation safety officer usually spends considerable time requesting, justifying, and oftentimes pleading with management for the necessary funds to fulfill his responsibilities. The degree of supervision of the activities of the radiation safety personnel by the radiation safety officer will depend upon the competency of such personnel, the complexity of the programs supervised, and the potential impact of decisions made.

Participating in Continuing Education Programs

Practices, procedures, and regulations change continuously in the radiation protection field. In order to effectively serve his employer, the radiation safety specialist must devote appreciable time to keeping up with the changes. New procedures and methodology for handling problems are constantly being developed. Regulations and regulatory guides are continually changing and require ever-increasing attention if an RSO is to remain current in the field. The certified health physicist is under additional obligation to accumulate continuing education credits in order to renew certification periodically.

PERSONNEL, FACILITY, AND EQUIPMENT REQUIREMENTS

The number of personnel required will be dictated by the scope of the operation, the decentralization of radiation sources, and the complexity of usage. For example, an operating nuclear power plant generally functions with a minimal number of personnel on site. The number of radiation areas entered are limited and access to contaminated areas are rigidly contolled or the contamination is contained in normally inaccessible areas. During an outage for repairs or refueling, protective covers and barriers may be removed, radiation sources may be moved to accessible areas, and the number of personnel requiring monitoring multiply. During such periods the potential for release of radioactivity, contaminating events, and personnel exposure will require a substantial increase in radiation protection personnel and supervision. Accidents, such as the one at Three Mile Island, require an extraordinary number of radiation protection personnel as well as other specialty personnel such as radiochemists, nuclear engineers, waste handlers, etc.

An industry that uses megacurie amounts of sealed gamma emitters, such as cobalt-60 for high-dose irradiation, may require fewer radiation protection personnel than a university radiation safety program that monitors the use of microcurie to millicurie amounts of unsealed radioisotopes in many different locations. This is true since the megacurie quantities must be contained within shielded fail-safe devices that automatically protect the worker. Safety procedures alone can not be relied upon for protection against exposure rates that could be lethal within short time periods.

The number of radiation protection personnel required will depend on the number of manhours necessary to perform the given responsibilities. Table 1 lists general guidelines for radiation safety staffing at medical institutions. Appendices C through F contain listings of operations and administrative functions of a radiation safety office as well as requirements for personnel, equipment, and space commitments. These documents and others[17-25,33] provide checklists of considerations in the design of facilities, equipment, and procedures for radiation safety operations in various kinds of facilities.

The number of personnel required will vary depending on the scope of the program and the complexity of the usage. Total man-hours required will also depend on the extent to which the various functions are performed by the radiation safety office and the availability of auxiliary support groups such as electronics laboratories for instrument repair and cali-

Table 1
RECOMMENDED MINIMUM RADIATION SAFETY STAFFING FOR VARIOUS CATEGORIES OF MEDICAL INSTITUTIONS[a]

Category	Radiation sources	Technician time	Professional (health physics) time
I	Low-level clinical and research laboratories[b] handling microcurie quantities of I-131, I-125, Cr-51, C-14, and H-3, plus radiographic units and fluoroscopes	6 man-hours/month	4 man-days/year (plus daily supervision by full-time qualified staff radiologist or other health professional)
II	Category I plus nuclear medicine	1 full-time radiation safety technician (possibly doing some minor part-time electronics maintenance)	1/2 time of health physicist (possibly including calibration of diagnostic X-ray units)
III	Category II plus teletherapy, radionuclide therapy, or units)		
III	Category II plus teletherapy, radionuclide therapy, or brachytherapy	1 full-time radiation safety technician[c]	1 full-time health or radiological physicist (possibly performing some diagnostic calibrations)
IV	Category III plus multi-megavolt therapy	2 full-time technicians — radiation safety and electronics[c]	1 full-time health physicist and 1 or more full-time radiological physicists with some radiation safety responsibilities

[a] All personnel are in addition to clinical radiological physics requirements. Also, for categories II—IV, the person serving as radiation safety officer (RSO) should be full-time member of the hospital staff.

[b] Major medical centers having larger research complexes may require larger radiation safety staffs just to meet survey requirements for the research laboratory areas. In some cases, medical research laboratories are serviced by university radiation safety offices when they are located in university medical complexes. Since situations vary, experience with the programs and organization of each institution is often needed to judge staffing requirements for surveying medical research uses of licensed radioactive materials (see Regulatory Guides 8.23 and 10.8).

[c] Plus proportionate secretarial-clerical assistance for correspondence and recordkeeping requirements.

Revised and adapted from Brodsky, A., Principles and Practices for Keeping Occupational Radiation Exposures at Medical Institutions as Low as Reasonably Achievable, NUREG-0267, U.S. Nuclear Regulatory Commission, Washington, D.C., 1982.

bration. Often overlooked initially but vitally important is the need for clerical support for the radiation safety office. Typical clerical and secretarial responsibilities are:

1. Maintaining good public relations associated with receptionist responsibilities
2. Locating and notifying radiation safety personnel during emergencies
3. Typing reports, surveys, office correspondence, license applications, research publications, lecture notes, handout training materials, and safety manuals
4. Distributing, collecting and processing personnel monitoring devices, e.g. film badges, TLD's, etc
5. Scheduling meetings, training programs and inspections of areas and operations
6. Preparing minutes for committee meetings
7. Preparing yearly reports for administration and governmental agencies
8. Initiating purchase requisitions and maintaining budget balances

9. Logging purchase orders for radiation sources
10. Supplying radiation safety information to requestors
11. Maintaining inventories and logging of supplies and equipment loaned to radiation workers
12. Conducting literature searches involved with research or specialty projects
13. Counting smears and completing survey forms
14. Inputting computer terminal information

Chain of Command

The responsibility and authority of the radiation safety officer (RSO) should be carefully considered and explicitly expressed in writing. Access to all areas in which radiation sources are used or stored and authority to order immediate cessation of such activities when in violation of established or acceptable safety practices should be granted to the RSO.

A condition of licensing is a firm commitment to radiation safety on the part of management. Therefore, the RSO should be answerable only to the upper levels of administration; he should not be put in a compromising situation where he must report administratively to potential violators of good radiation safety practices.

Space Requirements

The heart of the radiation safety operation is the radiation safety laboratory in which instruments are stored and samples are prepared and analyzed. Additional space is required for offices, secretarial and reception, instrument calibration, and waste processing and storage. Depending upon the scope and size of the operation, waste processing may require the greatest consideration and space allocation. With the ever-escalating cost of waste disposal and the uncertainties of burial capabilities, it may be economically advisable to install volume reduction and long term storage capabilities.[26,27] Provision for incineration, compaction, solidification, controlled space for short-lived radioisotope decay, and on-site burial should be considered. With the uncertainties regarding future availability of radioactive waste burial capabilities, many nuclear power plants are considering construction of on-site storage facilities that will house several years worth of radioactive waste.

Storage space for supplies such as protective gear, emergency decontamination supplies and equipment, solidification media, and waste shipping containers is necessary.

Equipment Requirements

In order to monitor and evaluate the radiation conditions in the work environment, the radiation safety office may require some or all of the following equipment:[28-31]

1. *Portable monitoring equipment* such as geiger counters, ionization chambers, neutron detectors, air sampling apparatus, velometers, etc.
2. *Sample collection and preparation* equipment such as air samplers, shielded containers, extraction columns, grab samplers, etc.
3. *Counting equipment* might include planchet counters, liquid scintillation counters, gamma spectrometers and computers for data analysis, calculations, cataloging, and inventorying.
4. *Specialized equipment* will vary from microwave detectors to whole body counting facilities.
5. *Calibration capabilities* range from calibrated plated or solution sources for use in calibrating sample counters or analyzers to sealed sources and associated space for the calibration of portable monitoring equipment.
6. *Instrument repair capabilities* may be required in-house, or contracted to outside agencies

7. *Sample preparation* can range from collecting representative wipe samples to extensive chemical separation for analysis of large-volume, low-activity samples.
8. *Clerical support and record keeping* may require transcription and even word processing equipment.
9. *Specialized vehicles or crafts* may be necessary when sampling or monitoring outside the work environment is required.
10. *Computers* (or terminals) for record retention or dose calculations.

The frequency of routine area surveys will be indicated by the quantity of radioactive material used, the hazard potential of the material, and the administered safeguards. Those individuals actually involved in the handling procedures should be capable of performing surveys after each handling procedure or suspected contaminating incident involving the material. The surveys performed by the radiation safety office should be of an auditing nature to insure adequacy of handling procedures and surveying on the part of the user. The frequency of such audits should be sufficient to insure absence of contamination, control of exposures, accountability of radiation sources, training and competency of personnel, and familiarity with handling and use procedures. The radiation safety office should perform those procedures which may be out of the capabilities of the user, e.g. airborne sampling, bioassay or isotope analysis.

Use of Consultants

When the radiation safety requirements are minimal or where advanced specialization is required infrequently, the needs may be supplied by consultation. Such programs are acceptable provided they result in an effective radiation safety program.

PERSONNEL SELECTION, TRAINING, AND SUPERVISION

The person who is designated as radiation safety officer should have sufficient education and training to permit effective fulfillment of the RSO responsibilities.[32] At times the radiation safety responsibilities may be secondarily assumed as in the case of the nuclear medicine physician who is responsible for the safe medical usage of radiopharmaceuticals, or as in the case of the industrial hygienist who assumes responsibility for safe usage of radiation sources in quality control devices such as thickness gauges.

When responsibility for radiation safety becomes a primary one, the requirement for specialized training and education increases and must be commensurate with the quantity, diversity, and extent of usage of radioactive materials. The professional health physicist has usually had extensive training and specialized radiation safety education at the graduate level.

The "qualified expert" is usually referred to as an individual who has the training and experience in radiation protection to (a) make the necessary radiation measurements, (b) evaluate their significance, and (c) institute any corrective measures called for by the evaluation. Such competence is readily recognized by those persons certified as having demonstrated such competence by such organizations as the American Board of Health Physics, the American Board of Radiology, or the American Board of Industrial Hygiene (Radiological Aspects).

Certification of competency at the technician level is granted by the American Board of Radiation Protection Technologists.

Sources of Trained Personnel

A listing of schools providing specialized programs in health or medical physics is contained in Appendix G. The advertisement of positions for radiation safety personnel is usually done through the newsletters of either the Health Physics Society, the American Association of Physicists in Medicine, or the local or regional chapters of these societies.

Training

In addition to the formal training obtained at the university level, radiation safety personnel can obtain continued and specialized training through participation in in-house training programs, specialized commercial training programs, seminars, symposia, and summer schools offered by the professional societies. Additionally, many individuals have received advanced training through military training programs such as those provided by the Nuclear Navy.

Operation of an effective radiation safety program requires a firm commitment of support on the part of management. The extent of the radiation safety program is dictated by the scope of radiation utilization. The competency and qualifications of the radiation safety personnel must be extensive enough to allow complete and effective coverage of all aspects of the radiation safety program.

APPENDIX A*
ORGANIZATIONS INVOLVED IN RADIATION PROTECTION

There are a number of national and international organizations that have published recommendations and guidance providing detailed methods, data, and scientific information for use in establishing radiation protection programs. The organizations and their addresses are listed below:

American Association of Physicists in Medicine (AAPM)
Radiation Protection Committee
335 East 45th Street
New York, NY 10017

American College of Radiology
6900 Wisconsin Avenue
Chevy Chase, MD 20815

American Conference of Governmental Industrial Hygienists
Committee on Industrial Ventilation
P.O. Box 453
Lansing, MI 48902

American Industrial Hygiene Association (AIHA)
66 S. Miller Road
Akron, Ohio 44313

American National Standards Institute, Inc. (ANSI)
345 East 47th Street
New York, New York 10017

Center for Devices and Radiological Health
Food and Drug Administration
Public Health Service
U.S. Department of Health and Human Services
Rockville, MD 20852

U.S. Department of Energy
Washington, D.C. 20585

International Atomic Energy Agency (IAEA)
Wagramerstrasse 5
P.O. Box 100
A-1400 Vienna, Austria

Publication orders from the U.S.A. should be addressed to UNIPUB, Inc., 345 Park Avenue South, New York, NY 10010

* Revised and adapted with permission from Brodsky, A., Principles and Practices for Keeping Occupational Radiation Exposures at Medical Institutions as Low as Reasonably Achievable, NUREG-0267, U.S. N.R.C. Washington, D.C., 1982.

International Commission on Radiation Units and Measurements (ICRU)
7910 Woodmont Avenue
Bethesda, MD 20814

Order publications from ICRU Publications, same address

International Commission on Radiological Protection (ICRP))

Order publications from Pergamon Press, Inc., Fairview Park, Elmsford, NY 10523, or through bookstores in the United States

International Labour Office (ILO)
Geneva, Switzerland

Joint Commission on Accreditation of Hospitals (JCAH)
875 N. Michigan Avenue
Chicago, IL 60611
Attention: Publications

Medical Internal Radiation Dose Committee (MIRD)
Society of Nuclear Medicine
475 Park Avenue South
New York, NY 10016

The MIRD committee has in recent years issued a number of excellent compilations of data and methods for calculating doses to humans from radionuclides used in medicine. These same data and methods are useful in monitoring and estimating both internal and external occupational exposures.

National Academy of Sciences — National Research Council (NAS-NRC)
2101 Constitution Avenue, NW
Washington, D.C.

National Council on Radiation Protection and Measurements (NCRP)
7910 Woodmont Avenue
Bethesda, MD 20814

Order publications from NCRP Publications, same address

National Institute for Occupational Safety and Health (NIOSH) and National Institute for Environmental Health Sciences (NIEHS) Department of Health and Human Services Washington, D.C.

Publications are available from the National Technical Information Service, Springfield, VA 22151

Standards Committee
Health Physics Society (HPS)
1340 Old Chain Bridge Road, Suite 300
McLean, Virginia 22101

World Health Organization (WHO)
Distribution and Sales Service
1211 Geneva 27, Switzerland

APPENDIX B
REPORTING REQUIREMENTS SUMMARIZED FROM 10 CFR 20

Under certain circumstances of incidences, licensees are required to report to the Director of the appropriate Nuclear Regulatory Commission Inspection and Enforcement Regional Office.

A. *Theft or loss of licensed material* in such quantities and under such circumstances that it appears to the licensee that a substantial hazard may result to persons in unrestricted areas.

a. Requires immediate report by telephone followed by written report within 30 days.

B. *Incidents* have varying reporting requirements dependent upon their seriousness:

IMMEDIATE NOTIFICATION:

a. Individual exposures of 25 rem or more whole body, 150 rems to skin of whole body or 375 rems to extremities.
b. Release of radioactive materials exceeding 5000 times the maximum permissible concentrations (when averaged over 24 hr).
c. Loss of one working week of any facility.
d. Property damage exceeding $200,000.

Notification must be made by telephone *and* telegraph, mailgram or facsimile and followed by a written report within 30 days.

24 HR NOTIFICATION;

a. Individual exposures of 5 rems or more whole body, 30 rems to skin of whole body or 75 rems to extremities.
b. Release of radioactive material exceeding 500 times the maximum permissible concentration (when averaged over 24 hr).
c. Loss of one day of any facility
d. Property damage in excess of $2000.

Notification must be made within 24 hr by telephone and telegraph, mailgram, or facsimile and followed by a written report within 30 days.

30 DAY NOTIFICATION:

a. Individual exposures exceeding the maximum permissible dose.
b. Exposures of individuals to concentrations in excess of the maximum permissible concentrations.
c. Exposure of minors in excess of the limits.
d. Levels of radiation or concentrations of radioactive materials in unrestricted areas in excess of 10 times the maximum permitted (whether or not they involve excessive exposure to an individual).

Report shall be in writing within 30 days.

Further clarification can be obtained from 10 CFR, 20.402, 20.403, 20.405 and Regulatory Guide 10.1.

APPENDIX C*
RADIATION SAFETY TASKS INVOLVED IN KEEPING OCCUPATIONAL EXPOSURES ALARA

1. Surveys of the following radioactivity areas:
   a. Nuclear medicine
   b. Radiation therapy
   c. Oncology
   d. Pathology
   e. Cardiology
   f. Pediatrics
   g. Radioactive waste disposal and storage
   h. Other research and clinical laboratories using radioactive materials

* Revised and adapted with permission from Brodsky, A., Principles and Practices for Keeping Occupational Radiation Exposures at Medical Institutions as Low as Reasonably Achievable, NUREG-0267, U.S. N.R.C., Washington, D.C., 1982.

2. Surveys of diagnostic and therapeutic machines and generators, including:
   a. Teletherapy sources and machines
   b. Computerized axial tomography scanners
   c. Interlock and safety checks
   d. Calibrations
   e. Fluoroscopes
   f. Radiographic X-ray
3. Personnel monitoring:
   a. Review of personnel exposure data and reports
   b. Preparation of reports required by regulations
   c. Filing, collecting, and mailing personnel monitoring devices (including late and lost)
   d. Special investigations of exposure and notifications to regulatory agencies as appropriate
   e. Calibration of personnel monitoring dosimeters, including commercially supplied film badge service
4. Radiation safety instrument calibration and maintenance:
   a. Calibration
   b. Battery replacement and adjustment
   c. Pocket chamber and TLD calibration
   d. Minor repair (electronic)
   e. Instrument selection and distribution
   f. Check-source calibration
5. Decontamination and waste disposal:
   a. Collection and packaging
   b. Surveying
   c. Recording
   d. Shipping arrangements
   e. Placarding
   f. Decontamination of surgical instruments, rooms, and laboratories
6. Leak-testing radioactive sources using the following techniques:
   a. Wiping
   b. Counting
   c. Calculation
   d. Recording
   e. Counter calibration
7. Evaluation of internal exposure by means of:
   a. Collection of samples, including air sampling when applicable
   b. Radiochemical or scintillation bioassay analysis
   c. Counter calibration
   d. In vivo counting
   e. Computer analysis of results
8. Special surveys of patients and rooms for implant, intracavitary, or unsealed radiopharmaceutical therapy, including:
   a. Room preparation and protective covering
   b. Labeling (bed, chart, door)
   c. Nursing staff and housekeeping staff briefings
   d. Background surveys
   e. Source insertion and afterloading surveys
   f. Surveys of patients in operating room and recovery room
   g. Placing of lead barriers
   h. Recovery of sources and wastes

   i. Survey of room cleanup and decontamination
   j. Instructions to patient and to family of patient as appropriate
   k. Measurement of radiation from cadavers and briefings to pathology staff and funeral directors as appropriate
9. Administration and consultation, including:
   a. Approval of facilities, equipment, and procedures used in areas where radioactive materials are handled
   b. Preparation of license applications and amendments
   c. Preparation of hazard evaluation reports for licensing
   d. Programming of routine required surveys
   e. Supervision of routine radiation safety operations
   f. Revisions to radiation safety manual
   g. Periodic radiation safety instruction for hospital staff and administration
   h. Training of residents and medical staff
   i. Conferences with physicians and other safety staff
   j. Coordination of radiation safety committee meetings and minutes
   k. Inspections and discussions with government regulatory agency representatives
   l. Professional meetings
   m. Selecting and ordering equipment and supplies
   n. Planning and budgeting
   o. Facility and shield design and meetings with architects
   p. Record maintenance and related computer programming
   q. Planning prompt effective response to incidents and emergencies involving radiation
   r. Providing instructional direction for outside persons (for example, firemen) who would respond to an emergency situation involving or potentially involving radiation
   s. Preparation of Radiation Safety Office reports to administration

APPENDIX D*
RESPONSIBILITIES AND PROCEDURES FOR KEEPING OCCUPATIONAL RADIATION EXPOSURES AT MEDICAL INSTITUTIONS AS LOW AS REASONABLY ACHIEVABLE

MANAGEMENT PHILOSOPHY AND ORGANIZATION

The radiation protection responsibility at a medical institution is to maintain exposures ALARA for employees, visitors, students, and patients not under medical supervision for the administration of radiation or radioactive materials for therapeutic or diagnostic purposes.

This responsibility should be carried out by means of:

a. Information and policy statements to the medical and hospital staff
b. Periodic management audit of operational efforts to maintain exposures ALARA
c. Continuing management evaluation of radiation safety staffing, program, and budget requirements
d. Management programs to ensure that all hospital staff and employees receive appropriate briefings and training in radiation safety, including ALARA concepts
e. Delegation of sufficient authority to the Radiation Safety Officer (RSO) to enforce regulations and administrative policies regarding radiation safety

* Revised and adapted with permission from Brodsky, A., Information Relevant to Ensuring that Occupational Radiation Exposures at Medical Institutions will be As Low As Reasonably Achievable, Regulatory Guide 8.18, U.S. Nuclear Regulatory Commission, Washington, D.C., 1977.

f. Administrative direction to ensure that any new hospital facilities or equipment that may affect radiation protection will be planned or designed in consultation with the RSO

STAFFING AND ORGANIZATION REQUIREMENTS

The time and effort required for each of the tasks discussed in Appendix C vary widely with the size of the hospital and the nature and extent of radioactive material usage. Each should be given careful consideration to ensure the functions are carried out completely and competently.

RADIATION SAFETY PERSONNEL QUALIFICATIONS

Management should select radiation safety personnel appropriate to the radiation safety program after careful review of the nature of the program and the extent of effort and expertise required to carry out the tasks noted in Appendix C.

ADMINISTRATIVE AUTHORITY

The Radiation Safety Office, supervised by the RSO, should have responsibility for carrying out the radiation safety program, including the tasks listed in Appendix C. This responsibility should be delegated in the Medical Staff Bylaws and should include authority for the RSO to communicate directly with the level of management that can take corrective action when needed to enforce rules and procedures pertaining to the institution's radiation safety program. Administrative authority to suspend certain activities temporarily should also be provided to the RSO when needed in emergencies to avoid immediate danger to life or health. However, the authority of the RSO to suspend activities should be exercised only when it is consistent with noninterference with life-saving medical procedures that warrant an overriding priority and that cannot await alleviation of the radiation safety problems.

MANAGEMENT AUDIT AND INSPECTION OF THE RADIATION SAFETY PROGRAM

Ultimate responsibility for the establishment and continuation of an adequate radiation safety program in a medical institution is with the governing body of the hospital. The administrator reporting to this governing body should be sufficiently informed at all times to be sure that all regulations are faithfully adhered to and that the use and safe handling of radioisotopes are properly carried out.

The hospital administration should consider an annual audit of the radiation safety program in cooperation with members of the Medical Isotopes Committee and the Radiation Safety Office. The results of this audit may then be discussed at an annual Medical Isotopes Committee meeting to ensure that all users and responsible staff are aware of current policies and procedures and methods for their improvement. A report containing the results of the audit should be maintained by the Radiation Safety Office for possible use in expediting any inspections by regulatory or accrediting agencies.

APPENDIX E*
RADIATION SAFETY SURVEYS AT PROCESSING AND MANUFACTURING PLANTS

Manufacturers licensed for radioactive materials should have a health physics staff capable of developing and implementing adequate survey programs.

Surveys performed should include those necessary to evaluate external exposure to personnel, concentrations of airborne radioactive materials in the facility, surface contamination levels, and radioactive effluents from the facility.

SURVEYS OF EXTERNAL RADIATION EXPOSURE LEVELS IN RESTRICTED AREAS

Radiation safety personnel should survey locations where individuals may be exposed to radiation intensities that might result in radiation doses in excess of 10% of the limits in any calendar quarter or where an individual is working with a source that could be used unshielded at any time to produce a gamma or beta dose rate exceeding 0.5 mrad/hr at 1 m.

Preoperational, routine, and special surveys of these areas should be performed by the radiation protection staff. Results of these surveys should be recorded. Also, workers should monitor themselves and their own individual activities if they are exposed to external radiation levels. These surveys by workers should consist of periodic instrument surveys during work with radioactive materials. Workers should be properly trained to conduct such surveys.

MEASUREMENTS OF RADIOACTIVE MATERIAL CONCENTRATIONS IN AIR

The radiation safety staff should perform measurements of radioactive material concentrations in air for areas where radioactive materials are handled or processed in unencapsulated form and when operations could expose workers to the inhalation of quantities of radioactive material exceeding the limits.

Collected air samples should be representative of the air in the workers' breathing zone. However, when obtaining representative samples from the breathing zone is not practicable, the samples should be obtained from a location at which the radioactivity concentration in air is known to be greater than that of the workers' breathing zone. For example, samples taken outside the breathing zone are acceptable if the sampler head is located so that the concentration of radioactive material in air at the location of the sampler head is equal to or greater than the concentrations in the breathing zone.

When measuring the quantity of radioactive material deposited on or in an air sample filter, the radiation safety staff should include appropriate corrections for alpha or beta absorption by the filter media and by material collected on the filter whenever these corrections may change results more than 10%. Filter media used for the collection of alpha emitters should retain collected material on the filter surface. Overestimates of the volume of air that has passed through the filter should be avoided by means of accurate calibration of the flow rate and by preventing or correcting for the loss of flow due to the accumulation of material on the filter.

Breathing zone or general air sampling should be conducted while work is in progress unless the results of continuous sampling verify that the concentration of radioactive material

* Revised and adapted with permission from Brodsky, A., Health Physics Surveys for Byproduct Material at NRC-Licensed Processing and Manufacturing Plants, Regulatory Guide 21, U.S. Nuclear Regulatory Commission, Washington D.C. 1979.

in the breathing zone is not likely to exceed 25% of the limits. The use of personal (lapel) samplers is acceptable for continuous air sampling as long as airflow rates are adequate to detect 25% of the limits during the sampling period. The air sampling frequency, if not continuous, and the times selected for sampling should be based on the nature of the manufacturing process involved and the probability that airborne radioactive material will be present. When assessing this probability is difficult, the frequencies listed in Table 1 are acceptable.

An air monitor may be needed to provide a warning signal if the possibility exists that the concentration of airborne radioactivity may become unexpectedly high. For each room or area where radioactive material is handled, an analysis should be performed to determine whether an air monitor is necessary. An air monitor should be provided if the analysis indicates that it is likely that, in the absence of an appropriate air monitor alarm, accidental conditions could cause an intake of radioactive material exceeding the intake that would result from inhaling such material for 40 hr at the concentration limits for air.

Workers should recognize that the principal function on an air monitor is to alert personnel to take immediate action to protect themselves from exposure to the unexpected release of airborne radioactive material. Inhalation exposures are in progress during the time between the release of the radioactive material and the sounding of the alarm. Thus, every reasonable effort should be made to minimize this period. In particular, the air inlet of the monitor should be located near the potential source of airborne radionuclides, preferably between the source and the workers. The use of long tubing or piping leading to the inlet should be avoided because of the high probability of alarm delay due to radionuclide deposition on the interior walls of the tube or pipe. The dose to personnel may be reduced by selecting a low-activity-level setpoint for the alarm; however, this may result in false alarms that weaken the workers' confidence in the monitor. These alternatives should be balanced to maximize safety.

The dose to personnel may also be reduced by providing a high flow rate of air through the detection chamber or filter. A device such as a limiting orifice that is intended to provide a constant flow rate should not be used with an air monitor when it reduces the flow rate to a level inadequate for sufficient warning of an accidental release. It is more important to maintain a high volume of air drawn through the filter, thus reducing the time of exposure before the alarm by using a higher flow rate, than to measure the concentration accurately. However, it is also important that routine intermittent and continuous releases be monitored.

SURFACE CONTAMINATION SURVEYS

Routine monitoring for radioactive contamination on surfaces of floors, walls, laboratory furniture, and equipment is a necessary part of the survey program. Failure to control surface contamination may result in unnecessary external or internal exposure of personnel to radiation. Although external radiation levels from radioactive contamination may at times be hazardous, the primary concern is to avoid internal exposure resulting from the intake of loose radioactive material by inhalation, ingestion, or skin absorption. Also of concern is limiting contamination to areas where it can be controlled and maintaining contamination levels low enough that leaks or failures in control equipment can be detected as early as practicable.

REMOVABLE CONTAMINATION

Removable contamination is that fraction of the contamination present on a surface that can be transferred to a smear test paper by rubbing with moderate pressure.

Methods and instruments used in surface contamination surveys should be sufficiently sensitive to detect the nuclides being monitored. Also, uniform methods for collecting and

Table 1
ACCEPTABLE FREQUENCIES FOR SURVEYS

Radionuclide group	External radiation surveys (nuclides with asterisks only)[a]		Amounts (curies) in process at any one time or placed into process in any 3 month period within any room requiring surveys					
			Air sampling[b]			Surface contamination		
	Weekly	Monthly	Weekly	Monthly	Quarterly	Weekly	Monthly	Quarterly
I: H-3, C-14, F-18,* K-42,* Cu-64,* Tc-99m,* In-113m*	If point source of activity could exceed 50 mrad/hr at 1m	If point source of activity could exceed 0.5 mrad/hr at 1 m	≥ 10	≥ 1 <10	<1	≥ 100	≥ 10 <100	<10
II: Br-82, Cr-51,* Fe-55, I-123,* Hg-197*			≥ 1	≥ 0.1 <1	<0.1	≥ 10	≥ 1 <10	<1
III: S-35, Au-198, Ca-47, I-132, Ce-141, Mixed fission products,* Sr-85, La-140, Nb-95, Zn-65, Co-58,* Fe-59,* Na-24,* Co-57,* Se-75,* Mo-99*			≥ 0.1	≥ 0.01 <0.1	<0.01	≥ 1	≥ 0.1 <1	
IV: Hf-181, Pm-147 P-32,* Ba-140,* Th-234, Kr-85, Ir-192,* Cl-36, Y-91, Ta-182, Ca-45, Sr-89, Cs-137, Co-60,* Ce-144,* 1-126, Eu-154, I-131,* I-125,* Tm-170, Na-22,* Mn-54,* Ag-110m,* Hg-203,* Rn-222,* Sn-113*			≥ 0.01	≥ 0.001 <0.01	<0.001	≥ 0.1	≥ 0.01 <0.1	<0.01
V: Tc-99, I-129, Ru-106			≥ 0.001	$\geq 10^{-4}$ <0.001	$<10^{-4}$	≥ 0.01	≥ 0.001 <0.01	<0.001
VI: Ra-223, Po-210 Th-227, Sr-90, Pb-210, Cm-242, U-253*			$\geq 10^{-4}$	$\geq 10^{-3}$ $<10^{-4}$	$<10^{-5}$	≥ 0.001	$\geq 0.10^{-4}$ <0.001	$<10^{-4}$
VII: Sm-147, Nd-144, Ra-226* Cm-244, Ra-228, Pu-241			$\geq 10^{-5}$	$\geq 10^{-6}$ $<10^{-5}$	$<10^{-6}$	$\geq 10^{-4}$	$\geq 10^{-5}$ $<10^{-4}$	$<10^{-5}$
VIII: Am-243, Am-241,* Np-237, Ac-227, Th-230, Pu-242, Pu-238, Pu-240, Pu-239, Th-228, Cf-252			$\geq 10^{-6}$	$\geq 10^{-7}$ $<10^{-6}$	$<10^{-8}$	$\geq 10^{-5}$	$\geq 10^{-6}$ $<10^{-5}$	$<10^{-6}$

[a] Nuclides with asterisks are those more likely to require external radiation surveys. [b] Assuming continuous sampling is unnecessary (see Section C.1.3).

analyzing smear samples should be used over extended periods of time in order to evaluate trends. Counting equipment used to analyze radioactive contamination on smear samples should be properly calibrated and maintained and should be capable of detecting the radiation from the smears. For example, smears containing low-energy radiation emitters (e.g., H-3, C-14, 1-125) should be analyzed with liquid scintillation or internal proportional counters. Check or calibration sources should be counted with each batch or daily workload of smear samples.

When contamination levels in restricted areas can potentially exceed 0.1% of the respective limits in line 2 of Table 2, the collection of smear samples should generally be preceded by a rapid overall survey with a portable, thin-window detector in order to:

a. Ensure that gross contamination levels are not already too high for counting in sensitive equipment
b. Minimize the chance for inadvertent spread of contamination by the smear survey or other activities to be performed in the meantime
c. Determine which areas require greater attention in smear testing

The instrument used should have a read-out system with as short a time constant as appropriate for the type of radiation to be detected and should be equipped with earphones or an external speaker system.

A standardized method for smear testing of a relatively uniform area should be used to aid in comparing contamination at different times and places. A dry smear taken from an area of about 100 cm^2 is acceptable to indicate levels of removable contamination.

A diagram of each routinely surveyed area should ordinarily be used for recording survey results. When appropriate, the diagram may be supplemented by or replaced by a detailed list of items and equipment surveyed. This procedure will provide radiation safety personnel with a method for identifying trends as well as satisfying regulatory requirements for survey records. The surveyor will find it helpful to specify key locations on the survey diagram that are smear-tested at each survey, in addition to other areas to be smear-tested in particular surveys, and also to provide a space reminding the recorder to include:

a. Contamination levels indicated during portable instrument survey
b. Make and model number of instruments used in the survey and in counting the smear samples
c. Disintegration rate of each sample
d. Background count
e. All counting times
f. Name of the person making the evaluation and recording the results and date

Provision should also be made on the diagram for recording an instrument check with an appropriate check or calibration source.

The surveys discussed above are regularly scheduled, conducted by radiation safety personnel, and recorded on the survey diagrams. In addition, whenever the manufacturing process is such that excessive contamination could occur between surveys by radiation safety personnel, more frequent, informal radiation surveys should be conducted by the radiation workers themselves; they need not be recorded. For example, a contamination survey can be made by collecting a smear sample and holding it within a few millimeters of (but not touching) a thin (less than 2 mg/cm^2) end-window detector while the detector is in an area where radiation levels are less than about 0.005 mrem/hr. At these levels, any appreciable surface contamination can be detected by simply holding the detector in a fixed position and moving the smear sample close to and away from the detector several times and noting

Table 2
RECOMMENDED ACTION LEVELS FOR REMOVABLE SURFACE CONTAMINATION IN MANUFACTURING PLANTS

	Type of radioactive material[a]			
	Alpha emitters			
Type of surface	High toxicity (μCi/cm^2)	Lower toxicity (μCi/cm^2)	Beta or X-ray emitters (μCi/cm^2)	Low-risk beta or X-ray emitters (μCi/cm^2)
1. Unrestricted areas[b]	10^{-7}	10^{-7}	10^{-6}	10^{-6}
2. Restricted areas[c]	10^{-4}	10^{-3}	10^{-3}	10^{-2}
3. Personal clothing worn outside of restricted areas	10^{-7}	10^{-7}	10^{-6}	10^{-6}
4. Protective clothing worn only in restricted areas	10^{-5}	10^{-5}	10^{-4}	10^{-4}

Note on Units: The above units of μCi/cm^2 have been used in this table since they are consistent with units adopted as national standards in several other nations and the IAEA (see Reference 6): the units of μCi and cm are already used to express concentration in 10 CFR Part 20, and they are readily convertible to SI units by the well-known relation: 1 μCi = 3.7×10^4 dis/sec = 3.7×10^4 Becquerels (Bq). They may also be easily converted to other frequently used units of radiation protection practice, i.e., disintegrations/minute/100 cm^2 = 2.22×10^8 $\times$ disintegrations/minute/100 cm^2 = 2.22×10^8 $\times$ (activity expressed in μCi/cm^2).
Note on Skin Contamination: Skin contamination should always be kept ALARA. Exposed areas of the body of persons working with unsealed radioactive materials should always be monitored and should be washed when any contamination is detected. It is important, however, that contaminated skin should not be so treated or scrubbed that the chance of intake of radioactivity into the body is increased. See Section 1.6 of this guide.

[a] High toxicity alpha emitters include Am-243, Am-241, Np-237, Ac-227, Th-230, Pu-242, Pu-238, Pu-240, Pu-239, Th-228, and Cf-252. Lower toxicity alpha emitters include those having permissible concentrations in air greater than that for Ra-226 (s) in 10 CFR Part 20, Appendix B, Table 1, Column 1. Beta or X-ray emitter values are applicable for all beta or X-ray emitters other than those considered low risk. Low-risk nuclides include those whose beta energies are less than 0.2 MeV, whose gamma or X-ray emission is less than 0.1 R/hr at 1 m/Ci, and whose permissible concentration in air in 10 CFR Part 20, Appendix B, Table 1, is greater than 10^{-6} μCi/mℓ.

[b] Contamination limits for unrestricted (noncontamination-controlled) areas in this table are considered to be compatible in level of safety with those for release of facilities and equipment for unrestricted use, as given in Regulatory Guide 1.86, "Termination of Operating Licenses for Nuclear Reactors," and in "Guidelines for Decontamination of Facilities and Equipment Prior to Release for Unrestricted Use or Termination of Licenses for Byproduct, Source, or Special Nuclear Material," which is available from the Division of Fuel Cycle and Material Safety, Office of Nuclear Material Safety and Safeguards, U.S. Nuclear Regulatory Commission, Washington, D.C. 20555.

[c] As adapted from Table 1 of Reference 4. Averaging is acceptable over inanimate areas of up to 300 cm^2 or, for floors, walls, and ceiling, 100 cm^2. These limits are allowed only in those restricted areas where appropriate protective clothing is worn.

the meter readings. This method may be used for the majority of radionuclides processed in manufacturing plants (excluding alpha and very low-energy beta emitters).

The contamination limits for restricted areas presented in Table 2 are the maximum that will be acceptable to the NRC staff. Limits established for a particular installation should generally be lower than those in Table 2 and should be ALARA for the particular operations involved.

FIXED CONTAMINATION

For the purpose of this guide, fixed contamination is defined as radioactivity remaining on a surface after repeated decontamination attempts fail to significantly reduce the contamination level. Since most detectors respond to both removable and fixed contamination, limits should be based on total contamination. Total contamination surveys, using instruments suitable for the radionuclides involved, should be conducted at least quarterly and simultaneously with a removable contamination survey. The limits appearing on line 2 of Table 2, multiplied by a factor of 5, are the maximum that will be acceptable to the NRC staff.

PROTECTIVE CLOTHING AND EQUIPMENT CONTAMINATION SURVEYS

Individuals working in areas where a potential for skin or clothing contamination exists should be provided with suitable protective clothing.

Potentially contaminated protective clothing and equipment should be surveyed, removed, and placed in suitable containers or lockers before the worker leaves the restricted area.

When protective clothing contamination levels exceed preselected limits, workers should be instructed to take care to avoid dispersal of contamination and to report the situation to the Radiation Safety Office. A member of the radiation safety staff should then survey and supervise any necessary decontamination or clothing disposal. The limits given on line 4 of Table 2 are the maximum that will be acceptable to the NRC staff.

Contamination levels observed and procedures followed for incidents requiring special surveys and decontamination should be recorded. The record should include the names of persons surveyed, a description of prior work activities, the probable causes, steps taken to reduce future incidence of contamination, times and dates, and the surveyor's signature. This information may be entered in a logbook. Individual worker surveys of themselves need not be recorded unless the limits on line 3 of Table 2 are exceeded. However, the radiation safety staff should maintain daily surveillance to ensure that the workers continue their own personal contamination surveys. Results of radiation safety surveillance should be recorded.

In restricted areas with little potential for surface contamination, personal clothing is often worn beneath protective clothing. Such personal clothing should be surveyed by the wearer before he or she leaves the restricted area (However, this is neither practicable nor necessary for employees working with only submicrocurie quantities of tritium or carbon-14). When personal clothing contamination levels exceed preselected limits, workers should be instructed to report the situation to the Radiation Safety Office. A member of the radiation safety staff should then survey and supervise any necessary decontamination or clothing disposal. The limits given on line 3 of Table 2 are acceptable to the NRC. Records should be maintained in the same manner as those for protective clothing contamination.

For individuals whose work is conducted in restricted areas with a potential for high surface contamination levels complete clothing changes are normally provided. In this case, personal clothing should be stored outside the restricted area. Surveys of personal clothing are not necessary, provided the area in which the clothing is stored is surveyed and the survey results are below the limits adopted for in-plant unrestricted areas. Particular attention should be paid to surveying the body, hair, bottoms of the shoes or feet, and the hands after removal of protective clothing and to washing before donning personal clothing.

PERSONAL SURVEYS

Individuals whose duties require work in restricted areas where radioactive contamination of body surfaces is probable should also survey all exposed areas of the body after showering and before donning personal clothing or leaving the restricted area. Workers should be required to report the detection of contamination on the body to the Radiation Safety Office. Decontamination attempts, under the direction of Radiation Safety Office personnel or a medical consultant, should be repeated until (a) such attempts cease to effect significant reductions or (b) such attempts threaten to damage the skin. When decontamination attempts are terminated, there should be no further concern if the residual contamination does not exceed preselected levels since the contamination would no longer present a significant ingestion hazard. If residual contamination exceeds the selected limits, the affected individual should be released but periodic surveys should be made until the limits are no longer exceeded. The resulting dose should be determined and entered in the individual's personnel dosimetry record. Complete records should be maintained of each incident of this nature.

Since manufacturing plants often process large quantities of unencapsulated radioactive material, bioassay programs may be required.

SURVEYS OF EQUIPMENT PRIOR TO RELEASE TO UNRESTRICTED AREAS

Surface contamination surveys should be conducted for both removable and fixed contamination before potentially contaminated equipment is released from restricted to unrestricted areas. If contamination is detected, decontamination procedures should be repeated until contamination is removed or additional efforts do not significantly reduce contamination levels.

INGESTION

Although it is highly unlikely that significant internal exposures will result from ingesting drinking water near work areas, any water fountains in areas where contamination of the fountains or water is possible should be smear-tested regularly, and the water should be sampled and analyzed at least quarterly. Also, surveillance should be included in the radiation safety program to ensure that workers observe rules to prevent ingestion of radionuclides, e.g., rules pertaining to eating, drinking, or smoking in work areas or while wearing potentially contaminated clothing, storing foods in work areas, or pipetting by mouth.

SURVEYS OF PACKAGES RECEIVED AND PACKAGES PREPARED FOR SHIPMENT

External radiation surveys and smear tests of external surfaces of packages received or packaged for shipment should be carried out near the receiving or packaging point to avoid unwarranted radiation exposures and inadvertent contamination of personnel or the facility. When many packages of a kind known to be generally free of contamination are received, smear testing of a suitable random sample should be considered in cases where smear testing of a large number of packages could increase external exposure of personnel. Delivery of packages within the plant should also be monitored when carried by personnel rather than mechanical conveyors. Surveys should be made to determine when carts rather than hand carrying should be used. Packages containing significant amounts of radioactive materials should not be surveyed or opened until the containers have been placed in the appropriate protective facility such as a radiological-type fume hood or hot cell.

No packages may be released for shipment or transfer when external radiation or surface contamination levels exceed limits set by the Department of Transportation in Title 49 of the Code of Federal Regulation. External radiation and contamination levels should be maintained ALARA.

CHECKS ON POSTING OF CAUTION SIGNS, LABELS, SIGNALS, CONTROLS, AND NOTICES TO EMPLOYEES

The radiation safety staff should perform surveillance at least weekly to ensure that signs, labels, signals, other access controls, and required Notices to Employees, copies of licenses, and other items are properly posted, legible, and operative. Radiation alarm signals and access controls should be tested to verify that they will operate properly under both the normal and abnormal conditions that might be expected to occur. Care should be taken to minimize exposure to personnel who are conducting the tests. Any signs, labels, or notices found to be missing should be promptly replaced.

SEALED SOURCE LEAK TESTS

Leak testing of sealed sources must be carried out in accordance with the terms and conditions of the manufacturer's materials license. Sealed sources containing

a. More than 100 mCi of a by-product material with a half-life of more than 30 days (except iridium-192 seeds encased in nylon ribbon) or
b. More than 10 mCi of an alpha emitter

must be leak tested for contamination or leakage at intervals not to exceed 6 months unless a different interval is specified for a particular manufactured source.

CALIBRATION OF RADIATION SAFETY INSTRUMENTS

Portable survey instruments should be placed on a routine maintenance and calibration program that will ensure that properly calibrated and operable survey instruments are available at all times for use by the health physics staff.

An adequate calibration of survey instruments cannot be performed solely with built-in check sources. Electronic calibrations that do not involve a source of radiation also do not determine the proper functioning and response of all components of an instrument. However, an initial calibration with a radiation source and periodic tests using electronic input signals may be considered adequate for high ranges that are not used routinely.

Daily or other frequent checks of survey instruments should be supplemented every 6 months with a calibration of each instrument at two points separated by at least 50% of each linear scale that is used routinely, or with a calibration at one point near the midpoint of each decade on logarithmic scales that are used routinely. Digital readout instruments with either manual or automatic scale switching should be calibrated as are linear readout instruments. Digital readout instruments without scale switching should be calibrated as are logarithmic readout instruments. Survey instruments should also be calibrated following repair. A survey instrument may be considered properly calibrated when the instrument readings are within ±10% of the calculated or known values for each point checked. Readings within ±20% are considered acceptable if a calibration chart or graph is prepared and attached to the instrument.

SURVEYS OF PROTECTIVE CLOTHING BEFORE AND AFTER LAUNDERING

All garments with contamination levels exceeding those given on line 3 of Table 2 should be either disposed of as radioactive waste or properly surveyed, packaged, and labeled and sent to a laundry licensed to process and handle radioactively contaminated clothing.

Each garment returned from a licensed laundry, or a sample of garments that are returned within a single package, should be monitored before use. If contamination levels on the garment exceed those given on line 4 of Table 2, the garment should not be used.

VENTILATION SURVEYS

Radiation safety personnel should conduct surveys monthly (or more frequently) to determine the face velocity of air at the entrance of radiological-type fume hoods in use to protect workers against the hazards from unencapsulated radioactive materials. Such surveys should be made by using a properly calibrated thermoanemometer, velometer, or a U-tube observation after the initial measurement of flow rate to determine whether the airflow has been reduced to unacceptable levels by filter loading or the malfunction of blowers, fans, etc. The minimum average face velocity for a fume hood with the sash in the operating position or for an opening in a special enclosure should be 100 ft/min, as determined from at least five different measurement points.

Corrective action should be taken as soon as possible when the face velocity is found to be deficient. Work should be terminated if the average face velocity falls below 100 ft/min.

In addition to these surveys, each enclosure should be equipped with a device that measures pressure drop across the hood filter. Workers should be instructed to maintain daily checks of these devices and to notify radiation safety personnel when the pressure drop exceeds a preset level.

At least annually, or when changes occur that might affect airflow, a survey should be made to determine the number or air changes per hour provided by the ventilation system in each room in which work with unencapsulated radioactive materials is conducted. A minimum of six changes per hour should be provided.

SURVEYS OF IN-PLANT UNRESTRICTED AREAS

Unrestricted areas should be surveyed periodically to ensure that radiation and radioactive material are adequately confined in restricted areas, except in cases where these materials must be transported between areas. Such transportation should be surveyed or planned with the radiation safety staff.

SURFACE CONTAMINATION SURVEYS

Removable surface contamination surveys in unrestricted areas should be performed and recorded at frequencies consistent with the potential for spreading contamination but not less frequently than quarterly. With the exception of lunch rooms and snack bars, random smear testing of floors and furniture is adequate. In lunch rooms and snack bars, equipment should also be surveyed. If such surveys reveal that radioactive contamination is being transferred out of restricted areas, immediate corrective action should be taken to eliminate such transfers, and decontamination efforts in the unrestricted areas should be repeated until it is evident that subsequent efforts would not significantly reduce contamination levels. If contamination is found in unrestricted areas, surveys should be performed on a more frequent schedule as necessary until the source of contamination is ascertained and corrected. The limits given on line 1 of Table 2 are acceptable to the NRC.

RADIATION SURVEYS

Radiation surveys in unrestricted areas should be performed and recorded at frequencies consistent with the types and quantities of materials in use but not less frequently than quarterly. These surveys should be made in areas adjacent to restricted areas and in all areas through which by-product materials are transferred and temporarily stored before shipment.

SURVEILLANCE

Health physics personnel should acquire detailed knowledge of each operation in order to (a) identify ways of preventing or minimizing exposures, (b) select appropriate times for making health physics measurements, and (c) adequately prepare for emergency conditions. Health physics personnel should be sufficiently familiar with each operation to explain it in detail, to describe potential hazards and the precautions taken to minimize exposures, and to discuss how this knowledge of the operation has influenced the selection of appropriate times for performing health physics measurement.

The surveillance program should include:

a. Regular inventory of radioactive materials and their locations
b. Frequent audits of radiation safety procedures and the uses and amounts of material in process compared to licensed possession limits
c. Discussions with personnel to ensure their continued awareness of safety procedures and the appropriateness of their instruction and training for the tasks they are performing.

These surveillance activities may be conducted during the performance of other survey measurements or tests. The radiation safety staff should conduct surveillance inspections in a manufacturing plant at least weekly. The surveillance should be performed at least annually by the Radiation Safety Officer in the presence of a management representative such as the plant manager to provide management with an awareness of the nature and importance of activities conducted for personnel protection and plant safety.

FREQUENCY OF SURVEYS

The frequency of routine surveys depends on the nature, quantity, and use of radioactive materials, as well as the specific protective facilities, equipment, and procedures that are designed to protect the worker from external and internal exposure.

Generally, surveys should be performed before radioactive materials are used in a new facility in order to establish a baseline of background radiation levels and radioactivity from natural sources, structural components of the facility (including radon and thoron emanation rates and concentrations), and any already existing operations with radiation sources in nearby rooms or facilities. These baseline surveys should be performed under the various conditions of containment, shielding design, and process heat loads to be expected under manufacturing conditions. Surveys of simulated process operations with nonradioactive reagents or smaller amounts of radioactive material should also be performed where appropriate to establish the performance of protective equipment and procedures before full-scale production using any new or untested facilities or processes.

Surveys should be repeated as soon as process operations begin with normal levels of radioactive material and with all potentially exposed workers present and carrying out their job functions. Surveys should also be conducted after any significant changes in the conditions that existed at the time of the most recent survey, including changes in the quantities of radioactive material handled or in protective equipment and procedures.

Routine and repetitive surveys are necessary to control the containment of radioactive materials within handling systems and to ensure the continued integrity of protective equipment and procedures. Surveys are also necessary for procedures in which sealed sources are handled outside shielded containers. For operations involving materials in gas, liquid, or finely divided forms, the survey program should be designed to monitor the continued adequacy of containment and control of the materials involved.

The minimum acceptable frequencies of surveys for manufacturing plants are given in Table 1.

RECORDS OF SURVEYS

Record retention requirements are that survey records be preserved for 2 years, except that records of air monitoring and (in the absence of personnel monitoring data) records of surveys to determine external radiation dose are to be maintained until the NRC authorizes their disposition.

Records may be maintained in logbooks or on special forms as long as they are clear, legible, understandable, and authenticated by authorized personnel. The signature of the person making the record and the date of the signature should be on the same page as the record and should immediately follow each record entry. Either the original or a reproduced copy or microform (duly authenticated) may be maintained to meet the storage requirements.

APPENDIX F*
SAMPLE CHECKLIST FOR RADIATION SURVEYS AT MEDICAL AND OTHER INSTITUTIONS

1. Initiate contamination survey report for each lab.
   a. Check previous survey results to determine patterns or problem areas.
   b. On survey form, fill in name of Authorized User, Department, Building and Room Number, and Survey Date.
   c. Sketch floor plan.
2. Ask lab personnel (and record answers on report form):
   a. What isotopes are being used? (Compare with what user is cleared for).
   b. Where in the lab are they used?
   c. Where are isotopes stored?
   d. What was last order? (Compare with card record).
   e. Is Authorized User available if needed? If not, give reason, e.g. on leave, out of country, terminated employment.
   f. In what other labs are isotopes used? (Compare with card record).
   g. Where is waste stored and disposed of?
   h. Have radioisotope users received instruction in safe handling procedures?
   i. Have people who visit the lab been instructed?
   j. Where appropriate, do radioisotope users have film and/or ring badges?
3. Check labeling
   a. Lab door — "Caution, Radioactive Material" (CRM)
   b. Liquid waste sink — "Contaminated Liquid Waste" (survey card should indicate radioactive sink — RS). Is sink log posted? Is it being used?
   c. Radioactive hood — "Caution, Radioactive Material" (survey card should indicate radioactive hood — RH). "Air Flow Check" label with date no older than 4 months required.
   d. Refrigerator and other storage areas — "CRM", including those in corridors.
   e. Radioactive waste containers — "CRM" or "Contaminated Waste" should be lined with plastic bag.
   f. Any area with external radiation over 2.5 mR/hr should be labeled with "Caution, Radiation Area" (CRA) and should be noted on survey form.
   g. Appropriate "Instruction to Workers" signs
4. Observe general laboratory conditions:
   a. Food and drink preparation and use in radioactive material areas?
   b. Waste container overfilled?

* Adapted from and reprinted with permission of the Education and Training Committee of the Health Physics Society, 4720 Montgomery Lane, Bethesda, Md., July 1980.

   c. Dosimeters being worn?
   d. Mouth pipetting?
5. Conduct laboratory survey using portable survey meter.
   a. Record external dose rate from accessible storage surfaces.
   b. Record exposure rate from contaminated surfaces.
6. Conduct smear survey:
   a. Take first smear near or in lab entrance.
   b. Take several smears from floor and benches and equipment as indicated by answers to earlier questions.
7. Discuss ''Instructions to Workers'' requirements.
8. Complete results:
   a. Count smears and list results on survey form.
   b. Notify lab personnel of contamination, and note on form who was called and date of notification.
   c. Identify all abnormal radiation safety conditions on survey form.
   d. Complete survey card, replace in file, and mail survey form copy to User.
   e. If lab has contamination (significant), call User, request cleanup and resmear.
   f. Resmear when notified or call User if no resmear was called for.
   g. File carbon copy of results form.

APPENDIX G
UNIVERSITY AND COLLEGE GRADUATE PROGRAMS IN HEALTH PHYSICS*

Institution and advisor	Program specialization[a]	Degree offered	Minimum requirements
University of Cincinnati			
Dr. James G. Kareiakes	MED	M.S.	
E-555 Medical Science Building			
University of Cincinnati			
Cincinnati, OH 45267			
Colorado State University			
Dr. Leslie Fraley, Jr. Chairperson	BIO	M.S., Ph.D.	[b]
Graduate Review Committee	ENV	M.S., Ph.D.	[b]
Department of Radiology and	PWR	M.S., Ph.D.	[b]
Radiation Biology	RHEALTH	M.S., Ph.D.	[b]
Colorado State University			
Fort Collins, CO 80523			
University of Colorado Medical Center			
Geoffrey S. Ibbott, Coordinator,	MED	M.S., Ph.D.	[b]
Graduate Program in Medical			
Physics			
Department of Radiology			
University of Colorado Health			
Science Center			
Denver, CO 80262			
Cornell University			
John S. Laughlin, Ph.D., FACR	BIO	M.S., Ph.D.	[b]
Professor of Biophysics	ENG	M.S., Ph.D.	[b]

* Revised and adapted with permission from Brodsky, A., Sample Checklist for Radiation Surveyor, Regulatory Guide 8.23, U.S. Nuclear Regulatory Commission, Washington, D.C. 20555, 1981.

Institution and advisor	Program specialization[a]	Degree offered	Minimum requirements
Cornell University Graduate School of Medical Sciences — SKI Division	MED	M.S., Ph.D.	[b]
	RPHARM	M.S., Ph.D.	[b]
	RHEALTH	M.S., Ph.D.	[b]
1275 York Avenue New York, NY 10021			
Emory University			
Dr. Richard C. Palmer, Director	MED	M.S.	[b]
Programs in Radiological Science	RHEALTH	M.S.	[b]
Division of Allied Health Professions Emory University School of Medicine P.O. Box 22991 Atlanta, GA 30033			
University of Florida			
Genevieve S. Roessler, Coordinator	BIO	M.S., Ph.D.	[b]
	ENG	M.S., Ph.D.	[b]
Radiological Sciences Program	ENV	M.S., Ph.D.	[b]
Department of Nuclear Engineering Science	PWR	M.S., Ph.D.	[b]
	MED	M.S., Ph.D.	[b]
University of Florida	RHEALTH	M.S., Ph.D.	[b]
223 Nuclear Sciences Center Gainesville, FL 32611			
Georgia Institute of Technology			
Dr. John W. Poston	ENG	M.S., Ph.D.	[b]
Associate Professor	ENV	M.S., Ph.D.	[b]
School of Nuclear Engineering	PWR	M.S., Ph.D.	[b]
Georgia Institute of Technology	MED	M.S., Ph.D.	[b]
Atlanta, GA 30332			
Harvard University			
Dr. Bengt Bjarngard	MED	M.S., Ph.D.	[b]
Department of Radiation Therapy 50 Binney Street Boston, MA 02115			
Dr. Dade W. Moeller	BIO	M.S., Ph.D.	[b]
Harvard School of Public Health	MED	M.S., Ph.D.	[b]
655 Huntington Avenue	RHEALTH	M.S., Ph.D.	[b]
Boston, MA 02115			
University of Illinois			
Louis R. Milavickas	ENG	M.S., Ph.D.	[b]
Nuclear Engineering and Bioengineering Programs	PWR	M.S., Ph.D.	[b]
214 NEL University of Illinois Urbana, IL 61801			

Institution and advisor	Program specialization[a]	Degree offered	Minimum requirements
University of Iowa			
J. W. Osborne, Director	BIO	M.S., Ph.D.	b
Radiation Research Laboratory	MED	M.S., Ph.D.	b
14 Medical Laboratory			
University of Iowa			
Iowa City, IA 52242			
University of Kansas			
Dr. Benjamin Friesen, Director	BIO	Ph.D.	b
Radiation Biophysics Program	MED	M.S., Ph.D.	b
University of Kansas	RHEALTH	M.S., Ph.D.	
140 NRC, West 15th Street			
Lawrence, KS 66045			
University of Kentucky Medical Center			
Dr. Joseph A. Sayeg	MED	M.S.	b
Department of Health Radiation Sciences	RHEALTH	M.S.	b
University of Kentucky Medical Center			
Lexington, KY 40506			
University of Michigan			
Dr. Phillip Plato	BIO	M.S., Ph.D.	b
School of Public Health	ENV	M.S., Ph.D.	
University of Michigan	PWR	M.S., Ph.D.	
Ann Arbor, MI 48109	RHEALTH	M.S., Ph.D.	b
University of Minnesota			
Dr. Donald E. Barber	ENG	M.S., Ph.D.	b
School of Public Health	ENV	M.S., Ph.D.	b
University of Minnesota	PWR	M.S., Ph.D.	b
1360 Mayo Memorial Bldg.	MED	M.S., Ph.D.	b
420 Delaware St., S.E.	RHEALTH	M.S., Ph.D.	b
Minneapolis, MN 55455			
University of Missouri — Columbia			
Dr. Stanley R. Bull	CHEM	M.S., Ph.D.	b
Nuclear Engineering	ENG	M.S., Ph.D.	b
University of Missouri —	ENV	M.S., Ph.D.	b
Columbia	PWR	M.S., Ph.D.	b
Columbia, MO 56201	MED	M.S., Ph.D.	b
University of North Carolina			
Dr. James E. Watson, Jr.	ENV	M.S., Ph.D.	b
Department of Env. Sci & Eng.	PWR	M.S., Ph.D.	b
School of Public Health	MED	M.S., Ph.D.	b
University of North Carolina	RHEALTH	M.S., Ph.D.	b
Chapel Hill, NC 27514			
Northwestern University			
Herman Cember	BIO	M.S., Ph.D.	b
Professor, Environmental Health	ENG	M.S., Ph.D.	b
Technological Institute	ENV	M.S., Ph.D.	b

Institution and advisor	Program specialization[a]	Degree offered	Minimum requirements
Northwestern University	PWR	M.S. Ph.D.	b
Evanston, IL 60201	MED	M.S., Ph.D.	b
	RHEALTH	M.S., Ph.D.	b
Oregon State University			
Dr. David L. Willis, Chairman	BIO	M.S., Ph.D.	
General Science Department	RHEALTH	M.S.	b
Oregon State University			
Corvallis, OR 97331			
University of Pennsylvania			
Dr. John Hale	MED	M.S.	b
Donner Center/G1			
Hospital of the University of Pennsylvania			
3400 Spruce Street			
Philadelphia, PA 19104			
University of Pittsburgh			
Dr. Joseph A. Watson	BIO	M.S., Sc.D.	
Department of Radiation Health	ENV	M.S., Sc.D.	
University of Pittsburgh	PWR	M.S., Sc.D.	
130 DeSoto Street	MED	M.S., Sc.D.	
Pittsburgh, PA 15261	RHEALTH	M.S., Sc.D.	
University of Puerto Rico			
Dr. Heriberto Torres, Head	RHEALTH	M.S.	b
Department of Environmental Health			
University of Puerto Rico			
P.O. Box 5067			
Rio Piedras, PR 00936			
Purdue University			
Paul L. Ziemer	ENV	M.S., Ph.D.	
Associate Head	PWR	M.S., Ph.D.	b
School of Health Sciences	MED	M.S., Ph.D.	b
Purdue University	RPHARM	M.S.,	
West Lafayette, IN 47907	RHEALTH	M.S., Ph.D.	b
Rensselaer Polytechnic Institute			
Dr. Donald Aulenbach	ENG	M.S., Ph.D.	
Department of Chem. & Environ. Eng.	ENV	M.S., Ph.D.	
	PWR	M.S., Ph.D.	
Rensselaer Polytechnic Institute			
Troy, NY 12181			
Rutgers University			
Dr. Francis J. Haughey	CHEM	M.S., Ph.D.	b
Radiation Science	ENV	M.S., Ph.D.	b
Rutgers University	PWR	M.S., Ph.D.	b
New Brunswick, NJ 08903	MED	M.S., Ph.D.	b
	RHEALTH	M.S., Ph.D.	b
San Diego State University			
Dr. Lester L. Skolil	RHEALTH	M.S.	b
Department of Physics			

Institution and advisor	Program specialization[a]	Degree offered	Minimum requirements
San Diego State University			
San Diego, CA 92182			
University of Southern California			
Dr. Walter Wolf	RPHARM	M.S., Ph.D.	[b]
Radiopharmacy Program, Sch. of Pharmacy			
University of Southern California			
1935 Zonal Avenue			
Los Angeles, CA 90033			
Texas A & M University			
Dr. R. D. Neff	BIO	M.S.	[b]
Radiological Safety Office	ENG	M.S., Ph.D.	[b]
Texas A & M University	PWR	M.S., Ph.D.	[b]
College Station, TX 77843			
University of Washington			
Dr. Kenneth L. Jackson, Chairman	BIO	M.S., Ph.D.	[b]
Radiological Sciences SB-30	ENG	M.S., Ph.D.	[b]
University of Washington	ENV	M.S., Ph.D.	[b]
Seattle, WA 98195	MED	M.S., Ph.D.	[b]
Washington State University			
Dr. Surinder K. Bhagat	BIO	M.S., Ph.D.	
Professor & Head of	CHEM	M.S., Ph.D.	
Environmental Engineering	ENG	M.S., Ph.D.	[b]
Sloan Hall 141	ENV	M.S., Ph.D.	[b]
Washington State University	PWR	M.S., Ph.D.	[b]
Pullman, WA 99163	RHEALTH	M.S., Ph.D.	[b]
University of Wisconsin			
Paul M. Deluca, Jr.	PWR	M.S., Ph.D.	[b]
Med. Physics Section, Dept. of Radiology	MED	M.S., Ph.D.	[b]
University of Wisconsin — Madison			
Madison, WI 53706			

Note: Prospective students should check into the program details of each university they may attend since programs vary significantly.

[a] Legend to categories of program specialization:

BIO = radiobiology; biological effects of radiation (molecular, cellular, systemic, organism, population, etc.)

CHEM = radiochemistry; effects of radiation on chemical systems, radiochemical techniques (including waste treatment)

ENG = engineering aspects of radiation protection (including facility design, instrument design, shielding, waste disposal, etc.)

ENV = environmental and ecological aspects of radiation protection (including surveillance, modeling, etc.)

PWR = health physics primarily related to the nuclear power industry (including reactors and other operations in the nuclear fuel cycle)

MED = medical applications of radiation (including radiology, radiation therapy, and nuclear medicine)
RPHARM = radiopharmacy
RHEALTH = radiological health

[b] The listed advisor stated that the MS program meets the minimim requirements as established by the Education and Training Committee of the Health Physics Society. No minimum requirements have been set for the Ph.D. programs.

REFERENCES

1. **Miller, K. L.,** A Radiation safety program for a new medical center, in Proceedings of the 9th Midyear Topical Symposium of the Health Physics Society on Operational Health Physics (Rocky Mountain Chapter, Health Physics Society, P.O. Box 3229), Boulder, Co., 1976.
2. **Ice, R. D.,** Establishment of a university radiation safety office, *Health Phys.,* 20, 444—447, 1971.
3. **Tolan, J. H.,** Organization of a small-scale radiation safety program, in *Health Physics Operational Monitoring,* Vol. 1, Willis, C. A. and Handloser, J. S., Eds., Gordon & Breach, New York, 1972, 321—327.
4. **Brodsky, A., Levin, S., and Durkosh, E.,** Staff and facility requirements for radiation safety in hospitals, presented at the 20th Annual Meeting of the Health Physics Society, Buffalo, New York, August 1975; abstracted in *Health Phys.,* 29, 924, 1975.
5. **Bradley, F. J.,** Administration of a radiation protection program, *Handbook of Radioactive Nuclides,* Wang, Y., Ed., CRC Press, Boca Raton, 1969, 795—798.
6. National Council on Radiation Protection and Measurements, Operational Radiation Safety Program, NCRP Report No. 59, National Council on Radiation Protection and Measurements, Washington, 1978.
7. U.S. Nuclear Regulatory Commission, Guide for the preparation of applications for licenses for laboratory and industrial use of small quantities of byproduct material, U.S. Nuclear Regulatory Commission Regulatory Guide 10.7, Revision 1, August 1979, Washington, D.C.
8. U.S. Nuclear Regulatory Commission, Guide for the preparation of applications for licenses for the use of gamma irradiators, U.S. Nuclear Regulatory Commission Regulatory Guide 10.9, April 1980, Washington, D.C.
9. U.S. Nuclear Regulatory Commission, Guide for the preparation of applications for use of sealed sources and devices for performing industrial radiography, U.S. Nuclear Regulatory Commission Regulatory Guide 10.6, December 1981, Washington, D.C.
10. U.S. Nuclear Regulatory Commission, Guide for the preparation of applications for special nuclear material licenses of less than critical mass quantities, U.S. Nuclear Regulatory Commission Regulatory Guide 10.3, Revision 1, April 1977, Washington, D.C.
11. U.S. Nuclear Regulatory Commission, Applications for Type A. License of broad scope, U.S. Nuclear Regulatory Commission Regulatory Guide 10.5, Revision 1, December 1980, Washington, D.C.
12. U.S. Nuclear Regulatory Commission, Guide for administrative practices in radiation monitoring, U.S. Nuclear Regulatory Commission Regulatory Guide 8.2, February 1973, Washington, D.C.
13. American National Standards Institute, Administrative Practices in Radiation Monitoring (A Guide for Management), ANSI Standard N13.2, 1969, New York.
14. International Commission on Radiological Protection, Recommendations of the International Commission on Radiological Protection, ICRP Publication No. 26, Pergamon Press, Oxford, 1977.
15. U.S. Nuclear Regulatory Commission, Code of Federal Regulations, Title 10, Part 20, Standards for Protection Against Radiation, Office of the Federal Register, National Archives and Records Service, General Services Administration, Washington, D.C., 1979.
16. U.S. Nuclear Regulatory Commission, Code of Federal Regulations, Title 10, Part 19, Notices, Instructions and Reports to Workers; Inspections, Office of the Federal Register, National Archives and Records Service, General Services Administration, Washington, D.C., 1980.
17. **Brodsky, A.,** Determination of facilities, equipment, and procedures required for various types of operations, *Handbook of Radioactive Nuclides,* Wang, T., Ed., CRC Press, Boca Raton, 1969, 664—710.
18. **Diegl, H. J.,** Guidelines for determining frequency of wipe surveys, in *Health Physics Operational Monitoring,* Willis, C. A. and Handloser, J. S., Ed., Gordon & Breach, New York, 1972, 385—396.

19. **Meinhold, C. B.,** Facility monitoring programs, techniques and problem solving, in *Health Physics Operational Monitoring,* Vol. 1, Willis, C. A. and Handloser, J. S., Eds., Gordon & Breach, New York, 1972, 363—371.
20. **Morgan, G. W.,** Laboratory design, *Radiation Hygiene Handbook,* Blatz, H., Ed., McGraw-Hill, New York, 1959, 9—2 to 9—12.
21. International Commission on Radiological Protection, The Handling, Storage, Use and Disposal of Unsealed Radionuclides in Hospitals and Medical Research Establishments, ICRP Publication No. 25, Pergamon Press, Oxford, 1976.
22. **Gallagher, F. E.,** A New Facility for Processing and Storage of Radioactive and Toxic Chemical Waste, in Proceedings of the 9th Midyear Topical Symposium of the Health Physics Society on Operational Health Physics (Rocky Mountain Chapter, Health Physics Society, P.O. Box 3229), Boulder, Co., 1976, 182—186.
23. U.S. Nuclear Regulatory Commission, Radiation Safety Surveys at Medical Institutions, U.S. Nuclear Regulatory Commission, Regulatory Guide 8.23, Revision 1, January, 1981, Washington, D.C.
24. U.S. Nuclear Regulatory Commission, Acceptable Programs for Respiratory Protection, U.S. Nuclear Regulatory Commission Regulatory Guide 8.15, October 1976, Washington, D.C.
25. **McConnon, D.,** A health physics program for a plutonium fuel fabrication facility, in *Health Physics Operational Monitoring,* Vol. 1, Willis, C. A. and Handloser, J. S., Ed., Gordon & Breach, New York, 1972, 89—108.
26. **Miller, K. L., Varano, L. A., and Brosey, B. H.,** A RAD Waste Compaction Program for a Medical Center, in Volume II of Proceedings, IRPA, IVth International Congress, Paris, France, April 24—30, 1977, 293—296.
27. **Bradley, F. J.,** Radioactive waste disposal, *Handbook of Radioactive Nuclides,* Wang, Y., Ed., CRC Press, Boca Raton, 1969, 781—794.
28. **Zuerner, L. V. and Kathren, R. L.,** Evaluation program for portable radiation monitoring instruments, in *Health Physics Operational Monitoring,* Vol. 2, Willis, C. A. and Handloser, J. S., Eds., Gordon & Breach, New York, 1972, 825—850.
29. **Schulte, H. F.,** Air sampling in operational monitoring, in *Health Physics Operational Monitoring,* Vol. 2., Willis, C. A. and Handloser, J. S., Eds., Gordon & Breach, New York, 1007—1027.
30. **Feldman, A.,** Factors and strategies in Selection of Instruments for radiation surveys Around Medical X-ray Installations, in Proceedings of the 9th Midyear Topical Symposium of the Health Physics Society on Operational Health Physics (Rocky Mountain Chapter, Health Physics Society, P. O. Box 3229), Boulder, Co., 1976, 151—153.
31. **Sommers, J. F.,** Sensitivity of G-M and ion chamber beta-gamma survey instruments, *Health Phys.,* 2, 775—761, 1975.
32. U.S. Nuclear Regulatory Commission, Qualifications for the Radiation Safety Officer in a Large-Scale Non-Fuel-Cycle Radionuclide Program, U.S. Nuclear Regulatory Commission Draft Regulatory Guide and Value/Impact Statement, April, 1982, Washington, D.C.
33. U.S. Nuclear Regulatory Commission, Guide for the Preparation of Applications for Medical Programs, U.S. Nuclear Regulatory Commission, Regulatory Guide 10.8, January 1979, Washington, D.C.

RADIATION EMERGENCY PLANNING AND DAMAGE CONTROL PROCEDURES

Robert G. Gallaghar

RADIATION EMERGENCY PLANNING

An emergency situation can arise from the use, storage, or transfer of radioactive material or from the misuse of equipment that can produce X-radiation or other forms of ionizing radiation. Incidents may involve the release of radioactive contamination as well as the accidental exposure of individuals to penetrating radiation. Sometimes the initial release of radioactivity in an uncontrolled manner goes undetected for long periods of time and at very low concentrations to produce "chronic" low-level contamination, as contrasted to a single episode in which a sealed radioisotope source fractures, releasing potentially serious amounts of radioactive contamination that may be inhaled, ingested, or absorbed into a person's body as well as spread to personal property and into the environment in an uncontrolled manner. The emergency measures that must be taken to cope effectively with these various types of situations are so broad in scope that we could not list every step that must be followed to remedy each emergency situation. Instead, we must place our confidence in the intelligence of mature, well-trained personnel who will apply their knowledge of radiological safety and use common sense to deal effectively with such emergencies. We hope that these individuals, who may be directly or indirectly involved in the management and documentation of radiation emergencies, will benefit from some of the experience we have gained over the last 30 years in the evaluation, control, and remedial action following a wide variety of emergencies involving radiation producing equipment and radioactive material.[1-5]

The best advice for protection against radiation accidents is to plan for them. The results of thorough accident investigations have invariably shown that most accidents could have been prevented had (1) the potential for that type of accident been recognized well in advance and (2) effective action been taken to eliminate the conditions that created the "ideal environment" for an unfortunate incident to have expanded into a full-scale radiation emergency.

All too frequently, we have found that *inhibited indecision* by those who are initially involved in a radiation incident is a major factor that directly affects the costs and severity of a radiation accident. There is no substitute for planning for radiation emergencies *before* an incident occurs. Planning for every conceivable adverse situation that might occur which could involve radiation can provide the best assurance that if and when a radiation incident occurs it will be controlled effectively.[6]

While planning for emergencies may have been done during the start-up of radiological operations to satisfy regulatory and licensing requirements, unfortunately, attention to updating and testing the emergency response plan often decays with a half-life that is usually inversely proportional to the magnitude of the routine use of the radiation sources. However, an audit by a qualified consultant health physicist or an experienced regulatory inspector may call attention to the need for periodic revisions of the radiation emergency procedures. Appendix A contains a suggested check list to be used in conducting an audit of an organization's radiation accident preparedness. The actual testing of the radiation emergency plans with an experienced person acting as an independent observer can produce a number of valuable recommendations and alternative plans for effective identification and control of emergencies involving radiation. An emergency plan should be documented, reviewed, and tested at least once a year.[7]

ORGANIZATION AND AUTHORITY TO CONTROL AN EMERGENCY

It is important that the administrative chain of command and channels of communication clearly authorize specific individuals to act *promptly* and *effectively* in the event of an incident that may involve radiation. The value of a concisely written policy statement that documents top management's concern for radiation safety is vital to the implementation of the practices and procedures that govern routine and *especially emergency* operations.[8,9] The responsibility for controlling radiation and complying with applicable regulations usually is delegated by top management to a specific individual who will be designated as ''Radiation Safety Officer'' (RSO). This person will be named in all applications to federal and state regulatory agencies for licenses, registrations, permits, etc., and should not be replaced by someone else without prior approval by the licensing agency. Rarely does an organization's Chief Executive Officer (CEO) realize the importance of selecting and providing the essential training and support for the individual appointed as RSO; nor does the appointee recognize the magnitude of the task of serving as RSO, which is usually assigned in addition to other full time duties. It is *essential* that the RSO have both the responsibility and the *authority* to control routine and emergency situations involving all aspects of radiological safety. The CEO cannot delegate or otherwise avoid direct *accountability* for effective control over licensed operations involving radiation.

It may seem trite to point out that in the event of a radiation emergency, *one* person must be clearly in charge of incident investigation and control. Presumably this will be the RSO; and hopefully there will be no doubt as to the RSO's authority to bring a radiation emergency situation under control even though the assignment as RSO probably is an additional responsibility to other duties. The actions taken to investigate, control, and document radiation incidents must be consistent with and indeed should be tangible evidence of the implementation of top management's policy to assure that all radiation risks will be controlled to *a*s *l*ow *a*s *r*easonably *a*chievable (ALARA).[10]

Responsibility

It is the responsibility of each manager to see that all personnel, including the RSO, have practical and well-understood plans that can be effective in controlling a radiation emergency. Regulations[11-13] specifically require that workers be instructed in all routine and emergency situations that may affect their health and safety. The legal liability of these ''Right to Know Acts'' may pose some significant and potentially devastating aspects when viewed as possible employers' negligence in the event of serious radiation accidents. The following (10 CFR 19.12) ''Instructions to Workers'' has been included with italics added to emphasize this essential aspect for controlling routine and emergency situations involving radiation:

> 19.12 INSTRUCTIONS TO WORKERS
>
> *All individuals* working in or frequenting any portion of a restricted area shall be *kept informed* of the storage, transfer, or use of radioactive materials or of radiation in such portions of the restricted area; *shall be instructed in the health protection problems associated with exposure to such radioactive materials or radiation, in precautions or procedures to minimize exposure,* and in the purposes and functions of protective devices employed; shall be instructed in, and instructed to observe, to the extent within the worker's control, the applicable provisions of Commission regulations and licenses for the protection of personnel from exposures to radiation or radioactive materials occurring in such areas; *shall be instructed of their responsibility to report promptly to the licensee any condition which may lead to* or cause a violation of commission regulations and licenses or *unnecessary exposure to radiation or to radioactive material;* shall be *instructed in the appropriate response to warnings made in the event of any unusual occurrence or malfunction that may involve exposure to radiation or radioactive material;* and shall be advised as to the radiation exposure reports which workers may request pursuant to 19.13. The extent of these instruction shall be commensurate with potential radiological health protection problems in the restricted area.[11]

The RSO has the responsibility to see that each radiation worker knows how to:

a. Recognize a radiation emergency situation
b. Prevent or confine the radiation accident
c. Exclude all personnel from possible risk of exposure
d. Immediately contact his supervisor and/or the RSO for assistance

Precautions must be taken, when evaluating the emergency, to minimize the potential hazards to individuals near the accident scene and to personnel performing the recovery or corrective measures.

Employee Orientation

"Think before you act!" is the most important order to give personnel in attempting to cope with a radiation accident. There have been numerous instances of a minor radiation incident becoming a major accident through misguided and impulsive actions. Indecision by supervisors and lack of initiative to promptly investigate and to control a suspected radiation risk is a major cause of additional losses following a radiation mishap. Unfortunately, to every list of causes of severe radiation accidents, such as equipment failure, human error, etc., must be added *"lack of emergency planning and training of personnel"*. Emergency planning is an essential item included in the initial application for a license to use any radioactive material and usually considered by regulatory officials when licensing other radiation sources. It is an important part of any Operating Procedures Manual and must be included in the initial, periodic, and on-the-job training that each radiation worker and his supervisor receives. However, the development implementation of any practical emergency plan should not be the sole responsibility of the RSO, but must also involve the help of all supervisors of radiological operations and other personnel who may be involved in the control of emergency situations such as fire, explosion, etc. These individuals should be asked to answer the following questions:

1. What can go wrong that might directly or indirectly create a radiation risk?
2. What action must be taken to avoid injury and unnecessary radiation exposures?
3. What can be done to eliminate or at least reduce the potential risks of a radiation accident?
4. In the event of an emergency, who must be called for help?

The orientation and training of employees, contractors, etc. will be a continuing task for the RSO and certain supervisors, the efficacy of which should be tested by the use of periodic radiation emergency drills. These exercises should be critiqued by an independent health physicist who is experienced in the management of radiation emergencies.

Orientation Information for Fire and Police Officials

It is difficult for fire and police officials to accurately evaluate the magnitude of a radiation risk at the time of an emergency without having had prior information about the user's operations, location of radiation sources, and the potential risks that may be involved during a fire emergency.[14] It is suggested that the RSO should invite local fire and police officers to attend an informal meeting and tour of all areas where radioactive materials are used or stored. The RSO and supervisors of the radiological operations should develop a form similar to Appendix B to document specific information that was given to these officials during the orientation session. Depending upon the magnitude of radiological operations, these visits and orientation sessions should be repeated every few years and soon after any significant changes in location or use of licensed materials have been made.

Supervisory personnel must have specific information available at home and at the office that will enable them to respond to an emergency situation effectively. Often their initial contact and coordination will be via telephone, and they will need to have an up-to-date list of emergency telephone numbers, current personnel roster with home telephone numbers, and some guidance as to the role they must play in any emergency. The following section is designed to provide practical information for the RSO and supervisors of radiation operations to use when they receive the first notification of an incident involving radiation.

NOTIFICATION, DOCUMENTATION, AND REPORTING OF RADIATION ACCIDENTS

It is the responsibility of the RSO to take whatever measures are necessary to cope with a radiation emergency, and to report the incident to his management and to regulatory authorities immediately or as soon as possible after the situation has been remedied, depending on the seriousness of the emergency. Any accident or abnormality in the operation of a device that can produce radiation or that contains radioactivity must be reported, so that the necessary corrective action can be taken by the manufacturer and by the regulatory agencies. Loss or theft of licensed devices, major spills, and some typical types of accident situations will be discussed briefly to illustrate the types of problems that can be expected, to suggest certain emergency control methods and sources of assistance to achieve effective control, and provide required notification and documentation.

During the first hectic hours following discovery of a radiation emergency, a steady stream of information must be sifted as efficiently as possible from those directly involved in the incident, from personal witnesses who may have different viewpoints (possibly involving guesses and personal emotions), and from health physicists' or radiation surveyors' measurements and observations. Based upon as many facts as can be established, evaluations must be made as to the magnitude of the accident, and certain decisions made to prevent further damage and to initiate remedial action. This is not a time conducive to documentations or scholarly reporting of information. Yet it is this period, immediately after the discovery of a radiation emergency, that certain documentation is vitally needed as a basis for specific reports which must be made to official regulatory agencies, top management, insurance carriers, and possibly to the news media.

The opportunity to obtain valid documentation of certain facts concerning an incident fades rapidly with time. The ability to recollect specific details about an accident suffers from the frailties of the human mind. Unfortunately, the tasks of notifying top management and official agencies and filling out required accident reports usually falls upon certain safety and management personnel at a time of maximum stress, when they can least afford the difficulty of extracting accurate data from feeble recollections. Furthermore, it is highly probable that top management may not be familiar with specific regulatory requirements on reporting of radiation emergencies and may be very reluctant to release any information until all aspects are known and some authorization has been given by the CEO or his designated assistant. Considerable savings in time, money, and reputations can be achieved by establishing emergency plans that specify personnel who will be responsible for obtaining data and complying with incident-reporting procedures by the use of some of the methods outlined below.

Initial Accident Notification

Invariably, the first notification of a radiation accident and the calls for help will be made by telephone. Hopefully, these calls will be made by someone who has received prior instructions concerning whom to notify and what information must be given. It is impossible in an emergency to expect an individual to remember and adhere to more than a few very simple rules. Thus, as a guide for reporting fires, accidents, and injuries, the use of a simple emergency notification procedure, similar to the one shown in Appendix C, is suggested. The procedure should be printed on brightly colored paper (e.g., pink or yellow) and posted in strategic areas, naturally, near a telephone. This form contains a few essential facts that have been reviewed and approved by several major municipal fire departments, physicians, and insurance carriers. Copies of this form are available from the author.

The person receiving an initial report of an accident involving radiation must be able to obtain essential information in order to evaluate the magnitude of the accident and institute remedial action, as well as to report the episode as required by specific regulations. To obtain these facts, the use of a form similar to that shown in Appendix D is recommended. This form contains a list of questions that have been found to be helpful in establishing the urgency of the situation and in determining the most effective methods of bringing the situation under control.

The use of a portable tape recorder or the aid of shorthand transcription to obtain a verbatim record of telephone and radio messages can be invaluable. An inexpensive battery-operated tape recorder can be used for this purpose. However, it is important to make certain that the electronic pick-up of the telephone or radio voice will be as clearly recorded as possible and that an adequate supply of blank tapes, batteries, etc. are available and used. When recording radiation emergency communiques, it is essential to indicate the time, date, and identity of the speakers; in some instances the location and origin of the call may also be useful. Care must be taken to identify the date and contents of tape cassettes containing recordings of important events, so that these tape cassettes can easily be used in the future without being lost or accidentally erased. Duplicate tapes can be made for use by investigators, but the original tapes should be placed in a vault or other secure location.

HAZARD EVALUATION AND REQUESTS FOR ASSISTANCE

Following the receipt of an initial report of radiation incident, certain key management personnel will review the information obtained in response to questions listed in Part A of Appendix D. These persons need to refer to recordings or transcriptions of the incoming emergency communiques that provide the facts on which to base a preliminary evaluation of the accident. Part B of Appendix D contains a list of some of the questions that must be answered as part of this hazard evaluation. Obviously, management's primary objective is to bring the emergency under control as effectively as possible, and then to institute remedial action so that routine operations can be resumed without delay. Radiological risks to individuals and potential costs of the accident will be primary considerations.

The severity of a radiation accident should never be underestimated. Avoid procrastination and inhibited indecision. More errors have occurred from inhibited indecision than from poor decisions!

Immediate action is taken to obtain outside help, such as fire, medical, police, and radiological assistance, if such is needed. An effective communications system is a prime necessity during this phase when efforts are being made to control the accident.

Effective communications systems should have been established within the organization prior to the accident, augmented by the necessary telephone, public-address, and radio equipment, to permit an uninterrupted flow of information to a communication center for interpretation, and for the issuance of instructions for radiation-risk control. An unlisted telephone number can be extremely valuable for such use. Access and knowledge of this unlisted telephone number should be carefully restricted to assure that this line will not be used except for the most essential purposes. All personnel should clearly understand and observe instructions concerning communications relative to the accident. All information should be channeled to one or two key personnel, and released, especially to outsiders, through one designated official. Warning: the use of radio communications can divulge information to outsiders, thus extreme caution must be exercised to maintain effective control over what information is sent by radio.

Certain officials, key employees, consultants, and trusted associates will be contacted in order to assist the organization to recover from the accident as safely, quickly, and economically as possible. Top management must be informed, along with the organization's legal counsel, physician, and health physics consultant. Each will be required to perform his or her services as needed in order to aid in recovery from the accident, and to coordinate and document such work with a responsible official with the organization. Insurance carriers must be notified relative to possible claims under existing workers' compensation, public liability, and physical damage coverage.

REPORTING OF RADIATION ACCIDENTS

Every organization has a policy according to which good or bad news concerning that organization is released to its own officials and to outside firms, official agencies, and eventually to the public. Unfortunately, many organizations fail to realize that they can have a radiation accident and may not be prepared administratively, technically, or financially to cope with such a situation; top management may not have recognized the need for an official of the organization to become aware of the legal responsibility for reporting a radiation accident within a prescribed period of time to certain official agencies, as required by law. One responsible individual within the organization must be clearly designated and briefed as to whom he is to notify, when, where, and how such reports must be transmitted, and what should be reported.

Naturally, a radiation accident is not the type of occurrence that an organization would want anyone to know about. In fact, it may be of interest to note that in our work on radiation accidents we have detected two, and possibly three cases of what psychologists refer to as "subconscious denial" on the part of the radiation workers that a radiation accident had occurred; that is, an individual refused to accept the fact that he had received a potentially serious exposure.

However, top management must make clear to each radiation worker that failure to notify certain designated personnel (e.g., an RSO or a corporate official) of an accident involving radioactive materials or radiation-producing equipment can be reason for dismissal. Furthermore, all radiation workers must be made aware of the responsibilities as specified by federal regulations[10-12] and other appropriate state and local regulations relative to their assigned duties, which involve radiation safety and the preparation of radiation reports. Usually these responsibilities are clearly defined in the operating procedures manual, and therefore the worker involved in a radiation accident should have received prior instructions as contained in the operating procedures manual, augmented by instructions on radiation emergencies.[11,13] He should know what to do to protect himself and his fellow workers in the event of an emergency, and whom to notify by using the procedure shown in Appendix C. The periodic use of the check list (Appendix A) will facilitate understanding and adherence to the emergency plan.

Notification of Regulatory Agencies

Certain regulations[10] require that official agencies be notified within periods ranging from immediately after discovery, in the case of the most severe accident, to 30 days following discovery of a minor accident.

The seriousness of the emergency will determine what notification requirements will be followed. Included as Appendix E are the Notification Requirements as specified in US-NRC Regulations Title 10, Code of Federal Regulations, Part 20. Immediately after evaluating the seriousness of the emergency, the RSO will report by telephone to his management any incident that caused, or threatened to cause, an emergency such as those listed in Appendix D.

Without delay, the company official whose name appears on the NRC or Agreement State license, or the designated representative of top management, should aid the RSO in determining the seriousness of the emergency. They should then notify the proper agencies by

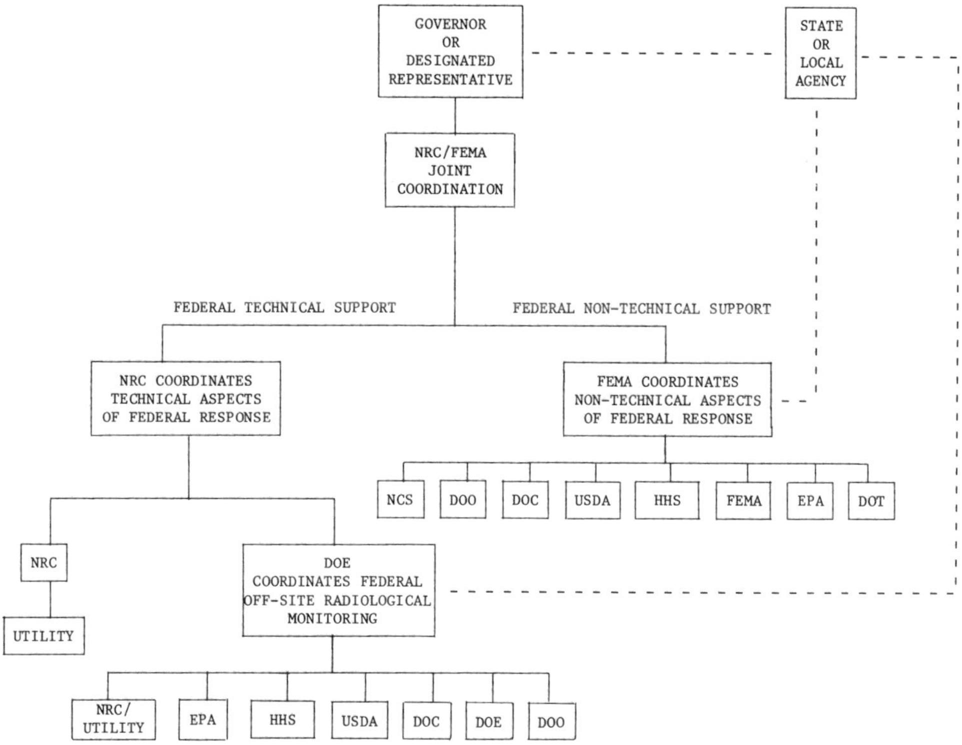

FIGURE 1. Federal response management diagram.

telephone and telegraph of the conditions that exist and of the corrective steps that will be followed. Final analysis of the episode will be made by the RSO, who will report the facts in writing to the proper agencies, such as the NRC or State Health Department, within 30 days, as prescribed by regulations.

Procedures to be followed when reporting radiation incidents are summarized in Appendix F. The locations and telephone numbers to be called are listed in appendix G for US-NRC licensees; Appendix H contains suggested state officials and their office and off-duty telephone numbers to be used to report emergencies involving Agreement State licensees and/or registered equipment and to request additional information, advice, or assistance. These regulatory agencies can provide valuable help, especially in the use of experienced personnel who are familiar with practical methods of coping with local authorities, news media, and the public. They will also evaluate the need to call upon the unique resources available from the Radiological Assistance Program (RAP) of the U.S. Department of Energy (see Appendix I).

RAP was originally established to provide emergency advice and assistance from the resources possessed by the national laboratories, Pittsburgh and Schenectady Naval Reactor Offices, Environmental Measurements Lab in New York City, the University of Rochester, and certain Department of Energy offices.[15] Currently, RAP supplies "back-up" personnel, sophisticated instrumentation, and emergency response capabilities to federal, state and/or local radiological health authorities as requested. In the event of a major nuclear accident, e.g., one involving a commercial nuclear power plant, they would coordinate off-site monitoring as described in the Federal Emergency Management Agency's (FEMA) National Radiological Emergency Preparedness/Response Plan as shown in Figure 1.[16,17]

It is important to note that there may be several official agencies (e.g., U.S. Nuclear Regulatory Commission, Occupational Safety and Health Administration (OSHA) of the

U.S. Labor Department, State and/or local radiation regulatory agencies) that must be notified in accordance with their specific regulations.[10,12] The content of such notification should state the facts as briefly and concisely as possible. If possible, mention of the names of individuals involved in the incident should be avoided. Since such notification can become a public record open to use by the news media, care should be taken in its preparation in order to comply with the existing regulations, yet not produce a severe public relations problem. Naturally, copies of any notification are a vital form of documentation and should be carefully kept as a permanent record.

Preparation and Releases to News Media

Obviously, the occurrence of a radiation accident will soon become known to a substantial number of people. Employees and their families may become concerned, and soon rumors may exaggerate the magnitude of the radiation risks. This is why the preparation and issuance of a concise factual statement in writing concerning the accident is recommended, and why one responsible individual should be officially designated to release all information concerning a radiation incident or accident. In fact, the NRC, as well as other regulatory agencies, have made it a practice to request the licensee to prepare a written press release, otherwise their public information officer will draft one for possible release to the news media. It has been our experience in the investigation and management of radiation emergencies that a short, concise, factual release is less likely to create headlines than the ill-advised practice of ''stonewalling'' or refusing to release any information. The employees and news media should be told what has happened, that steps are being taken by competent specialists to control any radiation risk, and that additional information will be released by the authorized spokesperson for the organization as it becomes available. All requests for information also should be directed to the individual designated to issue such information. All personnel involved in the investigation, control, and remedial action following an accident must be made to understand that *all* information concerning the incident will be released only by the designated spokesperson.

ACCIDENT INVESTIGATION AND DOCUMENTATION

One of the most significant facts that should be established concerning a radiation accident is the length of time that has elapsed since the accident occurred, especially if the accident involves the release of unsealed radioactive materials, a number of people, or personnel other than employees (e.g., public, personal property, subcontractor, or client personnel). The identity of such personnel and the description and location of property or equipment potentially involved in the accident must be obtained promptly. Appropriate action must be taken to evaluate and control any radiological risks and to avoid adverse public reactions resulting from the emergency. It has been found that the duration of time between the occurrence and the beginning of organized efforts to control the radiation emergency and abate undue alarm has a profound effect upon the total cost of the episode and its impact on reputations.

There is no substitute for qualified personnel experienced in the health physics and medical aspects of radiation emergencies.[18] Such personnel must be technically competent and certified by appropriate professional boards, so that their work and reports will satisfy future medicolegal requirements. Furthermore, they must be able to assume the technical responsibility and possible financial risks associated with the professional services offered. Prompt notification of such personnel by telephone can bring advice on the method for controlling the emergency, and assistance on some of the postemergency problems (e.g., public relations, insurance, regulations, and medicolegal aspects), through methods and contacts established and proven effective on prior radiation emergencies.

The initial phase of the radiation emergency has passed when effective action has been taken to control the emergency by quarantining the source of the radiation hazard along with all potentially affected areas and equipment. As a part of this procedure, prompt and effective medical attention must be obtained. References 19 and 20 contain information and advice that can be of considerable help to the physician.

Simultaneously with the detection and notification of the incident, radiological-safety surveys are made to determine the magnitude of the radiation risks. Essential health physics data must be gathered and interpreted. References 5,6,18,19,20, and 21 provide useful information for obtaining and utilizing such data.

Health Physics Data, Results of Radiation Surveys, and Medical Reports

Health physics data, results of radiation surveys, and medical reports on personnel involved in a radiation incident are essential forms of documentation. However, in a number of accidents the long-term value of these data has been overlooked in the process of concentrating upon the immediate use of the information to evaluate the situation and to restore the installation to normal operations quickly. Technical personnel who provide such data (1) will provide valid and pertinent information several years hence, (2) can easily be related to the episode and the individuals involved in the analysis and interpretation of the data, and (3) will be retained, identified, and easily accessible for review in the future.

At the present time we are without universally accepted standards for the preparation of health physics records. To completely describe and discuss the documentation of medical and health physics data is beyond the scope of this chapter. However, a few important items, which are the result of experience gained during the management of several radiation emergencies and during subsequent litigation, will be included.

Personnel Monitoring Data and Bioassay Results

Personnel monitoring data and bioassay results can be of much greater value if some additional facts concerning their use during and subsequent to a radiation emergency are documented.[22] For example, immediately following the discovery of an accident, personnel involved in the episode submit their film badges, thermoluminescent dosimeters (TLDs) or other types of dosimeters for processing. Film badges and TLDs must be processed without delay, especially if a self-reading dosimeter has gone ''off scale''. Some of the important facts that must be added to the reports of the personnel-monitoring results are:

1. The location of the body where the dosimeter and/or film badge was worn at the time of the accident
2. Time and date when these devices were first issued and dosimeters zeroed
3. The location of the individual during the accident and the route by which he or she left the accident scene
4. The time and date when the personnel monitoring equipment was turned in
5. The names of those who received and processed it

The circumstances under which the personnel monitoring devices were exposed should be documented by the use of a form letter similar to that shown in Appendix J.

It is just as important to document the fact that no radiation risks were present as it is to determine accurately the magnitude of such risks whenever and wherever they exist. This is especially true in the case of a radiation emergency involving potential exposure of personnel who are not employees of the licensed radiation user, or who are not considered radiation workers, but may have been in the area at the time of the accident.

Sometimes samples of clothing, metal buttons, jewelry, hair, or tissue may be collected for analyses, as in the case of neutron exposure. The location on the individual's body and his position relative to the source of exposure are essential pieces of information which must be adequately documented. The same applies to bioassay samples (e.g., urine, blood, breath, excised tissue, etc.).

The result of radiological analyses of samples of air, water, surface smears, etc., must be transmitted without delay to the health physicist. It becomes his responsibility to receive, plot, interpret, and utilize these data to control radiation risks. His responsibility for risk control does not end there; he must consider future interpretations, reviews, and possible litigation, which may necessitate the use of such data as evidence to establish, possibly years later in a court of law, certain facts concerning the accident. It would be desirable for such data to be reviewed by an individual experienced in the possible insurance and legal use of such documents before they are filed away following the radiation accident.

Eyewitness Accounts

Eyewitness accounts of a radiation accident provide essential documentation that can be extremely valuable, especially if they are obtained shortly after the incident, when facts are fresh in the person's mind. One of the best times to obtain such information is immediately after the required health physics and medical procedures have been completed and the individual has had a chance to regain his composure. Written statements should be obtained from any individual potentially exposed as a result of the radiation accident, or who claims to have been affected by it, as well as from those persons who may have pertinent information concerning the accident. These statements can be in the form of tape recordings or handwritten narrative reports of what the individual saw, did, or saw others doing, and where or when certain events relative to the accident took place. Such an individual should also describe how and why he believes the accident occurred. It is imperative that all those involved in the preparation of incident reports clearly understand that these statements and reports are not for the purpose of placing the blame but are purely to aid in gathering facts that can enable more accurate assessment of the risks and development of effective plans to prevent recurrences of such an incident. These accounts should not be prepared as a cooperative or "team" effort, nor should they be written under the "helpful" eye of a supervisor. They need not be in scholarly prose, but should be clear and accurate accounts in the individual's own words. Each should be signed and dated by the individual. Again, a tape recording of this report, which is later typed, signed by the individual, and dated, may be used. It is recommended that reports of this type be witnessed or notarized.

When such statements are reviewed by an experienced investigator, they sometimes produce clues that may be extremely important in reconstructing pertinent facts at the time of the accident and in determining its cause and practical methods of avoiding recurrences. Such statements have uncovered other undetected or unreported accidents that had occurred in the past. For example, in investigating the statement made by a radiographer during one radiographic accident, we learned about two others involving the same piece of equipment, but of lesser severity.

Videotape and Photographic Reenactments

Photographic and videotaped reenactments of the radiation accident are invaluable in establishing the location and identity of the individuals with respect to the radiation source. Eyewitness accounts are used to reconstruct the scene. A nonradioactive "dummy" radioisotope source is set up to duplicate the actual conditions during the radiation accident. Either the individuals involved in the incident or substitutes are asked to attempt to duplicate as closely as possible the actions that took place. We have used at least one motion picture camera, and sometimes several, as well as still cameras, to photograph such reenactments. Recent use of video equipment at the scene has convinced us that modern portable color video equipment is far more useful than motion pictures.

We have found it valuable to have a narrative account of the reenactment recorded on the video tape. The tapes also contain periodic time checks along with announcements of the running times; that is, while the narrator describes the actions being filmed, a timekeeper can be heard in the background counting off the seconds that have elapsed during each important phase of the reenactment. Thus, when the video recording is played back along with the movie or matched with sequence photographs, determinations can be made relative to the approximate times and distances where personnel may have received significant radiation exposures. Another very valuable technique is to include in the background of the picture at least one large electric clock that has been synchronized to start at an appropriate time during the reenactment in order to document the running time of the various stages of the reenactment.

Documentary photographs should also be taken of the equipment present in the incident. It is our practice to use a shielded periscope for photographing a source involved in a radiation accident. In some cases such photographs reveal wear or defects in the source or in the equipment. Radiation injuries should be photographed in color and properly labeled as to date and identity of the individual. The documentary, video tapes and photographs, together with the statements by personnel involved in the accident, enable the health physicist to reconstruct the scene for the purpose of obtaining radiation dosimetry data. Polaroid photographs can be very helpful during the dosimetry experiments as well as during the reenactment.

CONTROL OF RADIATION ACCIDENTS

The time to think about what to do about the control of a radiation accident is before it occurs. Take the time now to consider the following list of common radiation emergency situations and start to review and reconsider how to handle those types of emergencies that might require your assistance.

1. Loss or theft of radioisotope source or misuse of radiation producing equipment
2. Malfunction of radiation-producing equipment, radiation instruments, or services (e.g. warning lights, etc.)
3. Fire, flood, sprinkler deluge, other nonradiation catastrophe that may result in releasing radioactive contamination
4. Highway accident involving radioactive material
5. Accidents involving possible overexposure of personnel
6. Unauthorized or accidental entry into a radiation area

Some specific guidance for the management of each of these types of emergency situation will be given along with valuable references that should be reviewed for more detailed information.

Loss or Theft of Radioactive or X-Ray Equipment

Loss or theft of licensed radiation equipment or radioactive material requires that certain specific action must be taken without delay as soon as the loss or theft of a registered radiation device (e.g. portable or mobile X-ray unit) or a licensed source containing radioactive material becomes known to the owner or the RSO. If it appears likely that a substantial hazard may result to persons in unrestricted areas, the loss or theft of radioactive materials licensed by the U.S. NRC must be reported by telephone immediately to the nearest NRC Regional Office (see Appendix G). Prompt notification of the nearest state and local radiation control program director (Appendix H) is not only a requirement but can also bring valuable assistance and coordination of police, public health, and other services.

The RSO will also question personnel at the job location when the incident occurs and will advise local authorities of the nature of the hazards that may exist and aid them in recovery. The RSO must evaluate all facts reported to him, and attempt to locate the radioisotope equipment with the aid of a survey meter if at all feasible.

Fires, Explosions, or Major Emergencies

1. Notify all other persons in the area to leave at once.
2. Notify the fire department and other local plant safety personnel as well as the RSO. Give them the address of the location of the fire.
3. Upon their arrival, caution firemen where radioactive materials are stored or where radioisotopes were being used; give them the present location of the radioactive material, and advise them of the best entrance route to the radiation area and any precautions to avoid exposure or risk of creating radioactive contamination by use of high pressure water, etc.
4. Do not permit firemen to enter the radiation area after fire has been extinguished, until a thorough examination can evaluate the extent of the damage to the radioactive material.
5. Perform a thorough radiation survey of firemen and their equipment before they leave the controlled area. Decontaminate if necessary.

Minor Fires

1. Attempt to put out fires by approved means if fire safety or radiation hazards are not immediately present.
2. Govern fire fighting or other emergency acivities by the restrictions of the RSO. Avoid, if possible, the tracking of contamination or passing of contaminated equipment into clean areas by emergency workers.
3. Monitor all persons involved in combating the emergency.
4. Following the emergency, monitor the area, and determine the protective devices necessary for safe decontamination.
5. Decontaminate; follow a plan.
6. Permit no person to return to work without the approval of the RSO.
7. Prepare a complete history of the emergency and subsequent activity related thereto for the RSO.

Accidents Involving Possible External Radiation Overexposure

If radiation exposure has occurred, or is suspected to have occurred, proceed as follows:

1. Remove personnel involved from radiological operations immediately.
2. Have exposed individuals examined as soon as possible by a physician/radiologist.
3. Obtain and record all details of the incident.
4. Send TLDs or film badge to supplier for immediate processing. Complete preliminary report indicating type and energy of radiation in quadruplicate; and send two (2) copies with badge(s), one (1) to your consultant, and keep one (1) on file.
5. Have the person or persons complete a statement of facts on how exposure occurred and send it to the RSO.
6. Upon receipt of all facts and exposure results, the medical and health physics consultants and the RSO will determine what action must be taken before the person or persons can return to operations involving radiation.

Emergency Procedures for Incidents Involving Teletherapy Equipment

The emergency procedures to be used in case of shutter malfunction of a teletherapy unit depend on the individual installation. The following is an example.

If the warning signals indicate that the beam-control system has failed to terminate irradiation at the preset time, the following steps are to be carried out in a calm manner.

1. Turn off the main switch at the control (unless this interferes with the removal of the patient).
2. Open the door to the treatment room.
3. If the patient is ambulatory, direct him to leave the room. If the patient is not ambulatory, enter treatment room, avoiding exposure to the direct beam as much as possible, and try to close the manual emergency beam control; if not immediately successful, remove the patient from the treatment room.
4. Close and lock the door.
5. Notify the RSO.
6. No attempt to repair equipment should be made by inexperienced persons.
7. Repairs should be made only by experienced technicians under the control and/or supervision of the RSO.

Accidental Damage of Radiological Equipment

The RSO will determine the extent of the damage and analyze the recovery plan to repair damaged equipment. If it is obvious that the damaged equipment can be repaired without any risk to personnel, repair the equipment. A report must be prepared in writing. Note: Under no conditions can any repair be made to the encapsulated radioisotope source or actual housing, only to the accessories (e.g., cables, tubes, etc.).

Remember that the restricted area must be posted and kept under constant surveillance until the condition is remedied. The damaged device may be in such condition that special equipment may have to be constructed in order to retrieve the source safely.

Any radiological equipment or device must be thoroughly tested by the RSO and an authorized manufacturer's technical serviceperson before it is allowed to be used again following involvement in a fire, explosion, flood, collision, etc.

Malfunction of Equipment

X-ray equipment or devices containing licensed radioactive materials must be securely locked in a safe position and made inoperative as soon as they are believed to be defective. Only a licensed individual is authorized to repair defective radiation equipment. However, in an emergency, the RSO and/or the authorized user of the device can take such action as to retrieve the radioisotope source or to shield the gauge or deactivate the X-ray equipment. The person responsible for the use of the radiation device must restrict access to the radiation areas and equipment until the RSO arrives. The RSO must have and use one of at least two portable survey meters and immediately complete a detailed report in writing. The RSO will evaluate the incident thoroughly and will notify the NRC within 30 days, giving them details of the accident, provided it falls within their classification of a reportable accident.

Accidents Involving a "Free" Source (Open-Air Radiography Technique)

1. Check dosimeter pencil.
2. Using survey meter, locate source.
3. Develop a recovery plan.
4. Calculate exposure for approximate recovery time before attempting to make recovery.
5. Using remote-handling rod or improvised handling device (magnet on a pole, chewing gum on a stick, etc.), pick up source with rod and secure in exposure device.
6. Check dosimeter pencil.

Note: Free sources may contain as much as 1 Ci of ^{60}CO; radiation intensities will be quite high; the dosimeter pencil must be read frequently and carefully and personnel exposure limits must be watched.

7. If recovery cannot be made by the above method, then more consideration must be given to the emergency; a recovery plan must be developed, which must be approved by the RSO. Many complications may hinder safe recovery, but take the time to ensure safety.
8. If assistance is needed, the RSO will notify proper authorities. *Do not minimize the seriousness of the incident.* All facts must be considered for the maximum when evaluating the accident.

Highway or Railroad Accident Involving Radioactive Materials

Situations arising from this type of accident could vary tremendously, depending on the seriousness of the accident. However, maximum security must be maintained around the vehicle, and all bystanders must be excluded until the situation can be fully evaluated. Top priority must always be given to care of injured and to saving of human life.

The Materials Transportation Bureau of the U.S. Department of Transportation has prepared an excellent Hazardous Materials —1980 Emergency Response Guidebook (See Reference 23) for use by firefighters, police, and other emergency services as a guide for initial actions to be taken to protect themselves and the public when they respond to incidents involving all types of hazardous materials, including radioactive. Six guides (Potential Hazards Guides 61 to 66) provide radiological information on health hazards, fire or explosion, emergency action, firefighting, spill or leak, and first aid. Copies of this guidebook should be obtained and be kept accessible for immediate use in emergency service vehicles (fire, police, first aid, civil defense).

Immediate advice to emergency response officials can be obtained from the Chemical Transportation Emergency Center (CHEMTREC), a public service of the Chemical Manufacturers Association in Washington, D.C. CHEMTREC provides immediate advice for those at the scene of an emergency, then promptly contacts the shipper of the radioactive or other hazardous materials involved in the accident to obtain more detailed assistance and for necessary follow-up.

CHEMTREC operates a ''Hot-line'' 24 hr a day through a toll free, telephone service (WATS) number. In an emergency, dial 1-800-424-9300 (for calls outside the Continental U.S. call collect, Area Code 202-483-7616. Be prepared to provide as much of the following information as possible:

1. Name of caller and your call back number
2. Nature and location of the problem
3. Guide number (e.g. Guide 61 to 66 for radioactive materials)
4. Shipper or manufacturer*
5. Container type*
6. Hazardous material label or marking*
7. Rail car or truck number*
8. Placard on vehicle*
9. Carrier name*
10. Consignee*
11. Local Codition

Incidents involving shipments of hazardous material frequently occur at inconvenient locations making communication and coordination of emergency response efforts difficult. It is important that every effort should be made to keep a telephone line open so CHEMTREC

* This information can be found on the hazardous waste manifest and/or shipping papers. These documents must be in the cab of the motor vehicle, in the possession of a train crew member, in a holder on the bridge of a vessel, or in an aircraft pilot's possession.

or the shipper can make contact with the on-scene emergency response team leader to provide guidance and assitance.

If a vehicle accident involves radioactive material and there are no fire, explosion, spills, or injuries, a restricted area must be established, as specified in the following procedure.

1. If the survey meter is operable, use it to establish the perimeter of the restricted area.
2. If the survey meter is inoperable, use calculations to establish the perimeter of the restricted area, assuming that the source is in an exposed position inside of the vehicle. In case of a minor accident, where it can be visually determined that the source is safely stored in its container, no restricted area is required.
3. If the survey meter is operable, if no radiation hazard exists, and if the vehicle is movable, continue on to destination.
4. In any case, immediately after establishing the restricted area, have a responsible person notify your supervisor.
5. The RSO shall notify the NRC (when required by 20.402 and 20.403 of 10 CRF 20).
6. If the survey meter has been damaged, and if a visual examination detects any indication of damage to the source container, the vehicle shall be isolated and arrangements shall be made to secure an operable survey instrument.

Operable survey meters are available from a number of companies, from various colleges and universities, and from State Health Departments (see Appendix H). Survey instruments can be borrowed or rented in case of an emergency by calling 412-563-2242.

Radiation warning signs must be used in accordance with NRC and state regulation.

Unauthorized or Accidental Entry to Restricted Area

Gather all the facts and report to the RSO either (1) immediately by telephone, if possible overexposure is evident, or (2) in writing within 15 days, if no overexposure is evident.

The report must contain name and address, employer, telephone number, and the social security number of the unauthorized person or persons involved, as well as the description of the radiation source, by-product material, distance, time, and portion of body that was exposed.

Procedures for Radioactive Spills

Emergencies will generally be in the nature of spills, fires, or explosions, as a result of which radioactive materials are spread around the installation. Emergency procedures adopted from NCRP Report 48 are given here as a guide. It must be recognized that these procedures are general, and any specific emergency will call for further adaptations and changes in procedure.

Major Spills, Involving Radiation Hazards to Personnel

1. Notify all persons not involved in the spills to vacate the room at once. Limit the movement of displaced persons to confine the spread of contamination until they are monitored.
2. If the spill is liquid and the hands are protected, right the container; otherwise, use long tongs.
3. If the spill is on the skin, immediately flush thoroughly and monitor.
4. If the spill is on clothing, discard outer or protective clothing at once, monitor and decontaminate.
5. Turn off fans, try to avoid creation of airborne contamination.
6. Vacate the room but take care not to track or spread contamination.
7. Notify the RSO as soon as possible.
8. Take immediate steps to decontaminate personnel involved as necessary.

9. Decontaminate the area (personnel involved in decontamination must be adequately protected). The RSO will direct the decontamination.
10. Monitor all persons involved in the spill and cleaning.
11. Collect bioassay samples as specified by the RSO and/or medical consultant.
12. Permit no person to resume work in the area without the approval of the RSO and medical consultant.
13. A complete history of the accident and subsequent activity must be submitted to the RSO.

Minor Spills, Involving No Radiation Hazard to Personnel

1. Notify all other persons in the room and area at once.
2. Survey people before they become dispersed, and change clothes as necessary.
3. Permit only the minimum number of persons necessary to deal with the spill into the area.
4. Confine the spill immediately.
   A. Liquid spills
      a. Don protective gloves
      b. Drop absorbent paper on spill.
   B. Dry spills
      a. Don protective gloves.
      b. Dampen thoroughly, taking care not to spread contamination. Water may generally be used, except where chemical reaction with the water would generate an air contaminant; oil should be used instead.
5. Decontaminate; make a plan first.
6. A complete history of the accident and subsequent remedial or protective measures must be submitted to the Radiation Safety Officer.

Accidents Involving Radioactive Dusts, Mists, Fumes, Organic Vapors, and Gases

1. Notify all other persons to vacate the room immediately.
2. Hold breath and close air vents.
3. Vacate the room. Seal off area, if possible.
4. Notify the RSO at once.
5. Ascertain that all doors giving access to the room are closed. Post conspicuous warnings or guards to prevent accidental opening of the doors.
6. Monitor all persons suspected of contamination. Proceed with decontamination of personnel as directed by the RSO.
7. Report at once to the RSO all known or suspected ingestions or inhalations of radioactive materials.
8. Collect bioassay samples as directed by medical consultant.
9. Have thorough medical exam, possibly whole body gamma count performed as recommended by medical and/or health physics consultant before permitting exposed personnel to return to radiation work.
10. Evaluate the hazard and the safety devices necessary for safe reentry.
11. Determine the cause of contamination and rectify the condition.
12. Decontaminate the area only upon the advice of the RSO.
13. Perform an air survey of the area before permitting work to be resumed.
14. Submit a complete history of the accident and subsequent activities to the RSO.

Injuries to Personnel, Involving Radiation Hazard

1. Wash minor wounds immediately under running water, spreading the edges of the gash. If at all practical collect and retain cotton sponges, fluids, etc. for analyses.

2. Report all radiation accidents involving personnel wounds, over-exposure, ingestion, inhalation) to the RSO as soon as possible.
3. Call at once a physician qualified to treat radiation injuries and to collect additional bioassay samples; perform.
4. Permit no person involved in a radiation injury to return to work without the approval of the attendant physician and the RSO.
5. Prepare a complete history of the accident and subsequent activity related thereto for the RSO.

Appendixes 11 to 14 contain "Quick Reference Information" from NCRP-Report 65 which will be very helpful in evaluating and managing persons accidentally contaminated with radioactive materials. We highly recommend that this important booklet (Reference 16) be obtained and used in radiation emergency training courses.

SUMMARY

A radiation emergency can occur wherever radioactive materials or radiation equipment are used, stored, or transported. Plans for the prompt notification and documentation of essential facts should be established as part of the radiation emergency procedure. The value of such preparedness for the possibility of a radiation accident, however remote it may seem, will provide the radiation user with protection against unnecessary risks to personnel, facilities, and reputations. The value of proper documentation of a radiation accident should not be underestimated and the legal requirements of reporting such accidents within the prescribed reporting period must not be overlooked. In the case of individuals potentially exposed as a result of an accident, it is just as important to document the absence of such exposure as it is to measure it accurately. The methods of obtaining documentation and preparation of the necessary reports are described. Certain recommendations for reducing the possible risks resulting from radiation accidents are given.

REFERENCES

1. **Saenger, E. L., Gallaghar, R. G., Anthony, D. S., and Valear, P. S.,** Emergency Measures and Precautions in Radium Accidents, American Medical Association, Vol. 149, June 28, 1952.
2. **Gallaghar, R. G.,** Firemen must be protected against radiation hazards, *Occup. Health,* Vol. 3, 1953.
3. **Gallaghar, R. G., Zavon, M. R., and Doyle, H. N.,** Radioactive contamination in a radium therapy clinic, *Public Health Reports,* Vol. 70, No. 7, 1955.
4. **Gallaghar, R. G. and Saenger, E. L.,** Radium capsules and their associated hazards, *Am. J. Roentgenol. Radium Ther. Nucl. Med.,* Vol. 77, No. 3, 1957.
5. **Gallaghar, R. G.,** Radioisotope Hazards Evaluation, The National Insurance Buyer — (July), 1961.
6. **Gallaghar, R. G.,** Emergency planning and procedures, *Handbook of Radioactive Nuclides,* Wang, Y., Ed., CRC Press, Boca Raton, 1969.
7. NCRP (1978) National Council on Radiation Protection and Measurements, Operational Radiation Safety Programs. NCRP Report No. 59 (National Council on Radiation Protection and Measurements, Washington, D.C.).
8. International Atomic Energy Agency, Symposium on the Handling of Radiation Accidents, International Atomic Energy Agency, Vienna, Austria, 1969.
9. International Atomic Energy Agency, Evaluation of Radiation Emergencies and Accidents - Selected Criteria and Data, IAEA Technical Series Report No. 152, International Atomic Energy Agency, Vienna, Austria, 1974.
10. Code of Federal Regulations, Title 10, Atomic Energy; Part 20, Standards for Protection Against Radiation, *Fed. Regist.,* 1960.
11. Code of Federal Regulations, Title 10, Atomic Energy; Part 19. Notices, Instructions and Reports to Workers; Inspections, *Fed. Regist.,* 1978.

12. Code of Federal Regulations, Title 41-CFR-Part 50-204, Safety and Health Standards for Federal Supply Contracts, The Walsh-Healy Act, *Fed. Regist.*, 1964.
13. Working Safely in Gamma Radiography — A Training Manual for Industrial Radiographers, NUREG/BR-0024, U.S. Nuclear Regulatory Commission, Washington, D.C., 1982.
14. U.S. Atomic Energy Commission and HEW, Peacetime radiation hazards in the fire service, *Basic Course Resource Manual OE-84019*, U.S. Government Printing Office, Washington, D.C., 1961.
15. **Hull, A. P.,** The U.S. Dept. of Energy (DOE). Radiological Assistance Program: Personnel, Equipment and Resources, Safety Environmental Protection Div., Brookhaven National Laboratory. Upton, N.Y. 1983.
16. Federal Emergency Management Agency, National Radiological Emergency Preparedness/Response Plan Accidents (Master Plan), FR. 45248. p. 84910-17, 1980.
17. U.S. Dept. of Energy, Radiological Assistance Plan, Parts I (1975) and Part II. (updated every 6 months by Chicago Operations Office, Brookhaven Area Office, Upton, N.Y.
18. U.S. Atomic Energy Commission Clearing House for Federal Scientific and Technical Information, Radiological Emergency Operations, (Instructor's Manual TID-24918, Student's Manual TID 24918), National Bureau of Standards, U.S. Department of Commerce, Springfield, Virginia, 1969.
19. **Saenger, E. L., Ed.,** Medical Aspects of Radiation Accidents, U.S. Government Printing Office, Washington, D.C., 1963.
20. National Council on Radiation Protection and Measurements Management of Persons Accidentally Contaminated with Radionuclides NCRP Report No. 65, National Council on Radiation Protection and Measurements, Washington, D.C., 1980.
21. **Brodsky, A. and Beard, G. V.,** A Compendium of Information for Use in Controlling Radiation Emergencies, U.S. Atomic Energy Commission, Washington, D.C., 1960.
22. American Standards Association, American Standard for Administrative Practices in Radiation Monitoring. Subcommittee N2.6. Nuclear Standards Board, New York, N.Y. 1965.
23. U.S. Department of Transportation, Emergency Response Guidebook HAZARDOUS MATERIALS, DOT P. 5800.2. Materials Transportation Bureau, Research and Special Programs Administration, U.S. Department of Transportation, Washington, D.C., 1980.

APPENDIX A
A SUGGESTED CHECK LIST ON RADIATION ACCIDENT PREPAREDNESS

The following items are some, but not necessarily all, of the essential points that should be considered when formulating an emergency plan. These items should be included in periodic evaluations of radiation users and their readiness for an emergency that, either directly or indirectly, may involve radiation. The current status of each item should be designated as "Satisfactory" (S), "Marginal" (M), or "Unsatisfactory" (U), and appropriate action should be taken to achieve the desired degree of protection.

Item	Status (S,M,U)
Management	
1. Channel of command clearly established:	_______
2. Emergency Procedures well defined, understood and accepted:	_______
3. Copy of Emergency Procedures on hand, for key management personnel to use	_______
a. at office:	_______
b. at home:	_______
4. Communication channel established and posted:	_______
a. Plan designates *who* to call and gives office and home telephone numbers:	_______
b. Plan tells *what* information must be given:	_______
c. Plan specifies a key employee as Information Officer authorized to cope with all official communications (e.g., news media) other than emergency calls:	_______
5. Incident Evaluation Plan formulated and ready:	_______
6. Damage Control Plan formulated and ready:	_______
7. Medical Assistance Plan formulated and ready:	_______
8. Incident Notification Plan formulated and ready:	_______
9. Recovery Plan formulated and ready:	_______
10. Training and practice drill tested and critiqued:	_______
Health physics; safety and security	
1. Supervisor and radiation workers familiar with emergency procedures:	_______
2. Copies of Emergency Procedures on hand at office and at home:	_______
a. Emergency limits for radiation and contamination specified:	_______
3. Emergency equipment and instrumentation on "stand-by":	_______
a. Rescue equipment available and accessible:	_______
b. Portable instruments strategically stored:	_______
c. Emergency power for vital equipment:	_______
d. Extra personnel-monitoring equipment and protective clothing on "stand-by":	_______
e. Decontamination material ready:	_______
4. Evacuation plan	_______
a. Specific re-assembly areas designated:	_______
b. Methods for accounting for all personnel:	_______
5. Channel of command clearly understood:	_______
6. Emergency communications network planned and in readiness:	_______

Item	Status (S,M,U)
7. Radiation inventory current and radiation locations well-defined:	_______
8. Radiation Risk Evaluation Plan and data sheets formulated and ready:	_______
9. Orientation on possible radiation emergencies given to	
a. Supervisors and all radiation workers:	_______
b. Medical personnel to be called upon in an emergency:	_______
c. Local fire officials:	_______
d. Local police officials:	_______
e. Local public health officials:	_______
10. In the event of an emergency (e.g., after hours), the above (Item 9, a to e) know *what* to do, *whom* to contact, and *how* to cope with the incident as it pertains to their responsibilities:	_______
11. Auxiliary personnel available to assist:	
a. Health physics:	_______
b. Medical:	_______
c. Security:	_______
d. Services (temporary power, procurement, communications):	_______
Radiation workers	
1. Simplified Radiation Emergency Plan understood:	_______
a. Radiation warnings and alarms known:	_______
b. Evacuation signal and route known:	_______
c. Reassembly points (in safe area) specified:	_______
2. Channels of command clearly understood:	_______
3. Damage Control Measures clearly stated:	_______
4. Emergency Plan practiced at least once a year:	_______
5. Each worker has received safety training relative to his radiological safety responsibilities and is familiar with the written operating procedures and regulations governing the routine and emergency conditions affecting his work:	_______
Medical services	
1. Availability of medical assistance for the type of potential injuries from this installation:	_______
a. Specific M.D.'s have reviewed potential injuries, including those which may involve radiation:	_______
b. Plans are formulated and in readiness for	_______
i. removal of injured to specific hospitals:	_______
ii. Notification of physician, emergency medical facilities:	_______
2. Specific measures are to be taken to	
a. Provide prompt and effective medical aid for injured:	_______
b. Control radiation risks to medical team:	_______
c. Furnish radiation exposure evaluation data to physicians:	_______
3. Key management and health physicists have established communication network (e.g. unlisted telephone numbers for emergency calls to hospital officials, M.D., etc.):	_______
4. Adequate health physics assistance (certified health physicist or radiation physicist) is available, should the M.D. require a consultation:	_______

APPENDIX B
ORIENTATION SESSION ON RADIATION ACCIDENT PREPAREDNESS FOR FIRE AND POLICE OFFICERS

DATE__________________________ LOCATION__________________________

NAMES OF PERSONS ATTENDING:

__________________________ __________________________TITLE
__________________________ __________________________TITLE
__________________________ __________________________TITLE
__________________________ __________________________TITLE
__________________________ __________________________TITLE

SESSION CONDUCTED BY:

__________________________ __________________________TITLE

A. DESCRIPTION OF NORMAL OPERATIONS INVOLVING RADIATION

1. Radiation is used for:__________________________
2. Types of radiation emitted:__________________________
3. Description of radiation sources:__________________________
4. Location of radiation sources:__________________________
5. Radiation usage licensed by:__________________________
6. Radiological safety under direction of:__________________________
   Name__________________________ __________________________Title
7. Radiation safety inspections made by:__________________________
8. Frequency of surveys:__________________________
9. Date of last inspection by regulatory agency:__________________________
10. Security measures maintained on radiation sources:__________________________
    ____
11. Types of radiation warnings (alarm systems, interlock systems, warning signs, etc.):

B. RADIATION HAZARD EVALUATION DURING AN EMERGENCY

1. Are the containers used to shield radioactive material fire resistant?__________
   ____
2. Are all sources shielded?__________________________
3. Are the radioisotope containers apt to be affected by fire releasing radioactive air contamination?__________________________
4. Should the firemen wear self-contained breathing apparatus?__________
5. Should the firemen practice contamination control?__________
6. Is the radioactive material itself combustible or flammable material?__________
   ____
7. Will the radioactive material be affected chemically by smoke, heat, or water?_
   ____
8. Should the firefighters use radiation instruments before entering, or not?______
   ____
9. Types and locations of radiation instruments (at site):__________
10. Are spare instruments located outside radiation areas?__________
11. Auxiliary monitoring instrumentation can be obtained from:__________
    ____

12. If personnel-monitoring instruments (dosimeters and film badges) are required, they can be obtained from:____________________

C. THE FOLLOWING PERSONNEL ARE QUALIFIED TO ADVISE FIRE AND POLICE OFFICIALS:

Name	Telephone Day	Numbers Night

APPENDIX C
EMERGENCY NOTIFICATION INSTRUCTIONS

These instructions are to be read and followed by all employees in the event of an emergency.

Immediate notification of an emergency is to be given by telephoning in numerical order:

ORGANIZATION OR INDIVIDUAL	TELEPHONE NUMBER
FIRE	
1. Fire Department (Location)________	________
2. RSO________	________(Home)
3. Other________	________

INFORMATION GIVEN BY CALLER

1. Your name
2. Company name
3. Company address
4. Location of fire
5. Entrance firemen should use
6. Caution, if radioisotopes are involved
7. Warn, if airborne contamination, to use masks

INJURY

1. Regular Physician: Dr.________	________(Office)
	________(Home)
2. Alternate Physician: Dr.________	________(Office)
	________(Home)
or Emergency room of ________Hospital	________
3. Company Official________	________

INFORMATION GIVEN BY CALLER

1. Extent of injury
2. Present condition
3. First-aid measures taken

ACCIDENTS

1. No Injuries, No Radiation	
Company Official________	________
2. Radiation Involved	
RSO________	________
3. Off-Site Accidents	

If accident occurred off-site (highway, etc.), have someone maintain security over radiation source and keep personnel away while you call "collect" the individuals named above *plus* highway patrol and/or police.

INFORMATION GIVEN BY CALLER

1. What happened?
2. When?
3. Where?
4. Who was involved?
5. What has been done to control loss?
6. Current status?
7. Where you can be reached? (telephone no., location)

NOTE ALL OTHER PERTINENT INFORMATION ON REVERSE SIDE.

APPENDIX D
RADIATION-INCIDENT EVALUATION RECORD

In the event of a radiation accident, certain essential facts must be obtained as promptly and accurately as possible. These facts are needed to estimate the magnitude of the incident, limit the extent of the damage, and institute remedial measures. Try to obtain these facts calmly; use a tape recorder, if possible. Be sure to note specific details on this sheet, including the time the information was received and the name of the person who furnished it.

A. INITIAL EVALUATION RECORD

QUESTION	RESPONSE	BY	TIME
1. What happened?	________	________	________
2. When did it occur? (time, date)	________	________	________
3. Where did it happen? (building, floor, area)	________	________	________
4. Who was involved? (names, employer)	________	________	________
5. Who was exposed or injured? (name, extent of exposure or injury)	________	________	________
6. Where are the injured or exposed now?	________	________	________
7. How much damage to facilities?	________	________	________
a. Was damage confined to company property?	________	________	________
b. What damage was done to property of others?	________	________	________
8. Is radioactive contamination a problem?	________	________	________
a. If so, how extensive is contamination? (on-site, off-site)	________	________	________
b. What is being done to control the contamination?	________	________	________
9. Who, other than I, has been notified?	________	________	________
10. Where can you be reached, if you are needed?	________	________	________

B. PRELIMINARY EVALUATION BY THE RADIATION SAFETY OFFICER

1. Is outside help (fire, police, US-NRC, State Radiological Control) required? ________
2. Is medical assistance required? ________
3. Should personnel be evacuated? ________
   a. From the incident area or building? ________
   b. From the site? ________
   c. From the locations off-site? ________
4. Has the Radiation Emergency Plan been activated? ________
   a. Was the health physics consultant notified? ________
   b. If so, is additional help required? ________
   c. Were decontamination procedures mobilized? ________
5. What is the accident classification? ________

6. Have official agencies (NRC, state) been notified as required? ____________
7. What are the immediate problems? ____________
8. What are the long-range problems? ____________
   a. Off-site? ____________
   b. On-site? ____________
9. Estimate the duration of these problems. ____________
   a. Immediate ____________
   b. Long-range ____________
10. Have the families of the injured been contacted? ____________
11. What information should be given to the employees? By whom? ____________
12. Has a newspaper release been prepared by a company official authorized to disseminate information to news media?

NOTE *ALL* PERTINENT INFORMATION HERE AND ON REVERSE SIDE

APPENDIX E
NOTIFICATION REQUIREMENTS FOR INCIDENTS OR ACCIDENTS INVOLVING RADIATION

Accident description	Accident classification					
	For NRC licensees, per 10-CFR-20			For DOE operations, per DOE manual		
	A	B	C	A	B	C
Type A: Serious Incident, Immediate Notification Required						
For NRC licensees and/or DOE contractors						
1. Loss or theft of licensed radioactive material	x			x		
2. Exposure of individual's whole body to 25 rems or more	x			x		
3. Exposure of individual's skin of whole body to 150 rems or more	x			x		
4. Exposure of individual's hands and forearms or feet and ankles to 375 rems or more	x			x		
5. Release of radioactive materials in concentrations which, if averaged over 24 hr, would exceed 5000 times the limits specified in Appendix B, Table II of Title 10-CFR-20 (see Table 19, pp. 616 to 633)	x			x		
6. Loss of one workweek or more of the operation of any facility	x			x		
7. Damage to property exceeding $100,000	x			x		
In addition to the above, the following applies *only* to DOE installations and prime contractors:						
8. Any incident involving an atomic weapon that results in injury or damage to private property				x		
9. Any notice that an individual may have received 25 rems or more in a calendar year				x		
10. Any injury or illness diagnosed by an M.D. competent in nuclear medicine as having conceivably resulted from cumulative or massive radiation exposure				x		
11. Allegations the exemployees of the NRC, DOE, or its contractors are disabled as a result of exposure to toxic materials or radiation related to atomic-energy operations				x		
12. Any injury or industrial illness of 5 or more persons in DOE operation				x		
13. Any accident or radiation exposure that creates a significant public-relations problem				x		
14. Any off-site accident that involves vehicles carrying DOE shipments of radioactive materials				x		
Type B: Reportable Accident, 24-hr Notification Required						
1. Exposure of individual's whole body to 5 rems or more		x				
2. Exposure of individual's skin of whole body to 30 rems or more		x				
3. Exposure of individual's hands and forearms or feet and ankles to 75 rems or more		x				
4. Release of radioactive materials in concentrations which, if averaged over 24 hr, would exceed 500 times the limits specified in Appendix B, Table II, Title 10-CFR-20 (see Table 19, pp. 616 to 633)		x				

Accident description	Accident classification					
	For NRC licensees, per 10-CFR-20			For DOE operations, per DOE manual		
	A	B	C	A	B	C
5. Loss of one workday or more of the operation of any facility		x				
6. Property damage exceeding $1000		X				
7. Incident may not result in any of the above, but may create serious public-relations problems		x[a]				
Type C: Minor Reportable Occurrences, Notification Required Within 30 Days						
1. Radiation exposure of any individual in excess of limits specified in Title 10-CFR-20 or in NRC license conditions			x			
2. Radiation levels or radioisotope released in unrestricted areas, which have not resulted in excessive exposures, but have been in excess of 10 times any applicable limit set forth in Title 10-CFR-20 or in the conditions specified in an NRC license			x			
3. Bodily injury, property damage, or claim connected with the possession or use of radioactive material at a facility or in the course of transportation which would pertain to an indemnity agreement between the licensee and the NRC			x			

[a] NRC does not *require* notification, but it is suggested that they be notified.

APPENDIX F
RADIATION INCIDENT REPORTING PROCEDURES

REPORTING OF INCIDENTS

Type A incidents require *immediate* reports to the U.S. Nuclear Regulatory Commission, the U.S. Department of Labor, and, in certain states, to appropriate officials in the Health Department.

Type A-1

1. Immediately telephone the Director of the appropriate Nuclear Regulatory Commission Regional Compliance Office listed in Appendix D of 10-CFR-20.
2. Confirm the telephone report with a telegram.
3. Within 30 days, the licensee must make a formal written report of the incident to the Director, Division of Compliance, U.S. Nuclear Regulatory Commission, Washington, D.C. 20545, with a copy to the U.S. Nuclear Regulatory Commission Regional Compliance Office listed in Appendix D of 10-CFR-20.
4. It is also recommended that the licensee maintain a close liaison by telephone with the nearest U.S. Nuclear Regulatory Commission Compliance Office during the first few days following discovery of the incident

Type A-2

Refer to those requiring Department of Energy contractors and Department of Energy installations to report *immediately* to the Nuclear Regulatory Commission headquarters responsible for these operations. Specific instructions are contained in the Department of Energy Appendix 0502 of the U.S. Department of Energy Operational Safety Handbook. These procedures do not apply to the average radioisotope licensee.

REPORTING OF INCIDENTS REQUIRING REPORTS WITHIN 24 HR

1. The licensee must notify the Director of the appropriate U.S. Nuclear Regulatory Commission Division of Regional Compliance Office listed in Appendix D of 10-CFR-20. Within 24 hr after learning of an accident that may have caused, or threatens to cause, those effects listed in Part B, shall report as follows.

   A. Telephone the U.S. Nuclear Regulatory Commission Director of Compliance within 24 hr and report the incident.
   B. Confirm the telephone call by telegram within 24 hr.
   C. Provide a written report of the incident within 30 days to the Director of the U.S. Nuclear Regulatory Commission Regional Compliance Office, Washington, D.C. 20545, with a copy to the appropriate Nuclear Regulatory Commission Compliance Office. This written report must describe the extent of the exposures, levels of concentrations, cause of exposure, and corrective steps taken to avoid a recurrence.

MINOR INCIDENTS

Part C of the classification outline requires reports within 30 days. A report should be sent to the Director, Division of Compliance, U.S. Nuclear Regulatory Commission, Washington, D.C. 20545, with a copy to the appropriate Nuclear Regulatory Commission Regional

Compliance Office. This report must describe the extent of the exposures, levels of concentrations, cause of exposure, and the corrective measures taken to avoid a recurrence.

REPORTING TYPE B AND TYPE C INCIDENTS

The reporting of Type B and Type C incidents by Department of Energy contractors and Department of Energy operations is specifically covered in the Department of Energy Manual, Appendix 0502, Parts II and III, and should be followed as necessary.

OTHER ACCIDENTS AND OCCURRENCES THAT MUST BE INCLUDED IN ROUTINE REPORTS BY DEPARTMENT OF ENERGY CONTRACTORS (ALSO KNOWN AS TYPE C)

1. All accidents normally reported quarterly and annually.
2. Disabling occupational injuries.
3. Property damage or loss resulting from fires or other accidental causes.
4. All motor vehicle accidents (government vehicles only).

APPENDIX G
U.S. NUCLEAR REGULATORY COMMISSION REGIONAL OFFICES

	Address	Telephone: Daytime	Telephone: Nights and holidays
REGION I, U.S.N.R.C., OFFICE OF INSPECTION AND ENFORCEMENT			
Connecticut, Delaware, District of Columbia, Maine, Maryland, Massachusetts, New Hampshire, New Jersey, New York, Pennsylvania, Rhode Island, Vermont	631 Park Avenue King of Prussia, PA 19406	215-337-5000	215-337-5000
REGION II, U.S.N.R.C., OFFICE OF INSPECTION AND ENFORCEMENT			
Alabama, Arkansas, Florida, Georgia, Kentucky, Louisiana, Mississippi, North Carolina, Panama Canal Zone, Puerto Rico, South Carolina, Tennessee, Virginia, Virgin Islands, West Virginia	Suite 3100 101 Marietta Street Atlanta, GA 30303	404-221-4503	404-221-4503
REGION III, U.S.N.R.C., OFFICE OF INSPECTION AND ENFORCEMENT			
Illinois, Indiana, Iowa, Michigan, Minnesota, Missouri, Ohio, Wisconsin	799 Roosevelt Road Glen Ellyn, IL 60137	312-932-2500	312-932-2500
REGION IV, U.S.N.R.C., OFFICE OF INSPECTION AND ENFORCEMENT			
Arkansas, Colorado, Idaho, Kansas, Louisiana, Montana, Nebraska, New Mexico, North Dakota, Oklahoma, South Dakota, Texas, Utah, Wyoming	Suite 1000 611 Ryan Plaza Drive Arlington, TX 76012	817-860-8100	817-860-8100
REGION V, U.S.N.R.C., OFFICE OF INSPECTION AND ENFORCEMENT			
Alaska, Arizona, California, Hawaii, Nevada, Oregon, Washington, U.S. territories, and possessions in the Pacific	Suite 202 1990 N. California Blvd. Walnut Creek, CA 94596	415-943-3700	415-943-3700

APPENDIX H
STATE AND LOCAL OFFICIALS RESPONSIBLE FOR RADIOLOGICAL PROGRAMS (10/82)

State	Address	Name of official	Telephone No. Work	Off-Duty
Alabama	State Dept. of Public Health State Office Building Montgomery, AL 36130	Aubrey Goodwin (Dir., Div. of Rad. Health)	(205) 832-5990	272-6540
		Kirksey Whatley (Chief Licensing)	832-5590	288-7207
	Radiological Health Service Bureau of Environmental Health Jefferson County Health Dept. 1400 6th Avenue South Birmingham, AL 35233	Kenneth Thames	933-9110 ext. 1206	871-8251
Alaska	Dept. of Health & Social Science Pouch H-01 Juneau, AK 99811	Helen Beirne, M.D.	(907) 465-3030	
	Radiological Health Program Pouch H-06F Juneau, AK 99811	Sidney Heidersdorf	465-3019	789-9858
Arizona	AZ Radiation Regulatory Agency 925 South 52nd Street Suite 2 Tempe, AZ 85281	Charles Tedford	(602) 255-4845	FTS 765-4845
Arkansas	Department of Health 4815 West Markham Street Little Rock, AR 72201	E. Frank Wilson (Dir., Div. of Environmental Health Protection)	(501) 661-2301 -2302	753-2256
		Ruth, McBurney (Chief Licensing & Compliance, Rad. Health Sect)	661-2142	847-4448
California	State Dept. of Health Services 714 P Street Sacramento, CA 95814	Joseph Ward (Chief, Rad. Health Sect)	(916) 322-2073	391-7716
	County of Los Angeles Dept. of Health Services 313 North Figueroa Street Los Angeles, CA 90012	Joseph Karbus (Dir. Occupation & Rad. Management)	(213) 974-7891	368-3292
	Orange County Public Health & Medical Services Div. of Environmental Health Radiological Health Section 1725 West 17th St., Box 355 Santa Ana, CA 92702	James Hartranft (Public H.P.)	(714) 834-6884	728-4865
Colorado	Department of Health 4210 East 11th Avenue Denver, CO 80220	A. J. Hazle (Dir. Radiation & Haz. Waste Control Div)	(303) 320-8333 ext. 6246	422-4146
Connecticut	Department of Environmental Protection State Office Building Hartford, CT 06115	Arthur T. Heubner (Dir., Rad. Control)	(203) 566-5668	521-5050

State	Address	Name of official	Telephone No. Work	Telephone No. Off-Duty
Delaware	Department of Health & Social Services Jesse S. Cooper Memorial Bldg. Capitol Square Dover, DE 19901	Allan C. Tappert (Program Dir., Ofc of Rad. Health)	(302) 736-4731	
District of Columbia	Dept. of Environmental Service 415 12th Street, N.W. Washington, DC 20004	Herbert Wood, Ph.D. (Program Director, Bureau of Occup. & Inst. Hygiene)	(202) 724-4358	529-3349
Florida	Dept. of Health & Rehab. Svc. Ambassador Bldg., Suite 219 Tallahassee, FL 32301	Ulray Clark (Admin. Radiological Health Program)	(904) 487-1004	878-6754
Georgia	Dept. of Human Resources State Office Building 47 Trinity Avenue Atlanta, GA 30334	W. Scott Sprinkle (Acting Director, Rad. Health Sect.)	(404) 894-5144	
Guam	Bureau of Environmental Health Dept. of Public Health & Social Services Government of Guam P. O. Box 2816 Agana, GU 96910	Juan Rosario	(0) 734-9057	632-9122
Hawaii	Department of Health P. O. Box 3378 Honolulu, HI 96801	Thomas Anamizu (Noise & Radiation Branch)	(808) 548-3075	955-3666
Idaho	Idaho Department of Health & Welfare Statehouse Boise, ID 83720	Robert Funderburg (Program Mgr. Rad. Control Sect.)	(208) 334-4107	362-5260
Illinois	Department of Nuclear Safety 1035 Outer Park Drive Springfield, IL 62704	Maury Neuweg (Deputy Director Office of Rad. Safety)	(217) 546-8100	498-9798
Indiana	Indiana State Board of Health 1330 West Michigan Street Indianapolis, IN 46206	Hal S. Stocks (Chief, Rad. Health Sect.)	(317) 633-0150	253-6189
Iowa	Iowa Department of Health Lucas State Office Building Des Moines, IA 50319	John A. Eure (Dir., Rad. Health & Work Related Disease Sect)	(515) 281-4928	279-2208
Kansas	Bureau of Radiation Control Forbes Field, Bldg. 321 Topeka, KS 66620	Gerald W. Allen (Director)	(913) 862-9360 ext. 284	665-7153
Kentucky	Department of Human Resources 275 East Main Street Frankfort, KY 40621	Donald R. Hughes (Mgr., Radiation Control Branch)	(502) 564-3700	695-4321
		Roy P. Osborne (Sup. Registration Licensing &Cert. Sect)	564-3700	695-4321
Louisiana	Office of Environmental Affairs P. O. Box 14690 Baton Rouge, LA 70898	William H. Spell (Administrator, Nuclear Energy Division)	(504) 925-4518 (24 hr)	FTS 687-0598

State	Address	Name of official	Telephone No. Work	Off-Duty
Louisiana	Office of Environmental Affairs P.O. Box 14690 Baton Rouge, LA 70898	Steven C. Collins (Mgr. Nuclear Projects Sect)	(504) 925-4518 (24 hrs)	FTS 687-0598
		Ronald L. Wascom (Mgr. Radiation Control)	925-4518 (24 hrs)	FTS 687-0598
Maine	Radiological Health Program 157 Capitol Street Augusta, ME 04333	Wallace Hinckley (Manager)	(207) 289-3826	377-8834
Maryland	Department of Health & Mental Hygiene O'Conor Office Building 201 West Preston Street Baltimore, MD 21201	Robert Corcoran (Chief, Division of Rad. Control)	(301) 383-2744	823-8328
Massachusetts	MA Dept. of Public Health 600 Washington Street Boston, MA 02111	Robert Hallisey (Dir., Radiation Control Program)	(617) 727-6214 727-6248	729-5728
Michigan	Department of Public Health 3500 North Logan Street P. O. Box 30035 Lansing, MI 48909	Donald Van Farowe (Chief, Division of Rad. Health)	(517) 373-1578 373-0253	
		James Camburn (Chief, Invest. & Compliance Sect)	373-1578 373-0253	224-4457
		Dennis Hahn (Chief Licensing & Reg. Sect)	373-1578 373-0253	669-5777
Minnesota	Minnesota Dept. of Health 717 Delaware Street, S.E. Minneapolis, MN 55440	Alice T. Dolezal (Chief, Section of Rad. Control)	(612) 296-5323	890-7782
Mississippi	State Board of Health Felix J. Underwood Building 2423 North State Street P. O. Box 1700 Jackson, MS 39205	Eddie S. Fuente (Dir., Division of Rad. Health)	(601) 354-6657	982-2861
Missouri	Bureau of Radiological Health 1151 Christy Lane P.O. Box 570 Jefferson City, MO 65101	Kenneth Miller (Administrator)	(314) 751-2713 ext. 332	635-5489
Montana	Department of Health & Environmental Sciences Cogswell Building Helena, MT 59601	Larry Lloyd (Chief Occupational Health Bureau)	(406) 449-3671	442-1425
Nebraska	Department of Health 201 Centennial Mall, South P.O. Box 95007 Lincoln, NE 68509	H. Ellis Simmons (Chief, Division of Rad. Health)	(402) 471-2168	423-4947
Nevada	State Department of Human Resources 505 East King Street Carson City, NV 89710	John D. Vaden (Supervisor, Rad. Health Section)	(702) 885 4750	
New Hampshire	Bureau of Environmental Health P. O. Box 148 Concord, NH 03301	John R. Stanton (Chief)	(603) 271-4587	623-4743

State	Address	Name of official	Telephone No. Work	Telephone No. Off-Duty
New Jersey	Division of Environmental Quality Department of Environmental Protection 380 Scotch Road Trenton, NJ 08628	Frank Cosolito (Chief, Bureau of Rad. Protection)	(609) 292-5586	
New Mexico	Department of Health and Environment P. O. Box 968 Santa Fe, NM 87503	Al Topp, (Envir. Mgr., Radiation Protection Bureau)	(505) 827-5271	982-9224
		Benito J. Garcia (Health Program Mgr., Licensing & Registration Sect)	827-5271	FTS 476-5271
New York	Bureau of Radiation Control New York City Dept. of Health 377 Broadway New York, NY 10013	Leonard Solon, Ph.D. (Director)	(212) 556-7750	
	New York State Dept. of Labor 2 World Trade Center New York, NY 10047	F. J. Bradley, Ph.D. (Principal Radiophysicist)	488-7790	
North Carolina	Department of Human Resources P.O. Box 12200 Raleigh, NC 27605	Dayne Brown (Chief Rad. Protection Sect)	(919) 733-4283	787-5396
North Dakota	Division of Environmental Engineering North Dakota Dept. of Health Missouri Office Building 1200 Missouri Avenue Bismarck, ND 58501	Dana K. Mount (Director)	(701) 224-2348	223-6735
Ohio	Department of Health 246 North High Street P.O. Box 118 Columbus, OH 43216	Robert Quillin CHP (Radiological Health Program Director)	(614) 466-1380	486-8338
Oklahoma	State Department of Health P.O. Box 53551 Oklahoma City, OK 73152	J. Dale McHard (Chief, Occup. & Rad. Health Svc)	(405) 271-5221 (24 hr)	525-7824
Oregon	State Health Division P.O. Box 231 Portland, OR 97207	Marshall W. Parrott (Mgr. Radiation Control Sect.)	(503) 229-5797 (24 hr)	646-7694
		Ray Paris, HP (Emergency Response)	229-5797 (24 hr)	286-2451
Pennsylvania	Bureau of Radiation Protection 9th Floor, Fulton Building Third and Locust Streets P. O. Box 2063 Harrisburg, PA 17120	Thomas Gerusky (Dir., Bureau of Radiation Protection)	(717) 787-2480	783-8150
		Donald J. McDonald (Div. of Radiation Control)	787-3720	783-8150
	Philadelphia Dept. of Public Health 500 South Broad Street Philadelphia, PA 19146	Arthur Wallach (Asst. Commissioner of Health Environ. Health Services)	(215) MU6-5157	927-1476

State	Address	Name of official	Telephone No. Work	Off-Duty
Puerto Rico	Radiological Health Division G.P.O. Call Box 70184 Rio Piedras, PR 00936	David Saldana (Director)	(809) 767-3563	
Rhode Island	Department of Health Division of Occupational Health and Radiation Control Cannon Building Davis Street Providence, RI 02908	James E. Hickey (Chief)	(401) 277-2438	884-4732
South Carolina	South Carolina Dept. of Health & Environmental Control Bureau of Radiological Health 2600 Bull Street Columbia, SC 29201	Heyward G. Shealy (Chief)	(803) 758-8354	945-7694
South Dakota	State Department of Health Office of Air Quality & Solid Waste State Dept. of Water & Natural Resources Joe Foss Office Building Pierre, SD 57501	Joel Smith (Administrator)	(605) 773-3329	224-8427
Tennessee	Department of Public Health C2-12 Cordell Hull Building Nashville, TN 37219	J. A. Bill Graham (Director, Div. of Rad. Health)	(615) 741-7812	883-6445
		Charles P. West (Asst. Dir., Div. of Rad. Health)	741-7812	833-1695
Texas	Texas Department of Health 1100 West 49th Street Austin, TX 78756	David K. Lacker (Chief, Bureau of Radiation Control)	(512) 458-7760 Emergency (24 hr)	295-3026 458-7460
		Edgar D. Bailey (Dir., Div. of Licensing, Regis. & Standards)	458-7341 Emergency (24 hr)	926-1405 458-7460
		Richard Ratliff (Dir., Div. of Compliance & Inspection)	458-7750 Emergency (24 hr)	863-8520 458-7460
Utah	State Department of Health Bureau of Radiation and Occupational Health 150 West North Temple Box 2500 Salt Lake City, UT 84103	Larry Anderson (Director)	(801) 533-6734	295-3817
Vermont	Division of Occupational & Radiological Health Vermont Department of Health Administration Building 10 Baldwin Street Montpelier, VT 05602	Raymond McCandless (Director)	(802) 828-2886	223-5075
Virginia	Department of Health Bureau of Radiological Health 109 Governor Street Richmond, VA 23219	Charles Prince (Supervisor)	(804) 786-5932	323-2300

State	Address	Name of official	Telephone No. Work	Telephone No. Off-Duty
Virgin Islands	Natural Resources Management Division of Natural Resources Department of Conservation & Cultural Affairs P.O. Box 4340 Charlotte Amalie St. Thomas, VI 00801	Donald Francois (Director)	(809) 774-6420	774-1562
Washington	Department of Social & Health Services Airdustrial Park Olympia, WA 98504	Nancy P. Kirner (Supervisor, Radioactive Materials Control Unit)	(206) 753-3459	866-4747
	Environmental Monitoring and Emergency Response Unit 1409 Smith Tower Seattle, WA 98104	Robert Mooney	464-6840	
West Virginia	State Department of Health Industrial Hygiene Division 151 11th Avenue South Charleston, WV 25303	William H. Aaroe (Director)	(304) 348-3526 348-3427	776-4306
Wisconsin	Department of Health & Social Services Radiation Protection Section P.O. Box 309 Madison, WI 53701	Lawrence McDonnell (Chief)	(608) 266-1791	873-5483
Wyoming	Division of Health & Medical Services Hathaway Building 4th Floor Cheyenne, WY 82001	Martin Skinner, MD (Asst. Director & State Epidemiologist)	(307) 777-7951	

From Directory of Personnel Responsible for Radiological Health Programs. HHS Publication FDA 83-8027. National Center for Devices and Radiological Health, Food and Drug Administration, Public Health Service, U.S. Department of Health and Human Services, Rockville, Md., October 8, 1982.

APPENDIX I

DEPARTMENT OF ENERGY REGIONAL COORDINATING OFFICES FOR RADIOLOGICAL ASSISTANCE AND GEOGRAPHICAL AREAS OF RESPONSIBILITY

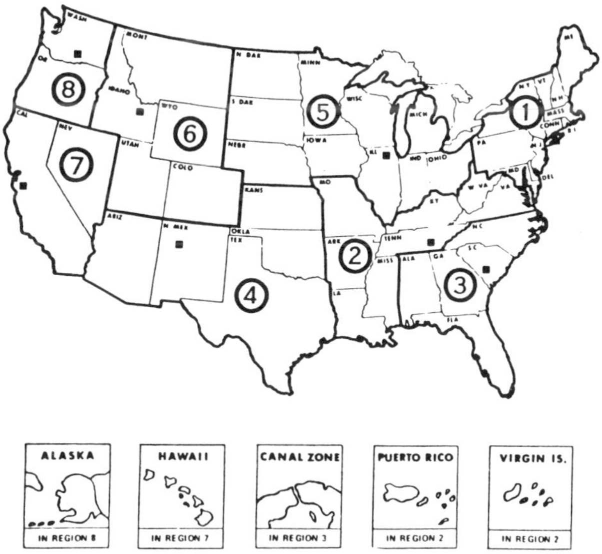

REGIONAL COORDINATING OFFICE	POST OFFICE ADDRESS	TELEPHONE for ASSISTANCE
1 BROOKHAVEN AREA OFFICE	UPTON, L. I. NEW YORK 11973	(516) 282-2200
2 OAK RIDGE OPERATIONS OFFICE	P. O. BOX E OAK RIDGE, TENNESSEE 37830	(615) 576-1005 or (615) 525-7885
3 SAVANNAH RIVER OPERATIONS OFFICE	P. O. BOX A AIKEN, S. C. 29801	(803) 725-3333
4 ALBUQUERQUE OPERATIONS OFFICE	P. O. BOX 5400 ALBUQUERQUE, NEW MEXICO 87115	(505) 844-4667
5 CHICAGO OPERATIONS AND REGIONAL OFFICE	9800 S. CASS AVE. ARGONNE, ILLINOIS 60439	Duty Hrs. (312) 972-4800 Off Hrs. 972-5731
6 IDAHO OPERATIONS OFFICE	550 SECOND ST. IDAHO FALLS, IDAHO 83401	(208) 526-1515
7 SAN FRANCISCO OPERATIONS OFFICE	1333 BROADWAY OAKLAND CALIFORNIA 94612	(415) 273-4237
8 RICHLAND OPERATIONS OFFICE	P. O. BOX 550 RICHLAND, WASHINGTON 99352	(509) 376-7381

Revised August 1981

APPENDIX J
INVESTIGATION OF PERSONNEL MONITORING RESULTS

MEMO TO: ______________________________

FROM: ______________________________

DATE: ______________________________

SUBJECT: Investigation of Radiation Exposure

The objective of personnel radiation monitoring is to measure occupational radiation exposures and to aid in the detection of unnecessary radiation dosages. The prompt investigation of any above-average exposure will be useful in determining methods of preventing unnecessary radiation exposures from recurring.

During the period from ____________________ to ____________________, your personnel radiation monitoring devices indicated an exposure of ______________ mR. The current permissible exposure level for X and gamma radiation is ____________ mR per quarter or ____________________ mR per year.

Please answer the following questions, and return this statement as quickly as possible, so that our records may be properly evaluated.

1. How did the exposure occur?

   ____

2. Why did the exposure occur?

   ____

3. What has been done to prevent recurrence of such an exposure?

   ____

4. Remarks:

   ____

   ____

   ____

   ____

SIGNED ______________________________ DATE ______________

(Employee)

FORWARDED ______________________________ DATE ______________

(Supervisor)

APPENDIX K
QUICK REFERENCE INFORMATION

A. On site emergency check list

Note: The sequence and priority of these actions will vary with different accident conditions.

- Provide emergency medical care immediately for serious injuries and preserve vital functions. Minor injuries can wait until after initial radiation survey has been completed.
- Remove individual from contaminated radiation area. Individual doses up to 100 rems may be permitted for life saving purposes or up to 25 rems for less urgent needs (NCRP, 1971). Teams may be used in relays to remove injured persons from very high radiation areas.
- Survey individual for surface contamination levels.
- Get nasal smears. Do this before showering (Sections 3.4.1 and 4.1.4).
- Remove contaminated clothes and replace with clean coveralls or wrap in blanket. Take individual to an area where skin decontamination or showering can be done.
- Decontaminate skin. Remove all transferable contamination if possible (Sections 3.7.4 and 7.1.5) by cleansing contaminated skin areas and showering.
- Cover contaminated wounds with sterile dressings before and after decontamination efforts (Section 7.2.5).
- Alert hospital and call for ambulance service as soon as it is determined that it is needed. Apprise them of situation if their help is required (Section 3.5.7).
- Identify radionuclide(s) involved in the accident and, if possible, ascertain its chemical form, solubility, and presumed particle size.
- Send personnel radiation dosimeters for processing.
- Get complete history of accident (Section 3.8.1), especially as it relates to the activities of the individual. Where was he? What was he doing? Exit path? Symptoms?
- Evaluate possibility of penetrating radiation exposure (Section 3.5.6).
- Advise individual on collection of all excreta (Section 3.5.8). Provide containers. Save other contaminated materials (Section 3.5.9).
- Be sure someone has assumed responsibility for management of the accident area. Is radiological assistance needed? Who will request it? From whom?
- Report your initial responses and evaluation to the plant manager (Section 3.5.4).
- Get names of supervisory and health physics personnel who will remain on call in case additional information is needed (Section 3.5.7).
- Take individual to the hospital if injuries require surgical care not available at plant or if further medical or dosimetric evaluation and treatment is required.
- Take precautions to prevent spread of contamination during transport and movement of the patient (Section 3.6). Have transport vehicles, attendants, and equipment checked for residual radioactive contamination before release from hospital area.
- If environmental contamination outside the plant has occurred, notify public health authorities (Section 3.9).
- Advise family and next of kin on the extent of injuries and exposure (Section 3.5.4). Plant management personnel and the medical department personnel should agree on the proper procedure.
- Find out where to send bioassay specimens and length of time required for analysis. Specify who will receive the results.

B. Identification tag information

Note: Each patient should be identified with as much of the following accident and treatment information as is available before sending to decontamination center or hospital. Health physicist or company physician should keep in contact with the hospital to supply additional information as needed.

a. Name of patient, employer, company number.
b. Physical injuries and treatment.
c. Skin surface contamination: its location, dose rate and/or count rate measurements initially and after decontamination, and description of decontamination methods and agents used.
d. Internal contamination.
    1. Radionuclide, its chemical form, probable solubility, and possible particle character.
    2. Suspected route of contamination.
    3. Nasal counts.
    4. Wound counts.
    5. Whole body counts.

6. Bioassay samples already collected.
7. Treatment initiated.

e. External exposure to penetrating radiation.
1. Precise location and position of the patient relative to the source of radiation at time of exposure.
2. Exact time and duration of exposure.
3. Was dosimeter being worn? Where? What types?
4. Has dosimeter been collected? By whom? Where is it now located?
5. Symptoms; type and time of occurrence.
6. Describe other dosimetric studies underway.
7. Treatment.

f. Name and phone number of company health physicist or physician for additional information.

C. Medical information check list

Note: These questions can be used by the attending physician at the hospital for obtaining historical information to assist in the early management of radioactively contaminated persons. The best information in industrial cases can probably be obtained from plant personnel, such as the health physicist or occupational physician familiar with the plant and accident details.

- When did the accident occur? What are the circumstances of the accident and what are the most likely pathways for exposure? How much radioactive material is involved potentially?
- What injuries have occurred? What potential medical problems may be present besides the radionuclide contamination?
- Are toxic or corrosive chemicals involved in addition to the radionuclides? Have any treatments been given for these?
- What radionuclides now contaminate the patient? Where? What are the radiation measurements at the surface?
- What information is available about the chemistry of the compounds containing the radionuclides? Soluble or insoluble? Any information about probable particle size?
- What radioactivity measurements have been made at the site of the accident, e.g., air monitors, smears, fixed radiation monitors, nasal smear counts, and skin contamination levels?
- What decontamination efforts, if any, have already been attempted? What success?
- Have any therapeutic measures, such as blocking agents or isotopic dilution been given?
- Was the victim also exposed to penetrating radiation? If so, what has been learned from processing personal dosimeters, e.g., film badge, TLD, or pocket ionization chamber? If not yet known, when is the information expected?
- Has clothing removed at the site of accident been saved in case the contamination still present on it is needed for radiation energy spectrum analysis and particle size studies?
- What excreta have been collected? Who has the samples? What analyses are planned? When will they be done?

D. Hospital decontamination procedures for protection of personnel and facilities

- Personnel should wear surgical scrub suits, surgical caps and gowns, and rubber gloves (surgical, household, or industrial depending upon duties).
- The team leader should be trained to recognize the rare instance when there may be a need for masks, respirators, or supplied airpacks due to the presence of high levels of alpha or beta radionuclides.
- Rubber or plastic shoe covers are desirable. Those performing the actual decontamination with water should wear plastic or rubber laboratory aprons. Good temporary shoe covers for dry areas can be improvised from brown paper bags held on with adhesive or masking tape.
- Air conditioning and forced air heating systems should be turned off so radioactive particulates are not carried into ducts or to other rooms unless a special filter system has been designed for use under these conditions.
- The floors should be protected with a disposable covering to reduce "tracking" by keeping cleaner surfaces and to aid the clean up tasks. The covering should be changed when significant contamination is present. Brown paper rolls (36 in. wide, 60-lb weight) are ideal where water is not used. Plastic sheets are useful where spillage of liquids is a problem, although ribbed or nonskid types should be used to reduce the chance of slips and falls.
- All contaminated clothing should be placed carefully into plastic or paper bags to reduce secondary contamination of area.
- Splashing of solutions used in decontamination should be avoided.
- Patients and other potentially contaminated personnel may move to clean areas only after surveys show satisfactory decontamination.
- All passage of persons and property between contaminated and clean areas must be surveyed and regulated by monitoring teams.

- Supplies are passed through monitoring stations from clean areas to contaminated areas. Reverse flow must not occur unless supplies are monitored and found clean.
- All individuals on the decontamination team shall be trained in radiological monitoring and decontamination techniques. Persons not working on the team should be excluded from the work area.
- Fiberboard or steel drums with tight fitting tops should be obtained for contaminated materials. Labels describing the contents should be affixed so that proper disposal can be carried out without reopening them. They may be sealed with masking tape or some other type of sealing tape.
- Personal dosimeters (pocket chambers, film badge or TLD dosimeters) should be supplied to all personnel working in the decontamination area. Personnel should be rotated after a dose of 5 rems (or less if possible) is received.
- The entry of all nonessential personnel including family, visitors, and administrative persons should be restricted.

From National Council on Radiation Protection and Measurements Management of Persons Accidentally Contaminated with Radionuclides, Report No. 65, National Council on Radiation Protection and Measurements, Washington, D.C., 1980.

PLANNING FOR AND MANAGEMENT OF RADIATION ACCIDENTS

Sydney W. Porter, Jr.

HISTORY OF RADIATION ACCIDENTS (CAUSES AND LESSONS LEARNED)

Acute Radiation Death Resulting from an Accidental Nuclear Critical Excursion on December 30, 1958

General Description of the Kelley Case[1]

This report is noteworthy because it involved the largest accidental dose of radiation received by man (to date) and because of the extremely professional and thorough workup of the case. This represents one of the best, if not the best, documented Acute Radiation Syndrome description that exists.

At 4:35 P.M. on December 30, 1958, an accidental critical excursion resulting in fatal radiation injury to an employee took place in the plutonium recovery plant at the Los Alamos Scientific Laboratory.

The time of the accident is quite important because a half hour earlier there had been about six other workers in the same room with Kelley. The date of the accident is important because the normal flow of fissionable material into the system was interrupted for year-end physical inventory. This interruption caused a routine procedure to become nonroutine and led to an accidential ''criticality'' of the Plutonium-rich solids that were accidently introduced into the system. The best estimate of K's average total-body exposure was probably between 3900 and 4900 rads, of which about 900 rads was due to fission neutrons. A considerably greater portion of the dose was delivered to the upper half of the body than to the lower half (see Table 1).

Clinical Course of Patient

In retrospect, the clinical course of patient K can be divided into four rather distinct periods, differing in duration, symptomatology, and response to supportive therapy. The first period (lasting about 20 to 30 min) was characterized by his immediate physical collapse and mental incapacitation, which progressed to semiconsciousness and severe prostration. The second period (lasting about 1 1/2 hr) began with his arrival by stretcher at the emergency room of the hospital and ended with his transfer from the emergency room to the ward for further supportive therapy. This second period was characterized by such severe cardiovascular shock that death seemed imminent during the entire time. During this period he seemed to be suffering severe abdominal pain. This third period was about 28 hr in length and was characterized by enough subjective improvement to encourage continued attempts to alleviate his anoxia, hypotension, and circulatory failure. The fourth period began with the unheralded onset of rapidly increasing irritability and uncooperativeness, bordering on mania, followed by coma and death in approximately 2 hr. The entire clinical course lasted 35 hr from the time of radiation exposure to death.

The most dramatic clinicopathological changes were observed in the hematopoietic and urinary systems. Lymphocytes were not found in the circulating blood after the 8th hr, and there was virtually complete urinary shutdown despite administration of large amount of fluids.

K's rectal temperature varied between 103 and 103.5°F for the first 6 hr and then fell precipitously to normal, where it remained for the duration of his life. This high initial temperature and its maintenance for 6 hr were considered in keeping with his suspected massive dose of radiation and were considered to be prognostically grave.

Table 1
SUMMARY OF ESTIMATES OF K'S RADIATION EXPOSURE

Region and conditions	Fast neutron dose (rads)	Gamma dose (rads)	Total dose (rads)
Head (incident)	2,600	7,800	10,400
Upper abdomen (incident)	3,000	9,000	12,400
Total Body (average)	900	3,000—4,000	3,900—4,900

Of all the various determinations made during the course of the illness, changes in white cell count were found to be the simplest and best prognostic indicator of severe irradiation. The virtual disappearance of lymphocytes from the peripheral circulation within 6 hr of exposure was considered a grave sign.

There were 16 different therapeutic agents employed in the symptomatic treatment of K over about a 30-hr period. In spite of this and continued oxygen administration, his heart tones became very distant, slow and irregular about 32 hr after irradiation. His heart then became progressively weaker and suddenly stopped 34 3/4 hr after irradiation.

Windscale Reactor #1 Accident of October 9 to 12, 1957

General Description of Windscale Reactor No. 1

Windscale Reactor No. 1 is an air cooled, graphite-moderated natural uranium-fueled plutonium production reactor. The core was partially ruined by fire on October 15, 1957. This fire resulted in a release of approximately 20,000 Ci I-131 to the downwind environment. According to the AEC Accident Information Report[2] about the Windscale Reactor incident, the accident was caused by operator judgement errors concerning thermocouple data, and was made worse by faulty handling of the reactor that permitted the graphite temperature to rise too rapidly. Also contributory was the fact that fuel temperature thermocouples were located in the part of the reactor which was hottest during normal operations rather than in the parts of the reactor which were hottest during a Wigner release. A second equipment deficiency was the reactor power meter which was calibrated for normal operations and read low during the annealing. As a result of the second heating cycle, the graphite temperature rose on October 9, especially in the lower front part of the reactor where some cladding had failed because of the earlier rapid temperature rise. Although there were a number of small Iodine releases on October 9, the releases were not recognized until October 10 when the stack activity meter showed a significant increase (which was not regarded as very important). Finally, on the afternoon of October 10, other monitoring areas (Calder site) showed activity was being released. Efforts to cool the reactor down by forcing air through the reactor failed, and only increased the magnitude of the radio-releases.

The estimated releases from the Windscale Accident were 20,000 Ci of I-131, 6000 Ci of Cs-137, 80 Ci of Sr-89, and 9 Ci of Sr-90. The highest off-site gamma level was 4 mR/hr of airborne activity. Air activity around the Windscale and Calder Plants measured often 5 to 10 times maximum permissible levels, with occasional peaks of 150 times permissible levels. The milk ban extended over approximately 260 miles.

During operations to bring the reactor under control, 14 workers received doses of greater than 3 R per quarter with the maximum exposures at 4.6 R per quarter.

Lessons Learned

1. There were many lessons learned concerning natural uranium reactor design and op-

eration. The inadequacies concerning reactor instrumentation and reactor operator training bring up points analogous to the TMI accident.

2. No guidelines existed for short-term permissible exposure to radioiodine in food. The British Medical Research Council performed a prompt and thorough investigation and analysis of short-term radioiodines in food. Much ingenuity was used in promptly deriving maximum permissible concentrations for I-131 in food. The emergency reference levels that resulted from this accident served as a basis for emergency planning guides[3] now used on a worldwide basis.
3. A useful correlation was derived for predicting significant radioiodine contamination in milk. It was found that gamma radiation levels in pastures which exceeded 0.035 mR/hr yielded milk which exceeded 0.1 μCi/ℓ.
4. Dose exposure from inhalation or plume exposure to radioiodines is negligible compared to drinking milk or eating dairy products. In an emergency, rapid gamma spectroscopy is preferable to radiochemical separation and subsequent samples.
5. There were 15 two-person teams used for performing radiation surveys and obtaining samples. It required 20 people for sample coordination and data reporting, and about 150 radiochemists were involved in sampling analysis.
6. Glass wool stack filters are not satisfactory under accident conditions.

Gulf Oil Accelerator Accident of October 4, 1967

General Description

A 3-MeV Van de Graaff Linear accelerator was being used by Gulf Oil Company technicians for the activation of soil samples on October 4, 1967. The combination of an interlock failure on the power key of the accelerator console and the taping of several of the interlocks on the safety tunnel door and the target room inside door produced three serious accidental exposures. One individual received approximately 100 rads whole body, a second individual received close to 300 rads whole body, and the third received approximately 600 rads whole body in addition to approximately 6000 rads to the hands and 3000 rads to the feet.

One of the accident victims reported to the medical department complaining of nausea, vomiting, and generalized muscular aches. His condition was first misdiagnosed as being due to the flu. When the second patient came in with approximately the same symptoms, it was decided that they may possibly have received a significant radiation exposure. Film badges were read and indicated that significant exposures had taken place. Dr. Neal Wald, of the University of Pittsburgh Radiological Health Division, supervised the dosimetry tests and also acted as coordinating physician in the work-up and treatment of the patients.

Dr. Wald very quickly and efficiently had absolute filter units flown in to a western Pennsylvania hospital in Pittsburgh where the three patients had been admitted. He set up these absolute filter/laminar flow filters to clean the patient's environment of all biological contaminants. These "reverse isolation" units were used on the 100-rad exposure patient for about 16 days, on the 300-rad exposure patient for about a month and half, and on the highest exposed patient also for about a month and half.

Dr. E. Donnal Thomas, from the University of Washington, was flown in to perform a bone marrow transplant on the 8th day after exposure. The patient's twin brother served as the bone marrow donor. Although this heroic medical treatment saved the 600-rad exposed patient's life, nothing could be done to save his arms and legs, each of which received thousands of rads exposure.

Lessons Learned

1. If the simple operating procedure of always using a survey meter when entering the exposure room had been followed, this tragic accident would have been avoided.

2. It was obvious that at least two of the interlocks had been taped closed for long periods of time prior to this accident. Such defeating of safety interlocks should never have been tolerated.
3. Regular maintenance checks should have been made on the key operated power interlocks for the accelerator.
4. Timely medical attention saved the life of the highest exposed person. The heroic procedure of a complete bone marrow transplant together with the use of reverse isolation room and quality medical care all were major factors in saving this patient's life.
5. Reverse isolation filters can be obtained in a matter of hours to set up any hospital to care for highly exposed patients.
6. In retrospect, medical authorities working with these patients recommended earlier amputation at a definitive level within 2 or 3 months after the exposure. They reasoned that the earlier amputation would have decreased the infection, would have resulted in a shorter period of severe pain, could have reduced the amount of pain medication for the patient, and possibly could have reduced the patient's hospital stay and led to an earlier rehabilitation. This earlier amputation would, of course, have been done by correlating the dosimetry information with the clinical observations.

The SL-1 Prototype Reactor Accident[4,5] (Idaho, January 3, 1961)

General Description

This is the first (and to date the only) fatal accident in the history of U.S. reactor operations. The SL-1 was a prototype of a small APPR (Army Package Power Reactor) designed for air transportation to remote areas for production of electrical power. This reactor was used for fuel testing and for reactor crew training. It was operated in the remote desert location of the National Reactor Testing Station in Idaho Falls, Idaho by Combustion Engineering for the U.S. Army.

It should be emphasized that the SL-1 was not a power reactor.

At the time of the accident, the SL-1 was loaded with 40 fuel elements and 5 control rod blades, and could produce a power level of 3 MW (thermal). It was a boiling water cooled and moderated reactor.

The accident resulted in the deaths of three military personnel. The accident was caused by the withdrawal of a single control rod at least several feet, which caused the reactor to go into prompt criticality. The reason why an experienced worker (licensed reactor operator with multiple refueling experiences) withdrew the control rod past its normal stop point will probably never be understood.

One of the three accident victims was still alive when the initial response personnel reached the scene of the accident. He was covered with (and his skin imbedded with) high activity fission products. Rescue and medical treatment were hampered by the fact that portions of the victim's skin exceeded 500 R/hr at 6″.

Lessons Learned

1. No reactor designed since the SL-1 accident can be brought prompt critical with a single control rod.
2. All reactors must have portable survey meters on-site that have ranges greater than 20 R/hr. Survey meters of 1000 R/hr range were recommended.*
3. Treatment facilities are required where a highly contaminated patient can receive definitive medical treatment with reasonable safeguards for attendant personnel. Since

* The TMI accident showed that 10K R/hr is the required range for gamma measurements, *and* for beta measurements.

most of these facilities will be in hospitals/clinics with ongoing missions, there must be provisions made for control of airborne and waterborne radiocontaminants.

X-Ray Machines, Industrial and Analytical[6–9]

Statement of the Problem

Accidental exposures from analytical X-ray machines are numerous and often involve extremely high exposures to small portions of the body. These exposures are well-documented in the four references cited above. It is not unusual for analytical X-ray machines to produce exposure rates of 500 R/sec at 10 cm from the tube focus. At shorter distances, 10,000 R/sec rates have often been measured. The beam is usually narrow, but even a few seconds exposure can result in severe local injury. Because of the fact that X-ray machines are often used in ''nonroutine'' circumstances, they lend themselves to the production of accidental exposures. The equipment used in normal operations appears to be reasonably safe and equipment failure has not been found to be a cause of severe exposures.

Lessons Learned From Accidental X-Ray Exposures

1. Most accidental exposures have occurred with nonroutine uses where equipment was demounted or shield covers removed.
2. In most serious exposures, adequate instruction for the staff and maintenance personnel has been lacking.
3. If simple and failsafe methods of ensuring that the tube was off during repairs and maintenance was in place, many accidental exposures would have been avoided.
4. Finger or wrist personnel dosimeters should be used for operators and maintenance personnel associated with these machines.
5. If the interlocks recommended by the ANSI Standard[9] N43.2 had been installed, many of the accidental exposures would have been avoided.
6. Operator error is a contributing cause in most of the accidents. Often this has been enhanced by lack of adequate enclosure or shielding design.

Industrial Radiographic Accidents

From the 1950's through the 1970's, the highest radiation accident rate for a single activity has consistently been with industrial radiographic operations.[10,11] The AEC/NRC has struggled over the years to improve the situation with a combination of improved regulations,[12] strict training requirements, and ever tougher inspection and enforcement policies. These Federal Government regulatory efforts have generally succeeded, but there are still many accidents associated with industrial radiography. The recent legislation enabling the NRC to levy huge monetary fines seems to be the most effective tool in keeping radiation safety focused in the minds of industrial radiographic management (and therefore in the workers minds as well).

Causes of Industrial Radiographic Accidents

1. Worker training — When one considers the constant use of radiation sources/machines on a daily basis, the industrial radiographer probably has lower specific education and training than any other type of radiation worker. Therefore, the training requirements[12] must be strictly enforced.
2. Worker production incentive — For years, the major incentive for industrial radiographers was based on the amount of successful radiographs per day that could be made. This practice lead to inadequate posting and monitoring, as well as occasional nonuse of personnel dosimetry so that the weekly 100-mrem limit would not be exceeded.

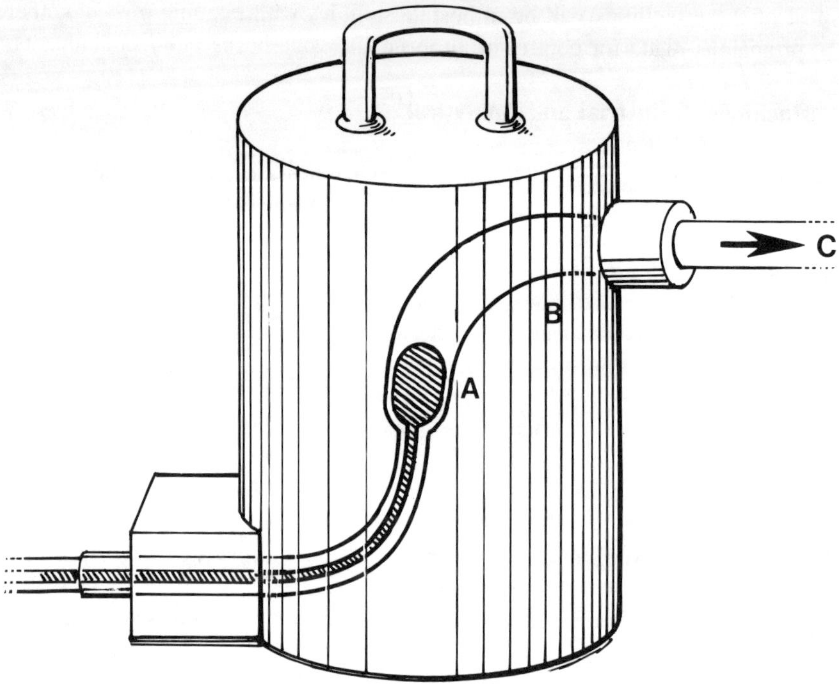

FIGURE 1. Industrial radiography camera. (A) Normal position of source when not in use, (B) channel leading from source storage to outside the shield, (C) source cable to exposure location.

3. Lack of proper monitoring — The thorough monitoring of the source pig (storage container) (Figure 1) after every exposure is most important. This single item is responsible for hundreds of unnecessary exposures, many of which are unrecorded, since industrial radiographers rarely use hand or finger dosimeters.
4. Equipment problems — Due to the heavy use of industrial radiographic cameras, the source-winding mechanism becomes loose, causing the source to incompletely retract into the safe storage position (Figure 1). There are also many instances of closet source interlock failure, causing accidental exposures.

DESIGN OF EMERGENCY PLAN

Many excellent guidelines[19-24] exist for the design of emergency plans. Less useful, but of help in specialized areas are References 25 through 41.

Initial Drafting of Emergency Plan and Procedures

First, one must assess the entire radioinventory for the subject facility. Then the maximum credible accidents must be analysed so that one can determine the probable maximum source release terms. Next, the plan and procedures must enable the facility operators to:

1. Recognize an accident situation
2. Classify the accident according to severity
3. Take steps to mitigate the accident
4. Make timely notifications
5. Call for help efficiently and quickly
6. Quantify releases

7. Keep track of exposures both on- and off-site, as well as to keep emergency exposures ALARA (as low as reasonably achievable)
8. Recover the facility as quickly as practical
9. Keep accurate and detailed records in case of ensuing law suits

Type of Accidents Associated with Nuclear Reactors (from most likely to least likely)*

1. Low level unexpected release of radiocontamination with little or no external radiation exposure to personnel. Usually occurs during major overhauls or in shipment of spent resin of spent fuel. Coolant system leakage and coolant sample sink spills are often causes of spread of radiocontamination.
2. Unexpected external exposure of personnel. Usually occurs during major overhauls or routine maintenance.
3. A combination of contamination spread, contamination of personnel and low level personnel external radiation exposure is the next most likely accident. These accidents occur under the same conditions as 1 and 2 above.
4. Gross surface contamination due to a major reactor coolant system leak or a leak of spent fuel coolant.
5. Chips or large particles of activated CRUD in skin, ear, or eye.
6. High level radiation exposure of plant personnel. Usually due to carelessness.
7. Release of small but greater than MPC quantities of radiowastes to outside of the plant boundary area. Usually associated with human failures.
8. Release of quantities of radionuclides to unrestricted environment which causes significant exposure of the general population. Probably associated with gross mechanical failure and incorrect reactor operator response.
9. Meltdown of reactor. Gross contamination offsite plus high personnel exposure would probably occur.
10. Reactor Excursion (SL-1 type of accident)

Radionuclides Expected from Water Cooled Reactor Accidents

1. Activated corrosion and erosion products (CRUD) in the coolant such as ^{60}Co, ^{58}Co, ^{59}Fe, ^{58}Mn, and ^{183}Ta.
2. Low level fission products are usually present in the coolant (^{131}I, ^{137}Cs).
3. Boiling water reactors have 1 and 2 above plus continuous offgassing of low levels of ^{3}H and noble radiogases such as ^{133}Xe, ^{135}Xe, ^{41}Ar, and ^{85}Kr.
4. Tritium is manufactured inside the core at the rate of 1.3×10^{-4} atoms of ^{3}H/fission. Only a fraction of this leaves the fuel.

Typical Nuclear Power Plant Emergency Plan Table of Contents

1.0 Introduction
2.0 Assignment of Responsibility
3.0 Emergency Organization
4.0 Emergency Response Support and Resources
5.0 Emergency Classification System
6.0 Notification Methods — Response Organization
7.0 Emergency Communications
8.0 Public Information
9.0 Emergency Facilities and Equipment
10.0 Accident Assessment

* The non-nuclear general industrial type of accident is by far the most likely type.

11.0 Protective Response
12.0 Radiological Exposure Control
13.0 Medical Support
14.0 Recovery and Reentry Planning
15.0 Exercises and Drills
16.0 Radiological Emergency Response Training
17.0 Emergency Plan Administration
18.0 Attachments — Letters of Agreement and Drawings

List of Typical Power Reactor Implementation Procedures
Refer to Appendix A.

RADIOLOGICAL ENVIRONMENTAL MONITORING DURING ACCIDENTS

This task is often called EREMP (Emergency Radiological Environmental Monitoring Program) at large facilities. One of the bitter TMI II accident lessons learned for the NRC and other U.S. Government Agencies was that one *cannot* successfully implement EREMP in 1 or 2 days without *extensive* prior planning which had *not* been performed by the NRC). The bottom line of the many millions of dollars spent by the U.S. Government monitoring the environment around the TMI nuclear station during the accident was that they measured less then 5% of the total releases. This was due to poor and *inadequate* prior planning.

Designing Environmental Radiological Emergency Monitoring Programs[9-19]

Thirty years of experience has shown this author that the only successful EREMP is one that is designed into the routine radiological environmental monitoring program. As the NRC learned the hard way, during the early days of the TMI II accident, one cannot successfully implement an EREMP in a day or two, no matter how much manpower and money are poured into the program.

Sampling Locations

All routine Radiological Environmental Monitoring Programs (REMP) locations will be utilized during long-term accident monitoring. In addition, a number of locations must be set up so that motorized survey teams have predetermined locations in each portion of each 22 1/2° sector (Figure 2 and Table 2). Obviously, there can be locations in areas with no roads, such as swamps or water. If there are trapper shacks or duck blinds, etc., or areas in which people travel by foot, the survey teams must find a way to perform surveillance if these areas exist in a downwind plume (within about 10 miles). NUREG 0654[23] which is the criteria for preparation and evaluation of Radiological Response Plans, Section 10, para J.10 of this document specifies requirements for designation of radiation and emergency monitoring locations. Table 2 specifies the sector and zone designation for radiation and environmental monitoring points. One is given the choice of designating 22 1/2° sectors by the cardinal directions (N, NNE, NE, etc.) or by simple letters A through R. However the use of simple letters A thru R should *not* be used because they are easily confused with the directional letters. For example, FEMA (Federal Emergency Management Agency) letter designation N stands for direction W. This is unnecessarily confusing. It is less confusing to use the directional W for west rather than the letter N. Each designated sample location should be utilized during a practice drill so that the people responsible for monitoring and sampling will be familiar with the location of each point and will be aware of radio blackouts, poor road conditions, problems with finding the locations in the dark, etc. Since no drill will cover all the predesignated locations within the 10 mile EPZ, one needs to design drills so that eventually all sample points have been covered. It is often very worthwhile to

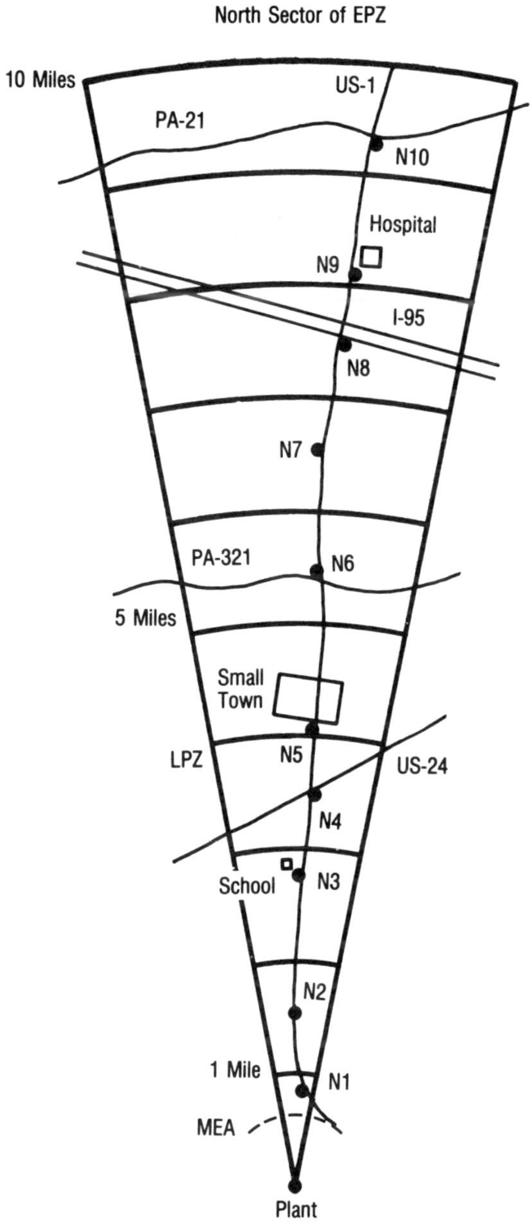

FIGURE 2. Example of a 221/2° sector.

predetermine the ability of the survey team vehicles to communicate with each predesignated point. The actual location of the sample point is chosen utilizing the same criteria as in the REMP, for example, line of site, minimum exclusion area, closest individual, closest community, closest school, hospital, nursing home, milch animal herd, garden, farm, etc.

Radiological Monitoring Survey Team

During a serious accident involving significant releases of radionuclides, radiological monitoring teams should be continuously monitoring in the field. They should, if possible, also continuously monitor on-site, depending on survey team exposure, and other considerations. Normally, these monitoring teams will be monitoring for ambient gamma and/or beta radiation, as well as taking air samples to measure the presence of radio-particulates

Table 2
SECTOR AND ZONE DESIGNATORS FOR RADIOLOGICAL SAMPLING AND MONITORING POINTS WITHIN EMERGENCY PLANNING ZONES

Sector nomenclature		Zone nomenclature	
Centerline of sector in degrees true north from facility	**22 1/2° sector**	**Miles from facility**	**Zone**
0 and 360	A[a]	0—1	1
221/2	B NNE	1—2	2
45	C NE	2—3	3
67 1/2	D ENE	3—4	4
90	E E	4—5	5
112	F ESE	5—6	6
135	G SE	6—7	7
157	H or SSE	7—8	8
180	J S	8—9	9
2021/2	K SSW	9—10	10
225	L SW	10—15	15
2471/2	M WSW	15—20	20
270	N W	20—25	25
2921/2	P WNW	25—30	30
315	Q NW	30—35	35
3371/2	R NNW	35—40	40
		40—45	45
		45—50	50

Area segment: An area is identified by a Sector and Zone designator. Thus, area NL is that area which lies between 348 3/4 and 11 1/4° true north from the facility out to a radius of 1 mile. Area SE4 would be that area between 123 3/4 to 146 1/4° and the 3- and 4-mile arcs from the facility.

[a] The letters I and O have been omitted from these sector designators so as to eliminate possible confusion between letters and numbers.

From NUREG-0654 FEMA-REP-1 Rev. 1, Criteria for preparation and evaluation of radiological emergency response plans and preparedness in support of nuclear power plants, U.S. Nuclear Regulatory Commission, Washington, D.C., November 1980.

and radiohalogens. These teams must be well trained in all monitoring procedures and must demonstrate the ability to succesfully monitor the environment, and accurately relay the data back to the base station. They must also be trained carefully to monitor their own exposure and relay this data back to the base station. Details such as survey meter, type and serial number, and open and closed window status must be carefully reported on well-designed log sheets.

At the beginning of an emergency, an emergency monitoring team may have to monitor for 12 hr continuously without a break. After the initial period, however, field time for the survey team should be decreased to 8 hr with at least one 1/2 hr break in the middle. Since continuous surveillance may be needed, appropriate procedures must be enforced to supply the survey teams with food and drink, instrument replacement, and for shuttling of air filter samples to the appropriate locations. Even though the survey teams will probably be working

12 hr, one needs 3 shifts a day to provide continuous surveillance. During the TMI accident, there was a minimum of 5 monitoring teams out at any one time for the first 2 weeks. The logistics of such an effort needs to be carefully thought out in the emergency planning stage.

Radiological Environmental Sampling Team

The types of environmental samples taken during an accident depend on the type of releases (airborne vs. water), direction of the wind, and time of year. Even in the dead of winter, soil samples and drinking water samples must be taken. Even though air monitoring devices may not detect radiohalogen releases, it is advisable to take milk samples because of the large bioaccumulation factor. Many food stuffs and environmental samples will have to be taken primarily for political reasons and to reassure the public, rather than for technical reasons only. During a significant release, it is important to build up a large base of "negative" data to show that the environment is not affected. This data is worth its' weight in gold during any subsequent legal proceedings. Predetermined log sheets utilizing carefully thought out off-site data procedures are a must for environmental samples.

All people taking environmental samples should have demonstrated a clear understanding of procedures and have documented field training. If it is at all possible, the off-site environmental sample data should be taken by an independent off-site group. It is also preferable for the routine environmental samples to be taken by the same off-site group, so that the valuable on-site group may be used for other data taking during an accident. It is noteworthy that during the TMI II accident, not one environmental sample failed to be taken that should have been taken, and not one environmental sample was lost, even though the sample rate increased by more than a factor of 10 in most cases.

Emergency Monitoring Equipment

The inventory of emergency monitoring equipment should be at least double for what one would need at any given time. Lockers should be placed around nuclear complexes in appropriate places so that no one accident will deny access to these lockers. To ensure readiness, the equipment should be inventoried and calibration-checked at least twice a year, and after each drill, to ensure readiness.

At large nuclear facilities, the van/trucks should be completely outfitted for both on- and off-site emergency surveillance. One needs to give some thought to the fact that during a serious emergency the on-site counting labs may be unusable. Therefore, an alternate counting lab or a portable counting lab is needed. This is a requirement[26] for nuclear power plants (refer to Reg. Guide 1.97, E Variable, Note 18, Rev. 3, May 1983).

The type and sophistication of environmental monitoring equipment should be designed for the nuclear facility's worst credible accident. Below is listed typical environmental monitoring equipment for nuclear power plants:

1. Air sampling equipment, battery operated for short-term samples, as well as 110 AC with strip chart recorders and alarm capabilities for longer term surveillance.
2. Liquid sample equipment should contain continuous samplers. In Northern climates the samplers must be environmentally hardened.
3. Portable gamma survey meters for in-plant work, with a range of 10kR/hr, and separate survey equipment used to measure beta up to 10 kR/hr. On-site, personnel dosimetry must include multi-filter beta capability as well as finger TLD's. Extremity dosimetry may be needed. Extra sets of controls are always needed in emergencies. It may be necessary to have a portable TLD reader so that it can be hooked up to the station computer via telephone modum in emergency locations. In-house survey teams, such as rescue and repair teams, should have low- and high-range pocket dosimeters as well as preset alarm dosimeters. Careful thought must be given to preestablished dose levels for teams that may be in high-range radiation areas.

5. Supplies of protective clothing should be supplied in emergency locations and in emergency vehicles/trucks. Extra back-up protective clothing should be available in case of an accident lasting for an extended period of time.
6. Respiratory equipment should be in all emergency lockers and vehicles. Lists of respiratory-trained personnel should be kept up-to-date and in each of the major emergency equipment storage areas.
7. Mobile vehicles equipped with radios are a must for emergency radiation monitoring survey teams. The location and availability of back-up vehicles must be known.
8. Environmental survey team equipment should be stored in a convenient place, preferably off-site, so that it is always available.
9. Emergency kits should be placed in the Technical Support Center (TSC) and the Emergency Off-site Facility (EOF) so that replacement survey teams need not go on-site in order to receive equipment prior to deployment.
10. For the severe airborne accident, preparations must be in place for the use of helicopters and/or single engine airplanes for airbourne surveillance.

Data Analysis

During a serious accident, as soon as possible, environmental data analysis should be shifted to off-site, such as the EOF. The data from environmental sample analysis should be collected and analyzed off-site. It is preferable that this should be wherever the normal environmental data is analyzed. Preset guidelines must be established as to when environmental sample data is to be reported to management. The method and frequency of promulgation of environmental sample data to State and Federal agencies should be agreed upon as early in the accident as practical.

TMI II ACCIDENT LESSONS LEARNED — HEALTH PHYSICS AND RADIOCHEMISTRY ASPECTS[46-50, 52,53]

Introduction

During the early hours of the March 29, 1979 TMI II accident, Porter Consultants, Inc. was assigned the following TMI activities:

1. *Radioeffluent release assessment (gaseous and liquid)* including sample collection, coordination of labs for sample counting, quality control of labs, data collection, data analysis, report generation, distribution of data to the State, NRC, and Utility.
2. *Dose assessment* including suspected and actual overexposure investigations, skin contamination and internal deposition investigations, significant exposure mockups and dose calculations.
3. *Radiological environmental monitoring program* including complete coordination of sample taking, data analysis, report generation and distribution, action point notifications, expansion of the program for the accident situation and then contraction of the program up to 1 year after the accident.
4. *Special beta dosimetry studies* including studies of the state of the art in beta personnel monitoring, modeling of the beta dose to skin from TMI contaminants, intercomparisons of all commercially available beta-gamma TLD personnel dosimetry systems (this assignment started in August 1979 as a result of the makeup valve room accidental overexposures).

The above list of activities gives a little insight into areas that the typical utility health physics staff cannot adequately accomplish during a serious accident. The TMI health physics staff was very experienced, knowledgeable, and capable. They worked 15 to 20 hr/day without a break for the first 2 weeks of the accident. Yet, the requirements of the accidents were so huge that they were unable to perform many important routine health physics tasks that ordinarily would be easily performed. It is difficult to describe the intense pressure and confusion, especially during the first 2 weeks of the accident. The other very surprising health physics aspect of the accident was the many knowledgeable, experienced professional plant personnel that disregarded their years of radiation safety training and experience and made judgment errors that contributed to overexposures and contamination, all with the intention of "saving the plant."

Lessons Learned — Aux Building Entry During Accident

1. All entries are to be on a new RWP reviewed by Senior H. P. on site and signed by the Unit Superintendent, or his alternate.
2. Appropriate Control Room should have absolute control over all Aux and Fuel Handling Building entries. No entries without a H.P. at the control point during the entry.
3. No entries without a properly operating survey meter of proper range (perform a spot check of meter response just prior to entry).
4. Obtain exposure history for all persons prior to entry into a high radiation area.
5. Designate allowable exposures during entry, no matter how important the task.

Lessons Learned — Primary Coolant Sampling During Accident

1. All samples to be taken on a new RWP reviewed by Senior H.P. on site and signed by Unit Superintendent or his alternate.
2. No coolant samples to be taken without extremity dosimetry.
3. No coolant samples to be taken without availability of tongs approximately 2 ft in length, and shielded gloves, in case sample is hotter than expected.
4. No coolant samples to be taken without a leaded glass personnel shield in place in case sample is hotter than expected.
5. Discontinue taking sample if exposure to extremity, or whole body, is likely to exceed preset levels which are clearly stated on the RWP.
6. Distribute significant exposures among a number of workers, if at all possible.
7. Review, within 24 hr, all cases of skin contamination in excess of action levels.

Lessons Learned — Make-up Valve Room Entry

1. Perform beta and gamma area surveys using a remote detector with appropriate range.
2. Initial entry in areas of more than 2 R/hr must have prior ALARA review.
3. Be aware of possible floor contamination when water leaks are suspected.
4. A consistent program for type and placement of personnel dosimetry must be put into operation.
5. When persons enter areas of more than 2 R/hr, do a readout of the TLDs immediately[52] upon exit from area.
6. Have a review and verification that all RWP requirements are being carried out *prior* to entry into areas of more than 2 R/hr.
7. Controlled time entries, into hazardous areas, must be carefully timed by H.P.

Lessons Learned — Protective Actions and Off-Site Environmental Surveillance from the State's Perspective[51]

1. Before you start a sampling regime, you had better have a criterion, so you have a recognized point for stopping it.
2. Guard against individuals and agencies who are not party to your plan interfering in it.
3. Have several confidential phone lines in place. Change the numbers after each crisis.
4. ARAC capabilities are better than most people thought.

5. Carry a tape recorder and talk to it regularly.
6. While the acute episode is in progress, do not read newspapers, watch television, or listen to the radio. Such activities will only make you schizoid.
7. Plan for food delivery and other niceties like sleeping facilities. You may not go home for a while.
8. Plan for alternate analytic capabilities. It does not take much of an accident to make your background go to pot.
9. More energy will be expended in heading off ridiculous decisions than in dealing with the real problem.
10. Emergencies cannot be managed from Bethesda (NRC Headquarters).
11. Protective action recommendations are not amenable to committee vote.
12. When something big happens there are many who think ''this is the chance of a lifetime. I may never again have the opportunity to affect the outcome. How can I screw it up.'' It is, they won't, and they do in many ways.
13. Do not be afraid to put nonessential calls on hold or to hang up on ridiculous calls.
14. The Federal response by RAP teams and tech grunts was great. The same cannot be said about some appointed officials who attempted to participate.
15. From the perils of a new administration, deliver us, O Lord.

REFERENCES

1. *J. Occup. Med.*, (Special Supplement) 3, 3, 1961.
2. *The Windscale reactor incident*, U.S. AEC Accident Information Bulletin, Issue 73, December 1957.
3. **Bryant, P. M.,** Data for assessments concerning controlled and accidental releases of I-131 and Cs-137 to the atmosphere, *Health Phy.*, 17, 1.
4. U.S. Atomic Energy Commission, Investigation board report on the SL-1 accident, U.S. NRC, Washington, D.C., 1961.
5. American Nuclear Society, Special report on SL-1 accident, Nuclear News, Feb. 1961.
6. **Lubenau, J. O., Davis, J., McDonald, D., and Gerusky, T.,** Analytical X-ray hazards: A continuing problem, the 12th Annual Meeting of the Health Physics Society, Washington, D.C., June 1967.
7. **Lindell, B.,** Occupational hazards in x-ray analytical work, *Health Phys.*, 15, 481—486, 1968.
8. **Haynie, J. S. and Olsher, R. H.,** A summary of X-ray machine exposure accidents at the Los Alamos National Laboratory, LALP 81—32; March 1981.
9. American National Standards Institute, Standard #N43.2, Radiation safety for X-ray, diffraction and fluorescence analysis equipment, 1977.
10. Symposium on the Handling of Radiation Accidents, IAEA, Vienna, 1969.
11. Symposium on the Handling of Radiation Accidents, IAEA, Vienna, 1977.
12. Code of Federal Regulations, Title 10, Part 34, Licenses for radiography and radiation safety requirements for radiographic operations.
13. USEPA, Environmental Radioactivity Surveillance Guide, ORP/SID 72-2, June 1972.
14. IAEA Safety Series #18, Environmental monitoring in emergency situations, Vienna, 1966.
15. IAEA Safety Series #41, Objectives and design of environmental monitoring programs for radioactive contaminants, Vienna, 1975.
16. IAEA Safety Series #46, Monitoring of airborne and liquid radioactive releases from nuclear facilities to the environment, Vienna, 1978.
17. U.S.N.R.C. Regulatory Guide 4.1, 4.2, 4.6, 4.13, and 4.16.
18. ASTM, STP 698, *Effluent and Environmental Radiation Surveillance*, Kelly, J. J., Ed., 1980.
19. **Reimig, W. C., Ed.,** Environmental surveillance in the vicinity of nuclear facilities, H. P. Society Symposium Proceedings, Charles C Thomas, Springfield, Ill., 1970.
20. **Eisenbud, M.,** *Environmental Radioactivity*, Academic Press, New York, 1973.
21. **Goldbud, B. and Jones, J.,** Radiological Monitoring in the Environment, Pergammon Press, Elmsford, N.Y., 1965.
22. IAEA Proceedings, Radioactive contaminants of the marine environment, Vienna 1973.

23. NUREG 0654-FEMA-REP-1, Rev. 1, Criteria for preparation and evaluation of radiological emergency response plans and preparedness in support of nuclear power plants, NRC, 1980.
24. Code of Federal Regulations Title 10, Part 50, Appendix E, Emergency Planning and Preparedness for Productin and Utilization Facilities.
25. U.S. NRC Reg. Guide 1.101, Emergency planning for nuclear power reactors, Rev. 2, October 1981.
26. U.S. NRC Reg. Guide 1.97, Instrumentation for light-water-cooled nuclear power plants to assess plant and environs conditions during and after and accident, Rev. 3, May 1983.
27. U.S. NRC Reg. Guide 2.6, emergency planning for research and test reactors, March 1983.
28. EPA-520/1-75-001, Manual of protective action guide and protective actions for nuclear incidents, June 1980.
29. 43FR58658, Planning basis for the development of state and local government radiological emergency response plans in support of light water nuclear powerplant, December 1978.
30. 43FR8790, Accidental radioactive contamination of human food and animal feeds, December 1978.
31. 43FR58789, Potassium iodine as a thyroid-blocking agent in a radiation emergency, December 1978.
32. 44FR75344, Development plan-issuance of protective action guides for airborne releases of radioactivity as federal guidance, December 1979.
33. 45FR55402, Nuclear regulator commission, emergency planning, August 1980.
34. 45FR84910, National radiological emergency preparedness/response plan for commercial nuclear power plant accident (master plan), December 1980.
35. NUREG-0092, radiological emergency response planning, *Handbook for Federal Assistance to State and Local Government,* January 1979.
36. NUREG-0728, NRC incident response plan, September 1980.
37. EPA 520/1-78-001A, Protective Action Evaluation, Part 1, The effectiveness of sheltering as a protective action against nuclear accidents involving gaseous releases, April 1978.
38. EPA 520/1-78-001B, Protective Action Evaluation, Part II, The effectiveness of sheltering as a protective action against nuclear accident involving gaseous releases, April 1978.
39. FEMA-REP-2, Guidance on offsite emergency radiation measurement systems, Phase 1, Airborne Release, September 1980.
40. NUREG/CR-1745, Analysis of techniques for estimating evacuation, (BHARC-40/80-017), Times for emergency planning zones, November 1970.
41. Personnel dosimetry for radiation accidents, IAEA Symposium, Vienna 1965.
42. Evaluation of radiation emergencies and accidents. Selected criteria and data, IAEA Technical Report #152, 1974.
43. NCRP Report #55, Protection of the thyroid gland in the event of releases of radioiodine, August 1977.
44. NCRP Report #54, Management of persons accidently contaminated with radionuclides, April 1980.
45. **Purington, R. and Patterson, W.,** *Handling Radiation Emergencies* National Fire Protection Assoc., 1977.
46. Report of the President's Commission on the Accident at Three Mile Island, John G. Kemeny, Chairman, October 1979, Washington, D.C.
47. Technical Staff Analysis Report on Chemistry to the President's Commission on Three Mile Island, English, Robert, E., October 1979, Washington, D.C.
48. Technical Staff Analysis Report on Technical Assessment of Operating, Abnormal and Emergency Procedures to the President's Commission on Three Mile Island, Eytchison, Ronald, M., October 1979, Washington, D.C.
49. Report of the Office of the Chief Counsel on Emergency Preparedness to the President's Commission on Three Mile Island, Gorinson, Stanley, M., et al., October 1979, Washington, D.C.
50. Report of the Office of the Chief Counsel on Emergency Response to the President's Commission on Three Mile Island, Gorinson, Stanley, M., et al., October 1979, Washington, D.C.
51. Personal communication of 7/79 from M. Reilley, Bureau of Radiological Health, PA State.
52. **Sherbini, S. and Porter, S. W.,** A Review of the Current Deficiencies in Personnel Beta Dosimetry, with Recommendations, NUREG/CR-3296 U.S. Nuclear Regulatory Commission, June 1983.
53. President's Commission on the Accident at T.M.I., Report of the Task Group on Health Physics and Dosimetry, October 31, 1979, Washington, D.C.

APPENDIX A
List of Typical Power Reactor Implementing Procedures

Section I — On-site Procedures

EP I-0	Accident Classification Guide Part 1 Radiological Part 2 Operational Part 3 Fire/Natural/Security Part 4 Miscellaneous Flow Chart
EP I-1	Notification of Unusual Event/Significant Event
EP I-2	Alert
EP I-3	Site Area Emergency
EP I-4	General Emergency
EP I-5	Personnel Emergency
EP I-6	Radioactive Spill
EP I-7	Station Fire
EP I-8	Personnel Accountability
EP I-9	Search and Rescue Operations
EP I-10	Conducting an Inventory of Emergency Equipment
EP I-11	Communications Equipment
EP I-12	Site Evacuation
EP I-13	Post Accident Low Pressure Injection Monitoring
EP I-14	Initiation of Recovery Operations
EP I-15	Stable Iodine Thyroid Blocking
EP I-16	Recall of Evacuated Site Personnel
EP I-17	Radiation Protection — Emergency Action
EP I-18	Operations Support Center Activation
EP I-19	Activation/Evacuation of the Technical Support Center

Section II — Off-site Procedures

EP II-1	Emergency Response Manager Preparation to Assume Responsibilities
EP II-2	Site Support Manager Preparation to Assume Responsibilities
EP II-3	Radiological Support Manager Preparation to Assume Responsibilities
EP II-4	Notification of Corporate Emergency Response Personnel
EP II-5	Emergency Paging of Corporate Emergency Response Personnel
EP II-6	Off-Site Administrative Support
EP II-7	Testing of Emergency Procedure EP II-4

Section III — Security Emergency Procedures

EP III-1	Opening of the Technical Support Center
EP III-2	Opening of the Emergency Operations Facility
EP III-3	Personnel Accountability
EP III-4	Site Evacuation — Security Support
EP III-5	Emergency Vehicle Support

SECTION IV — RADIATION PROTECTION/CHEMISTRY EMERGENCY PROCEDURES

EP IV-101	TSC Initial Response
EP IV-102	Control Room Initial Response
EP IV-103	Control Point Initial Response
EP IV-104	TSC Evacuation
EP IV-105	Control Point and Equipment Evacuation
EP IV-106	ALARA Task Review and Emergency Exposure Authorization
EP IV-107	Radiation Monitor Evaluation
EP IV-108	Protective Action Recommendations
EP IV-109	Plume Tracking by Helicopter
EP IV-110A	Field Monitoring by TSC

EP IV-110B	Field Monitoring by EOF
EP IV-111	Effluent Dose Calculations
EP IV-112	Emergency Operations Facility — Radiological Assessment
EP IV-113	Computerized Dose Calculations
EP IV-114	Computerized Dose Calculations on Programmable Calculator
EP IV-115	Personnel and Vehicle Survey
EP IV-116	Fire Brigade Escort
EP IV-117	Reentry Team Radiation Protection
EP IV-118	High Activity Sample Analysis
EP IV-119	Personnel Decontamination
EP IV-120	Equipment Decontamination
EP IV-121	Containment Atmosphere Remote Sampling
EP IV-122	Emergency Staffing Guide
EP IV-201	Radiation Protection Senior Supervisor Response
EP IV-202	Chemistry Senior Supervisor Response
EP IV-203	Administrative Assistant Response
EP IV-204	Short Term Environmental Response
EP IV-205	Material and Instruments Supervisor Response
EP IV-206	Dosimetry-Counting Room Supervisor Response
EP IV-207	Rad Waste Supervisor Response
EP IV-208	Dose Assessment — ALARA Supervisor Response
EP IV-209	In-Plant Supervisor Response
EP IV-210	Procedures-Training Supervisor Response
EP IV-211	Radiation Protection Communications Guide
EP IV-212	Radiation Protection Emergency Inventory Control
EP IV-301	Interim Post Accident Primary Coolant Sampling
EP IV-302	Emergency Sampling Procedure for the Plant Vent

SECTION V — ENGINEERING DEPARTMENT EMERGENCY PROCEDURES

EP V-1	Notification of Engineering and Construction Department
EP V-2	Corporate Engineering Support Manager Response (CHERC)
EP V-3	Site Engineering Support Manager Response (EOF)
EP V-4	Corporate Engineering Team Leader Response (CHERC)
EP V-5	Corporate Quality Assurance Department Response (CHERC)
EP V-6	Site Quality Assurance Department Response (EOF)
EP V-7	Site Engineering Team Leader Response (TSC)
EP V-8	Methods Department and Engineering Department Divisional Representatives Response (CHERC)

SECTION VI — PLAN ADMINISTRATION

EP VI-1	Revision and Approval of Plans and Procedures
EP VI-2	Distribution of Plans and Procedures
EP VI-3	Review of Plans and Procedures
EP VI-4	Procedures Format
EP VI-5	Conduct of Drills and Exercises

SECTION VII — PUBLIC INFORMATION

EP VII-1	Public Information Notification
EP VII-2	General Manager — Information Services Response
EP VII-3	Public Information Manager Response
EP VII-4	Public Information Technical Liaison Response
EP VII-5	Public Information Technical Assistant Response
EP VII-6	Internal Information
EP VII-7	Media Relations
EP VII-8	Emergency News Center Activation/Public Information Coordinator Response

ADDENDUM

FIGURES

EMERGENCY RESPONSE DECISIONS IN THE PLANNING PROCESS — PREDETERMINED CONDITIONS FOR PREDETERMINED ACTIONS*,**

James A. Martin, Jr.

INTRODUCTION

One objective of emergency planning should be to make as many protective action decisions as possible before emergency situations occur, thereby minimizing the number of decisions that would have to be made in an emergency. Most radiological emergency response plans today forego protective action decision making until an incident is in progress. In contrast, current emergency planning guidance calls for certain key response decisions to be made in the planning process. Herein, various facets of this action planning will be explored, radiological bases will be developed from this perspective, the action planning that is feasible in a preincident time frame will be bounded, and the application of the decision process will be illustrated by examples. The emphasis will be on public protective action decisions for nuclear power plant accidents, including nonaction decisions as well as action decisions made in the planning stage.

Some of the following points will be disconcerting for some readers, at least initially. The art is developing and is incomplete. The emphasis on the provisions of nonradiological, in-plant bases for public protective actions has been found to be especially unsettling for planners more familiar with older recommendations which were based exclusively on off-site monitoring as a precursor to protective action decisions. Their forebearance is requested.

Major impediments to the implementation of this art exist at two ends of the protective action spectrum. At the lower end, health physicists find it difficult to decide today that for some levels of future radiological releases, no protective actions in the public domain would be warranted. Nuclear engineers have little difficulty in this regard; indeed this aspect meets with favorable response.

At the upper end of the protective action response spectrum, when public evacuation decisions are to be made in the planning process, obstacles to decisions are abundant. Many nuclear engineers believe, in good faith and perhaps correctly, that evacuations by the public would never be necessary. Health physicists, meteorologists, and radiological monitoring specialists are disconcerted here, also, for two reasons: (a) basing planned initial protective actions on plant parameters, even in the absence of radiation to be measured in the environment, is counter to the prevailing ''monitor first, then act'' planned (postponed) decision process and (b) under the current concept the facility operators could cause the initiation of precautionary protective actions, including evacuations, in the public domain. This appears to place the plant operator in the position of possibly usurping the role of public health officials. As will be seen, this is not the case. Rather, under highly restricted circumstances the plant operators would implement protective action decisions made earlier, perhaps years earlier, by plant and public health and safety officials.

The currently developing art leads to very simple, yet not simplistic, immediate protective action criteria. Under the current scheme, initiation of protective actions in the public domain, because of accidents at nuclear power plants, should be extremely rare. Yet, if such were ever necessary or desirable, public protective action should commence early should a major

* Based in part on a presentation at the Health Physics Society Annual Meeting, San Francisco, CA., June 27— July 2, 1976.

** The opinions, findings, conclusions, and recommendations of the author do not necessarily reflect official policy of the Nuclear Regulatory Commission.

accident scenario ever develop. It is possible that predetermined protective actions, including evacuations, would be completed at some future time well before public health officials would assemble, or even be aware of a problem, and even in the total absence (postaccident assessment) of a major radiological release to the environment. Such occurrences should also be extremely rare to nonexistent.

Thus, under this scheme the public should not be called upon for protective actions unnecessarily, perhaps never. But if precautionary protective action is ever necessary or desirable, such action should occur early, well before radiological exposures in the environment would occur. This is the balance being sought.

In the following, basic radiation protection bases will be explored first. Examples to illustrate the current art will follow.

PROTECTIVE ACTION GUIDES

One decision aid for radiological emergency planning is a Protective Action Guide (PAG), which is a projected absorbed dose to individuals in the general population which would warrent protective action following a contaminating event.[1,2] It can be helpful to make such projections for events which are only postulated. One can, for example, estimate the activity that would have to be released to the atmosphere, without a significant wind shift during the release period, to result in doses equal to PAGs offsite. A comparison of these calculated activities and inventories of radionuclides in plant systems can then be made to predetermine those system failures which could possibly lead to PAGs and those that could not, as a means to assess the light water nuclear power reactors (LWR) system implications of PAGs. The general approach can be extended easily to other fuel cycle activities and applied to specific sites.

At the outset a few basic perspectives are worth stating explicitly. First, it must be recognized that a Protective Action Guide is not an observable parameter. By its very definition a PAG is a *projected* dose. There are no projected dose meters or instruments. PAGs are conceptual guides rather than operational tools. Protective actions are undertaken based on observables related to what is occurring at a given time and the rate at which observables are changing. Current emergency planning emphasizes emergency action levels (EALs) rather than the protective action guides on which the EALs are based. EALs are predetermined observables which should prompt the initiation of specific predetermined actions should they ever be observed. The actions would not necessarily be protective; they could be simply notification actions, or assessment, corrective or mobilization actions, depending on the predetermined level or scoping of the threat or problem related to particular EALs. In fact, for many EALs developed to date it has been predetermined that protective actions in the public domain would *not* be warranted; this is an important emergency management decision made in the planning stage.

References 1 to 5 provide various protective action guidance for emergency planners. Table 1 lists doses presented in these references that do or could have the connotation of being a trigger level for emergency protective action, should they ever be observed. The British Emergency Reference Levels (ERLs) are independent of the pathway from source to individual. The U.S. Federal Radiation Council (FRC) doses are for the milk and food pathways. The U.S. Environmental Protection Agency (EPA) doses are for the external gamma and inhalation pathways. The U.S. Food and Drug Administration (FDA) doses are proposed for human food and animal feed. (The FDA also provided EALs for I-131, Cs-137, Sr-89, and Sr-90 for environmental contamination levels). Herein, only the whole body and thyroid doses due to atmospheric releases will be considered, and PAGs of 5 and 25 rem, respectively, will be used as representative of the guidance available. An appropriate caveat will acknowledge the important preventive PAG proposed by the FDA (see footnote for Table 1).

Table 1
DOSE COMMITMENT GUIDES FOR EMERGENCY PLANNING[a]

	EPA PAGs	FRC PAGs	British ERLs	FDA[b] PAGs
	Category 1			
Whole body	1—5	15	10	0.5—5
Thyroid	5—25	30	30	1.5—15
Bone				
Endosteal tissue	—	—	30	0.5—5
Marrow	—	15	10	0.5—5
Skin (beta)	—	—	60	0.5—5
Gonads	—	—	10	0.5—5
Lung	—	—	30	0.5—5
Other	—	—	30	0.5—5

[a] Dose commitments in rem.

[b] FDA PAGs are for food and agricultural pathways. At the lower PAG, milk-producing animals should be removed from pasture. At the higher PAG, milk should be removed from commerce.

Table 2
MINIMUM ACTIVITY INVENTORIES (CURIES) UNDER POOR METEOROLOGICAL CONDITIONS FOR PAGs OF 5 REM (WB) AND 25 REM (THY)

Isotope	Pathway	Dose Factor[a] (rem-m^3/Ci-sec)	Source term (Ci)[b,c] corresponding to 25 rem (Thyroid)	5 rem (Whole body)
I-131	Milk	115,000	2.2	
	Inhalation	395	630.	
I-133	Milk	8280	30.	
	Inhalation	174	440.	
	Cloud gamma	0.033	7,550,000.	1,510,000.

[a] Rem/Ci-sec/m^3 concentration-exposure in air. Childs thyroid dose commitment factors. Factor for cloud gamma dose taken as 1/6 semi-infinite cloud model dose factor for 0.8 MeV gammas.[6]

[b] At $X/Q' = 10^{-4}$ sec/m^3 (e.g., 10 m release height, F stability, 2 m/s wind, 2 km downwind).

[c] Typical annual releases (for comparison):

BWR 100,000 Ci noble gases; 1 Ci radioiodine.
PWR 200 Ci noble gases; 20 mCi radioiodine.

PAGs AND ACTIVITY RELEASES

Table 2 lists the total activities of noble gases and radioiodines which, if released under extremely adverse atmospheric dispersion conditions, could lead to offsite dose commitments of 5 rem whole body or 25 rem thyroid *via* the external (cloud) gamma, inhalation and milk pathways. For this example a dairy farm was assumed at 2 km downwind from a release point. In application, site-specific calculations would be made. The calculational procedure used to derive these inventories is presented and discussed briefly in Appendix A.

Table 3
TYPICAL INVENTORIES FOR A 1000-MW(e) NUCLEAR POWER REACTOR

	Inventories (curies)	
Location	**Fuel**	**Gaps**[a]
Core with 0.5-hr decay	8×10^9	1.4×10^8
Spent fuel storage pool	3.6×10^8 (AV)	3.8×10^6 (AV)
	1.3×10^9 (MAX)	1.3×10^7 (MAX)
Shipping cask	2.2×10^7	3.1×10^5
Fuel assembly with 3-day decay	2.2×10^7	2×10^5
PWR waste gas storage tank		9.3×10^4
BWR waste gas decay line		5.5×10^3

[a] "Gap" is a euphemism for the gas spaces in the fuel pellets and between the fuel pellets and the tube (cladding) holding the fuel pellets.

Except for the cloud gamma dose, the semi-infinite cloud model[6] was used for the calculations. For the cloud gamma dose under the assumed meteorological dispersion conditions (Class F atmospheric dispersion with a ground level release), the semi-infinite cloud dose factor for 0.8 MeV gamma rays was reduced by a factor of 6 to account for the finite extent of the cloud[6] and the decrease of dose with depth in the body. All other assumptions used are listed in the table. As shown in the table, releases of about 2.2 or 630 Ci of I-131 could lead to doses of 25 rem (thyroid) *via* the milk and inhalation pathways, respectively. A release of 1,510,000 Ci of gamma emitters could lead to a 5 rem (whole body) dose *via* the cloud gamma pathway under the assumed poor dispersion conditions. This presumes that no shelter or other protective measures were to be taken and that the exposed individual was to remain on the centerline of the cloud during its entire passage. For the milk pathway, dairy animals were presumed to graze uninterrupted on pasture contaminated by the center of the cloud. These are all very conservative assumptions, such that, for average meteorological conditions, considerably greater radioactivity would have to be released for a PAG to be exceeded at about 2 km. Inventories of these radionuclides in plant systems which are less than those noted would not induce doses greater than PAGs.

RADIONUCLIDE INVENTORIES IN LWR SYSTEMS

Estimates of inventories in LWR systems were collected for comparison to the activities listed in Table 2. These are displayed in Tables 3 and 4. Many of these data were taken directly from tables in References 7 through 10. Those estimated by this author, using data in these references, are as follows. The activity in a boiling water reactor (BWR) waste gas treatment system (WGTS) was calculated using the condenser off-gas radionuclide mix and release rates (2 Ci/sec total) presented in Reference 9. It was assumed that no gases escape from the WGTS and the resulting equilibrium activity is listed in Tables 3 and 4. All other data in Table 3 were obtained from Reference 7. In Table 4, the core gap activity was taken to be 1% of the total noble gas and radioiodine inventory in Reference 7; this is consistent with assumptions in Reference 7. The maximum radioiodine activity in the demineralizer in a pressurized water reactor (PWR) after a primary coolant purge (after shutdown) was estimated to be identical to that in the primary coolant with 0.1% being passed to the waste gas storage tank (WGST). For the noble gases, it was assumed that only 0.1% would remain in the demineralizer, with virtually 100% being passed to the WGST. The radioiodine activity listed in Table 4 for the BWR steam line was estimated from measured steam line concentration data presented in Reference 10 for four operating BWRs. These data were normalized

Table 4
TYPICAL NOBLE GAS AND HALOGEN INVENTORIES FOR A 1000-MW(e) NUCLEAR POWER PLANT

Location	Inventories (curies)	
	Noble gases	Halogens
Core with 0.5-hr decay	3.4×10^8	7.2×10^8
GAPS (1% Core)	3.4×10^6	7.2×10^6
Spent fuel storage pool	5.8×10^5 (Av.)	1.8×10^5 (Av.)
	4.6×10^7 (Max)	5.3×10^7 (Max)
GAPS	1.7×10^4 (Av.)	$9. \times 10^5$ (Av.)
	1.4×10^6 (Max)	2.6×10^5 (Max)
Fuel assembly with 3-day decay	4.1×10^6	2.7×10^6
GAPS	4.1×10^4	2.7×10^4
PWR waste gas storage tank after primary coolant purge	9.5×10^{4}[a]	1.
PWR demineralizer after primary coolant purge	9.5×10^1	$1. \times 10^{3}$[a]
BWR steamline (10^7 lb/hr)	10^4 Ci/hr	25 Ci/hr
BWR waste gas treatment system	5500	0.25
Shipping cask — gap activity	1.7×10^4 (Av.)	1 (Av.)
	1.4×10^6 (Max)	3.4×10^2 (Max)

[a] Primary coolant inventories.

to a 1000 MW (electric) power plant. All other system inventories are expected to be less than those listed in Tables 3 and 4.

LWR SYSTEM IMPLICATIONS OF PAGs

By comparing the data in Tables 2 and 4 one can conclude that at a light water reactor only the failure of irradiated fuel and fuel cladding could lead to off-site doses in excess of PAGs *via* all three pathways considered herein, i.e., the external cloud gamma, inhalation and milk ingestion pathways. Release of the gap activity in one fuel bundle within a few weeks after reactor shutdown could lead to off-site doses in excess of whole body and thyroid PAGs *via* the inhalation and milk ingestion pathways, but not *via* the external gamma pathway. However, spent fuel resides under about 30 ft of water, which can provide very efficient scrubbing of a release, except for relatively innocuous noble gases.

Only thryoid PAGs could be exceeded given gross failures of a selected few systems other than irradiated fuel. The BWR steam line break and the PWR steam generator failure accidents, which may release primary coolant, if not promptly terminated by appropriate corrective action, could lead to a thyroid PAG *via* the milk pathway. The appropriate immediate protective action in such a case would be to protect milk by removing selected dairy herds from pastures in nearby downwind areas.

In this light, only a loss-of-coolant accident (LOCA) with the release of coolant directly to the atmosphere, and damage to irradiated fuel could lead to off-site doses clearly exceeding PAGs. Only in the core of the reactor is there clearly enough energy to provide a driving force necessary to project the requisite activity into the atmosphere in a short time. As discussed in Appendix B the primary coolant (water, steam) would be the principal motive force.

These perspectives are succinctly summarized in Table 5. Emergency planners can use

Table 5
POTENTIAL FOR LWR SYSTEM TO CAUSE A DOSE EQUAL TO A PAG AT 1 MILE OR BEYOND (ATMOSPHERIC RELEASES)

System	Cloud gamma whole body PAG (5 rems)	Child's thryoid PAG	
		Via inhalation	Via milk[a]
Core fuel			
UO_2	X	X	X
Gaps	X	X	X
SFSP[b]			
UO_2 (total)	?	X	X
Gaps (total)	—	X	X
Fuel bundle UO_2	—	X	X
Fuel bundle gaps	—	X	X
Primary cooling water	—	?	X
Other systems	—	—	—

Note: X = Necessary inventory clearly available.
? = Necessary inventory available on occasion.
— = Necessary inventory not available.

[a] For FDA Emergency PAG of 15 rems. Both the PWR and BWR waste gas treatment system could occasionally contain enough radioiodine for the FDA preventive PAG of 1.5 rems (thyroid) to be exceeded if it were all released, especially during periods of rainfall.

[b] Spent fuel storage pool. Relatively cool used fuel stored under 30 ft or so, of water.

such information to predetermine the timing, type, and extent of predetermined protective actions appropriate for the postulated system failure(s). Some protective actions would be warranted based solely on in-plant observables. Although the strict FRC definition of a PAG addresses actions to be taken *following* a contaminating event, for selected events, e.g., on-site evidence of major core damage, immediate predetermined protective actions could be planned to be initiated even before an actual release occurs, if the planners can predetermine and agree on the necessary and sufficient conditions.

PREDETERMINED VS. AD HOC PROTECTIVE ACTIONS

The distinction between predetermined actions for predetermined conditions and ad hoc actions based on what may be observed at some future time is important. The word "initiate," as in "initiate protective actions," is also important. What may be planned to be initiated at some future time based on predetermined action levels can be changed on an ad hoc basis at any time, *for good cause*. The word "warrant" is also important, as in "initiation of predetermined protective action(s) would be warranted." "Warrant" implies a very strong recommendation that is not to be dismissed lightly. But it is not an irrevocable command. Further, protective actions can be initiated at any time based on what is actually occurring, or is perceived to be occurring at the time.

DICHOTOMY AND ITS RESOLUTION

The foregoing discussion is somewhat dissonant. Apparently, protective action decisions can be made now, which would be warranted for implementation at some future time. But *ad hoc* decisions can be made at any time. Until recently, the second option has been overriding in the planning process. Either covertly or overtly, in the past emergency planners have opted for today's protective action decision to wit: we will appraise each situation as it unfolds at the time and make our protective action decision then. This is a common management decision made in the face of major uncertainties regarding the future.

However, at the outset it was noted that one objective of emergency planning should be to make as many protective action decisions as possible before events occur, so as to minimize the number of decisions that would have to be made in an emergency. There exists today sufficient radiation protection guidance and knowledge of nuclear power plants to resolve the apparent dichotomy, remove the major uncertainties, and provide for management of future initial protective action decisions in today's time frame. The pertinent guidance will be discussed in the following two sections. Practical applications will then be discussed.

STOCHASTIC AND NON-STOCHASTIC RADIATION EFFECTS

Two basic radiation protection objectives are fundamental: in a controlled radiation environment (1), *avoid* nonstochastic effects, and (2) *reduce* stochastic effects to a level which is as low as reasonably achievable (ALARA).[11] Nonstochastic radiation effects appear at doses generally above 25 to 100 rem for total body irradiation and well above such doses for individual body organs. These effects would be manifest within hours or days after the dose is delivered. (Delivery of the dose over a short time is presumed, i.e., in days or less.) The effects include readily observable changes in blood cell counts at the low end (i.e., 25 to 100 rem whole-body dose), to death within a week to 60 days at the high end (i.e., 500 rads whole-body dose or greater). The 100 to 500 rad range is very narrow on the scale of possible doses, but it would require a truly momentus accident to induce such doses off-site.

Stochastic effects are those for which no dose thresholds for damages are presumed. These damages (effects) would occur randomly throughout the population of late survivors of an exposed population. Usually, the effect does not become manifest until after a delay (latent period) of 1 to 10 years, or so, and can occur at any time later. Leukemia is an example of this type of effect. The incidence rate of the effect is usually so low compared to "naturally" occurring effects that it would be extremely difficult or impossible to ascribe an effect in a particular individual to the earlier radiation exposure as a cause-effect relationship. Further, many of the effects may not actually occur at very low doses; they are, indeed, presumed.

As will be illustrated below, the potential for the induction of nonstochastic effects is limited as a practical matter to the area within 10 miles of a nuclear power plant. Conceptually, such effects are possible beyond 10 miles, but with vanishingly small probability and only by using bizarre assumptions (such as presumptions of disasters without even leisurely emergency response).

Stochastic effects, however, have no range (distance) limit under the assumption of no radiation dose threshold for such effects. Further, stochastic effects are in proportion to the number of people exposed. For most LWRs the product of population and dose (not shown) increases monotonically with distance from the source, with half or more of the population dose (sometimes called the collective dose) being accumulated beyond 50 miles in almost all cases.[12] This is true for any release occurring during dry weather. The bulk of the stochastic effects could be accumulated within shorter distances for releases of particulates and water soluble materials during periods of intense precipitation. Such materials could appear in surface waters after being washed out of the atmosphere and be transported long distances (over periods of at least weeks) to ocean waters. At any rate, stochastic effects are far-field effects, predominantly, and protective actions in the near field would seldom, if ever, be mitigating for them. As will be explained below, little, if any, radiation protection guidance is available to aid the emergency planner with regard to the far field and no predetermined criteria have been developed.

Thus, basic radiation protection objectives: *avoid* nonstochastic effects and *reduce* stochastic effects using ALARA, drive the emergency planners' primary attention to the near field as a practical matter, i.e., to within about 10 miles of a light water reactor.[13] These basic radiation protection objectives were formulated explicitly for controlled situations in the workplace, but they are transferrable to the postulated or conceptualized uncontrolled accidental release situation. Indeed, they are transferred in current emergency planning guidance, although seldom explicitly stated as such.

RADIATION PROTECTION GUIDES AND PROTECTIVE ACTION GUIDES

The concepts of ALARA and PAGs for unplanned releases were clarified in the U.S. in three guidance documents sponsored by the U.S. Federal Radiation Council and promulgated as guidance for Federal agencies by Presidents Eisenhower, Kennedy, and Johnson in 1960, 1961 and 1964.[2,14,15] The earlier Radiation Protection Guides dealt with the actions recommended for normal operations involving radioactive materials and with unplanned releases of radioactivity in quantities of a few to many multiples of routine planned releases.

The later Protective Action Guides were promulgated as thresholds for predetermined actions in the public domain. These thresholds are often taken as limits. PAGs clearly were not intended as limits: "If the projected dose *exceeds* the PAG, protective action is indicated" (emphasis added).[2]

Thus, PAGs are trigger levels for action, not limits on doses. Nevertheless, the FRC also said: "The PAG represents the Council's judgment as to where this (risk vs. benefit) balance should be for the conditions most likely to occur. If in a particular situation, there is available an effective action with low total impact, initiation of such action at a projected dose lower than the PAG may be justifiable. If only very high impact action would be effective, initiation of such action at a projected dose higher than the PAG may be justified." (Parenthetical remark added.)

These apparently conflicting directions are fundamental to the problem being addressed here.

The Radiation Protective Guidance was promulgated "for the guidance of Federal agencies in activities designed to limit exposure of members of population groups to radiation deposited in the body as a result of their (sic) occurrence in the environment." The Radiation Protection Guides (RPGs) are expressed as annual dose rates and concentrations of radioactive materials in the general environment. The RPGs are 1.5 rem/year for the thyroid, 1.5 rem/year for bone, and 0.5 rem/year for the bone marrow.

In addition, the FRC established graded scales of action for three ranges of transient rates of intake of radionuclides:

Range	Action(s)
I	Periodic confirmatory surveillance as necessary
II	Quantitative surveillance and routine control
III	Evaluation and application of additional control measures as necessary

Except in a very general sense, the FRC did not specify the meaning of the phrase "control measures", other than to state that "the character and import of these actions could vary widely, from those which (would) entail little interference with usual activities, such as monitoring and surveillance, to those which (would) involve a major disruption, such as condemnation of food supplies." It did not address at all the phrase "as necessary" in the

RPG guidance. This was not done until the Protective Action Guide concept was established later by the FRC, in 1964. As discussed above, it was then that the FRC limited the uncertainty to some extent when it established PAGs which would warrant protective actions. The principal thrust of the RPG guidance dealt with situations for which greater than normal surveillance and monitoring would be warranted.

It is necessary to interpolate between the RPG and PAG guidance to discover where control measures including disruption of the public would begin to be warranted. Clearly, within RPG Ranges I and II, such disruption would not be warranted. Here, controls on the source would be indicated. Clearly, at or above PAG levels, protective (vs. other) actions would be warranted. Thus, Range III marks the demarcation range.

To quantify this range, the FRC provided the following ranges of transient intakes for use with respect to the graded scale of actions:

Radionuclide	Range III (μCi/day intake)
I-131	0.0001—0.001[a]
Sr-90	0.0002—0.002
Sr-89	0.002—0.02

[a] For small children. For adults, the intake rate would be ten times higher.

For Range II, the daily intake ranges were established as a factor of 10 lower than for Range III. Range I encompasses zero intake to the lower limit for Range II.

The upper limits for daily intake for Range III of the RPGs can be compared to derived preventive environmental emergency action levels provided by the U.S. Food and Drug Administration.[5] These action levels are for monitored levels of radioactive contamination in the environment:

Nuclide	Preventive PAG (monitored variable) (μCi/ℓ in milk)	Total intake in body (infant) (μCi)
I-131	0.015	0.09
Sr-90	0.009	0.2
Sr-89	0.14	2.6

The protective action appropriate at these levels would be to remove grazing dairy herds from contaminated pasture to protect the sensitive milk pathway. Removal of such herds from pasture would cut this pathway at its source, the pasture, and if instituted at an appropriate early time could virtually eliminate the necessity for impounding milk supplies a few days later.

Comparison of the FRC Range III levels and the FDA preventive PAG derived levels shows that protective actions for the milk pathway would not be warranted until the FRC Range III levels were exceeded by a considerable factor, i.e., of the order of a factor of 10 or more (This assumes a nominal intake rate of 1 ℓ of milk per day.) Thus, an interpolation between the RPGs and the PAGs clearly indicates that throughout the RPG ranges, from I through III, controls on sources would be indicated actions. Protective actions would not be warranted until contamination levels well exceed the Radiation Protection Guides. This conclusion is a logical interpolation of existing Federal guidance, however, and cannot be attributed directly to a Federal body.

UNFINISHED BUSINESS (PAGs)

Before turning to the practical application of these radiological protection concepts in the emergency planning (vs. response) phase, it is well to consider explicitly two important aspects of the emergency planning problem which are not discussed in current protective action guidance. First, neither the total area nor the total population that might be affected by an accidental release is addressed in current guidance. This is unfortunate.

Clearly, what might be reasonably achievable over a small area or by a small number of persons might be extremely difficult or practically impossible to achieve over a large area or by a large number of persons. If one farm is ever contaminated to a low level (e.g., FRC Range III), protective (preventive) action might well be prudent under ALARA. If a whole state or region of the U.S. were to be contaminated at the same level, removal of all grazing dairy herds from pasture could be very disruptive. Such contamination could occur because of atmospheric weapons fallout, for example.

As a result, current emergency planning throughout the world is incomplete as regards definitive plans for controls over the very large areas that could be contaminated by a major nuclear power plant accident, or by weapons fallout. The planning for the food pathways today is limited to predetermined conditions for surveillance and monitoring and the establishment of control points. It is weak in addressing the major problems that would be associated with the disruption of large areas of commerce by the institution of protective and preventive actions on a massive scale.

This problem awaits resolution. In the meantime, ad hoc rather than predetermined actions would be instituted if the need ever arises. In essence, decision-makers are forced to decide today to delay some major projective action decisions regarding the far field until later.

The second problem regards the method or approach of the use of PAGs in the planning process. The focus on projected doses is nearsighted, at best, in the planning stage. The result is the prevalence of plans for environmental monitoring as a precursor to protective actions, regardless of the magnitude of an accident. In such cases the planners avoid protective action decisions in the planning stage. Such decisions are left for the response stage. The result is a patent, fundamental weakness: little is added to the provisions for safety since monitoring and ad hoc decisions would surely be performed in a response situation even in the absence of a special plan to do so.

This problem may have its source in the FRC definition of a PAG, which concludes with the phrase "... following a contaminating event." For many conceptual cases the phrase may be appropriate. But for some easily visualized cases it is inappropriate. For example, for fallout from atmospheric nuclear weapons tests, there is no *a priori* need to plan to await actual contamination of grazing herds in the eastern U.S. before fallout arrives from the west, especially where rainfall is intercepted. Grazing dairy herds could well be removed from pasture beforehand. Such a minimal protective action could be planned for appropriate cases, especially when stored feed is abundant. At this time no such decision has been made beforehand. Rather, the planning decision is to monitor first and act later.

This problem is even more visible for the case of plans for responses to accidents at nuclear power plants. In this case, the potential problems are well known, the locations of the plants are known, and the necessary conditions for the potential for PAGs to be exceeded are also known. Yet, many plant, federal, state, and local agency emergency plans call for protective action decisions to be made solely on an *ad hoc* basis, based on projected doses and radiological monitoring information at the time.

The emphasis on environmental monitoring as a precursor to protective action has its place, i.e., for smaller accidents.[16] But, for a major accident involving core melt, which should be an extremely rare event, the reactor containment should isolate the event from the outside world, so there should be little or no radioactivity emanating from the plant into the environment at the time, or ever, perhaps. Based on the prevalent current concept, projected doses would be less than PAGs; thus, no protective action would be indicated.

Yet, by hypothesis, the core would be melting,* a grave prospect. By prevalent concepts, protective action would not be indicated unless the containment failed with the possible release of large amounts of radioactivity to the environment in a puff. Patently, this would be somewhat late for protective actions to be initiated. This is a direct result of the use of the literal definition of the PAG, the reluctance of planners to predetermine when protective actions would be warranted (and unwarranted), and the emphasis on radiological monitoring as a precursor to protective action.

That the latter position is untenable for LWRs can be illustrated by a very simple example. Presume that the U.S.E.P.A whole body PAG of 5 rems would be the trigger level for protective action during an emergency, which it is touted to be in most LWR emergency plans. For argument's sake, take this absolutely literally. Operationally, during an emergency it would require a measured dose rate of the order of 1 rem/hr projected to be sustained for 5 hr for the PAG to be exceeded, or 5 rems/hr projected to be sustained for 1 hr, or 500 mrem/hr projected to be sustained for 10 hr, or a similar combination. All of this without a projected wind shift during the projected release period. Using the example inventories, presented earlier, required to induce a PAG at 2 km (1.25 miles) downwind, it is obvious that at least megacuries per hour of radioactivity would have to be in the effluent stream at the source, projected to be sustained for hours. On a normal day, scores of megacuries per hour would have to be in the effluent stream. In brief, there would have to be an accidental release of ominous proportion before protective action would be recommended to the public, under this concept. Although such a response scenario is conceivable, a *plan* to respond in such a manner is not a prudent plan. It provides little in the way of a potential benefit for the public over and above what would surely occur without a plan. In short, it is not much of a plan.

As will be explained in the next section, at this time the attention of emergency planners is being focused on predetermined *plant* conditions that *should and should not* prompt the initiation of predetermined protective actions offsite. As will be seen, under this scheme the operators at the plant would become the implementers of protective action decisions made years earlier by planners. This ''act first, monitor later'' concept was described succinctly and to the point by the National Council on Radiation Protection and Measurements in Appendix C to NCRP Report No. 55:[17]

MILK CONTROL

Countermeasures to avoid milk contamination and the risk of radiation exposure to milk users resulting from a nuclear facility accident must be implemented immediately after an accident if they are to be effective. The protective actions to be considered require breaking the cycle through which contamination spreads, namely, the pasture-cow-milk-man pathway.

Since the potential for accidental radiation exposure of the population through milk may extend for many miles from the accident site; and since the magnitude of exposure through milk may be 400—700 times greater than through inhalation, the need for appropriate (early) protective action is of paramount importance.

First, a predetermined emergency communications plan must be set in motion on an area-by-area basis whereby dairy farmers in the (likely) affected land area are alerted immediately and instructed by the appropriate state and local officials to move their cattle from pasture to stored feed. This breaks the cycle of transmission of radioactivity contamination at the root and must be accomplished immediately.

Within 48—72 hours, contaminated land areas can be identified by ground and aerial surveillance. Only those farmers in contaminated land areas would be required to keep their cattle on stored feed. This obviously reduces the possibility of fluid milk contamination ...'' The parenthetical words were added by this author.

This eminently reasonable ''act first, monitor later'' plan to protect the milk pathway

* Core melt should be distinguished from fuel melt. Core materials (steel, silver, zirconium) have much lower softening and melting points than uranium oxide fuel.

Table 6
EMERGENCY CLASSIFICATION SCHEME

Class	Plant operator action	Offsite agency action
Notification of unusual event	Notifications	Awareness
Alert	Mobilize plant resources	Standby
Site area emergency	Full mobilization	Mobilize and inform public
General emergency	Full mobilization	Recommend predetermined protective actions off-site

illustrates the simplicity, practicality and potential efficiency and efficacy of the result. The introduction of an analogous planning concept for the protection of people also is the principal thrust of current emergency planning.

EMERGENCY CLASSIFICATION SCHEME — PREDETERMINED ACTIONS FOR PREDETERMINED PLANT CONDITIONS

Based in part on the foregoing concepts, a four-level emergency classification scheme is currently being implemented for nuclear power plants.[18] Each class of emergency would require predetermined types of actions appropriate to the import of the classification. The four levels, in increasing order of severity, are called (1) unusual event, (2) alert, (3) site area emergency, and (4) general emergency.

This nomenclature is standard in the U.S. industry to assure the commonly understood import of an emergency classification, i.e., the very names scope the extent or magnitude of an emergency and predetermined actions. The operator, utility, and off-site agency actions for each class are succinctly described in Table 6. Fuller descriptions of the classes and examples of predetermined events are presented in Table 7. The preponderance of nonradiological initiating conditions is noted. Individual plants must develop observables (emergency action levels) which would indicate the presence of the initiating event. The operators must declare and announce the appropriate emergency class within 15 min of the observation of the predetermined action levels, or within 15 min of an *ad hoc* decision to declare an emergency based on other observations of similar import. (It is presumed that the reader will pause to study Tables 6 and 7.)

The general emergency is the only class for which protective actions in the public domain have been predetermined. Indeed, it has been predetermined that immediate predetermined protective actions would *not* be warranted for the lower classes of emergencies. These are fundamental scoping decisions made in the planning stage, long before emergencies would occur.

General emergencies would be called for a core melt or for plant conditions clearly leading to core melt. A core melt condition should be obvious to the operators. For conditions clearly leading to core melt, no unusual radiological indications need be present. The projected dose offsite at either time could well be zero (see Appendix B). Yet protective action would be warranted, as planned years earlier. For example, a general emergency would be called should physical control of a nuclear power plant ever be lost to intruders. In this case, no unusual plant parameters need be present, radiological or not. (Security plans and alarms should be activated at the time, of course, but the point is with regard to the other

Table 7
FOUR LEVEL EMERGENCY CLASSIFICATION SCHEME

Emergency class	Class description	Example initiating conditions[a,b]
Unusual event	Events are in progress or have occurred which indicate the potential degradation of the level of safety of the plant. No radioactive releases requiring off-site responses expected.	Loss of off-site power or on-site ac power capability. Fire lasting more than 10 min. Security threat or attempted sabotage. Contaminated patient transported to hospital. Radiological effluent technical specifications exceeded. Reactor scram (unplanned shutdown).
Alert	Events are in process or have occurred which involve an actual or potential substantial degradation of the level of safety of the plant. Any radioactive releases expected to be small fractions of EPA PAG exposure levels.	Increase in radiation levels in-plant by a factor of 1000. Complete loss of any function needed for plant cold shutdown. Fire potentially affecting safety systems. Ongoing security compromise. Loss of all on-site dc power. Primary coolant leak rate greater than 50 gal/min. High radiological effluent release rate (>5Ci/sec).
Site area emergency	Events are in progress or have occurred which involve actual or likely major failures of plant functions needed for the protection of the public. Any releases not expected to exceed EPA Protective Action Guide exposure levels except possibly near the site boundary.	Fire compromising the functions of safety systems. Loss of all vital on-site dc power for more than 15 min. Loss of off-site power and loss of on-site ac power for more than 15 min. Loss of coolant accident (LOCA) greater than makeup pump capacity. Degraded core with possible loss of coolable geometry. Evacuation of plant control room and control of shutdown systems not established from local stations in 25 min.
General emergency	Events are in progress or have occurred which involve actual or imminent substantial core degradation or core melt.	Loss of physical control of the facility. Any major internal or external event which could cause massive common damage to plant safety systems (e.g., major uncontrolled fires in safety systems; major earthquakes). Loss of two of three fission-product barriers with clear potential for loss of the third. Extremely high levels of radiation in containment (e.g., 10,000 R/hr or greater). For pressurized water reactors (PWRs) Small and large LOCAs with failure of emergency core cooling system (ECCS). Loss of feedwater and condensate systems, followed by loss of emergency feedwater. Containment isolation and failure of containment heat removal systems for several hours. For boiling water reactors (BWRs) Transient with failure to control reactor power (e.g., failure to SCRAM). LOCA with ECCS failure. Reactor shutdown (e.g., SCRAM) but decay heat removal systems fail to function for several hours.

Table 7 (continued)
FOUR LEVEL EMERGENCY CLASSIFICATION SCHEME

[a] These example initiating conditions are not EALs. EALs are the predetermined observables associated with the initiating conditions.

[b] These are specific predetermined examples only, presented as aids in scoping possible events and associated emergency classes. Other conditions may occur for which the plant operators must decide an emergency class on an ad hoc basis, using these examples as guides. Other predetermined conditions can be developed as warranted.

plant aspects.) The plant could well be operating normally, i.e., producing electric power. Yet, the nearby public would be requested or ordered to leave the area. This has been decided now.

Patently, general emergencies should be extremely rare events. Indeed, they should never occur. Concommitantly, initiation of predetermined protective actions should never occur. Conversely, should a general emergency ever be declared, such would be an event of grave import and world-wide notoriety. Precautionary evacuation of at least nearby areas, where feasible, should commence, and even larger areas would be impacted. This should result from the very declaration of the general emergency. Yet, so long as the containment remains intact, little or no contamination of the environment would occur, *a la* the infamous accident at Three Mile Island. The predetermined initial protective actions for this class are precautionary in intent. Predetermined evacuation and shelter scenarios for the general emergency class are elaborated on below.

The radiation protection basis for the General Emergency class is very simple. As shown above, if a reactor core is not damaged or threatened, protective action guides should not be exceeded in the near term and the immediate initiation of predetermined protective actions would not be warranted. If a reactor core is damaged at some future time, the operators would have 15 min to correct and control the situation; if they could not, the planners say today that the situation then would be so grave that predetermined precautionary protective actions would be warranted. We are unwilling to plan to await coincident containment failure. *Early* initiation of protective action is planned, well before an actual major release. Yet the action level is so high it should never be reached.

The importance of the operator in this scheme cannot be overemphasized. The operators are first on the scene, they are always present. They must scope their problem. The operators are instructed (and protected) by emergency operating procedures which they are charged to follow. The action levels for general emergencies have been predetermined by plant management and agreed to by state and local agencies before the event. The state and local agencies agree to the predetermined action levels and predetermined actions, also long before the event. Indeed, the planners and decision-makers who made the initial decisions may no longer be in evidence or in positions of authority at the time. The plans are laid with the understanding that protective actions off-site will not be initiated without grave cause, and will be initiated *early* (i.e., well before a major release) for sufficient cause.

The other three emergency classes have equally well-founded bases. The unusual event class was developed in response to numerous state and local agency requests to receive information regarding unusual conditions at a plant before these come to the attention of the media (and then the public). To minimize even the appearance of "not knowing what is going on" and to assure the exercise of emergency organization notification schemes, the unusual event "emergency" class was established. For this class, notifications of various preselected individuals is the predetermined action. This "emergency" class also has the potential to stop rumors of events of greater import. Noteworthy, no protective actions would be recommended to the public for events in this class. This has been decided now.

The alert emergency class would require additional staffing of on-site emergency centers as the predetermined action. The purpose of this emergency class is very simple: source control. For this class, events threatening irradiated fuel would be in progress which the operators could not control within 15 min of their awareness, and which would involve significant degradation of plant systems needed for control of irradiated fuel. Radiation levels could be normal. An uncontrolled fire in plant secondary safety systems would be an example for this class. The immediate predetermined actions would require the addition of a number of preselected individuals of various expertise to the plant staff within about 30 min of the alert declaration. This assures (but does not guarantee) that a variety of skills would be called to the plant, or made available, in a timely fashion to help control whatever situation occurs, of the noted type. State and local agencies would also be notified for this class; simple awareness is all that would be required of them for this class. No public notifications are planned for this class.

The site area emergency class would require the staffing of both on-site and off-site emergency centers. A high level of emergency preparedness is predicated. Radiation levels may be normal. An uncontrolled fire in a primary plant safety system is an example of an event which could trigger this class. If radiation levels were or could be elevated, radiological monitoring teams would be dispatched both on-site and off-site. Notification of the public would not be mandatory, but could commence in order to control rumors that might be caused by the planned high level of activity (not necessarily radioactivity) in the area, as by interception of shortwave radio signals, for example. If radioactivity in small to moderate levels is actually released, low impact protective actions may be instituted but on an *ad hoc* rather than a predetermined basis, based predominantly on environmental monitoring data. Removal of dairy herds from pasture in nearby areas to protect milk may be recommended, for example, especially where rainfall would be intercepted. This class corresponds closely to the classical emergency response plan.

This predetermined, graded response, emergency action scheme conforms in both letter and spirit to the basic radiation protection guidance discussed above.

SHELTER AND EVACUATION PLANS

The predetermined protective action scheme for a general emergency calls for graded scales of timing and sizes of off-site areas that would be affected.[18] Initially, persons in all areas within 10 miles of plant would be notified to take shelter as available, shut windows and doors, and listen to radio and television for further instructions. Prompt notification means must be in place continuously, and periodically exercised, to assure the capability to provide the initial notification of the public within 15 min of the general emergency declaration.[19] These means include administrative and physical means. (These *prompt* notification means should not be confused with the *early* notification scheme.)

It should be noted that this is not a ''hair trigger'' scheme, 30 min could elapse between the onset of extensive core damage and the notification of the public. These 30 min would be available for assessment and corrective actions by the operators and reduction of the emergency class. If, in 30 min from the onset of the action levels, the conditions for a general emergency were to persist, predetermined notifications of the public for protective actions would be initiated. These 30 min are not provided by design, however; rather, the planning recognizes that it would require such elapsed times to carry out various necessary actions by plant and notification officials.

With these comments as background, the predetermined immediate and early evacuation and shelter plans[18] can be scoped succinctly as follows:

1. If irradiated fuel is not damaged, no public notifications would be warranted.
2. If spent (used) fuel is damaged, no immediate predetermined protective actions offsite would be warranted.

3. If significant core damage, or the clear threat thereof, occurs (e.g., ten to thirty percent cladding failure), the public within about 2 miles should be instructed to evacuate where possible as a precautionary measure. All other persons would be instructed to remain in available shelter. (At a few highly congested, high population density sites, only those persons within the 2-mile radius might receive the earliest notification, although provisions for the warning capability would extend for about 10 miles.[19])
4. After the immediate notifications of the public, if the operators cannot assure that the situation is under control, persons within 5 miles would be instructed to evacuate, when feasible before a major puff release. If control is assuredly established, all persons beyond 2 miles would be instructed to remain in available shelter.
5. If a major puff* release of radioactivity actually occurs, the following instructions should be provided to the public: those evacuating should continue; those in shelters should remain in shelters; those stalled in traffic should take the best shelter available. In addition, radiological monitoring teams, aided by meteorological projections, would locate and identify areas of high contamination left in the wake of the puff. Areas of rainfalls and calms should be identified quickly. Immediate evacuations, where at all possible, of areas of identified high contamination would be recommended. Television would be very helpful in this situation. Evacuation in directions perpendicular to the puff traverse should be recommended, where possible, as this would require the least amount of time.[20]

These would be the immediate, predetermined actions. After these actions were accomplished, the designated emergency response organizations would proceed on an *ad hoc* basis using information available at the time. Note that actions 1, 2, and 3 would be initiated solely on the operator's assessment, as predetermined. The other steps would require more complex and coordinated emergency responses. In all but extremely rare circumstances, step 3 should be completed well before the necessary coordinations could be reasonably accomplished.

SHELTER AND EVACUATION DISTANCES

The basis for the predetermined evacuation and shelter distances is informed judgment. There is no guiding formula or equation. In the remainder of this section various facets of the considerations that led to these distances will be explored, but the following is not to be taken as a classical argument of proof.

For core melt accidents at nuclear power plants, the potentials for stochastic and nonstochastic radiation effects in individuals can be illustrated using Figures 1 through 3. In Figure 1 the qualitative relationship between dose and distance for an atmospheric release is shown. The upper curve in Figure 1 shows the theoretical relative reduction in dose with downwind distance (not necessarily line-of-sight distance). The lower curve shows the relationship as it most often occurs as a practical matter. These curves are normalized to a distance of 0.5 mile, which is the average distance from a LWR to the site property line. As illustrated in Figure 1, there is a major reduction in dose potential between 0.5 and 2 miles, with a smaller dose reduction potential between 2 and 5 miles. This reduction is due to atmospheric dilution.

At all but a very few nuclear power plant sites, there are relatively few persons within 2 miles of the plant. This area is included in what are called the "Exclusion Area" and the "Low Population Zone" required by the siting regulations of the Nuclear Regulatory Commission.[21] Except in the most unusual circumstances there should be few impediments to immediate evacuations of these areas. The coincidence of a core melt and serious impediments to a speedy egress of such small areas should be extremely rare to nonexistent. In the rare

* All life threatening releases would be puff releases. See Appendix B for a discussion of major accident sequences.

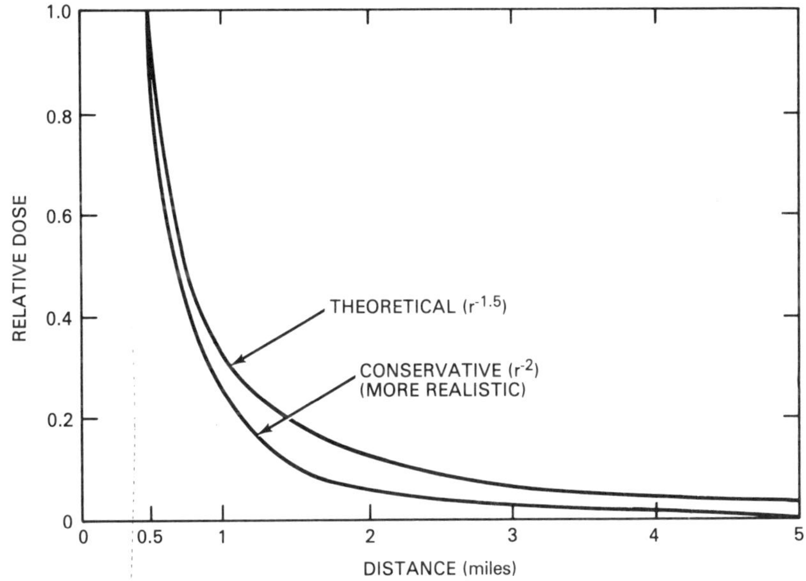

FIGURE 1. Dose potential as a function of distance along actual track of a puff. A ground level release is assumed. The lower curve is a $1/r^2$ relationship.

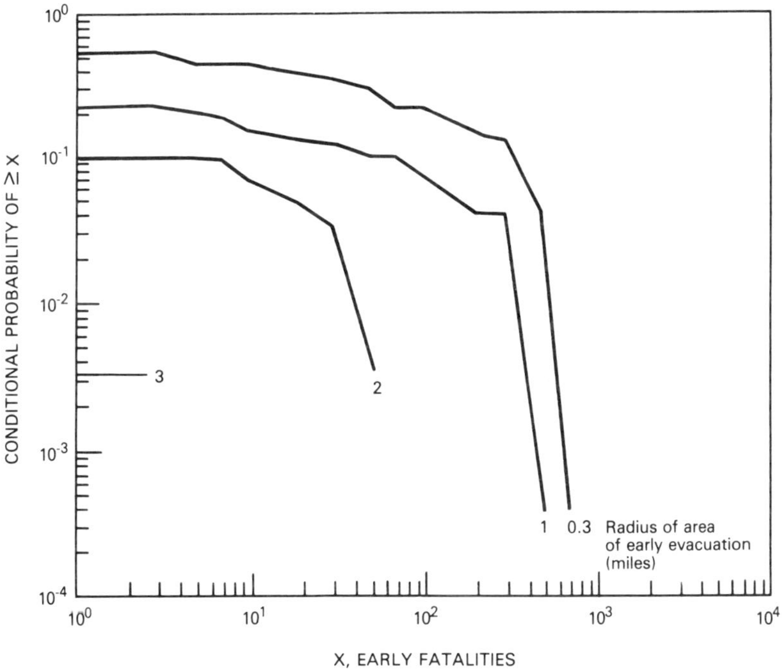

FIGURE 2. Illustration of the potential for reduction of early fatalities assuming early evacuation within various distances. A major atmospheric release and sheltering beyond the noted distances for 4 hr after the passage of a puff was assumed.

case where the low population zone (LPZ) does not extend to 2 miles, the predetermined immediate evacuation area could be limited to the LPZ, with shelter elsewhere.* Shelter

* NRC Regulations allow a staged (by area) public notification scheme.[19]

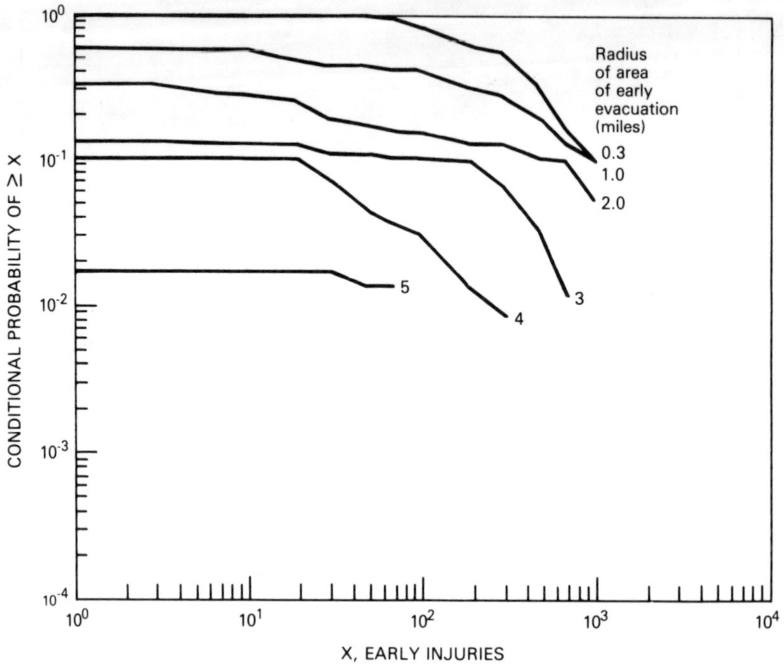

FIGURE 3. Illustration of the potential for reduction of early injuries assuming early evacuation within various distances. A major atmospheric release and sheltering beyond the noted distances for 4 hr after the passage of a puff was assumed.

should be more efficacious in high population density areas, as compared to low population density areas.

The potential for avoidance of nonstochastic effects in the event of a major nuclear power plant accident is illustrated in Figures 2 and 3. The assumptions made for the calculated results in these figures were: population density of 1000 persons/square mile (a very high density); sheltering for 4 hr after passage of a puff by the population outside various early evacuation zones; early evacuation (before a release) by persons within various distances of the plant; and the propulsion of major fractions of the inventory of radionuclides in the core of a 1000-MW -electric reactor (highest power level) into the atmosphere, at ground level, in a puff, with very short warning time (1 hr). The calculations were made using the Consequences of Reactor Accidents Code (CRAC) developed for the Nuclear Regulatory Commission.[22,23]

The sensitivity tested in these calculations was the probability and numbers of early fatalities and injuries as a function of the distances within which early evacuations were conducted. The results are shown in Figures 2 and 3.

As illustrated in Figure 2, for even this extreme accident early evacuations of areas within 2 miles of a plant would substantially reduce the chance of an early fatality. As discussed further below, early fatalities at the longer ranges would be caused by a coincident rainfall.

As illustrated in Figure 3, early evacuation within 2 miles would reduce the probability of an early injury by a factor of nearly ten as compared to the immediate shelter assumption. Early evacuation of areas within 5 miles reduces this relative probability by a factor of fifty. But, at one-third of the LWR sites in the U.S. the number of residents within 5 miles is large, 10,000 to 100,000.[24] Evacuation by such large numbers of persons is infrequent (see below) and would be very disruptive, and could require a few hours to accomplish. At these sites, especially, any predetermined evacuation action levels for the five mile radius must be appropriately qualified, as they are in 4 and 5 above.

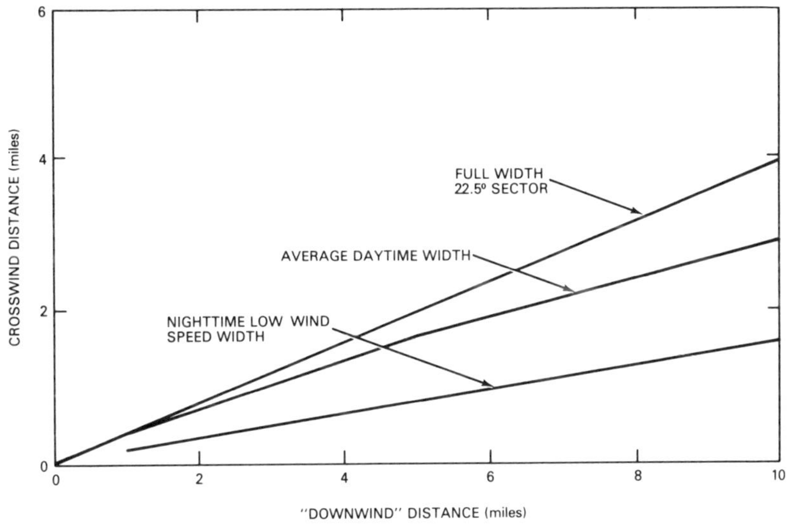

FIGURE 4. Theoretical full widths of puffs at 1% of maximum concentration vs distance along track of puff.

Two observations are helpful to the planner in this regard. First, all of the calculated early injuries beyond 2 miles (illustrated in Figure 3) resulted from rainfall situations and were due to the high ground level dose rates resulting from heavy deposition of radionuclides on the ground after plume (puff) passage.[12,23] Second, the area of heavy contamination would not be wide. Normally, it would be possible to walk out of the contaminated area in a reasonably short time. This potential is illustrated in Figure 4 in which the full width of a puff is shown as a function of distance along it's track, for two atmospheric dispersion conditions. For reference, the width of a 22.5° sector (1/16 of a circle, corresponding to the width of sectors for the sixteen cardinal compass directions, N, NNE, NE, etc.) is also shown in the figure.

As illustrated in Figure 4, at 5 miles the ''footprint'' of a puff should be less than 2 miles wide. At 10 miles along the trajectory, the width would be less than 4 miles. In either case, the average person normally could walk easily out of a highly contaminated area in a relatively short time (an hour or so). Interestingly, given early warning and clear instructions, a person could walk away cross-wind from plumes and avoid plume exposures entirely,[20] but this would be an idealized case most often. However, in those instances when the plume could be seen (see Appendix B), walking away from a plume could occur as a natural reaction for some persons.

Thus, evacuation of contaminated areas between 2 and 5 miles should be quite feasible normally for most persons in the vicinity of at least two-thirds of the LWR sites in the U.S. At the remaining sites sheltering in the area between about 2 and 5 miles might be preferred as a predetermined measure until after passage of a puff, after which people in highly contaminated areas could be requested or ordered to leave. Shelter factors should be more substantial in highly congested areas. Early identification of areas of calms and precipitation would be extremely important in the event of an actual major release; there is no practical limit on the distance to which such effects could be manifest.

PERSPECTIVES ON EVACUATION

A few perspectives regarding evacuations of historical record are noteworthy. Emergency evacuations by thousands of persons are not uncommon. Indeed, in the U.S. sizeable evacuations occur with a frequency of 1/week to 10 days.[25-27] Noteworthy is the fact that injuries and deaths due to the evacuations, per se, are rare; historically, a risk of about one death per million persons moving is observed.[25] Trauma and fright are normally observed, but panic is rare.[25-29] Widespread panic has not been observed in evacuations. Often, more time is consumed by authorities in coming to a decisions to order an evacuation than by the evacuees leaving an area. Indeed, the latter observation was one of the principal motivating factors for the development of predetermined action criteria.

Precautionary evacuations are common.[25-30] Some cryptic information regarding evacuations which occurred during the period March 1976 through June 1978 is presented in Table 8. These were compiled from news clippings by this author. The observation that no deaths or injuries due to the evacuations, per se, is often made in news accounts. Other compilations confirm these general observations.[25-30] Coincidentally, as this is being written (December 14, 1982) 17,000 evacuees are returning to a "5 mile area" (sic, CBS News) in the southern U.S. and 5000 persons are leaving an area in the western U.S. No injuries were observed in the former incident, at least. The 17,000 evacuees live near a nuclear power plant currently under construction; the plant was not the cause of the evacuation.

The dynamics of the evacuation process can be complicated. Analyses of the process most often center on roads, intersections, and queueing theory. But the complications should not hide the facts of the matter. The process of leaving an area is common. A helpful perspective on the matter can be obtained by perusal of the information in Figure 5, which illustrates road capacities using the three assumptions noted in the figure caption. Curve A in this figure is for the case of the National Safety Council safe driving admonition: maintain a 2-sec separation time between vehicles. As illustrated in Figure 5, road capacities exceed 1000 vehicles/hr/lane at speeds as low as 10 mph. In fact, using the 2-sec rule, speeds over 10 mph add little to the road capacity. A capacity of 2000 vehicles/hr/lane is common in a heavy traffic situation (see curve C of Figure 5).

From this perspective, one can easily understand the observation noted in a U.S.E.P.A. study[25] that evacuations of up to 15,000 persons/hr/road have been observed in evacuations by large numbers of persons (the average occupancy per vehicle was observed to be four). It is also understandable why many thousands of persons have been observed to evacuate an area in a few hours or less. The emptying of a sports stadium is a common example.

It has long been known[28,29] that warning time and motivation of the public are the key elements of a successful evacuation. Provisions in an emergency plan for reduction of warning times and for strong motivating instructions are the key elements of an evacuation plan. Extremely inclement weather, e.g., a heavy snowfall on the roads, would present a severe impediment to evacuation, or course (see the following section on entrapment scenarios). Such major impediments to evacuation could be identified quite easily at any time and a contingency immediate shelter recommendation would be the obvious choice at such a time. However, in the light of the fact that the public, *itself*, would implement either an evacuation or shelter plan, the provisions for early and prompt warning and motivation would be the same in either case. In essence, the public protects itself in an emergency, by and large. Regardless of what one would want members of the public to do to protect themselves from something they could not sense, one would have to tell them. And the earlier they would be told, the better, in a clear and imminent threat situation. Thus, an evacuation plan reduces to a notification plan,* as does a shelter plan.

One final note regarding the matter of roads: to empty something, the funnels must be kept open. Much attention is often paid to the intricacies of road networks within areas to be evacuated. This is a myopic viewpoint. The important roads are those leading from the

* The distinction between early evacuation and relocation is noted. Early evacuation should be planned to occur in low population areas *before* serious exposure to a puff. Relocation would be a later protective action to reduce exposures in localized heavily contaminated areas.

Table 8
SELECTED EVACUATIONS OF RECORD

News date	Time	Place	Number of persons	Incident
4/26/78		Bowling Green, Ky.	1,500	Tank car containing poisonous gas ruptured.
5/15/78		Nacogdoches, Tex.	1,000	Chemical explosion — train wreck.
6/21/78	11 p.m.	Salonika, Greece	600,000	Earthquake.
6/30/78		Destrehan, La.	3,000	Rail car gas leak (styrene gas).
4/8/78		Brownson, Neb.	1,500	30-car derailment — tank car exploded (phosphorous).
4/8/78		Pineville, Ky.	2,000	Liquid propane tank car leak.
4/1/78	p.m.	Kingsburg, Ind.	2,500	Fire at chemical plant — toxic fumes.
3/15/78	p.m.	Steubenville, Ohio	2,000	Chemical plant explosion — toxic chlorine gas.
3/8/78	Day	Vicksburg, Miss.	1,200	Insecticide tank at chemical plant exploded.
3/2/78		Galax, Va.	200	1600 gal liquified propane spill.
2/27/78		Youngstown, Fla.	250	Ruptured railway car — chlorine gas — wind shift noted.
2/27/78		Waverly, Tenn.	2,000	Derailed tank car explosion — volatile propane.
1/28/78	a.m.	Damascus, Ark.	500	Leak from fuel tank (nitrogen tetroxide).
1/17/78	a.m.	Pond Eddy, Pa.	52	11,000 gal acetaldehyde spill.
12/29/77		Goldonna, La.	800	Chemical freight train crash.
11/29/77	3 a.m.	Norfolk, Neb.	1,000	Tank car carrying propane gas ruptured.
11/28/77	Night	Battle Creek, Neb.	771	Propane gas leak from tank car.
11/8/77	Noon	Marion, Ia.	1,000	Tank car carrying propane gas ruptured.
10/15/77		St. Marys, Kan.	600	Toxic fumes — unknown origin.
10/13/77	Day	Chattanooga, Tenn.	800	Gas fumes — elementary school.
10/8/77	Day	Midland, Mich.	2,000	Poisonous chlorine gas leak — from chemical plant.
10/4/77	Day	Kansas City, Mo.	160	Elementary school — carbon monoxide leak.
9/19/77	3 a.m.	Berryville, Ark.	2,600	Fire — fertilizer warehouse — ammonia and nitric acid.
9/5/77	9 p.m.	Watseka, Ill.	2,000	Railroad car derailed — ethylene oxide.
7/13/77	3 p.m.	Rockwood, Tenn.	5,200	Chemical truck wreck.
5/17/77	3 a.m.	International Falls, Minn.	2,000	Rail car leaked chlorine gas.
12/11/76	3 p.m.	Baton Rouge, La.	10,000	Chlorine gas leak — chemical plant.
5/29/76		Centerville, Ill.	500	Toxic fumes released — 2 tank cars. Chlorosulfonic acid and sulfuric acid.

Table 8 (continued)
SELECTED EVACUATIONS OF RECORD

News date	Time	Place	Number of persons	Incident
5/16/76	4 a.m.	Glen Ellyn, Ill.	1,000	Tank car leaking toxic ammonia fumes.
4/13/76	4 a.m.	Dwight, Ill.	3,800[a]	Liquid bromine leak — truck.

[a] Included the evacuation of 209 severely retarded and handicapped children only nine of whom could walk; 92 elderly patients from a different center, also. Total time consumed by the evacuation was 2 hr, and little confusion was noted. Public officials complained about the lack of resources.

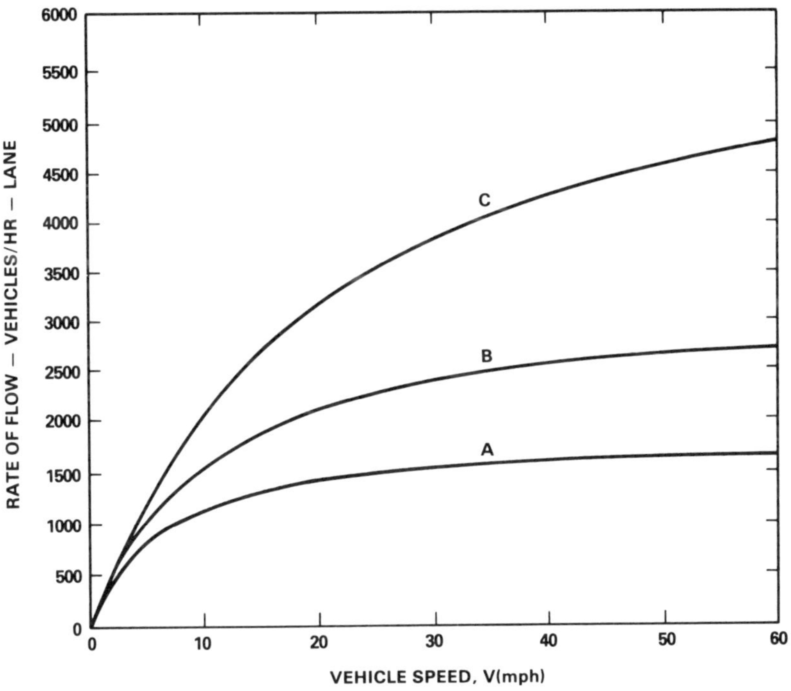

FIGURE 5. Rate of flow of vehicles per lane of road; (A) 2 sec separation time; (B) separation distance of 1 vehicle length/10 mph of speed; and (C) separation distance of 1 vehicle length/20 mph of speed. Average vehicle length of 16 ft assumed.

periphery to open areas. Bottlenecks and dead ends outside the area to be evacuated would be the major roadway impediments during normal weather conditions. Further, it would be helpful to stop traffic intent on entering from distances two to five times the radius of the area to be evacuated. Only about 330 vehicles can occupy one lane-mile of road.

This information is not presented to make a case for the cavalier treatment of evacuations. Evacuations should not be ordered without grave cause. However, given grave cause, such as a core melt at a nuclear power plant, trauma and fright in the public domain would be expected and understandable, but broadcast panic would not be expected. The expeditious movement by up to at least many thousands of persons should be a low-risk activity. Contrary, false impressions by many radiological emergency planners are a serious impediment to the development of evacuation criteria and plans.

ENTRAPMENT SCENARIOS

Objections to this predetermined protective action and emergency management scheme can be raised. Indeed, it is not perfect. There is no guarantee that all persons would receive exposures at levels as low as reasonably achievable given their particular situations at all times. Evacuation is not a panacea. In retrospect, after an accidental release, it could well be determined that some persons left a perfectly safe area only to have arrived at an unsafe area during transit. The special case of intercepting and traveling with a puff is discussed in some detail in Appendix C. Many such scenarios can be readily conceptualized for which the predetermined action scheme would not be the best, or an available, response. However, coincidences of core melt and major impediments to speedy egress of small areas by most people should be extremely rare. Expedient shelter of some sort is always available. Morever, most state and local emergency planners have identified population groups for whom special assistance would be provided during an emergency for which evacuation would be warranted.

Entrapment scenarios are simple to postulate. A major release of radioactivity without warning is conceptually possible, as a major earthquake which causes a reactor accident. A major snow and ice storm coincident with a major LWR accident can be postulated, and is possible. In these cases, many people could be harmed. For the most part, such scenarios are entrapment by definition: by postulate there is no way out. These postulates are most disturbing to those who seek absolute guarantees of safety, no matter what the circumstances.

Absolute guarantees are not available and are not given. Rather, these action plans are of the nature of a limited warranty. They have been devised based on an extensive background of radiation protection concepts and practices, knowledge of plant systems, investigations of thousands of potential accident scenarios, and abundant information regarding the response of the public in threatening situations. They call for early, normally feasible protective actions. They offer an excellent chance for avoidance of unnecessary disruption of the public, for avoidance of nonstochastic radiation effects, and for maintaining stochastic effects to reasonably achievable levels, even under major nuclear power plant accident conditions. They meet the primary objectives of an emergency response plan.

SUMMARY

The management of emergency preparedness for the nuclear power industry centers around the concept of predetermined actions to be initiated for predetermined conditions. The predetermined conditions and actions are embodied in four scoping emergency classes. The plant operators would have 15 min to control predetermined situations after they become aware of them, or officially declare the appropriate emergency class. For plant conditions which exclude the clear potential for core melt, notification, assembly, and corrective actions are predetermined. For actual or imminent core melt conditions immediate precautionary evacuations of nearby areas are planned, even in the absence of effluent radioactivity. The latter should be extremely rare to nonexistent events. Immediate protective actions are predetermined to be unwarranted for noncore melt events. After the initiation of the predetermined actions, augmented staff would proceed as necessary based on actual conditions at the time. This is an "act first, monitor later" scheme for major accidents and a "monitor first, act later" scheme for lesser accidents.

Under this scheme the plant operators would be the key individuals in the initial phase of an emergency response. This is appropriate. Those first on the scene must scope the magnitude of a problem. By predetermining the actions appropriate for predetermined conditions, the emergency planners have provided the operators with the authority and responsibility to implement a graded scale of predetermined actions appropriate for a wide spectrum of predetermined possibilities. Appropriate actions should be initiated early under this scheme. For slowly developing events, the early availability of expert assistance for the site should assuage a deteriorating situation before it becomes serious. For situations which would threaten the public, the predetermined action levels should prompt the initiation of feasible protective actions by the public *early*, well before a release occurs, to provide the nearby public with time for an appropriate protective response.

This scheme is not perfect. But it was developed on a rational, logical basis after carefully considering fundamental radiation protection guidance, applying a good deal of common sense, and with the recognition that timeliness would be the essence of a response to an emergency. The requirements for appropriate, early and predetermined responses of a graded scale, provide a high degree of assurance that emergency responses, at licensee, federal, state and local levels will be timely and in proportion to the levels of the threat at the time.

REFERENCES

1. Federal Radiation Council, Background material for the development of radiation protection standards, report No. 5 (July 1964) and 7 (May 1965), USGPO, Superintendent of Documents, Washington, D.C.
2. Federal Radiation Council, Radiation protection guidance for federal agencies — memorandum for the President, *Fed. Reg.*, 64-8590, 12056, August 22, 1964.
3. Medical Research Council, Criteria for controlling radiation doses to the public after accidental escape of radioactive material, Her Majesty's Stationary Office, London, September 1974.
4. U.S. Environmental Protection Agency, Manual of protection action guides and protective actions for nuclear incidents, EPA-520/1-75-001, Office of Radiation Programs, Washington, D.C., September 1975, revised July 1979.
5. U.S. Food and Drug Administration/Department of Health and Human Services, Accidental contamination of human food and animal feeds — recommendations for state and local agencies, *Fed. Reg.*, 43, 242, December 15, 1978; 47, 205, October 22, 1982, 47073.
6. U.S. Atomic Energy Commission, Meterology and Atomic Energy — 1968, D. Slade, Ed., (n.b. pp. 329 and 347). Availability: NTIS, Springfield, Va. 22161.
7. U.S. Nuclear Regulatory Commission, Reactor Safety Study, Appendix V, WASH-1400 (NUREG-75/014), October 1975. Availability: NTIS, Springfield, VA. 22161.
8. **Dyer, N. C. and Baston, J. E.,** PWR Waste gas treatment system dose evaluations under upset conditions — final report, Aerojet Nuclear Co., Idaho Falls, Idaho, June 1975.
9. **Dyer, N. C., Schultz, R. J., Killian, E. W., and Baston, J. E.,** BWR Waste gas treatment system dose evaluations under upset conditions, Aerojet Nuclear Co., Idaho Falls, Idaho, May 1974.
10. **Pelletier, C. A.,** Results of independent measurements of radioactivity in process systems and effluents at boiling water reactors, Environmental Programs Branch, USNRC, Washington, D.C., May 1973.
11. International Commission on Radiological Protection, *Recommendations of the International Commission on Radiological Protection — Radiation Protection*, ICRP No. 26. Pergamon Press, New York, January 17, 1977.
12. U.S. Nuclear Regulatory Commission, Technical guidance for siting criteria development, NUREG/CR-2239. USNRC, Washington, D.C., December 1982.
13. U.S. Nuclear Regulatory Commission and U.S. Environmental Protection Agency, Planning basis for the development of state and local government radiological emergency response plans in support of light water nuclear power plants, NUREG-0396; EPA 520/1-78-016, USNRC, Washington, D.C., December 1978.
14. Federal Radiation Council, Radiation protection guidance for federal agencies — memorandum for the President, *Fed. Reg.*, 60-4539, 4402—4403, May 18, 1960.
15. Federal Radiation Council, Radiation protection guidance for federal agencies — memorandum for the President, *Fed. Reg.*, 26, 9057—9058, September 26, 1961.
16. **Martin, Jr., J. A.,** Perspectives on the role of radiological monitoring in an emergency, *Trans. Am. Nucl. Soc.*, 34, 727—729, June, 1980.
17. National Council on Radiation Protection and Measurements, Protection of the thyroid gland in the event of releases of radioiodine, NCRP Report No. 55, August 1977.
18. U.S. Nuclear Regulatory Commission and U.S. Federal Emergency Management Agency, Criteria for preparation and evaluation of radiological emergency response plans and preparedness in support of nuclear power plants, NUREG-0654/FEMA-REP-1, Revision 1, November 1980 (n.b. Appendix I.)
19. Nuclear Regulatory Commission, Emergency planning — final regulations, *Fed. Reg.*, 45, 162, August 19, 1980.
20. **Martin, Jr., J. A.,** Doses while travelling under well established plumes, *Health Phys. J.*, 32, 305—307, April, 1977.
21. Code of Federal Regulations, Title 10 (Energy), Part 100 — Reactor site criteria. USNRC, Washington, D.C.
22. U.S. Nuclear Regulatory Commission, Overview of the reactor safety study consequence model, NUREG-0340, USNRC, Washington, D.C., June 1977.
23. Personal communication, Dan Albert and Dave Aldrich, Sandia National Laboratories, Albuquerque, N.M.
24. U.S. Nuclear Regulatory Commission, Demographic statistics pertaining to nuclear power reactor sites, NUREG-0348, USNRC, Washington, D.C., October 1979.
25. U.S. Environmental Protection Agency, Evacuation risks — an evaluation, EPA-520/674-002, Office of Radiation Programs, USEPA, Washington, D.C., June 1974.
26. **Hilbert, G. O., Berkley, J. H., and Quinn, F. M.,** Mississauga: lessons in large scale evacuation, NUS Corporation, Rockville, MD. In 1982 Hazardous Materials Spills Conference (Proceedings), April 19—27, 1982, J. Ludwigson, Ed. Avail: Government Institutes, Inc. 966 Hungerford Drive, Rockville, MD 20850. December 1982.

27. **Gant, K. S. and Schweitzer, M.,** Protective actions as a factor in power reactor siting, Oak Ridge National Laboratory, Oak Ridge, TN, draft October 1982.
28. Defense Civil Preparedness Agency, a perspective on disaster planning, TR-77, U.S. Federal Emergency Management Agency, Washington, D.C., December 1972.
29. **Perry, R. W., Lindell, M. K., and Greene, M. R.,** *Evacuation Planning in Emergency Management,* D.C. Health & Co., Lexington, MA, 1981.
30. **Kreps, G. A.,** Individual and societal effects of peacetime and wartime nuclear disasters, in Proceedings of a Sypmposium: The Control of Exposure of the Public to Ionizing Radiation in the Event of Accident or Attack, April 1981, National Council on Radiation Protection and Measurements, Bethesda, MD.

APPENDIX A
DERIVATION OF EQUATIONS

The radionuclide inventories listed in Table 2 in the main text were derived using the following approach: Dose rate (D) is related to radionuclide concentration (χ) by the relationship:

$$\dot{D} = (\chi)\ (DRF) \tag{1}$$

where DRF is an appropriate dose rate factor. The state of the art today of environmental dose and pathway models is such that dose rate ractors are tabulated for important radionuclides, body organs and pathways.[1,2] For atmospheric releases χ is derived from the relationship:

$$\chi = (\chi/Q')\ (Q') \tag{2}$$

where χ/Q' is the aeolian dilution factor, the ratio of concentration (χ) of a pollutant at a point downwind of a release occurring at a rate Q'. Then,

$$\dot{D} = (\chi/Q')\ (Q')\ (DRF) \tag{3}$$

Thus, dose rate $\dot{D}$ is proportional to release rate, Q'. χ/Q', may be obtained from equations or, more easily, from graphical displays.[3] A consistent set of units for these parameters must be used, of course. One consistent set would be $\dot{D}$ in rad/sec, χ in curies/m^3, Q' in curies/sec, and DRF in rad/sec per curie/m^3.

In these units, χ/Q' is in sec/m^3. It is helpful to picture the inverse of χ/Q', i.e., Q'/χ, which has units of m^3/sec, i.e., a volumetric flow rate. If a pollutant is mixed with a large volume of fresh air (high flow rate, or high m^3/sec), then χ/Q' is small, and vice versa. Thus, χ/Q' is simply a measure of dilution. Good mixing of a pollutant with fresh air leads to a low χ/Q'. Values of χ/Q' are in the range 10^{-4} to 10^{-6} sec/m^3 between 1 and 10 miles from a ground level release.[3]

Assuming that χ/Q' is constant over the period of release, Equation 3 can be integrated to obtain an equation for the total does (D):

$$D = (\chi/Q')\ (Q)\ (DRF) \tag{4}$$

Here, total dose, D, is proportional to total Curies released, Q. The values of Q tabulated in Table 2 in the main text were derived by simply equating D to a protective action guide for the pathway of interest, assuming a particularly adverse χ/Q' (i.e., 10^{-4} sec/m^3), and selecting a tabulated DRF appropriate for the particular pathway of interest. Q was then calculated using the last equation, above. The DRFs used to derive the Qs in Table 2 are listed in Table 2. Although other tabulations may provide slightly different values of DFRs than those used herein, the principal insight would not change significantly.

REFERENCES

1. U.S. Atomic Energy Commission, Final environmental statement: numerical guides to meet the criterion "as low as practicable...", WASH 1258, Vol. 2, U.S. Nuclear Regulatory Commission, Washington, D.C., 1973.
2. U.S. Nuclear Regulatory Commission Regulatory Guide 1.109, U.S.N.R.C. Washington, D.C., 1977.
3. **Turner, D. B.** Workbook of atmospheric dispersion estimates, AP-26 U.S. Environmental Protection Agency, Office of Air Programs, Research Triangle Park, N.C., revised 1970.

APPENDIX B*,**
LWR ACCIDENT SPECTRUM-RELEASE CHARACTERISTICS AND CONSEQUENCES

Possible releases of radioactive materials from light water nuclear power reactors (LWRs) range from the routine and benign to the catastrophic and deadly, with likelihood (or probabilities) ranging from unity (routine releases) to very small (catastrophic releases). Before TMI the latter types of accidents were not explicitly considered in the AEC and NRC licensing process. Since TMI, the potential for the high (off-site) consequence accidents are being considered explicitly in numerous licensing areas, notably in off-site emergency planning. The demarcation is the current explicit consideration of those accidents which include major or massive containment failures.

The problem, of course, is the enormous amount of volatile radioactive species present in the core of an operating LWR and the power in the decay heat (after shutdown) available to drive this material from the core into the environment. Shutdown decay heat is of the order of 3 to 5% of full power during the first hour after shutdown. For a 3300 megawatt-thermal (MWT) reactor, initial decay heat is an impressive 150 MWT, a substantial driving force if not controlled (vaporization of water at a rate of about 1000 gal/min could remove this decay heat and protect the core, by the way). The in-core activities of volatile species are impressive also. The billion, or so, curies of these species ($^1/_2$ hr after shutdown) can be broken down roughly as follows: 300 million (M) Ci of noble gases; 600 M Ci of radioiodines; 130 M Ci of tellurium-132; 30 M Ci of ruthenium-106; 20 M Ci of radiocesiums; and a host of other radioisotopes in substantial abundance. These are the potential radiological source terms.

It is instructive to compare these inventories to the activity required to be released to induce doses equal to Protective Action Guides. For a X/Q' of 10^{-4} sec/m^3, the following table can be constructed:

PAG (rem)	Q (curies)	Organ/pathway
5	1,500,000	Whole body/cloud (external) gamma
25	600 (I-131)	Thyroid/inhalation by child
15	2 (I-131)	Thyroid/air-pasture-cow-milk-ingestion by child

Thus, a release of only very small fractions of the core inventory would be needed to result in doses exceeding PAGs in the near field off-site. However, only irradiated fuel and primary cooling water contain the requisite inventories. No other system failures would induce a PAG. Thus, where current PAGs are planned as triggers for protective actions off-site, only the reactor core, the spent fuel storage pool, and the primary water should be of concern and a loss of coolant accident (LOCA) or the significant threat thereof would be a necessary precursor to protective action off-site. The fuel in the fuel storage pool is cool to start with, or course, so the primary concern from a PAG perspective is the core.

One caveat is important: The U.S. Food and Drug Administration (FDA) has proposed a preventive PAG of 1.5 rem for the milk pathway, for which dairy animals should be removed from likely or actually contaminated pasture. Catastrophic accidental releases of I-131 from the waste gas storage tank at a PWR site, or the effluent treatment system at a

* Combines Mr. Martin's two Workshop presentations: "Consequence Scenarios and Sensitivities", and "Release Characteristics from a Spectrum of Accidents".

** Reprint from NUREG/CR-0032, Proceedings of the Workshop on Meteorological Aspects of Emergency Response Plans for Nuclear Power Plants, Dec. 1—3, 1981, Menlo Park, CA, August 1982, U.S. Nuclear Regulatory Commission, Washington, D.C.

BWR, could result in pasture contamination leading to such a PAG, especially during a period of precipitation.

The masses of various materials that could be involved in a core melt accident may be of interest also:

H_2O	2×10^5 kg
UO_2	10^5 kg
Zr (clad)	2.0×10^4 kg
Sn (clad)	300 kg
Fe (structure)	2.5×10^3 (in core)
	2.5×10^4 kg (core + bottom structure)
I	18 kg
Cs	255 kg
Ba, Sr, Mo	416 kg
Zr (fission product)	276 kg
Ru, Rh, Pd, Te	318 kg

and smaller masses of other radionuclides. (Silver in control rods is receiving increased attention currently because of its low melting point and volatility at high temperatures).

Many chemical forms of these materials would be present in a core melt scenario; gases, vapors, particulates, soluble, and insoluble forms are possible in many combinations. The radioiodines and cesiums are of special concern because of volatility and high consequence potential. (Noble gases are relatively innocuous). A noteworthy complicating factor in this regard is the decay chain Te, I, Xe, Cs, Ba, La; a halide (I) decays into a noble gas (Xe), which decays into an alkali metal (Cs). The matter is extremely complicated, but an important current consensus is that in an aqueous environment, even at high temperatures, I and Cs would exist as I^- and Cs^+ ions dissolved in water and in a dry system I_2 would be the dominant form of iodine. Many interesting reactions involving steel, paint, hydrogen, lubricants (oils), steam, and high temperatures which produce organic iodines (e.g. gaseous CH_3I) have also been noted. If released to the atmosphere, CH_3I could decompose in sunlight to form I_2, however; the phenomenon has been observed, but little is known about it.

The distribution of particle sizes is also of interest. Very little hard data is available in this regard. What is known can be succinctly stated: insoluble materials rapidly agglomerate to diameters in the range 0.5 to 2. μm, with log-normal distributions of geometric standard deviation in the range 1.5 to 1.8. In an aqueous (steam) environment in a containment these particles act as condensation nuclei for the formation of water droplets, the sizes of which are in the range 10 to 20 μm. Settling of larger droplets acts to cap the size. This information pertains to intact containments and the atmosphere within a steamy containment. Interestingly, fog and a definite violet tinge has been observed at high I_2 concentrations in such an environment. Very little is known in the reactor community regarding the particle size distributions that would be evident in the atmosphere in failed containment scenarios. Evaporation of droplets of hot water released (blown out) to the atmosphere would leave residual particles of speculative size but probably less than several microns. For intact containments, only very small (submicron) sized particles would be released to the atmosphere; most likely, only the noble gases would be released in significant abundance, over a long term, a la the TMI accident.

Before proceeding to a discussion of major accident sequences and consequences thereof, it is worthwhile, even necessary, to establish a perspective regarding their probability or likelihood. Succinctly, the likelihood is very low for a single reactor and for the industry in any year. The calculated probability per reactor year projected over the lifetime of the current industry is also low, but there is a large uncertainty in the current estimates. The current status is illustrated in Figure 1, in which release fractions of the core inventory for various accidents are plotted against the calculated probability of such releases. The data points displayed are taken from the Reactor Safety Study (WASH-1400) and are illustrative

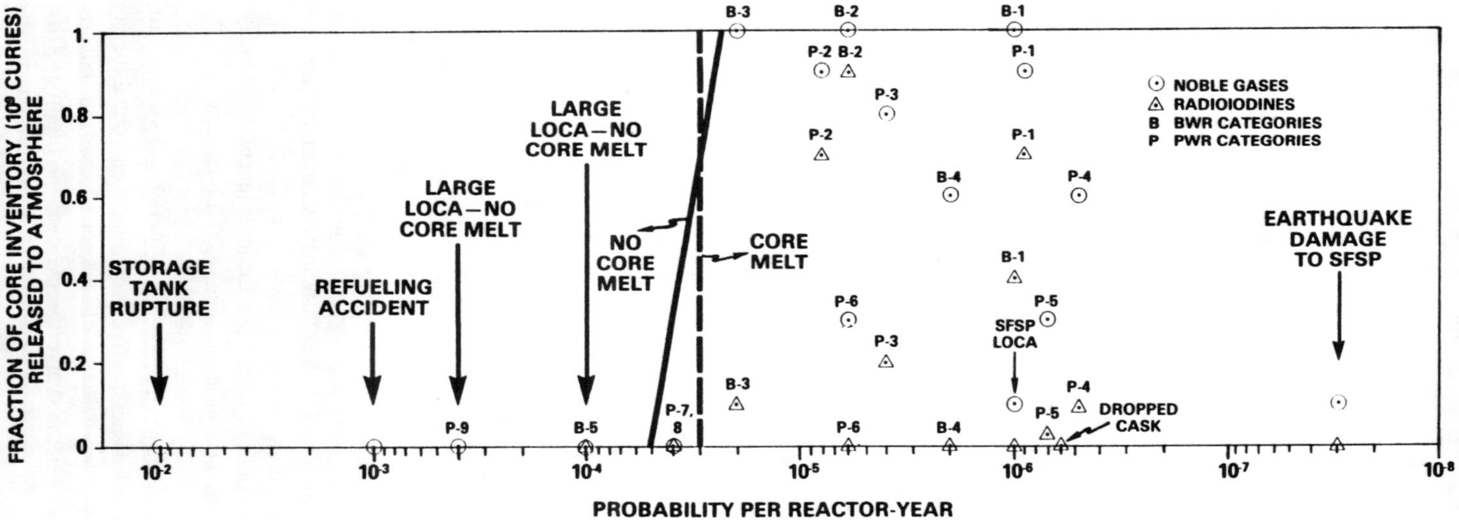

FIGURE 1. Release fractions vs. probabilities for nuclear power plant postulated accidents. From Tables V2-1 and V2-2 of Wash-1400 (Reactor Safety Study).

only since they may or may not truly represent the current industry, post-TMI fixes. The following comments on this data and its importance are a fair representation of the current estimates, nonetheless. It is obvious from the figure that the probabilities of major release fractions are at or below about 2×10^{-5}/reactor year. It is extremely difficult to cope with such small numbers. Assuming 100 reactors of current vintage operating for 40 years each (the current industry), and a probability of a major release of 2×10^{-5}/reactor year, the probability of a major release during the life of such an industry would be 0.08, or 12:1 against such an occurrence. This is a not uncomfortable prospect. Unfortunately, the uncertainty in the basic probability estimate is very large, off-times quoted as at least an order of magnitude either way. Thus, the calculated chance of a major release in the U.S. over the life of the industry is in the range between virtual certainty and at least 100:1 against. This estimate does not include considerations of sabotage and certain external events, e.g., massive earthquakes.

It is also worth noting that the large release fractions (0.1 to 0.8) of the core inventory as presented in Figure 1 have been strongly attacked as being unrealistically high. Considerable efforts are underway at this time (ca. early 1982) to assess the potential release fractions more realistically. For scoping purposes, it is merely noted here that certain potential release fractions can hardly increase significantly (from, e.g., 0.8) and that a reduction by a factor of ten to twenty would virtually eliminate the chance of early death and injury as consequences of LWR accidents, assuming only a modicum of leisurely protective actions off-site.

Catastrophic decompression of a containment would result in the release of large amounts of water, at least, at sonic velocities (choked flow). Depending on the location of the break and the initial trajectory of the release (up or down), plume rise up to 600 m, or so, is possible, but the range 10 to 200 m is more likely. Release rates as high as 2×10^5 g/sec (H_2O) have been estimated. It is not known whether or not the water would flash to vapor in the atmosphere, or agglomerate into drops large enough to settle out. Mass loadings could be as high as 20 g (H_2O)/m^3 (air) at a mile or so, i.e., at the saturation point at STP. (A deep sea fog contains 1 to 3 g H_2O/m^3 air). Explosive decompression would be spectacular, or course. The leading puff release could last from minutes to tens of minutes, depending primarily on the magnitude of the driving pressure and reservoir. The puff release of water could contain anywhere from very little of the core inventory to major fractions of the core inventory of radionuclides, depending on the accident sequence (loss of water before or after core damage or melt).

Patently, if a containment does not fail catastrophically, longer duration releases (a la TMI) would result. These releases would be gases and vapors, predominantly. However, daughter products of the noble gases and condensible vapors would be attracted to atmospheric particles, most likely in the submicron range (0.1 μm or less) where the available number density and surface area (for condensation) is highest. These daughter products are relatively short lived (40-min half-life, or less, e.g., Rb-88 and Cs-138). The capture of these particulate daughter products in air samplers could prove misleading to the unwary.

Many containment failure/core melt scenarios can be postulated, but four sequences encompass the various possibilities:

1. Core melt/melt-through of basemat
2. Core melt/containment failure by overpressure
3. Containment failure by overpressure/core melt
4. Containment bypass/core melt

The first two of these are notorious. The first is the "china syndrome" accident where the core melts through the concrete base and enters the ground. Pressure relief is via tunneling of water, steam, etc. to the surface, with a ground level release, or only a small plume rise.

This would be a dirty release and should be obvious. There is a good chance, however, that only invisible noble gases would percolate to the surface. Time delays after melting of the core through the steel pressure vessel to the basemat could range from hours to days, and never in some cases. Failure of containment heat removal systems during this sequence could (would in small containments) result in containment fracture, or catastrophic failure resulting in a rapid blowdown. A 1 ft^2 hole, e.g., a 2″ × 6′ crack, would result in a blowdown (blowout) in a $^1/_2$ hr or less. Operability of containment sprays and filters would influence (reduce) releases to the environment, but the results would be messy, nonetheless, because of flashing of steam and water aerosols carrying radioactivity. A very large (200 m) visible plume rise could result if the release were to be directed upward. Rainout from the plume (puff) is possible. Substantial deposition near the source and a moderate plume rise could result for a downward directed release. Major fractures below the water line would release the largest fraction of the available activity (curies). The smaller the crack or opening above the water line the larger the resulting ratio of noble gas to other species of materials, and the slower the release. In general, the less water that is flashed or otherwise projected to the atmosphere, the greater should be the ratio of noble gases to other species, and the less the consequences off-site.

The last two sequences listed above would involve containment failure before core melt. Both would involve major losses of low activity coolant to the atmosphere initially, but with possibly significant differences in off-site consequences due to the different potentials for internal scrubbing via natural processes. The third sequence could result from a failure to scram (trip, shut off) the reactor upon containment isolation, the dumping of large amounts of power into the containment (more than the containment heat removal systems could handle), and containment failure due to overpressure. The resulting massive loads could cause a massive LOCA, or LOCAs, and core melt. Relatively large fractions of the radioactive materials released from the core could remain in containment deposited on various surfaces because of the relatively lower driving force (i.e., loss of pressure before melt). Major releases at ground level could result, nevertheless, but less than that produced when a strong driving force exists on radioactive material per se.

The fourth scenario is called the interfacing systems LOCA, or Event V in the Reactor Safety Study where it was first identified. In this scenario the primary cooling water blows down via a failure in isolation valves separating the 2000 psi primary system (PWR, BWR pressure is 1000 psi) and a low pressure system (e.g., RHR system at 100 psig). This blowdown by-passes containment entirely. There is enough potential energy to actually destroy the auxiliary building if released in a short time ($^1/_2$ hr or less). The core then melts, releasing materials at a rate proportional to volatility (i.e., in sequence, noble gases, iodines, and cesiums, etc. with some mixing). It is currently assumed that because of the high heat these volatiles escape to the atmosphere without significant plateout in the plumbing. There is a possibility being investigated, that the driving forces for these volatiles would not be sufficient to prevent substantial plateout, resulting in a smaller (yet substantial) source term. Vapors released to the atmosphere would eventually condense on atmospheric particles (and possibly some core matter). This would be a short duration, also spectacular, accident with potentially very high consequences because of the short (no) warning time before release. Although the initial blowdown could result in a moderate plume rise of the relatively low activity water, the high activity releases could be near or at ground level. Since the identification of this sequence, quality assurance on the interfacing systems has been intensified to reduce its likelihood substantially.

Many other types of accidents can occur, of course, but unless irradiated fuel is damaged, radiation exposures off-site should be well below that necessary to induce a dose for which there would be a detectable radiation effect in the human body. As noted above, PAGs should not be exceeded unless damage to irradiated fuel or a LOCA occurs. Nevertheless, emergencies may well be declared for non-LOCA or fuel damage accidents, hearings may be held, fines assessed, and reports written in response to such accidents of lesser importance. Part of the record may be an assessment of doses and contamination levels in the environment, for which meteorological information will be used, at least in part. It must be recognized, however, that for such events the collective (population) dose, i.e., the man-rem, or person-rem, may well be the prime issue. Latent cancers and genetic effects are functions of the collective dose. It is important to recognize that such doses occur predominantly where the people are, which is predominantly far from the source of the release, often between 20 and 100 miles from the source. Thus, regional meterology during the period of release and subsequent transport, rather than site meteorology, would be the prime meteorological concern. Site meteorology during the period of release would be used, in part, to assess conformance with pertinent regulations regarding doses at or near the site boundary, i.e., 10 CFR Part 20, Appendix I to 10 CFR Part 50, 10 CFR Part 100 (NRC Regulations), and 40 CFR Part 190 (EPA Regulation). For such assessments, numerous dosimeters are currently required in the site environs to provide a direct measurement of external (cloud) gamma dose (and "shine" dose). Air samplers are also required in the environs, but there is an excellent chance that any release would miss these fixed samplers. Many small accidents would result in puff releases, and would be long gone before portable air samplers could be fielded. Thus, site meteorology would be important to assess inhalation exposures nearby resulting from small releases. Since small accidental releases are virtually certain, whereas large releases are speculative, it may well be the case that the site meteorological data will find its most important use in demonstrating that pertinent regulations are not violated.

Given an accidental release in-plant or on-site, which results in a release to the atmosphere, there may or may not be a measured release or release rate available (i.e., a source term). Consequences of noncore-melt accidents will be discussed first. Most releases in-plant should be released, if at all, through engineered safety features (e.g., filters) and past or through radiation detectors. Two aids would be available in this case: source terms should be small and dominated by noble gases, and a measured release rate would be available. An exception could occur if the source of a release is aged spent fuel in the spent fuel storage pool (SFSP). In this case weak gamma and beta emitting longer-lived noble gases (Xe-133 and Kr-85, respectively) could be mixed in roughly equal proportions (curies) with other volatile species (I, Cs) and a source term may not be known, especially in older LWRs. Normally, if a source term has been measured, that release can be assumed (at least initially) to have passed through engineered safety features, lacking any evidence to the contrary.

Some smaller accidents could result in a release that by-passes monitored release paths. Most of the potentially more serious noncore-melt accidents would fall in this category. The consequences of such accidents are assessed using very conservative assumptions in Safety Analysis Reports (SARs) for all but the very oldest LWRs. A typical table in an SAR could appear as follows:

		Dose (rem) at 2206 m[a]	
Infrequent accidents	**Duration of release**	**Thyroid**	**Whole body**
Radioactive waste system failure	2 hr	0.1	0.1
Steam generator tube rupture[b]	2 hr	13	1.0
Fuel handling accident	2 hr	2.1	0.044
Limiting faults[b]			
Main steam line break	2 hr	79	1.0
Large-break LOCA	2 hr	85	1.2

[a] The site boundary distance which yields the highest radiological dose following the postulated accident.

[b] These presume some fuel failures as part of the scenario.

Table 1
CONTRIBUTION OF DIFFERENT EXPOSURE PATHWAYS TO LATENT CANCER FATALITIES FOR A PWR-2 RELEASE CATEGORY[a]

	Percentages							
	Leukemia	Lung	Breast	Bone	GI Tract	All other	Total	Whole Body
External cloud	0.2	0.1	0.5	0.1	0.1	0.1	1	1
Inhalation from cloud	0.5	4	0.7	0.2	0.4	0.2	6	3
External ground (<7 days)	3	2	7	0.7	0.9	3	16	16
External ground (>7 days)	12	8	28	3	4	11	66	68
Inhalation of resuspended contamination	0.2	1	0.2	0.4	0.2	0.1	3	2
Ingestion of contaminated foods	2	1	3	1	1	1	9	10
Subtotals	18	16	39	5	6	16	100	100

[a] Except thyroid cancer, which is calculated separately.

Such information could be used to scope the potential consequences, recognizing the extreme conservatisms in the assumptions and calculations performed before the fact. The various assumptions are listed in SARs. One conservatism, the use of the "semi-infinite" dose factor for external (cloud) gamma whole body dose is noteworthy. The use of this dose model tends to overestimate the whole body dose by a factor of 5 to 20 for the meterological conditions assumed during the release period (e.g., Pasquill Class F stability, 1 m/sec wind speed). Consequences of accidents of this ilk would involve the inhalation and contamination pathways predominantly. From a meterological standpoint, the trajectory of such releases, ground level puffs for the most part, would be of paramount concern, mostly for the initial direction of site and off-site radiological survey terms. Diffusion should be of secondary concern initially, since the lack of a source term would prohibit an accurate dose calculation. (Although this is certainly true, guesstimates of dose would undoubtedly be made to satisfy craving appetites. For such gross estimates visual observation of local weather conditions should suffice to estimate the stability class at the time and precalculated doses and dose rates for various scenarios would be useful assessment aids).

Consequences of releases of major fractions of the core inventory of volatile radioactive species to the atmosphere would be severe, widespread, far-reaching and long lasting. From a meterological and protective action standpoint, it is extremely important to recognize the high worth of the ground contamination pathways as compared to the cloud (external) gamma and inhalation pathways. An appreciation of this perspective can be gained by a perusal of the information displayed in Figure 2 and Table 1. Figure 2 illustrates the calculated contribution of various nuclides to whole body dose, by three major pathways at a range of $^1/_2$ mile, for one postulated core melt scenario (the BWR-1 release from the Reactor Safety Study). Average whole body dose contributions are displayed, as calculated for 91 different weather sequences. The time scale on the horizontal axis pertains to the inhalation pathway only, and merely indicates that the whole body dose after inhalation monotonically increases somewhat over a period of time as the radioactive material in the body releases its energy. The important meteorological perspective is that the contributions of dose via the three pathways (inhalation, cloud (external) gamma, and ground contamination) are about equal (1/3 each) on the average at short range for these scenarios. This is for a 4 hr exposure to

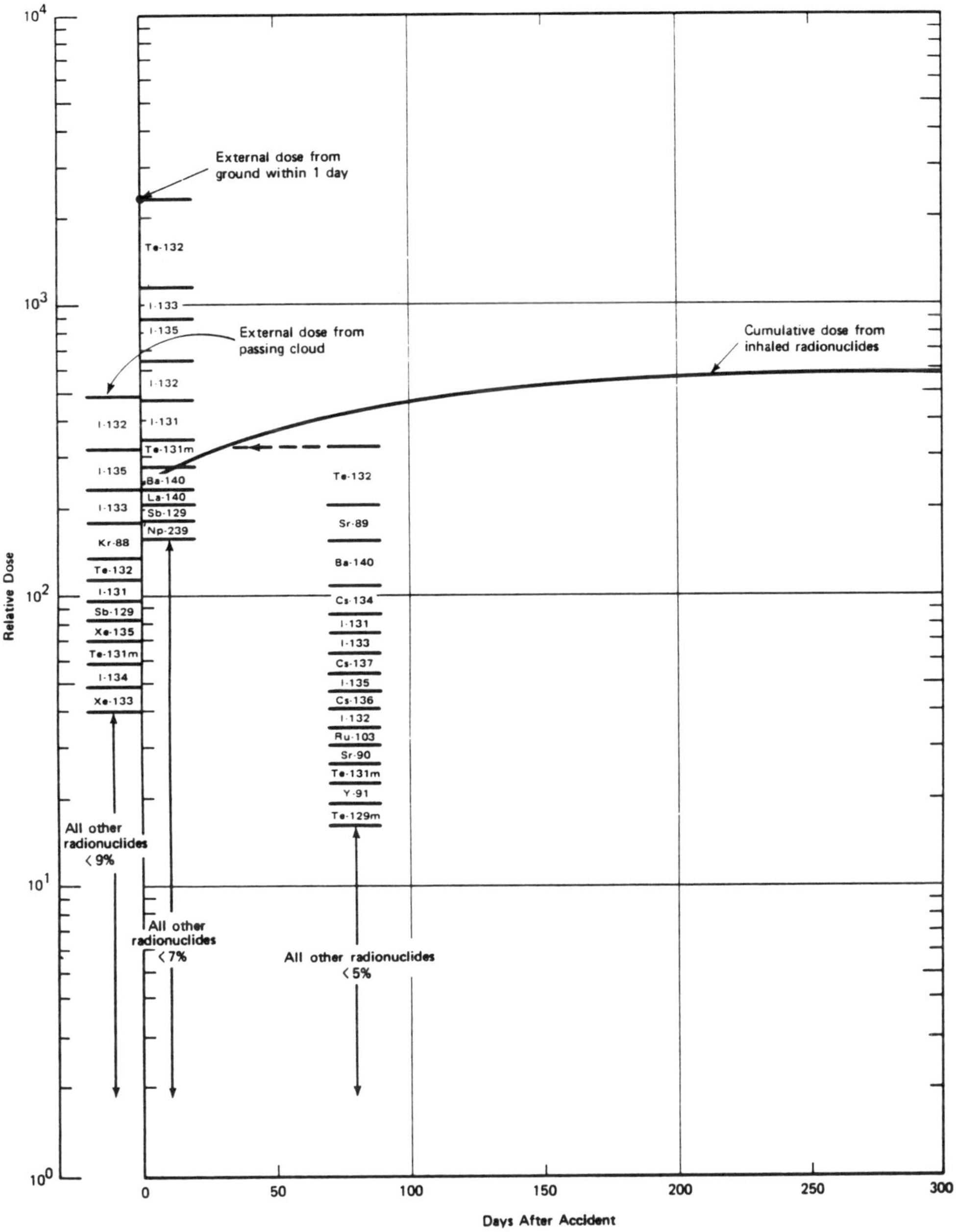

FIGURE 2. Relative doses to bone marrow at 0.5 miles from reactor.

ground contamination. Patently, the longer the ground exposure, the larger the relative worth of the ground contamination pathway.

The relative importance of deposition from the atmosphere to the ground pathways, for releases of mixed chemical species, increases with distance from the source. This is illustrated in Table 1 which shows the various contributions to latent cancer production by various organs and pathways for another postulated accident (the PWR-2 release of the Reactor Safety Study). Perusal of the data in this table will impress the significance of the ground pathways. Even for the immediate period of plume (puff) traverse, the cloud gamma pathway contributes only about 5% of the total calculated latent cancers. In the long term this pathway

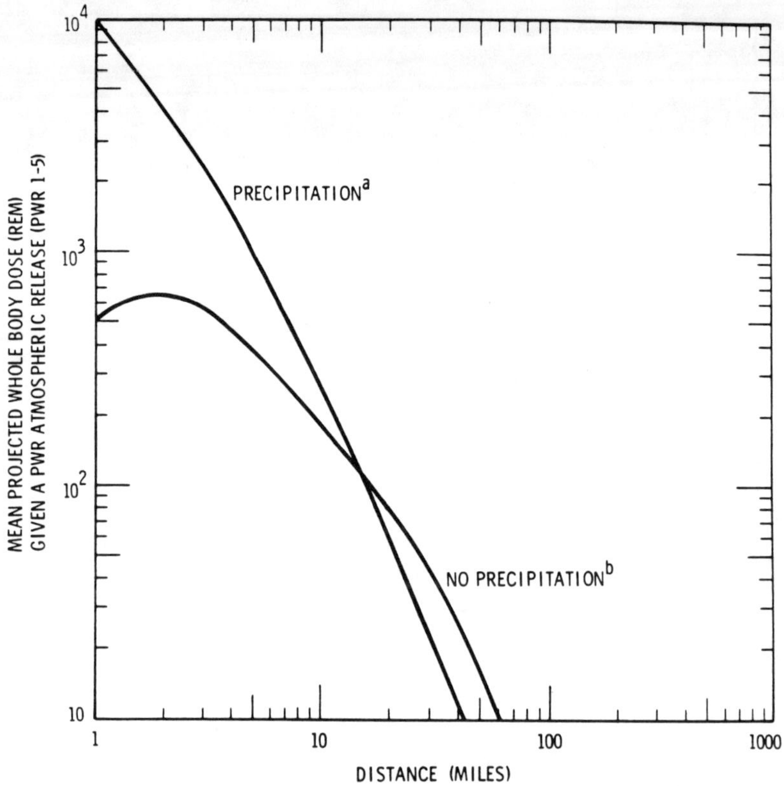

FIGURE 3. Comparison of mean projected whole body dose vs. distance for accidents in which precipitation* and no precipitation** conditions exist at the start of release. Projected doses are for an individual located outdoors,*** and are conditional on a PWR "atmospheric" release (PWR 1-5).

contributes only about 1% of the insult. These are long range and long term affects; the ground pathways dominate the insult because of the long exposure times involved.

Intercept of precipitation and plume (puff) traverse could increase the relative worth of the ground pathways for a mixed species release. After the composition of the source term and the release trajectory, precipitation could well be the next most important parameter of concern in an actual release situation. As illustrated in Figures 3, 4, and 5, precipitation within 10 miles of a release point could dominate the magnitude of the consequences, as compared to many other meterological variables.

Although not shown explicitly in any of these displays, the coincidence of a major mixed species release, precipitation, a calm and a major populated area would induce among the highest consequences in accident/release scenarios, in terms of the number of persons affected and the value of the property damaged. Calms at the point of a release could be beneficial. A calm after some traverse at nominal wind speeds (5 to 10 mph) could result in high consequences. In some respects, a calm downwind of a release, or precipitation, could be beneficial, e.g., if they occur in unpopulated areas. But precipitation along the plume traverse has the clear potential for contaminating surface and ground water, as well as surfaces. Surface waters could carry contamination hundreds of miles from a release point, requiring,

* Accidents in which it is precipitating (rain or snow) at the start of release.

** Accidents in which it is not precipitating (rain or snow) at the start of release.

*** Shielding factor for airborne radionuclides = 1.0. Shielding factor for radionuclides deposited on ground = 0.7. 1-day exposure to radionuclides on ground.

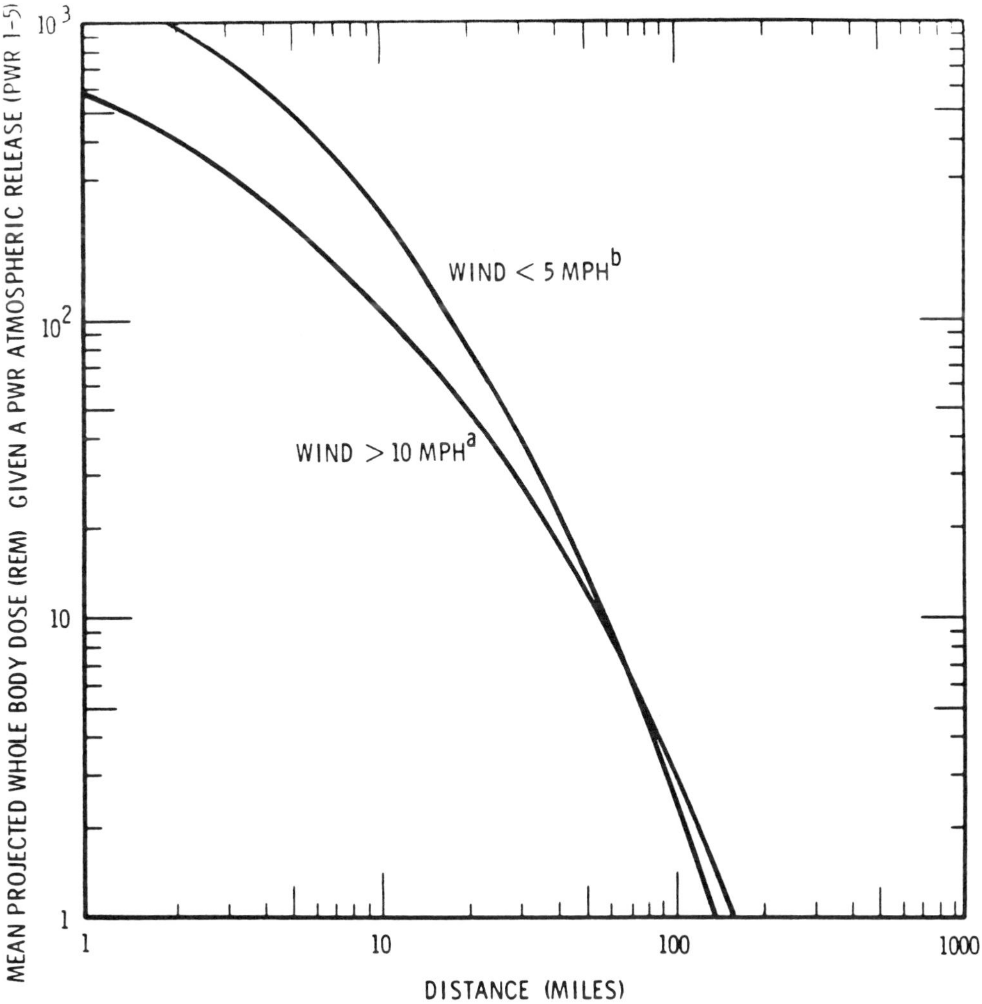

FIGURE 4. Comparison of mean projected whole body dose vs. distance for accidents in which high wind* and low wind** conditions exist at the start of the release. Projected doses are for an individual located outdoors,*** and are conditional on a PWR "atmospheric" release (PWR 1-5).

as a minimum, sequential shutdown of water intake pumps at municipalities downstream. (Restart of pumps after a short period might well be possible for a slug impact).

From an overall perspective standpoint, the insensitivities of certain important consequences to annual average meteorology is worth noting. To examine this matter, hourly data from 29 weather stations across the U.S. were used for consequence calculations. Consequences were calculated assuming a mix of major release core melt scenarios (10^{-4} to 10^{-5} per reactor year probabilities). The results are summarized in the three figures in Figure 6. In these figures, the magnitudes of the calculated consequences are displayed as a function of the probability of a consequence of certain magnitude. The calculations were performed for two sites: the heavily populated Indian Point site about 35 miles north of New York City on the Hudson River, and the Diablo Canyon site near Santa Barbara, California, for which

* Accidents in which the windspeed is greater than 10 mph at the start of release.

** Accidents in which the windspeed is less than 5 mph at the start of release.

*** Shielding factor for airborne radionuclides = 1.0. Shielding factor for radionuclides deposited on ground = 0.7. 1-day exposure to radionuclides on ground.

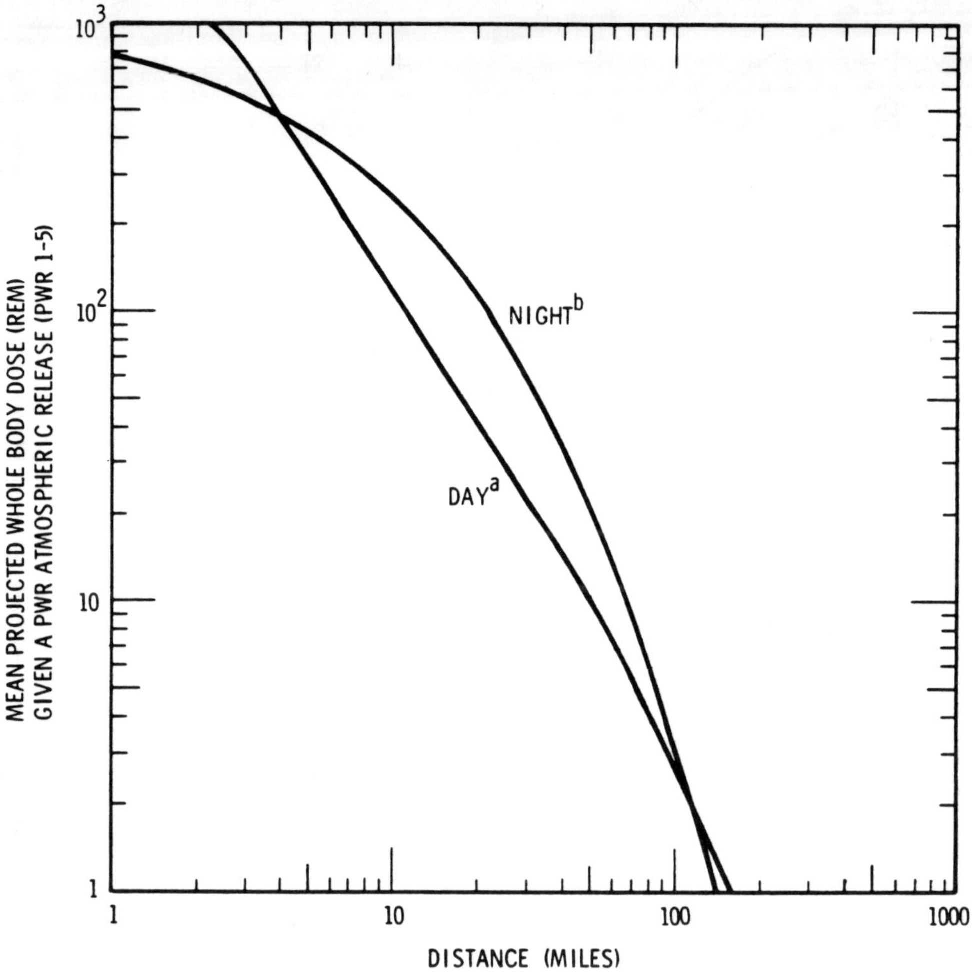

FIGURE 5. Comparison of mean projected whole body dose vs. distance for accidents that begin during the day* and night.** Projected doses are for an individual located outdoors,*** and are conditional on a PWR "atmospheric" release (PWR 1-5).

there are no residents within 5 miles of the site. As is readily apparent from the Indian Point figures, the results of the early death and latent cancer fatality calculations are particularly insensitive to weather sequences except at the low probability, higher consequence portions of the curves. Because of the lack of residents close to Diablo Canyon, the conditional probability of an early death is much lower than that at Indian Point, by two orders of magnitude, in fact. Since the chance of an early death beyond 5 miles is low to begin with, the Diablo Canyon results are in many ways an amplification of the tails of the Indian Point figures, where low probability coincidences of population, calms, and precipitation (as well as the source term) govern the results. Note that the conditional probabilities in the figures should be reduced by a factor between 10^{-4} and 10^{-5} to arrive at an absolute probability estimate. These are indeed low probabilities. As displayed in the latent cancer figure, different meterological sequences produce very little differences in latent cancer production, as noted

* Accidents in which the release starts between 7:00 a.m. and 7:00 p.m.

** Accidents in which the release starts between 7:00 p.m. and 7:00 a.m.

*** Shielding factor for airborne radionuclides = 1.0. Shielding factor for radionuclides deposited on ground = 0.7. 1-day exposure to radionuclides on ground.

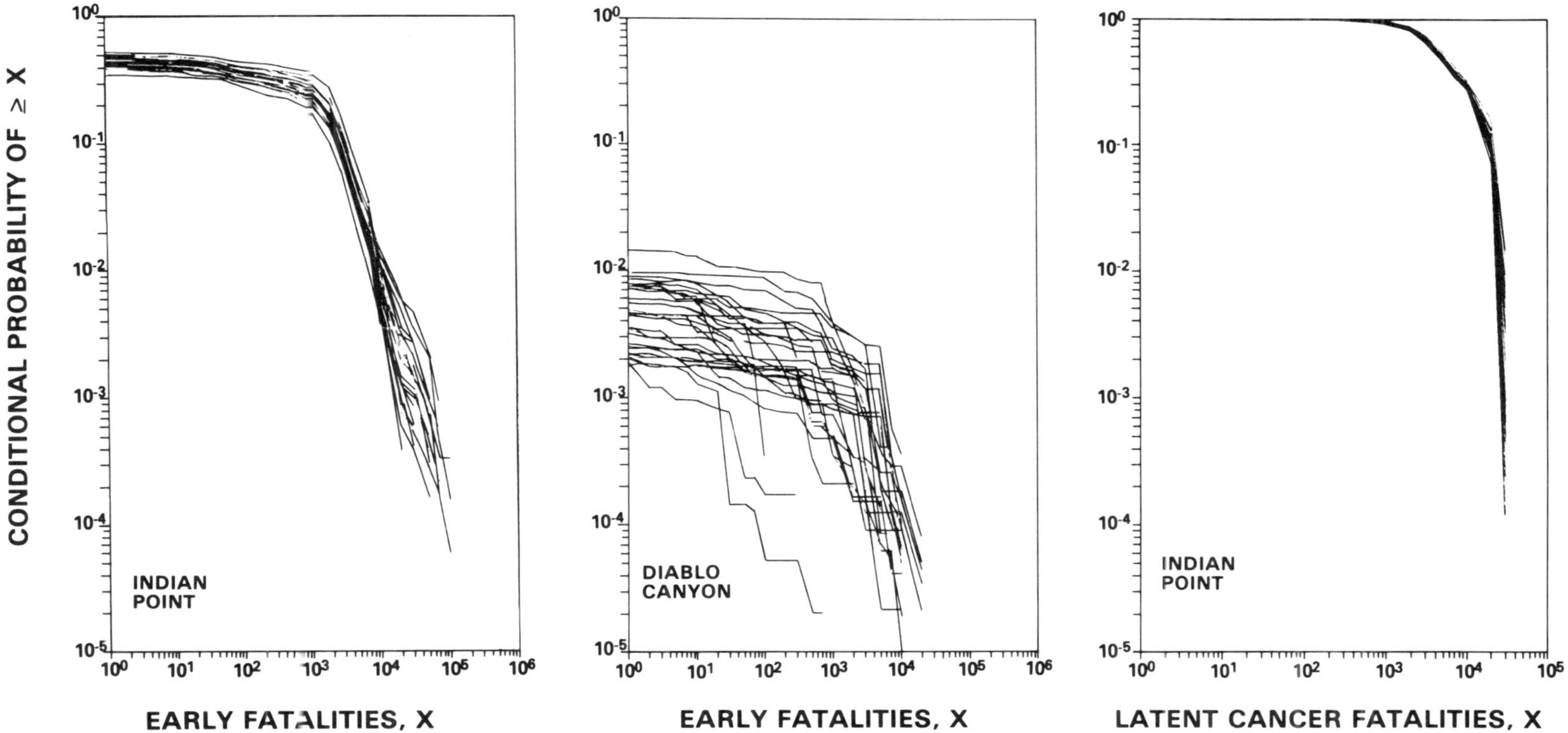

FIGURE 6. Probabilities of early and late fatalities for two sites, assuming: 1120 MW (electric) reactor, large release fractions, 1 hr warning before release, leasurely evacuation within 10 miles. Meteorological data from 29 NWS weather tapes were used to generate the statistics, using 91 start times for the accident throughout a year, for each NWS type. Probabilities conditional on the accident occurring.

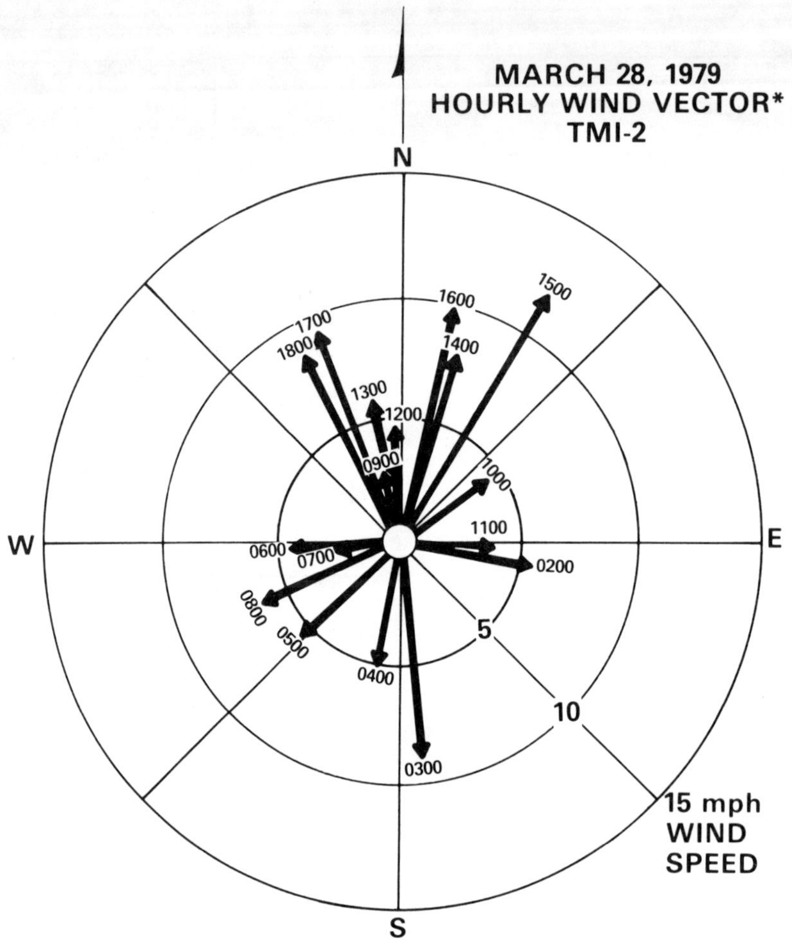

FIGURE 7. Direction to which the on-site wind was blowing.

above. The same result pertains for chronic releases; annual collective dose depends almost solely on curies released and total population, and has little to do with annual wind roses or weather sequences. It's also a far-field (long range) effect; man-rem accumulates where the people are.

Thus, consequences depend predominantly on the magnitude of a release and the release trajectory during transport, and where the people are located. Calms and precipitation are important also. For release scenarios which do not begin until a few hours after the declaration of an emergency, the meteorological information of importance would be weather projections, for the most part, rather than the site meterological information per se.

All-in-all, site meterological information would be of most value in the event of a selected few accident sequences or scenarios for which it would be possible to project or calculate a near-field dose (one objective), i.e., a source term would be available. Otherwise, the dose and dose rate objectives would be accomplished by utilizing near-field dosimetry augmented by data collected by monitoring teams. To satisfy the second dose objective, the collective dose (far-field) calculation, regional meterology and transport codes would have to be used, also supplemented by data from mobile radiological monitoring teams. This would not be a short term need, however.

Finally, certain aspects of the hourly wind rose and accident and protective action sequences during the TMI accident are worth discussion. Figure 7 presents the hourly wind vector as measured at the site during the first day. Because of a computer crash, this data was not obtained until several days after the accident even though verbal reports from the site were obtained throughout the time period. Note that the wind direction at the site varied continually for over 12 hr before becoming steady during the night. The variability of direction is characteristic of the light (wispy) winds during the day. It is especially noteworthy that between 7:30 a.m. and 8:00 a.m. warnings of imminent evacuations to the west of the site were made by the State (PA). At 8:10 a.m. this preparedness was reduced to a standby notice because dose rate measurements to the west were "only" 1 mR/hr. This was just at the time the core was uncovered by several feet, or so! Further, even had an evacuation to the west of the site been initiated at 8:00 a.m., or so, by 9:00 a.m. the wind had shifted to the north! As noted by the NRC Special Inquiry Group, the evacuation of the Low Population Zone (2.5 radius area surrounding the site) should have been completed based on in-plant observations, as was set forth in the emergency plans, and as emphasized in current NRC emergency planning guidance. This is especially noteworthy because the current NRC protective action guidance is based on two imminently reasonable guidelines: do not plan to send people outside if heavily laden plumes are in the area, and do not plan to await an actual major release to the atmosphere before recommending protective actions to people. These two fundamentals underlie the Emergency Action Level and predetermined protective action concepts developed before and since the TMI accident. From a dose projection meterological standpoint, this means that the plans are laid with the explicit understanding that projected doses would most likely not be known or very low when protective action would be recommended. This fundamental perspective limits both dose projection and meterological needs for short-term, short-range protective action decisions. These needs would have to be satisfied for longer term, longer range projections, however. During TMI, the evacuation recommendation which did occur was made predominantly on the basis of in-plant uncertainties and public concern as compared to dose projections (and meterology). The assessment of projected health effects, calculated the first day and reported days and weeks later, did utilize site and regional meterological data to buttress the off-site dosimetry data. This sequence is virtually planned for the future, albeit with (hopefully) better coordination and more timely actions and results, if needed.

REFERENCES

Reactor Safety Study, WASH-1400 (NUREG-75/014), USNRC, October 1975 (n.b. Appendix VI, Calculation of reactor accident consequences).

Wall, I. B., et al., Overview of the Reactor Safety Study Consequence Model, NUREG-0340, USNRC, June 1977.

Technical basis for estimating fission product behavior during LWR accidents, NUREG-0772, USNRC, June 1981.

Aldrich, D. C., et al., Sandia National Laboratories, Examination of offsite radiological emergency protective measures for nuclear reactor accidents involving core melt, NUREG/CR-1131, USNRC, June 1978.

Aldrich, D. C., Impact of dispersion parameters on calculated reactor accident consequences, SAND79-2081, Sandia National Laboratories, Albuquerque, N.M., November 1979.

Martin, J. A., Jr., Perspectives on the role of radiological monitoring in an emergency, *Trans. Am. Nucl. Soc.*, 34, 727—729, June 1980, (available from author, USNRC).

Technical guidance for siting criteria development, NRUEG/CR-2239, USNRC, in preparation, January 1982, (estimated availability date May 1982).

Hilliard, R. K. and Coleman, L. F., Natural transport effects on fission product behavior in the containment systems experiment, BNWL-1457, Battelle Memorial Institute, Pacific Northwest Laboratories, Richland, WA., December 1970.

Nuclear aerosols in reactor safety, Nuclear Energy Agency/Organization for Economic Co-Operation and Development. 2, rue André-Pascal, 75775 Paris Cedex 16, France, (in english), June 1979.

Proceedings of the CSNI Specialists Meeting on Nuclear Aerosols in Reactor Safety, NUREG/CR-1724, USNRC, Washington, D.C. (in english), October 1980.

Dennis, R., Ed., Handbook on Aerosols, TID-26608. NTIS, U.S. Dept. Commerce, Springfield, V.A., 1976.

APPENDIX C
DOSES WHILE TRAVELING WITH A PUFF

Under the guidance discussed in the main text of this chapter a precautionary evacuation of areas within 2 to 3 miles of a LWR would be recommended before containment failure for a core melt accident sequence. It is possible that some persons could be outside traveling should a major puff release occur while they are in transit. This Appendix will provide some insight on the relative worth of traveling while caught in a puff, as compared to the case where a person remains stationary and is exposed to the full puff.

The analysis will emphasize the worst case of actually being caught in a plume. Thus, it is presumed that the planned emergency response scenario does not work for some reason. As a point of reference, only 6 min is required to travel 3 miles at a nominal country speed of 30 mph. The implications of this statement are obvious. In this light, the following might be described as an elegant analysis of trivia, but some interesting insights are obtained. Two cases are considered: traveling downwind with a puff and traveling upwind through a puff.

TRAVELING DOWNWIND WITH A PUFF

From the equations in Reference 20 of the main text the following equation can be developed for the case of a person traveling downwind with a puff when the dose rate is proportional to inverse distance squared (realistic, conservative case):

$$D_{dw} = \dot{D}_o r_O / w$$

where: r_O is the distance from the starting point to the release point; $\dot{D}_o$ is the dose rate at r_O; D_{dw} is the dose accumulated while traveling downwind in this unfortunate manner, and w is the speed of travel.

Note that the traveler's speed is equal to the wind speed. If the wind speed is less than w a person can outrun a puff and the equation does not hold. If one starts earlier than the release or at the instant of release, and travels faster than the wind speed (nominal 5 to 10 mph) the dose can be avoided altogether. If the puff does not follow the road, doses would be lower than that indicated by the equation. If one is overtaken by the puff, which passes over the traveler, the traveler would be exposed to a lower dose than the stationary person at the closer distance, and to a lower dose than calculated here. If the release is of long duration, the person traveling would be exposed to only a fraction of the release as compared to the stationary person. In the noted reference it is shown that doses while traveling at a moderate speed across a puff would be less than if one were to travel downwind with a puff. Thus, this analysis is on the worst case side and pertains generally to a very unlikely evacuation scenario. It could pertain to a valley situation with an unfortunate delay in warning time, however.

Now, the stationary person at r_O would be exposed to a dose D_s given by:

$$D_s = \dot{D}_o T$$

where T is the duration of the puff. This person would also be exposed to ground contamination, but this dose will be ignored here. Thus,

$$\text{Thus, } D_{dw}/D_s = r_O/(wT)$$

T is speculative, of course, and would be difficult to predict during an emergency, much less ahead of time. Under the puff assumption, let T = 0.5 hr, which is the shortest duration

Table 1
TRAVELING TO STATIONARY DOSE RATIOS (TRAVEL DOWNWIND WITH A PUFF)[a,b]

Starting distance r_O (miles)	Traveler's speed[c]			
	5 mph	10 mph	20 mph	30 mph
1	0.4	0.2	0.1	0.07
2	0.8	0.4	0.2	0.17
3	1.2	0.6	0.3	0.20
4	1.6	0.8	0.4	0.27
5	2.0	1.0	0.5	0.33

[a] Puff duration assumed to be 0.5 hr. Longer duration releases will decrease the calculated dose to the traveler.
[b] Exposure to ground contamination by the stationary traveler is neglected. Inclusion of this would reduce the ratios shown in the table.
[c] Traveler's speed assumed equal to the wind speed, and starting time assumed equal to the time that the puff reaches r_O. (Nominal wind speed is 5 to 10 mph.)

puff estimated in the Reactor Safety Study for a core melt accident. This will tend to conservatively maximize the ratio.

The results using these assumptions are shown in Table 1. The dose ratios are generally much less than one for persons starting at close range (r_O less than 3 miles) and traveling at moderate speed. The trends in the data comport with intuition: traveling faster lowers the dose to the traveler and leaving nearby areas provides relatively greater benefit than leaving areas further away. Interestingly, traveling at slow speeds with the puff, from distances further away, could conceivably be worse than staying in place.

TRAVELING UPWIND INTO A PUFF

Assuming that dose rate increases with inverse distance squared as one approaches the source, it can be shown that the dose accumulated while traveling upwind into a puff is given by:

$$D_{uw} = \dot{D}_o r_O (r_O - r_1)/(r_1 w)$$

and the ratio of this dose to D_s is:

$$D_{uw}/D_s = r_O(r_O - r_1)/(wr_1T)$$

Where r_1 is the closest distance of approach to the source.

Let T = 0.5 hr, as before, and r_1 = 0.5 mile, which is a nominal LWR site boundary distance. Then the calculated ratio D_{uw}/D_s is given in Table 2 for some example conditions.

As shown in Table 2, traveling from long distances toward the source would be far from beneficial under the assumed conditions. (But recall, the time required to travel 5 miles at 20 mph is only 10 min. This re-emphasizes the extremely pessimistic assumptions used to derive the ratios in Table 2. This also emphasizes the potential value of an early warning). On the other hand, even traveling into a puff could be beneficial for persons starting from

Table 2
TRAVELING TO STATIONARY DOSE RATIOS (TRAVELING UPWIND INTO A PUFF[a]

Starting distance r_O (miles)	Traveler's speed 5 mph	10 mph	20 mph	30 mph
1	0.4	0.2	0.1	0.07
2	2.4	1.2	0.6	0.4
5	—[b]	9.0	4.5	3.0

[a] Puff duration = 0.5 hr. Site boundary distance = 0.5 mile. Travel starts when puff reaches r_O. No ground contamination exposures.

[b] Ratio not calculated; the travel time would be longer than the puff duration and the equation does not hold for this case.

short range and traveling at moderate country speeds, as compared to staying in place and being exposed to the full puff and any ground contamination.

In brief, it would be better to go rapidly through a puff than to stay in place and be exposed to all of it. And the greater the warning time, the better.

TRANSPORTATION OF RADIOACTIVE MATERIALS

Frank J. Bradley

INTRODUCTION

The occasional transport of radioactive materials (ram) prior to 1940 led to certain restrictions being placed on their transport. The main reason for the restrictions was the fogging of undeveloped film that was also in transit. From these simple regulations there has grown a complex set of regulations as ram has developed into an important commodity in commerce with an estimated 2.2 million ram shipments made in 1975 and a projected 5.6 million ram shipments in 1985.[1]

The number of shipments underestimates the total amount of ram that may be in transit at any time because it does not include most private private carriers, such as radiographers and well loggers who are also hauling ram from one job to another.

The basic framework for the regulations was set in 1947[2] to protect film and, somewhat incidentally, man. The resultant exposures to transport workers and to the public have been investigated in recent years[3] and in most instances the estimated annual exposures were within the recommended dose for an individual member of the public (0.5 rem/year). This was partially fortuitous since one might have expected with the vast increase in number of ram shipments to see higher doses to the transport workers. So long as the transport worker is only occasionally handling ram packages, his nonradiation worker status appears to hold. In special cases transport workers become radiation workers. This occurs among transport workers with certain freight forwarders who handled large numbers of ram packages on a daily basis. It is estimated[4] that for a transport worker handling between 100 and 1000 transport index (TI) units (label) per year the average and individual worker doses would be within recommended limits; however, for workers handling between 1000 and 10,000 TI units (label) per year, an individual will occasionally exceed the recommended dose value but the average dose will be within the population dose limits. In handling greater than 10,000 TI units (label) per year, the transport workers become radiation workers who require monitoring and specialized training.

REGULATIONS

Ram transport regulations applicable to the shipper, carrier, and consignee define in considerable detail what can be transported, how it can be transported, where it can be transported, and how it is received. These regulations are published in the *Federal Register* by the U. S. Department of Transportation (DOT) and the U. S. Nuclear Regulatory Commission (NRC). Besides the federal regulations many state and local jurisdictions have passed rules and regulations to further insure safety in transporting ram. Finally there are bridge, tunnel, and turnpike authorities who levy their own requirements which are partially dictated by insurance and bonding rules.[5] The federal ram transport requirements contain exemptions for such items as industrial gauges containing ram, certain low specific activity ram, escorted ram shipments, etc.

The changing regulatory framework arises from attempts to correct defects as they show up in ram transport incidents and also to remain compatible with the International Atomic Energy Agency (IAEA) transport regulations, which aids the free flow of commerce across national borders.

In 1976 the U.S. Department of Transportation consolidated all radioactive material transport regulations into one body of regulations. The pertinent sections of the Code of

Federal Regulations, applicable to the shipper, to which we will refer in the following sections, are as follows:

- Title 49, Part 172 — "Hazardous Materials Table and Hazardous Materials Communications Regulations" (see Appendix B).
- Title 49, Part 173 — "Shippers-General Requirements for Shipments and Packagings" (see Appendix C).
- Title 49, Part 178 — "Shipping Container Specifications" (see Appendix H).

In addition, under the broad authority of the Atomic Energy Act of 1954, the U. S. Nuclear Regulatory Commission has promulgated regulations covering packaging of radioactive material but only applicable to source material, by-product material and special nuclear material as follows:

- Title 10, Part 71 — "Packaging of Radioactive Material for Transport and Transportation of Radioactive Material Under Certain Conditions" (see Appendix K).

The shipper also must be familiar with the DOT Regulations governing the carriers since packaging and shipping requirements are a function of the carrier mode — rail, air, vessel, or highway.

The carrier regulations are as follows:

- Title 49, Part 174 — "Carriage by Rail" (see Appendix D).
- Title 49, Part 175 — "Carriage by Aircraft" (see Appendix E).
- Title 49, Part 176 — "Carriage by Vessel" (see Appendix F).
- Title 49, Part 177 — "Carriage by Public Highway" (see Appendix G).

The U.S. Department of transportation's regulatory authority does not extend to the consignee. Consequently, as a result of a 1971 airplane contamination incident,[6] the NRC amended its regulations to place requirements on the consignee for timely receipt and checking of ram packages. These are as follows:

- Title 10, Paragraph 20.205 — "Procedures for Picking Up, Receiving, and Opening Packages" (see Appendix I).

Regulations basically of a performance type and applicable to shippers and consignees are found in State Radiation Regulations, some of which are reproduced in the Appendixes (Appendixes M, N, O, P, and Q).

Many state transportation departments or their equivalents issue hazardous material regulations applicable to intrastate movement of such commodities and should be consulted. Title 10 CFR, Part 71 makes the requirement explicit that intrastate ram packages must be transported in accord with interstate requirements.

The impact of these regulations on the shipper, carrier, and consignee is covered in the following sections.

SHIPPERS

General

A shipper is generally one who prepares radioactive material (ram) for shipment. He will turn over the ram-containing package to a private, contract, or common carrier for transport to its destination. In some cases, the shipper may be a broker who acts as middleman between the actual shipper (or generator) and the consignee. The broker may never see the ram package and the broker relies on the actual shipper to perform all the tasks as enumerated below, but the broker's name might be listed as the shipper. Today, especially in cases of waste shipments, the consignee, if a waste site operator, may want the generators name listed as well. In other cases, a "drop shipment" may be made. This occurs in commerce when one firm receives an order and gives the order to a second firm to fill and make the shipment, but the shipper is listed as the original firm taking the order.

The shipper is responsible in broad terms for the following:

1. Package the ram in such a manner that the dose received by the transport worker and public while the package is in transit is within permissible limits.
2. The external radiation will cause minimal or no fogging to film in transit.
3. That external removable contamination will not cause injury to persons or damage to goods in transit.
4. In case of an accident, the probability of an injury from radiation to the transport worker or public or contamination of persons, goods, or property is kept within acceptable limits.

Since the transportation of hazardous substances is commonplace in a technical society, complex transportation regulations exist for substances such as poisons or explosives and radioactive materials have been grafted onto them. Originally, ram was classified as a Class D Poison for transport purposes, but today the term radioactive is sufficiently common to have a category of its own in the regulations.

The shipper in the transportation system which consists of the shipper, carrier, and consignee is normally the most knowledgeable about what it is that is being shipped. Consequently, the regulations place the main responsibility on the shipper to ensure the safe transit of the radioactive material. Many of the requirements are based on the physical, chemical, and biological characteristics of radioactive material. In the regulations as presently constituted, radioactive materials are divided into two broad classes: (1) Radioactive White I, emitting minimal external penetrating radiation and (2) Radioactive Yellow, emitting various levels of external penetrating radiation. These classes are based on external dose rate measurements as follows:

Label	At any point on accessible surface of package (X) (mrem/hr)	At 3 ft from external surface of package (transport index:T.I.) (mrem/hr)
Radioactive-White	≤0.5	0
Radioactive-Yellow II	0.5<x≤50.0	0<.I.≤1.0
Radioactive-Yellow III[a]	50.0<x≤200	1.0<T.I.≤10.0

[a] Mandatory label for Fissile Class III and "large quantity" package

There is another potential "hazard" associated with the radionuclides U-233, U-235, and Pu 239 called special nuclear material (SNM). These radionuclides in sufficient mass become critical, i.e., create more radioactive material through the fission process. Since this property is a function of the mass of SNM and other matter present, such as, hydrogen, another separate class of fissile radioactive materials are included in the regulations designated Fissile Class I, Fissile Class II and Fissile Class III.

Preparation and Packaging of Radioactive Material for Shipment

The regulations cover the shipment of ram in any physical state: solid, liquid, or gas.

For shipping purposes, the physical form of ram is divided into two broad categories: normal form and special form ram. Special form ram must meet the criteria as given in

Table 1
ACTIVITY RANGES FOR VARIOUS RADIOACTIVE MATERIAL CATEGORIES

Group/form	Limited or exempt quantity[a,b] (Ci)	Type A quantity (Ci)	Type B quantity (Ci)	Large quantity (Ci)
Group I/normal form	<0.00001	0.00001 < A < 0.001	0.001 < A < 20	>20
Group II/normal form	<0.0001	0.0001 < A < 0.05	0.05 < A < 20	>20
Group III/normal form	<0.001	0.001 < A < 3	3 < A < 200	>200
Group IV/normal form	<0.001	0.001 < A < 20	20 < A < 200	>200
Group V/normal form	<0.001	0.001 < A < 20	20 < A < 5,000	>5,000
Group VI/normal form	<0.001	0.001 < A < 1,000	1,000 < A < 50,000	>50,000
Group VII/normal form	<25	25 < A < 1,000	1,000 < A < 50,000	>50,000
All/special form	<0.001	0.001 < A < 20[c]	20[c] < A < 5,000	>5,000

[a] 49 CFR 173.391(a) specifies these quantities including footnotes b and c limited quantities.
[b] Not more than 15 g, U-235
[c] Except Cf-252 which is <2 Ci

173.398(a) and designates ram in nondispersable form. Normal form ram includes all other ram. Normal form is further divided into seven transport groups as given in 173.390(a). These transport groups are based on the radiotoxicity of the radionuclide and are based on the maximum permissible body burden of ram. If a particular radionuclide is not listed, or for mixtures of radionuclides use 173.390(b) or 173.390(c) respectively.

Table 1 summarizes the activity range for categories designated limited quantity (basically an exempt quantity as far as the regulations are concerned), Type A quantity, Type B quantity, and large quantity. Each category must meet increasingly restrictive requirements with respect of packaging, carriage, notification, and routing (a new requirement). There is an additional category called low specific activity (LSA), such as, natural uranium and natural thorium. Additionally, a lot of ram waste generated in laboratories, nuclear reactors, and industrial processes utilizing ram can be classified as LSA.

Historically, many Radiation Safety Officers (individuals designated by management to implement a Radiation Safety Program) have classified all waste as ram waste independent of half-life and specific activity. The present economics of ram waste disposal have now made this approach prohibitively expensive. In addition, the U. S. Nuclear Regulatory Commission, after some criticism, has formulated a policy for H-3 and C-14 LSA which has eased considerably the requirements for their disposal. These requirements are given in Title 10, parts 20.301 and 20.305 (see Appendix J).

Source material comprising U-natural, U-depleted (in U-235), or Th-natural is LSA material. Since this is the raw material of the nuclear fuel cycle, there is a large quantity of this material shipped each year in various chemical forms including ores, refined products, such as, "black oxide" (U_3O_8), "green salt" (UF_4), "yellowcake" (UO_2), and uranium hexafluoride" (UF_6), as gas. Uranium and thorium in elemental state are metals and similar in their physical properties to lead. In a finely divided state such as machine turnings and dust, they are pyrophoric, i.e., they spontaneously oxidize in air. A recent fire in a truck of ram waste was traced to elemental uranium that was very difficult to extinguish. Elemental U-natural, U-depleted, and Th-natural in a finely divided state must be oxidized chemically or by combustion before packaging unless they are covered and surrounded by an inert, nonoxidizing gas or liquid. Massive elemental U-natural, U-depleted, or Th-natural in form such as metal bars oxidizes on the surface, but such oxidation does not proceed any further, or if it does only at slow rate. Further surface oxidation can be controlled by surface treatment. The various chemical forms of uranium classified as LSA are usually shipped in 17H drums (178.118).

The requirements for LSA material are given in 173.392 and may be summarized as follows:

1. It must be packaged in a Type A quantity container such as a 17H steel drum, or a Type B container as applicable for the radioactivity of the LSA material shipped.
2. The package must be marked and labeled in accord with 172.300 and 172.400 except as noted in Item 3 below.
3. LSA material shipped in exclusive-use vehicles (except aircraft) are exempt from specification packaging, marking, and labeling provided they are packaged in strong tight packages so that there will be no leakage of ram under conditions normally incident to transportation and packages must have no significant removable contamination. Such packages must have external dose levels of:

    a. $\leq$1000 mrem/hr at 3 ft (closed transport vehicle only).
    b. $\leq$200 mrem/hr at any point on external surface of car or vehicle (closed transport vehicle only).
    c. $\leq$10 mrem/hr at 6 ft from vertical plane as determined by external surface of car or vehicle or if the load is transported in open vehicle, at any point 6 ft from vertical plane as projected from outer edge of vehicle.
    d. $\leq$2 mrem/hr in any normally occupied position in car or vehicle, except that this provision does not apply to private motor carriers.

Ram as by-product material, accelerator-produced material, or naturally occurring radioactive material (except U-natural and Th-natural) are prepared for shipment classifying the material into normal form or special form. The criteria for special form ram material are given in 173.398(a) and are summarized as follows:

1. The ram must be either in massive solid form or encapsulated; it must not dissolve or convert into dispersible form to the extent of more than 0.005% by weight during immersion for 1 week in water at pH 6 to 8 and 68°F and maximum conductivity of 10 μmhos/cm.
2. In massive solid form, the ram must not break, crumble or shatter if subjected to the percussion test as specified in regulations.
3. It must not melt, sublime, or ignite at temperatures below 1000°F.
4. If encapsulated, the capsule must retain its contents when subjected to the free drop, percussion, heating, and immersion tests as specified in the regulations. The capsule must not melt, sublime, or ignite at temperatures below 1475°F.

When a shipper classifies ram as special form, he must maintain a complete certification on file for at least 1 year after the last shipment and be prepared to supply it to the DOT with supporting safety analysis that ram meets the requirements as specified in regulations and summarized above. In case of export shipments of ram as special form the shipper must obtain a "Certificate of Competent Authority" for the ram from "Office of Hazardous Materials Regulation, U. S. Department of Transportation, Washington, D.C. 20590" (as of March 1981). Radioactive materials that do not meet special form criteria are normal form which is classified into 7 transport groups. Knowing the following variables:

1. A radioactive species and whether or not it is fissionable material
2. Activity
3. Form of ram, special or normal, if normal form what is its transport group
4. Transport mode and if by highway whether it is by exclusive use vehicle, then the appropriate ram package can be selected.

The selection of a few examples will serve to demonstrate the selection of the proper package.

Example #1 — 100 Ci, Ir-192, Special Form

Such an activity source is typically used for field radiography and on any given day there are hundreds of such sources being transported throughout the U.S. As noted in Table 1, such a source falls in column # 4 and requires a Type B package. A typical Type B package for such a source is given in Figure 1. This package is usually fabricated with depleted uranium which makes a compact shield for Ir-192 sources due to the excellent gamma ray absorption properties of uranium.

Example #2 — 5 Ci, Mo-99/Tc-99m Generator

Such generators are used in nuclear pharmacies and Tc-99m is "milked" off (eluted) for use in the formulation of radiopharmaceuticals. Since Mo-99 is a fluid mixture on a resin bed, it is normal form. From the list of radionuclides in 173.390, (Appendix C) we find that Mo-99 is in Transport Group IV. Table 1 indicates this is a Type A quantity which requires a Type A package.

A typical Type A package for Mo-99/Tc-99m is given in Figure 2 in Appendix U. Also as with the Ir-192 radiography container the inner shipping container serves in the pharmacy as a storage and dispensing set-up for the Tc-99m; consequently, the packing and unpacking instructions are extremely important to get the maximum use out of the container.

Example #3 — 500,000 Ci, Co-60 Special Form

From Table 1 we see that such a source is classified as a large quantity source. The shipping container for this source must be approved and certified by the U.S. Nuclear Regulatory Commission. The standards for such containers are given in the NRC. Regulations in Part 71 of Title 10 of the Code of Federal Regulations (Appendix K). The only specification container for large quantity sources is a spec 6M which could not be used for this size source. The NRC publishes a "Directory of Certificates of Compliance for Radioactive Material Packages" (NUREG-0383) and should be consulted for an appropriate package for this size source.

Example #4 — 5 Ci, Co-60; 1 Ci, Bi-210, and 2 Ci, Cs-137, Normal Form

Going to the list of radionuclides in 173.390 and Table 1, 5 Ci, Co-60 is Transport Group III, Type B quantity; 1 Ci, Bi-210, Transport Group II, Type B quantity; 2 Ci, Cs-137 Transport Group III, Type A quantity. The criteria for handling mixtures of radionuclides is given in 173.390(c). For this case taking Type B quantities the ratios of actual activity to permissible activity must be less than or equal to unity.

The ratios are:

$$\frac{5}{200} + \frac{1}{20} + \frac{2}{200} < 1 \text{ and a Type B package is permissible.}$$

A specification Type B package is a Spec 6M drum and would be acceptable under the general license of 71.12 of Title 10, provided the shipper has a quality assurance program whose description was submitted and approved by U. S. Nuclear Regulatory Commission as satisfying the regulations.

Package Measurements

Depending on the radionuclide, either one, two, or three radiometric measurements are necessary on each ram package. For a Radioactive White I labeled package with a radionuclide which emits a nonpenetrating radiation, (e.g. Po-210, a pure alpha emitter or C-14, a weak beta emitter) only an external contamination survey by wipe or smear technique is required by 173.397. This requirement specifies a smear must be taken over an average 300 cm^2 of the package area. For Po-210 (α) the maximum allowed contamination is 220 dpm/cm^2 which equates to 30,000 pCi over the 300 cm^2. A relatively high contamination value by some standards. For packages transported in exclusive use vehicles the maximum permitted removable contamination is 10 times this value or 300,000 pCi. The external radiation criteria for Radioactive White I packages given in above is a radiation dose rate of less than or equal to 0.5 mrem/hr on the surface of the package.

For any activity of any radionuclide, it is theoretically possible to make the package Radioactive White I by using the proper amount of shielding.

There are economic and physical limitations which restrict the use of this label to modest quantities of alpha and beta emitters or small quantities of other ram.

The other two measurements involve the penetrating radiation emanating from the package. These are a surface measurement and a measurement taken at 3 ft. Readings are in units of millirem per hour. The 3 ft reading is also the transport index which gets entered on the Radioactive Yellow II or Radioactive Yellow III labels. The two types of penetrating radiation are X- or gamma rays and neutrons. The X- or gamma rays are usually measured in roentgen or rad units and converted directly to rem (since the quality factor is 1 for X- or gamma rays the millirad reading is the same as millirem reading) (rigorously, if a meter is calibrated in milliroentgen units then it should be multiplied by 1.11 to convert to millirad units and multiplied again by 1 to convert to millirem units). Neutrons are considerably different from X- or gamma rays in that different energy neutrons have different quality factors. This situation can be alleviated by using neutron survey instruments that read directly in millirem units. There are very few nuclides that decay by emission of a neutron and they have a relatively short half lives and are usually found only in a reactor. Neutron sources found in commerce arise from spontaneous fission, such as, Cf-252 and alpha sources mixed with beryllium, such as, Am-241 + Be, Pu + Be and Ra + Be sources. The neutrons emitted by these sources have a distribution of energies from 1 to 10 MeV.

Other important neutron sources encountered in transit are spent fuel rods from a nuclear reactor. The neutron dose rate is a function of degree of fuel burn up, time out of reactor, and shipping cask design. The simplest approach is to use a neutron dose rate meter measuring in mrem/hr, for example, one based on the Hurst-type detector.

Special nuclear material in single packages have a fissile transport index as given in 173.396. It is conceivable that a package will have a ram TI and a fissile TI. The fissile TI is based on the rams potential for neutron multiplication. The governing TI is the higher of the two. Compounding the problem is the ratio of hydrogen to fissile material (H/X present) and the regulations must be consulted to insure that the correct fissile TI is assigned to the package.

Marking, Labeling, and Sealing of Ram Packages

Hazardous material packages must be *marked* with the proper shipping name as prescribed in 172.300. The proper shipping name for radioactive material are as follows (172.101):

- Radioactive device, nos
- Radioactive material, fissile, nos
- Radioactive material, LSA, nos
- Radioactive material, nos
- Radioactive material, limited quantities, nos
- Radioactive material, special form, nos
- Plutonium nitrate solution
- Thorium metal, pyrophoric
- Thorium nitrate
- Uranium hexafluoride, fissile (containing more than 0.7% U-235)

- Uranium hexafluoride, low specific activity (containing 0.7% or less U-235)
- Uranium metal, pyrophoric
- Uranyl nitrate hexahydrate solution
- Uranyl nitrate, solid

Besides the proper shipping name for the ram in the package, the following items may need to be marked on the package, if applicable:

1. If the gross weight of package exceeds 110 lb then the gross weight must be marked on the package
2. If the package conforms to Type A or Type B performance standards or is a DOT specification container then this fact must be marked on the package
3. If the package has a NRC or DOT Certificate of Compliance this must be marked on outside of the container
4. The package must be marked with name and address of shipper or consignee
5. If the ram package contains low specific activity ram and is shipped in sole use vehicle, then each package must be marked with a hazardous material designation, ''Radioactive Material, LSA'' (173.392(c)(8))

While it might appear redundant, besides the marking with shipping name on the package, each ram package must have 2 labels (affixed to opposite sides) which contains additional specific information regarding the nuclide(s) in the package. These labels are designated Radioactive White I (172.436), Radioactive Yellow II (172.438) and Radioactive Yellow III (172.444). As noted, the distinction between Radioactive Yellow II and Radioactive Yellow III is based on the surface and 3 ft dose rate. The numerical value of the dose rate at 3 ft is also the package transport index or TI. Radioactive Yellow II packages are limited to a dose rate at 3 ft from package of less than 1.0 mrem/hr and a surface dose rate of less than 50 mrem/hr. Also to be filled in on the label are the package contents, i.e., radionuclides and number of curies of each.

Radioactive White I label permits a maximum dose rate of 0.5 mrem/hr on the surface.

A recent amendment to Title 49 DOT Regulations permits labels that are compatible with IAEA Regulations.

A seal must be provided on outside of ram package 173.393(b) in order to detect if the package was ''illicitly opened''. A wire lead seal for bolted drums is acceptable. The type of seal for cardboard boxes is often debated, but usually acceptable is a seal which indicates if it has been tampered with.

Shipping Papers

The shipping papers for radioactive materials must contain a description of the hazardous material and other information as follows (172.202):

1. Proper shipping name (172.101).
2. Hazard class (172.101) when the same as shipping name except for n.o.s. it does not have to be repeated.
3. Quantity by weight, volume or as otherwise appropriate.
4. Type of packaging.
5. Name of radionuclide if listed in 173.390.
6. Physical state and chemical name if in normal form.
7. Activity contained in each package in units of curies, millicuries, or microcuries (abbreviations Ci, mCi, and μCi respectively are acceptable).
8. Category of label for each package in shipment, i.e., Radioactive White I, Radioactive Yellow II, and Radioactive Yellow III.

9. In case of Radioactive Yellow II and Radioactive Yellow III the transport index of each package.
10. For fissile radioactive material, i.e., Pu-238, Pu-239, and Pu-241, U-233, and U-235:

    a. "Fissile Exempt" (see 173.396(a))
    b. Fissile Class I, or Fissile Class II, or Fissile Class III.
    c. In case of Fissile Class III shipment the following statement must be included: "Warning-Fissile Class III Shipment-Do Not Load More Than *** (insert correct number for each shipment) Packages Per Vehicle" and "In Loading and Storage Areas, Keep at Least 20 Feet (6 meters) From Other Packages Bearing Radioactive Labels".
    d. In case of Fissile Class III shipment by water the statement "For Shipment By Water, Only One Fissile Class III Shipment is Permitted in Each Hold".

11. If ram package has a U.S. Department of Energy (or ERDA, AEC), or NRC approval, the package identification marking (173.393(a)).
12. If export shipment, package identification marking as prescribed by IAEA.
13. In case of ram shipment offered and accepted for transportation within U.S. under the provisions of 171.12(e) the shipping paper shall state: "This Shipment Contains Packages of Type A/Low Specific Activity Radioactive Materials Limited in Accordance with the 1973 IAEA Regulations Persuant to 171.12(e)".
14. In case of empty packages, the notation "EMPTY" or "EMPTY-Last Contained XXX" insert hazardous material name as given in 172.101 in place of X.
15. In case of transportation by air, if the package is prohibited abroad passenger carrying aircraft the statement "Cargo-Only Aircraft".
16. In case of rail transportation, the shipping paper must include the statement "Placarded" followed by the name on placard — for ram this would read "Placarded-RADIOACTIVE".
17. In case of water transportation the additional entries:

    a. Identification of the type package, i.e., barrels, drums, cylinders, boxes,
    b. Number of each type of package,
    c. Gross weight of each type of package.

Placarding Motor Vehicle, Rail Car, or Freight Container

Each motor vehicle, rail car, and freight container transporting one or more Radioactive Yellow III labeled packages must be placarded on each side, front and rear with placard specified in 172.556. No placarding of a ship or plane is required. In the case of low specific activity (LSA) radioactive material which is being shipped in sole-use or exclusive-use transport vehicle without the regular labels except for Radioactive-LSA package label, placarding of transport vehicle is required pursuant to 173.392(c)(7).

In the case of radioactive material in form of uranium hexafluoride, fissile (>0.7% U-235) or uranium hexafluoride, LSA (≤0.7% U-235) placards "RADIOACTIVE" and "CORROSIVE" are required. The "CORROSIVE" placard is not required for shipments of less than 1000 lb gross weight.

In the case of highway transport it is the responsibility of the shipper pursuant to 172.506 and 172.508 to provide the proper placard to the motor carrier and in case of rail transport to provide and affix the proper placard to the rail car.

In case of freight containers with a capacity of 64 ft^3 or more the radioactive placard must be attached to the container by the shipper whether the container is to be transported highway, rail, air, or water. The regulations are very specific as to the construction, size, durability and visibility of the placard. The specifications are given in 172.519 reproduced in Appendix B in this chapter.

Insurance

Two types of insurance are available: first-party property damage or personal injury insurance; it is usually obtainable from conventional insurers or is available from specialized nuclear insurers, such as, Nuclear Energy Property Insurance Association (NEPIA), as members of the Mutual Atomic Energy Reinsurance Pool (MAERP), or for electric utilities with nuclear power reactors, the Nuclear Mutual Limited (NML).

First-party insurance is similar in concept to fire insurance that one might take out on one's house. The second type of insurance is third-party coverage for damage or contamination of someone else's property or personal injury to another person arising from one's own nuclear activities.

Because the federal government, through the Price-Anderson Act, requires and provides, in part, insurance for operators of nuclear reactors, fuel reprocessors and others processing special nuclear material; (Pu, U-233, or U-235 in amounts above certain limits) many insurance policies carried by shippers and carriers possess the ''Nuclear Energy Liability Exclusion Endorsement'' (See Appendix T). This endorsement basically excludes coverage by any insurance covered by the Price-Anderson Act and in many instances excludes all radioactive contamination and injuries arising therefrom. Therefore, many firms obtain insurance from nuclear energy liability insurance pools (NELIA or MAELU) for this type of coverage. Since this type of coverage is highly specialized, it is suggested that a shipper or carrier contact his insurance broker to determine the type of coverage that he needs to assure coverage for transport incidents involving radioactive material.

CARRIERS

Responsibilities of Carrier

Carriers are unique in the ram transport system. They shoulder the most responsibility, but they are not licensed to handle ram as is the shipper and consignee. Common carriers are licensed by the Interstate Commerce Commission (ICC) for general carriage with certain conditions. This situation is changing as more specialized carriers are serving the nuclear industry, for example, to transport ram waste and nuclear reactor fuel. If the carrier is licensed to handle ram, there is more assurance that persons actually handling and transporting ram are trained in the requirements of the regulations. This is not to recommend that common or contract carriers must be licensed (private carriers usually are licensed) to handle ram since the thrust of the regulations is to obviate this need. The carriers overall ram safety record is good, but the public's concern over ram safety places a ram incident in a special category. This concern about the lack of control over the carrier has led many local and state jurisdictions to issue their own regulations covering the carrier. Some of these regulations will be discussed later in the section entitled ''Routing (DOT Dockett HM-164)''.

The carrier regulations will be discussed in the following sections, but there are broad areas that are common to the mode-specific regulations. Some common areas are loading of ram onto transport vehicles, receipt of shipping paper from shipper, problems associated with commingling ram with other hazardous materials and passengers also in transit, expedited shipments, lost and astray ram shipments, pick-up and delivery of ram shipment to consignee, accidents, and clean up following spills. Each of these create different problems in the different transport modes.

There are three different types of carrier

1. Private carrier, where the shipper uses his own transport vehicle and drivers to transport ram; ram transport is only incidental to shippers main line of work. Field radiography

involves this type of ram transport wherein the radiography firm transports the radiography source usually in company owned van and the driver is the radiographer.

2. Contract carrier, the shipper contracts with a carrier to carry his ram shipment, generally in sole-use vehicle, from point A to point B.
3. Common carriers are licensed by Interstate Commerce Commission to handle certain goods between selected points over specified routes. These carriers are regulated carriers and must accept hazardous materials if the shipment is otherwise in accord with the regulations.

The U. S. Department of Transportation publishes regulations to ensure the safe transport of hazardous materials in interstate commerce. They have inspection staffs which inspect carriers in each transport mode, rail, air, water, or highway, to determine compliance with hazardous materials regulations. Water transport is regulated by the U. S. Coast Guard which in peacetime is part of the U. S. Department of Transportation.

Intrastate shipments, those that originate and end in the same state without crossing any state border, are covered by each state's transport regulations usually promulgated by the state's Department of Transportation. The state regulations may or may not conform to DOT regulations.

Appendix N in this chapter includes a summary by state and local jurisdiction indicating whether they have passed DOT regulations for hazardous materials.

The U. S. Nuclear Regulatory Commission has promulgated 10 CFR 71.5 which specifies that intrastate ram transport must conform to DOT ram transport regulations.

It is the carrier's job to transport ram from consigner to consignee. The shippers job is prologue and the consignee' job is epilogue to ram transport task performed by carrier.

Carriage by Rail, 49 CFR 174

Two main categories of ram shipments move by rail. One is bulk low specific activity source material shipments usually uranium ore and refined mill products. The other is power reactor spent fuel rods which require massive shielding. Today, uranium mills are placed close to uranium mines and much of the ore and mill shipments move by truck. There is no commercial fuel rod reprocessing, consequently, there is little actual ram movement by rail. But transport economics could change where it would again become important.

Regulations place responsibility for compliance with Part 174 on the carrier and the carrier must instruct his employees in the requirements of the regulations.

Section 174.12 requires the originating carrier or freight forwarder to keep on file a copy of the certified shipping paper accompanying the ram shipment.

The rail carrier must expedite and forward the ram shipments according to 174.14 within 48 hr after acceptance (excluding Saturdays, Sundays, and holidays) with the exception for lines with intermittent service in which case the ram shipment must be moved on the first available train.

The regulations (174.16) require the consignee to pick up ram shipments within 48 hr (excluding, Saturdays, Sundays, and holidays) of its arrival at the destination depot of the carrier, after notice was sent or given to the consignee of its arrival. If the consignee does not remove the ram shipment (in carload lot size) then the carrier can:

1. Store on his property or another person's property (presumably with concurrence of other person) if safe storage on carrier's property is not available, or
2. By sale at expiration of 15 days after notice of arrival was sent or given to the consignee and provided shipper was notified of nondelivery within a 48-hr period and orders for disposition were not received. In case of ram, it is not that simple since ram can only be sold and physically transferred to a licensed person.

If the ram shipment is in less than carload lot size, then the carrier can:

1. Return to the shipper if notice of nondelivery was requested and given to the shipper and orders to return to the shipper were received, or
2. Store on the carrier's property, or
3. Store on another person's properties, if safe storage on carrier's property is not available, or
4. By sale at the end of 15 calendar days after arrival notice was sent or given to the consignee and provided the shipper was notified of nondelivery at the end of the 48-hr waiting period, and orders for disposition were not received (note restraint as given above on this sale).

The regulations (174.24) specify no carrier can accept a ram shipment unless accompanied by a properly executed shipping paper and certificate if required. Each waybill, switching ticket, switching order, or other billing used must indicate which trailer or containers on railcars contain ram and which must be placarded (174.25).

The marking and placarding of rail cars are covered in 174.59 and requirement for removal of placard after unloading is covered in 174.69.

The restrictions on commingling ram with other hazardous material are given in Table in 174.81. For example, ram may not be loaded or stored with low explosives or black powder, high explosive, initiating or priming explosives, wet blasting caps, ammunition for cannon with explosive projectiles, explosive projectiles, detonating fuses, Class A, etc., but can be loaded or stored with ammunition for cannon with empty, inert loaded or solid projectiles, propellant explosives, Class B, fireworks, small arms ammunition, primers for cannon or small arms, percussion fuses, time fuses, cordeau detonant fuse, flammable liquids, flammable solids, corrosive liquids, nonflammable gases, poisonous gases, and other ram.

Rail cars placarded "RADIOACTIVE" may not be placed next to another placarded car (except if placarded "COMBUSTIBLE"), engine, occupied caboose, or carload of undeveloped films (174.89).

There is a separate Subpart K to Part 174 to cover the specialized requirements attached to ram shipments. The Table in 174.700(c) stipulates minimum separation distance between ram packages and persons, or undeveloped film as a function of TI unit as follows:

Total TI	Minimum distance between ram package and undeveloped film	Minimum distance between ram package and persons
0	0	0
0. to 10.0	15 ft	3 ft
10.1 to 20.0	22 ft	4 ft
20.1 to 30.0	29 ft	5 ft
30.1 to 40.0	33 ft	6 ft
40.1 to 50.0	36 ft	7 ft

The maximum TI for all ram packages per rail car or stored together in one location are 50 TI units. The exception to this requirement is in case of sole-use or exclusive-use shipments using the whole rail car. In the case of Fissile Class III ram shipments in which nuclear criticality controls are necessary during the shipping phase there must be no combining this shipment with other fissile ram packages in the same rail car. In loading and storage areas, Fissile Class III packages must be separated by at least 20 ft from other ram-labeled packages.

A flatbed rail car can transport ran packages weighing 15,000 lb or more. A gondola can transport any of the following:

1. Ram packages overweighing 5000 lb or more or,
2. Strong wooden boxes with inside containers of solid ram secured, braced and cushioned or,
3. Ram in concrete filled metal drums or in concrete vaults weighing 700 lb or more. Regulations (174.715) stipulate that after a ram shipment is transported in an exclusive-use rail car, that rail car must be surveyed and decontaminated to 0.5 mrem/hr or less at any accessible surface and no significant surface contamination per the limits in 173.397(a). In case of rail cars in continuous exclusive-use ram service a survey must be conducted after each use to ensure that interior surfaces are less than or equal to 10 mrem/hr at surface and 2 mrem/hr at 3 ft from the interior surface. The rail car must be stenciled with wording "FOR RADIOACTIVE MATERIALS USE ONLY" in 3 in. high letters on both sides of the rail car.

In case of rail accidents involving ram packages the carrier must notify the shipper as soon as practicable if there has been any break in ram packages and possibility of ram contamination exists. In case of ram contamination, all contaminated rail cars, areas, and roadbeds must be decontaminated to less than a 0.5 mrem/hr external dose rate on surface and removable contamination to less than limits in 173.397(a). The ram package should be segregated from personnel and if assistance is needed, immediately notify the nearest U.S. Nuclear Regulatory Commission Regional Office and U.S. Department of Energy Regional Offices. Both addresses with phone numbers are given in Appendix Y).

Carriage by Aircraft (49 CFR 175)

A well-publicized incident involving the contamination of a passenger aircraft and exposures to passengers almost put an end to this convenient transport mode. The incident involved short lived radionuclides Mo-99/Tc-99m.

The leakage and contamination were not immediately discovered and by the time the airline was alerted, the plane had made several additional trips involving more luggage and people. Fortunately, the short half lives: $T^1/_2$ = 66 hr for Mo-99 and $T^1/_2$ = 6 hr for Tc-99m reduced the need for extensive decontamination. But it dramatized the potential and caused some airline pilots and airlines to refuse ram shipments until more assurances regarding their safety were forthcoming. The real need of shipment via aircraft is for short lived radionuclides and there was a dramatic rise in the use of these short lived radionuclides in nuclear medicine in the last 10 years. Fortunately a tightening in the regulations on transporting ram packages via passenger aircraft and a realization by industry (the shippers) of the need for better quality control on ram packages and tightening packaging procedures has led to a restoration of the public's confidence in this transport mode. Initially, the only way important short lived radionuclides could reach many cities in useful quantities was by passenger carrying aircraft. Since 1970, there has been a rise in cargo only aircraft usage which do not have the same restrictions as passenger aircraft.

The transport system for short lived radionuclides used in nuclear medicine has generally worked in the following way.

The ram packages are taken to a freight forwarder, the freight forwarder assembles groups of packages going to one area into overpacks and turns the overpack over to airline for transport to another city. At the other end, the above procedure is reversed. Overpacks are broken down and distributed to local users.

Appendix E, Section V, contain Sections of 49 CFR 175 pertaining to ram. Section 175.10, Exceptions included an exemption from this Part for ram in limited quantities (see Table 1) manufactured articles containing ram or uranium or thorium metals, other than in fuel rods. These exemptions are routinely extended. Subsection 175.30 stipulates that the carrier need not accept ram packages unless:

Table 2
MINIMUM DISTANCE BETWEEN RAM PACKAGE AND PEOPLE AND UNDEVELOPED FILM

	Minimum distance between undeveloped film and ram packages by duration of flight					Minimum distance between ram packages and persons or dividing partition separating person from ram package
TI units	0—2 hr (feet)	2—4 hr (feet)	4—8 hr (feet)	8—12 hr (feet)	12 hr (feet)	(feet)
0	0	0	0	0	0	0
0.1—1.0	1	2	3	4	5	1
1.1—5.0	3	4	6	8	11	2
5.1—10.0	4	6	9	11	15	3
10.1—20.0	5	8	12	16	22	4
20.1—30.0	7	10	15	20	29	5
30.1—40.0	8	11	17	22	33	6
40.1—50.0	9	12	19	24	36	7

1. Ram is authorized and within quantity limitations given in 172.101.
2. Ram must be described and certified on shipping paper and one copy of shipping paper must be retained by originating carrier for 90 days.
3. Ram packages are properly labeled, marked, and sealed.
4. Labeled ''CARGO ONLY'' if ram package is not authorized aboard passenger-carrying aircraft.
5. Carrier must inspect package for holes, leakage, and other indications of its integrity.

The pilot-in-command of the aircraft must be notified (175.33) in writing before take off when ram packages and other hazardous materials are placed aboard his aircraft including description of ram as given in shipping papers, location aboard his aircraft, and results of inspections as specified in item 5 above.

In section 175.79, there is a requirement to orient hazardous material packages as specified on the package. Packages with markings ''This Side Up'' or arrows pointed in an up direction must be oriented in this direction. The package that leaked Mo/Tc-99m mentioned above was apparently placed on its side during part of its transit and since the seal on the package had not been maintained the liquid leaked out. Subpart 175.79(b) requires that packages containing hazardous material liquids must be oriented with closures in the up direction.

Regulation 175.85 stipulates that ram packages cannot be carried in the cabin of passenger-carrying aircraft although this requirement was recently amended. For nonmedical and nonresearch ram packages that must be carried on cargo-only aircraft, the ram package may be placed in the cargo location inaccessible to a crewmember during flight. Until a recent amendment to regulations, the ram package had to be in an accessible location.

Specific requirements peculiar to ram packages are given in 175.700. These involve the minimum separation distance between ram package and areas continuously occupied by people or animals and undeveloped film. These distances are as follows for various durations of flight are found in Table 2.

According to 175.700(b) the air carrier must notify shipper in case of ram package breakage, spillage, or suspected ram contamination. The aircraft in which there was ram contamination cannot be returned to normal use until accessible surfaces in normal use are decontaminated to less than 0.5 mrem/hr external radiation and removable surface contamination reduced to limits in 173.397(a). If the carrier wants radiological advice, he can contact the NRC and the Department of Energy. Section 175.75 specifies a maximum of 50 TI units aboard any single aircraft. There is an explicit prohibition in 175.700(c) against transporting large quantity ram (see Table 1) aboard passenger-carrying aircraft. Exception to this provision can only be obtained from the Director, Office of Hazardous Materials Regulation, Materials Transportation Bureau, DOT. As a result of the Mo/Tc-99m incident described above 175.700(d) was added prohibiting ram packages aboard passenger-carrying aircraft except for ram, "intended for use in, or incident to, research or medical diagnosis or treatment". Up until May 3, 1981, this prohibition did not apply to limited quantities of ram as defined in 173.391(a), (b), or (c).

Section 175.710 gives special requirements for fissile Class III ram packages. They cannot be carried aboard any aircraft except if they are: (1) carried on cargo-only and exclusive-use aircraft and (2) there can be no other ram-labeled package on board.

Carriage by Vessel (49 CFR 176)

Vessel refers to the transport vehicle used in water. Within the continental U.S., there is little ram movement by water, except in special situations. Movement of radiography and wireline (logging) sources to offshore oil and gas fields is one example. The movement of spent fuel rods off the eastern end of Long Island by ferry due to routing restrictions through New York City is another example. The main carriage by water is to and from overseas ports and would involve bulk shipments, of uranium ore and the refined product, LSA shipments, spent reactor fuel elements, and large radioactive sources.

The applicable regulations are given in Part 176 and are enforced by U.S. Coast Guard.

Segregation from other hazardous materials aboard vessels other than the ferry vessel is specified for ram in Table II of 176.83. The table recommends that ram be stored on cargo vessels and passenger vessels *separated from* explosive A, B, and C, flammable compressed gases, flammable or combustible liquids, flammable solids labeled spontaneously combustible, flammable solids labeled dangerous when wet, organic peroxides, corrosive materials, and *away from* nonflammable compressed gases, oxidizers, and Class A poisons.

Separated from and *away from* have specialized meaning and the regulations must be consulted to determine their precise meaning in individual situations. For example *separated from* means in separate holds when stowed under deck and *away from* means the hazardous materials can be stored in same hold provided a minimum horizontal separation of 10 ft is provided. Special rules, applicable to ferry vessels and barges are also included.

In 176.700 special storage requirements for ram aboard vessels are given. These regulations specify that "Radioactive White" and "Radioactive Yellow" labeled packages must be stored separately from living space and any space continuously occupied. Mail bags may not be stored with ram packages; a ram package that is a significant heat source must not be overstowed with other cargo and if stored under deck the hold must be ventilated.

Each Fissile Class III shipment must be stowed with a minimum separation distance of 20 ft from all other ram packages with "Radioactive Yellow" labels.

The ram package stowage must be handled and managed in such a way that no person will receive a dose of more than 100 mrem in any 6-day period or more than 500 mrem/year (assumes a nonradiation worker population). The dose rate in any occupied area must be less than 0.5 mrem/hr; if the ram package requires special handling the shipper shall supply a copy of special handling requirements to the vessel master or person in charge of vessel. Special handling requirements as a function of the transport index are as follows (176.700(h)):

1. Maximum TI units of stored ram packages in any group is 50 TI units. Each group of ram packages must be separated by at least 20 ft from another group of ram packages. The separation requirement does not apply to LSA shipments or full-load shipments if shipper has the exclusive-use of the vessel and Fissile Class II packages do not exceed 50 TI units.

2. Maximum TI units aboard any vessel is 200 TI units without prior authorization by the DOT.
3. Minimum separation distances between the ram packages and occupied area and undeveloped film are given in 176.700(h) as a function of travel time and amount of cargo providing shielding around ram packages.

In case of accidents that may lead to ram package breakage or leakage, there must be no unnecessary contact with ram packages until handling damaged packages is supervised by a qualified expert. The exception to this requirement is in the case of LSA ram shipments. In case of ram leakage, all vessel surfaces must be decontaminated to less than 0.5 mrem/hr external radiation and removable contamination reduced to less than or equal to limits in 173.397(a).

Carriage by Public Highway (49 CFR 177)

Rail, air, and vessel shipments of ram are usually remote from our daily lives but ram shipments via the public highways can pass outside our front door. Public concern over the impact of such highway shipments on their lives has led to support for banning certain types of ram shipments through certain locales. Banning of a ram shipment through one locale and its diversion to another locale has logically lead to the banning of the ram shipment by the second locale as well. The pyramiding regulations are best exemplified around New York City. Finally, this has led to a national routing regulation issued as DOT Docket HM-164. This regulation will be reviewed in the next section and is reproduced in Appendix W).

The purpose of these regulations as stated in 177.800 is the promotion of safe transit of hazardous materials by private, contract, and common carriers in interstate and foreign commerce. It requires the carrier to follow rules and train his employees in the rules.

Section 177.801 stipulates that a carrier may accept hazardous material if in compliance and certified to be in compliance with Parts 170 to 189 for carriage but must reject hazardous material not in compliance with the referenced parts. This section also authorizes the inspection by a representative of the initial carrier or Bureau of Explosives of the ". . . methods of manufacturer, packing, and storage so far as they affect safety in transportation. . ."

The regulation also states that when the initial carrier accepts a ram package for carriage over public highway and subsequent loading onto a vessel or rail car that pertinent regulations as given for these transport modes must be complied with as well as with the motor vehicle requirements.

Motor carriers must comply with 44 CFR Parts 390 to 397 in as far as these requirements are applicable.

Section 177.807 states that each carrier must report incidents involving hazardous materials as required by 171.15 and 171.16. Section 177.810 grants continuing authority to state and municipal jurisdiction to regulate the flow of hazardous materials through urban vehicular tunnels used for transportation within their jurisdiction. Section 177.815 requires a carrier to maintain a supply of hazardous material labels to replace lost or destroyed labels based on information in shipping papers. For ram packages, this means a supply of Radioactive White I, Radioactive Yellow II, and Radioactive Yellow III labels.

A carrier in accepting ram packages for shipment must receive shipping papers properly executed in accord with 172.201, 172.202, and 172.203. In addition, the carrier must obtain a shipper certification except in case of a private carrier. In case of an accident or inspection of a vehicle carrying ram packages, the driver must provide or have easily accessible the properly executed shipping papers.

The total number of TI units is limited to 50 TI units per motor vehicle except that this limitation does not apply in those cases where the sole commodity in the motor vehicle are ram packages. The limitations on sole-use shipments are those given in 173.393(j).

The separation distances between ram packages, occupied areas, and undeveloped film (177.842)(b) are the same as those listed in Table 2.

For ram packages in storage depots each ram package storage shall have no more than 50 TI units and the minimum distance between storage areas is 20 ft.

Section 177.842(d) stipulates that ram packages placed on motor vehicles must be blocked and braced so that they do not move under conditions normally incident to transportation. This is a relatively mild requirement as it might have required bracing for accident conditions as well.

Section 177.842(f) is a broad requirement that Fissile Class III ram shipments are transported in accord with the regulations. One of the main requirements for such shipments is repeated by explicitly stating that no other Fissile ram package is commingled with Fissile Class III ram shipment. Also no other radioactive-labeled packages are stored, loaded, or placed closer than 20 ft to a Fissile Class III shipment.

Each vehicle used to transport LSA ram must be surveyed after each use and decontaminated to less than 0.5 mrem/hr external radiation from all accessible surfaces and removable contamination to less than limits specified in 173.397(a). This requirement does not apply to a motor vehicle if it is used solely in transporting ram. If sole-use vehicles are contaminated they must be stencilled in lettering at least 3 in. high "For Radioactive Material Use Only" on both sides and they must be kept locked at all times except during loading, unloading, and inspection. The maximum contamination limits are less than or equal to 10 mrem/hr on interior surface or 2 mrem/hr at 3 ft from interior surfaces.

Ram packages must not be loaded, transported, or stored with other hazardous materials as follows (177.848): black powder, high explosives, initiating or priming explosives, blasting caps, ammunition for cannon, etc.; explosive projectiles and detonating fuses. Ram packages may be stored with ammunition for cannon with empty projectiles, propellant explosives (Class B), fireworks, small arms ammunition, primers for cannon, percussion fuses, time fuses (Class C), cordeau detonant fuse, fireworks (common), flammable liquids and gases, flammable solids, corrosive liquids, nonflammable gases, poisonous gases, and other ram packages except as noted above for Fissile Class III shipments.

In case of fire, accident, breakage, or unusual delay involving ram packages, the carrier must (177.843(c), 177.861):

1. Follow procedures given in 171.15 and 171.16.
2. Notify shipper.
3. Vehicles, building areas or equipment shall not be placed back in use until all accessible surfaces are less than 0.5 mrem/hr external radiation on surface and removable contamination is decontaminated to less than limits given in 173.397(a), (state or local ram regulations would apply to highway, bridge, or tunnel contamination and the carrier must comply with such regulations).
4. Not stated but the state or local radiation control officers should be informed of incidents or unusual ram package delay.

Routing (DOT Docket HM-164)

The highway routing requirements are not finalized to date (July 1981) and are therefore kept separate from Part 177 requirements enumerated in the preceding section. The new routing requirements for placarded motor vehicles carrying ram packages would supersede state and local rules and would permit transportation through vehicular tunnels if the tunnel is part of a preferred route. A new proposed Section 177.825 "Routing and Training Requirements For Radioactive Materials" stipulates that the carrier is required to ensure that a placarded motor vehicle with ram packages takes a route which minimizes the radiological risk. The route selection shall be based on accident rates, transit time, population density, activities day and night on date of transit. The carrier must inform the driver that ram packages are in the shipment and select a general route to follow. This requirement does not apply in the following cases.

1. Only one practicable highway route available, or
2. Motor vehicle is operated on a preferred highway under conditions given below.

If the ram package contains a large quantity of ram as defined in Table 1, then the driver shall operate the motor vehicle over a preferred route selected to reduce time in transit, except that an interstate system by-pass or beltway around a city shall be used when available.

A preferred route is:

1. Interstate system highway for which no alternative route is designated by the State Routing Agency as provided by regulations.
2. A state designated route selected by the State Routing Agency in accord with DOT "Guidelines for Selecting Preferred Highway Routes for Shipments of Large Quantity Radioactive Materials".
3. When a deviation from the preferred route is necessary then the route selected shall be in accord with criteria given above for ram routes.
4. Deviation from preferred routes is permitted under following conditions:

    a. Emergency conditions
    b. Necessary rest, fuel, and vehicle repair stops
    c. To extent necessary to pick up, deliver, or transfer large quantity ram package.

The carrier of a large quantity ram package shall prepare a written preferred route plan and give a copy to his driver and a copy to shipper.

The route plan shall contain:

1. Origin and destination points, route selected, planned stops, estimated departure and arrival times
2. Telephone numbers which will access emergency assistance in each state to be entered
3. The carrier must use a trained driver

Training provided the driver must be:

1. Given within prior 2 years
2. Material in the training course must cover:

    a. Properties and hazards of ram
    b. Pertinent regulations, especially Parts 172, 173, and 177 of Title 49
    c. Emergency procedures

The driver must have in his possession a certificate of training and route plan. In case of irradiated reactor fuel shipments, the carrier must also comply with Part 73 of Title 10 which covers the physical security of the irradiated fuel and variations from routing requirements are permitted in this case.

To ensure national consistency between these route plans, an Appendix A is included which defines the ground rules for state and local requirements to be consistent with the new highway routing requirements in Part 177 of Title 49.

Postal Service (39 CFR 21 and 124)

Surprising to some, ram does move through the mails and there are regulations which specify the conditions for such mail, both domestic and foreign. Domestically, there are a large number of sealed sources in use and one of the conditions of use involves a periodic leak test. This test normally involves wiping the sealed source in a prescribed manner with some type of absorbent material, such as filter paper or absorbent cotton. Normally, the counting of the wipe for ram is done in-house but there are also authorized leak test kits wherein the user will send the kit back to a service firm for radiometric analysis. Since the maximum permitted leak is 5000 pCi except in the case of teletherapy sources which is 50,000 pCi, the normal leak test can be mailed. There is always the finite probability that the leak test will identify a leaker in which case the regulations on mailing ram freight might be exceeded. Therefore, many leak test kits require the checking of the wipe with an appropriate GM type survey meter and then sending the kit, if the results indicate that it is permitted, through the mails.

Besides such sources, calibration and the standard source can be sent through the mails within the limits as specified.

The only authorized mailable radioactive materials are those which are classified as "small quantities" of radioactive materials or "radioactive devices" as prescribed in 49 Code of the Federal Regulations 173.391. Thus, those ram which are mailable are as follows:

1. Small Quantities (49 CFR 173.391 (a))

Transport Group (173.389 (h)), (173.390)	Maximum quantity per package
I	0.01 mCi
II	0.1 mCi
III, IV, V, or VI	1.0 mCi
VII	25.0 Ci
Special form RAM (173.389 (g))	1.0 mCi
Tritium oxide in aqueous solution	0.5 mCi/mℓ (3 Ci/package limit)
Fissile radioactive material (173.389 (a))	15 g[a]

[a] The total radioactivity may not exceed either the applicable activity limit for the appropriate transport group or the special form radioactive material limit.

a. The above materials must be securely contained in strong, tight packages to prevent leakage of the contents during normal postal handling. Liquid ram must additionally be packaged within a leak-resistant and corrosion-resistant inner container, surrounded by sufficient absorbent material to absorb at least twice the volume of the liquid radioactive contents.
b. The radiation dose rate at any point on the external surfaces of the package must not exceed 0.5 mrem/hr.
c. There must be no significant radioactive material on the external surface of the package (173.397 (a)). Contamination levels when averaged over an area of 300 cm^2 must not exceed any of the following:

Contaminant	Maximum permissible level	
	$\mu Ci/cm^2$	$dis/min/cm^2$
Natural or depleted uranium and natural thorium		
Beta-gamma	10^{-3}	2200
Alpha	10^{-4}	220
All other beta-gamma emitting radionuclides	10^{-4}	220
All other alpha emitting radionuclides	10^{-5}	22

d. The outside of the inner container must be marked "Radioactive".

2. Radioactive devices (49 CFR 173.391 (b)).

Manufactured articles such as instruments, clocks, electronic tubes, or apparatus, or other similar devices, having ram (other than liquid) in a nondispersible form, as a component part, are mailable providing that the following conditions are met:

a. The ram must be securely contained within the devices, or securely packaged in strong tight packages, such that there will be no leakage of ram under conditions normally encountered in postal handling.
b. The radiation dose rate at 4 in. from any unpackaged device must not exceed 10 mrem/hr.
c. The radiation dose rate at any point on the external surface of the outside container does not exceed 0.5 mrem/hr.
d. There must be no significant ram on the exterior of the package (as per 1.c. above).
e. The total radioactivity content of a single package containing radioactive devices must not exceed the following:

	Quantities in curies	
Transport group	**Per device**	**Per package**
I	0.0001	0.001
II	0.001	0.05
III	0.01	3.0
IV	0.05	3.0
V or VI	1.0	1.0
VII	25.0	200.0
Special form RAM	0.05	20.0
Fissile RAM	15 g[a]	15 g[a]

[a] The total radioactivity may not exceed either the applicable activity limit for the appropriate transport group or the special form radioactive material limit.

For foreign mail service the restrictions given above are applicable and in addition:

a. Shipments must be sent in a registered airmail letter package (however, not all countries accept registered mail. This should be checked with the postal service in advance).
b. The address side of each package containing a ram must bear a white label bearing the French words ‘‘MATIERES RADIOACTIVES’’.
c. The package wrapper must also bear a label reading: ‘‘Return to Sender in Case of Nondelivery’’.

CONSIGNEE

A. Introduction

As a result of the investigation by the National Transportation Safety Board of a Delta plane contamination incident on December 31, 1971 and January 1, 1972, the Board made some observations and also some recommendations. It observed that there was adequacy of transport regulations for radioactive materials. What it did find, however, was that there was totally inadequate inspection of the shipper and carrier to determine their compliance with the regulations. There was also a multitude of agencies involved in the promulgation and enforcement of regulations, including the U.S. DOT, U.S. NRC (at the time, U.S. AEC), and FAA. Finally, the U.S. DOT had no jurisdiction over the consignee who it turned out had a great deal to do with alerting the carrier and shipper of the Mo Tc-99m contamination problems. Since the consignee, under normal circumstances, must be licensed by U.S. NRC or an Agreement State, it is the responsibility of these agencies to issue regulations binding on the consignee. The Board recommended regulations to ensure expedious pick-up and checking of packages containing Type B and large quantities of ram. These recommendations were accepted by addition of 10 CFR 20.205 to the NRC regulations and subsequent changes in agreement with state regulations.

The NRC has issued Regulatory Guide 7.37 which further expands on the consignee requirements in the regulations. This guide states that the record indicates an unusually good record with respect to leaking ram packages. From 1940 to 1974 millions of ram packages were shipped millions of road, vessel, and rail miles with only 100 ram packages known to have leaked. Doubling this figure (to account for under-reporting in the early years) still leaves an impressive safety record. More recent studies[8] indicate that the record of contamination-free ram packages in transit continues to be the norm.

The regulations with respect to Type B and large quantity ram packages are logical and only codified what was standard practice in the industry. Contaminated ram packages and higher than normal dose rates on ram packages would lead to in-house health physics problems. Therefore, many programs for receiving and surveying of ram packages were in existence at the time this was made a regulation.

The regulations and procedures involve some increased workload on radiation safety or health physics staffs. They involve also a considerable amount of paper work to maintain records which can be checked by regulatory agencies to ensure compliance with the regulations. All of this is necessary to reassure the public that ram packages can be transported safely without injury or threats of injury.

Specific Regulations for Consignee

The consignee must have a ram license to receive, possess, and use ram. To this general rule, there is an exception: ''NARM'' radionuclides, naturally occurring (except U-nat and Th-nat) and accelerator-produced radioactive material, do not come under the provisions of the Atomic Energy Act of 1954 and as such are not regulated by the U.S. Nuclear Regulatory Commission, but in all cases are regulated by agreement states.

The nonagreement states (those states in which the NRC still exercises licensing and inspection authority) present a mixed regulatory pattern. Some nonagreement states require a license for NARM users, while others require registration of NARM users. The varied requirements for each state are summarized in Table 3. At present, the distribution and use of naturally occurring ram (except U-nat, U-depl, and Th-nat) is decreasing but the use of accelerator-produced radionuclides is increasing particularly in the field of nuclear medicine where some accelerator-produced radionuclides have found important uses. Whether a state requires licensure or registration of NARM, it is the responsibility of the receiver, possessor, and user to be aware of and adhere to the appropriate requirements.

The federal regulations for picking up, receipt, and opening of ram packages are contained in 10 CFR 20.205. Subpart 20.205 (a) covers pick-up or receipt by the consignee of Type B and large quantity ram packages. To assist the consignee in the pick-up receipt and unloading of such ram packages, the shipper is required (71.55) to notify the consignee of (1) the date of shipment, (2) expected arrival date, and (3) any special loading/unloading instructions.

In case of the delivery of such a ram package to the consignee by a carrier, the consignee must make arrangements to be on hand to receive and check the ram package.

In case the consignee is to pick-up the package at the carrier's terminal, the consignee must make arrangements with the carrier in order that he can pick-up the ram package expeditiously upon receipt of notice from the carrier of ram package arrival.

Subpart 20.205(b) requires the consignee to monitor most ram packages upon receipt for ram leakage, but there are a list of exemptions as follows:

1. If the ram package contains an exempt quantity of ram as defined in Table 1.
2. If the ram package contains activity less than or equal to 10 mCi of H-3, C-14, S-35, or I-125 (or one presumes any combination of activity of these four radionuclides adding up to 10 mCi or less).
3. If the ram package contains only ram gases or a special form ram.

TABLE 3
STATUS OF RAM CONTROL BY STATE, TERRITORY, AND DISTRICT OF COLUMBIA

State	NRC agreement state status	NARM regulatory control
Alabama	Agreement state	License
Alaska	Nonagreement state	
Arizona	Agreement state	License
Arkansas	Agreement state	License
California	Agreement state	License
Colorado	Agreement state	License
Connecticut	Nonagreement state	Registration
Delaware	Nonagreement state	Registration
District of Columbia	Nonagreement state	
Florida	Agreement state	License
Georgia	Agreement state	License
Hawaii	Nonagreement state	Registration
Idaho	Agreement state	License
Illinois	Nonagreement state	License
Indiana	Nonagreement state	Registration
Iowa	Nonagreement state	Registration
Kansas	Agreement state	License
Kentucky	Agreement state	License
Louisiana	Agreement state	License
Maine	Nonagreement state	Registration
Maryland	Agreement state	License
Massachusetts	Nonagreement state	Registration
Michigan	Nonagreement state	
Minnesota	Nonagreement state	Registration
Mississippi	Agreement state	License
Missouri	Nonagreement state	Registration
Montana	Nonagreement state	Registration
Nebraska	Agreement state	License
Nevada	Agreement state	License
New Hampshire	Agreement state	License
New Jersey	Nonagreement state	License
New Mexico	Agreement state	License
New York	Agreement state	License
North Carolina	Agreement state	License
North Dakota	Agreement state	License
Ohio	Nonagreement state	Registration
Oklahoma	Nonagreement state	Registration
Oregon	Agreement state	License
Pennsylvania	Nonagreement state	License
Rhode Island	Agreement state	License
South Carolina	Agreement state	License
South Dakota	Nonagreement state	Registration
Tennessee	Agreement state	License
Texas	Agreement state	License
Utah	Nonagreement state	
Vermont	Nonagreement state	Registration
Virginia	Nonagreement state	License
Washington	Agreement state	License
West Virginia	Nonagreement state	Registration
Wisconsin	Nonagreement state	Registration
Wyoming	Nonagreement state	Registration
Puerto Rico	Nonagreement state	Registration

4. If the ram package contains ram in other than liquid state, e.g., Mo-99/Tc-99m generator, and not exceeding Type A quantity.
5. If the ram package contains ram with a half-life less than or equal to 30 days and ram activity is less than 100 mCi.

Removable surface contamination monitoring must be done upon receipt, or at least within 3 hr of receipt if received during normal working hours or within 18 hr at all other times. The removable contamination limit is 10,000 pCi/100 cm^2 (defined as significant contamination in 173.397). If the smear results exceed this value then the consignee must *immediately* notify the final deliverying carrier and the U.S. Nuclear Regulatory Commission Regional Office by telephone or telegraph.

The consignee should have emergency procedures which would specify what the carrier must do with the information which he is relaying. The carrier is obligated upon notification of leaking package pursuant to 177.861 (for land carriage) to isolate vehicles, building areas, or equipment where the ram was spilled and not place in operation again until the external dose rate is less than 0.5 mrem/hr on any accessible surface and the removable surface contamination is less than the limits given in 173.397(a). These actions could cause considerable disruption of the carrier's activities and should be, if possible, coordinated with the shipper and the U.S. Nuclear Regulatory Commission or the agreement state personnel.

The immediate objective is to determine the extent of contamination. Except for a few air carriers, most common and contract carriers do not have the necessary expertise nor equipment to make an immediate determination of such contamination.

A suggested procedure for the consignee is to notify all carriers in the chain and to recommend isolation of potentially contaminated areas until they are checked by qualified personnel. The urgency of the countermeasures is a function of the radionuclide and activity that leaked out. This requires professional judgement concurred in by the regulatory personnel in whose jurisdiction the contamination has occurred. In addition, 20.205(c) requires that all ram packages containing Type B and large quantity of ram must be checked to determine the external surface and 3-ft dose rates, except for those packages shipped in exclusive-use transport vehicles. If readings in excess of 200 mrem/hr on the surface or 10 mrem/hr at 3 ft are found then the nearest NRC regional office and final delivering carrier shall be *immediately* notified. What the final delivering carrier would do with this information is not obvious. Certainly, if there exists the possibility that carrier personnel received greater than 0.5 rem then the carrier has an obligation to inform his personnel, but in the absence of external removable contamination and the probability that carrier personnel received or will receive less than 0.5 rem total dose, the carrier should be told that this is for informational purposes only. When the probability exists that carrier personnel may have received significant external doses that might require medical attention, the consignee in cooperation with the NRC and the responsible agreement state personnel have to notify and advise the carrier.

Good Operating Procedures

Examples of the specialized procedures needed to remove ram from a shipping container are given in Appendixes U and V for Tc-99m from an Mo-99m/Tc-99m generator. Similar generators are in common use in nuclear pharmacies for dispensing Tc-99m. The shipping container combines as a shielded shipping and storage container and the Tc-99m is "milked" or eluted from the ion exchange column only when needed. Within 3 hr of receipt of the ram package (assuming activity is greater than 20 Ci), the generator shall be monitored for the removable contamination using smears. A quick check can be made of the smear by checking with a GM survey meter with a 30 mg/cm^2 or less thick window on a GM tube. A more accurate determination can be made later if there is any indication of leakage. The maximum permissible upper limit for removable contamination is sufficiently high that a portable GM survey meter can determine if the limit is exceeded for most radionuclides. For weak beta emitters, e.g., C-14 and S-35, a thin end window GM tube with less than 2 mg/cm^2 will detect a sufficient number of beta particles to be useful. The exception is tritium (H-3) whose weak beta particles require a windowless gas-flow counter operating in GM or the proportional region or liquid scintillation counter.

For the external surface and 3-ft measurements an appropriately calibrated ion chamber instrument or GM-type survey meter are used.

The training of personnel for receipt, unloading, and opening of ram packages will depend on how the radiation safety program functions at a given facility. In many institutions, the Radiation Safety Officer serves basically in an audit function. The actual health physics work is carried out by personnel in each individual laboratory or department working with ram. In this case, a more extensive training program for each laboratory must be conducted to conform to the regulations. In addition, the individual laboratory or department must document that the monitoring actually took place.

In other institutions the radiation safety program has trained personnel centrally located and all ram is centrally received and distributed to the individual labs and departments. In this case the ram package monitoring is an added function to their daily monitoring and documentation is still necessary. This type of centralized health physics staff is common at nuclear power stations.

Finally, the consignee is obligated to have written procedures for the receipt and opening of ram packages and an internal audit program to determine whether the procedures are being followed by the consignee personnel (20.205)(d).

Subpart 10 CFR 71.55 requires the shipper to provide the consignee any special instructions necessary for the safe opening of the ram package. In some cases, this could be critical in reducing exposures to consignee personnel. The wide variety of ram package design and their effect when unloading on the gamma ray dose to consignee personnel makes it imperative that appropriate precautions upon receipt of a ram package be taken utilizing the instructions provided by the shipper.

Agreement states have enacted comparable regulations to 20.205. The New York State Labor Department requires its licensees acting as consignees (see Appendix O) to establish procedures to ensure that receipt and opening of the ram package is done safely. Also that the licensee has procedures for unloading the ram package from the carrier's vehicle in a safe manner. These requirements are phrased in more general terms than 20.205 permitting somewhat more latitude to the licensee in establishing his own procedures. The Suggested State Regulations simply state that procedures must be established for the opening of a ram package in a safe manner (see Appendix M).

REFERENCES

1. U.S. Nuclear Regulatory Commission, NUREG-0170, December, 1977.
2. **Evans, R.,** Problems Associated with the Transportation of Radioactive Substances, NAS-NRC Publication 205, 1951.
3. **Shapiro, J.,** Exposure of Airport Workers to Radiation from Shipments of Radioactive Materials, NUREG-0154, January, 1977.
4. **Bradley, F. J., Jones, A., and Kelly, K.,** Transport Worker Radiation Exposures Handling Air, Shipments of Radioactive Materials, Proc. of 4th Int. Cong. of IRPA, April, 1977.
5. Compendium of Regulations-Shipments of Radioactive Materials over Toll Roads, Bridges, and Tunnels-International Bridges, Tunnels, and Turnpike Association, Inc., February, 1972.
6. National Transportation Safety Board, NTSB-AAS, April, 1972.
7. U.S. Nuclear Regulatory Guide 7.3, Procedures for Picking Up and Receiving Packages of Radioactive Material, Washington, D.C., May, 1975.
8. **Bradley, F. J., Jones, A., and Kelly, R.,** Transport Worker Radiation Exposures Handling Air Shipments of Radioactive Materials, Proc. of 4th Int. Cong. of IRPA, April, 1977.

ADDENDUM
PROPOSED AMENDMENTS TO U.S. DOT RAM REGULATIONS-49 CFR PARTS 171, 172, 173, 174, 175, 176, 177, AND 178

To become consistent with the International Atomic Energy Agency (IAEA) regulations the U.S. DOT has proposed amendments to the existing ram regulations which are included in this addendum. The proposed amendments became effective July 1, 1983. The main difference between existing ram transport regulations and the new IAEA-type amendments lies in the elimination of Transport Groups with Type A and Type B activities and replaced by A_1 and A_2 activities. The A_1 activity is defined as the maximum activity of special form radioactive material permitted in a Type A package and A_2 activity is defined as the maximum activity of normal form (ram other than special form or low specific activity) radioactive material permitted in a Type A package. As given in Table 1, the rather cumbersome Type A, Type B, and Large Quantity activity classification scheme divided into normal form and special form by Transport Groups has been rationalized somewhat. Whether the transport industry will transport ram any safer after 25 years under the old system will remain to be seen.

The term "large quantity" of radioactive materials which is important in the existing regulations will be dropped. This term which refers to radioactive material activities requiring special approved packaging by the U.S. Nuclear Regulatory Commission and the special highway routing of the shipments is replaced by the term "highway route controlled quantity".

The new term "highway route controlled quantity" is 3000 times A_1 or A_2 or 30,000 Ci whichever is least.

Under the new regulations all ram exceeding A_1 activity for special form or A_2 for normal form must be shipped in a Type B container. The upper activity limit for a Type B package is spelled out in the regulations or in the package approval.

The MTB believes that it is prudent to both accept this new pathway as necessary to provide a complete system for setting Type A values and to minimize unnecessary fluctuations in the Type A limits.* While there is some uncertainty as to the exact values which will result from the final, accepted new IAEA system the MTB is confident that the values now available are conservative and will most probably not be lowered. Therefore, for those nuclides which are limited by the skin exposure pathway values have been selected as follows:

Case 1: The transport group values are adopted as the new A_2 values.
Case 2: The values now available are adopted in lieu of the 1973 IAEA values.

The radionuclides which are affected in Case 1 are:

Ag-111	Nd-147	Si-31
As-77	Nd-149	Sm-153
Au-196	Os-193	Te-127M
Cd-115	Pd-109	Te-127
Ce-143	Pm-149	Te-129
Dy-165	Pr-143	W-187
Er-171	Pt-197m	Zn-69m
Gd-159	Pt-197	Zn-69
In-115m	Re-186	
Mo-99	Sc-47	

The radionuclides which are affected in Case 2 are:

* The rest of this section is from the *Fed. Reg.*, 48(48), 10223, 1983.

Au-199	Eu-155	Rh-105
Br-77	Hf-181	Ru-103
C-14	Hg-203	S-35
Ca-45	I-133	Sb-125
Ce-141	In-111	Sr-89
Cl-36	Ir-192	Tb-160
Cs-134m	K-43	Tc-99
Cs-135	Lu-177	Te-129m
Cs-137	N-13	Th-231
Cu-64	Np-239	Tl-204
Cu-67	Os-191	Tm-170
Er-169	Pm-147	W-185
Eu-152	Rb-81	Yb-175

In both cases the values adopted herein are no lower than the previously existing transport group values and yet are lower than the previously proposed 1973 IAEA A_2 values. For the radionuclides listed under Case 1, the A_2 is set at the old limit of 20 Ci as each nuclide was previously in transport group IV which had this limit. The nuclides listed in Case 2 have been assigned the currently available values under the new IAEA system. These values are between the old transport group and the 1973 IAEA values. When the new IAEA system is fully implemented by the IAEA and the skin exposure pathway is taken into due account then MTB expects to complete the alignment of A_2 values between the U.S. and the IAEA.

CLASSIFICATION OF RULE; REPORTING REQUIREMENTS; AND IMPACT ON SMALL ENTITIES

Nonmajor rule

The Materials Transportation Bureau has determined that this regulatory amendment is not a major rule under terms of Executive Order 12291 or significant under DOT regulatory procedures (44 FR 11034) and does not require a Regulatory Impact Analysis, nor does it require an environmental impact statement under the National Environmental Policy Act (42 U.S.C. 4321 et. seq.).

This determination is made on the basis that: (1) the final rule will have an annual effect on the economy not exceeding $100 million, (2) there will be no major increase in costs or prices for consumers, individual industries, federal, state, or local governmental agencies, or geographic regions, and (3) it will not result in significant adverse effects on competition, employment, investment, productivity, innovation, or the ability of the U.S.-based enterprises to compete with foreign-based enterprises in domestic or export markets.

The Department has determined under Council of Environmental Quality guidelines not to prepare an environmental impact statement for the amendment herein.

Concurrently with the publication of this rule-making document, the Department is making available in its Dockets Branch at the address indicated above, an ''Environmental Impact Assessment of Changes to Radioactive Materials Transport Regulations'' intended to support a negative declaration. This assessment was prepared by the U.S. Nuclear Regulatory Commission in support of its changes to 10 CFR Part 71 which are to be published in a subsequent issue of the Federal Register. Its analyses and conclusions are considered directly applicable to the proposals by the Department herein, in support of this negative declaration.

Paperwork Reduction Act

In accordance with the Paperwork Reduction Act of 1980 (P.L. 96-511), certain reporting or record-keeping provisions that are included in this regulation have been submitted for approval to the Office of Management and Budget (OMB). They are not effective until OMB approval has been obtained and the public notified to that effect through a technical amendment to this regulation. Other information collection requirements contained in this regulation (§§ 173.471(a), (d), and (f), 173.472 (b) and (e), 173.473(a), 173.476(a) and (b), and 173.478(a)) have been approved by OMB and assigned control numbers indicated in the regulatory text of this document.

Impact on Small Entities

Based on limited information available concerning size and nature of entities likely to be affected, I certify that this amendment will not, as promulgated, have a significant economic impact on a substantial number of small entities. Small businesses potentially affected include manufacturers, distributors, carriers, and users of (1) radiopharmaceuticals; (2) measuring, detecting, and calibrating devices which employ radioactive materials; and (3) packagings specifically designed for use in the transportation of radioactive materials. The economic impact on such small entities will be minimal.

List of Subjects

- 49 CFR Part 171 — Exports, hazardous materials transportation; imports.
- 49 CFR Part 172 — Hazardous materials transportation; labeling.
- 49 CFR Part 173 — Hazardous materials transportation; packaging and containers.
- 49 CFR Part 174 — Hazardous materials transportation; railroad safety.
- 49 CFR Part 174 — Hazardous materials transportation; railroad safety.
- 49 CFR Part 175 — Hazardous materials transportation; air carriers, radioactive materials.
- 49 CFR Part 176 — Hazardous materials transportation; maritime carriers.
- 49 CFR Part 177 — Hazardous materials transportation; motor carriers.
- 49 CFR Part 178 — Hazardous materials transportation; packaging and containers.

In consideration of the foregoing, Parts 171, 172, 173, 174, 175, 176, 177, and 178 of Title 49, Code of Federal Regulations are amended as follows:

Part 171 — General Information, Regulations, and Definitions

1. In § 171.7, paragraphs (c) (15), (d) (10) and (d) (11) are revised to read as follows, and paragraph (c) (25) is removed and reserved.

§171.7 Matter incorporated by reference

(c)* * *

(15) IAEA: International Atomic Energy Agency, Wagramerstrasse 5, P.O. Box 100, A-1400, Vienna, Austria

(25) (Reserved)

(d)* * *

(10) IAEA ''Regulations for the Safe Transport of Radioactive Materials, Safety Series No. 6, 1973 Revised Edition (as amended).''

(11) United States Nuclear Regulatory Commission (USNRC) 10 CFR Part 71, ''Packaging of Radioactive Material for Transport and Transportation of Radioactive Material Under Certain Conditions.''

2. In § 171.8, the entry for ''full load'' is removed, a definition for ''IAEA'' is added

in its proper alphabetical sequence, and the following definitions are revised to read as follows:

§171.8 Definitions and abbreviations

"IAEA" means International Atomic Energy Agency.

"Package" or "Outside Package" means a packaging plus its contents. For radioactive materials, see § 173.403 of this subchapter. "Packaging" means the assembly of one or more containers and any other components necessary to assure compliance with the minimum packaging requirements of this subchapter and includes containers (other than freight containers or overpacks), portable tanks, cargo tanks, tank cars, and multi-unit tank car tanks. For radioactive materials, see § 173.403 of this subchapter.

"Preferred route" or "Preferred highway" is a highway for shipment of "highway route controlled quantities" of radioactive materials so designated by a State routing agency, and any Interstate System highway for which an alternative highway has not been designated by such State agency as provided by § 177.825(b) of this subchapter.

"Radioactive materials" See § 173.403 of this subchapter for definitions relating to radioactive materials.

2a. In § 171.11, paragraph (d)(6)(ii), is amended by removing section reference "§173.393(b)" and inserting in its place "§173.471, 173.472 and 173.473"; paragraph (d)(6)(iii) is amended by removing section reference "173.393 (p)(q) and (r)(3)" and inserting in its place "173.448(e)(f) and (g)(3)"; paragraph (d)(6)(iv) is amended by removing section reference "§173.391" and inserting in its place "§§173.421, 173.422 or 173.424, as appropriate"; and paragraph (d)(6)(v) is revised to read as follows:

§171.11 Use of ICAO Technical Instructions

(d)* * *

(6)* * *

(v) Type A package contents shall be limited in accordance with §173.431 of this subchapter.

3. In §171.12, paragraph (e) is revised to read as follows:

§171.12 Import and export shipments

(e) Radioactive materials being imported into or exported from the U.S., or passing through the U.S. in the course of being shipped between places outside the U.S., may be offered and accepted for transportation when packaged, marked, labeled, and otherwise prepared for shipment in accordance with IAEA "Regulations for the Safe Transport of Radioactive Materials, Safety Series No. 6, 1973 Revised Edition (as amended)", if:

(1) The radioactive material is offered and accepted in accordance with the requirements of Subparts C and F of Part 172 of this subchapter pertaining to shipping papers and placarding

(2) For fissile materials and Type B packages, the competent authority certification and any necessary revalidation is obtained from the appropriate competent authorities as specified in §§173.471, 173.472 and 173.473 of this subchapter; and all requirements of the certificates and revalidations are met

(3) Type A package contents shall be limited in accordance with §173.431 of this subchapter

(4) The country of origin for the shipment has adopted the IAEA "Regulations for the

Safe Transport of Radioactive Materials, Safety Series No. 6, 1973 Revised Edition (as amended).''

Part 172 — Hazardous Materials Tables and Hazardous Materials Communications Regulations

4. The Hazardous Materials table (shown below) to § 172.101 is amended as follows:

§172.101 Purpose and use of hazardous materials table

5. In §172.203, paragraph (d)(1)(i) is amended by removing section reference ''§173.390'' and inserting in its place ''§173.435''; paragraph (d)(1)(vi)(A) is amended by removing section reference ''§173.396(a)'' and inserting in its place ''§173.453''; paragraph (d)(1)(vi)(B) is amended by removing section reference ''§173.389(a)'' and inserting in its place ''§173.455'; paragraph (d)(1)(vii) is amended by removing the phrases ''U.S. Energy Research and Development Administration (ERDA)'' and ''ERDA'', and inserting in their appropriate place ''U.S. Department of Energy (DOE)'' and ''DOE'', and by removing section reference ''§173.393a'' and inserting in its place ''§173.471''; paragraph (d)(1)(viii) is amended by removing section reference ''§173.393b(a)(3)'' and inserting in its place ''§173.473''; paragraph (d)(1)(ix) is removed; and the last sentence of paragraph (d)(1)(iii) is amended to read as follows:

§172.203 Additional description requirements

(d)* * *

(1)* * *

(iii)* * * For the shipment of a package containing a highway route controlled quantity of radioactive materials (see §173.403(1) of this subchapter), the words ''Highway route controlled quantity'' must be entered in association with the basic description.

§172.204 [Amended]

6. In §172.204, paragraph (c)(4) is amended by removing section reference ''§173.391(a)(b) or (c)'' and inserting in its place ''§§173.421, 173.422, 173.424.''

§172.310 [Amended]

7. In §172.310, paragraph (a)(2) is amended by removing section reference ''§§173.389(j) and (k) and 173.398(b) and (c)'' and inserting in its place ''§173.403''; and paragraph (a)(3) is amended by removing section reference ''§§173.393a and 173.393b'' and inserting in its place §§173.471, 173.472, and 173.473.''

8. In §172.400, paragraph (b)(10) is revised to read as follows:

§173.400 General labeling requirements

(b)* * *

(10) Package of low specific activity radioactive material, when being transported in a transport vehicle assigned for exclusive use of the consignor under §173.425(b) of this subchapter.

9. In §172.403, paragraph (a) is amended by removing section reference ''§173.391 or §173.392'' and inserting in its place ''§§173.421 through 173.425''; paragraph (g)(1) is amended by removing section reference ''§173.390'' and inserting in its place ''§173.435''; paragraph (g)(2) is amended by removing the phrase ''Number of curies'' and inserting in its place ''Activity''; paragraph (g)(3) is amended by removing the section reference ''§173.389(i)'' and inserting in its place ''§173.403''; paragraph (d) is removed and reserved; and paragraphs (b) and (c) are revised to read as follows:

+EAW	Hazardous materials descriptions and proper shipping names	Hazard class	Identification number	Label(s) required (if not excepted)	Packaging		Maximum net quantity in one package		Water shipments		
					Exceptions	Specific requirements	Passenger carrying aircraft or railcar	Cargo only aircraft	Cargo vessel	Passenger vessel	Other requirements
					(a)	(b)	(a)	(b)	(a)	(b)	(c)
	Deletions										
	Plutonium nitrate, solution	Radioactive material	NA9185	Radioactive (See 172.403)	173.393	173.396			1,2	1,2	
	Radioactive device, n.o.s.	Radioactive material	UN2911	None	173.391				1,2	1,2	
	Revisions										
	Radioactive material, empty packages	Radioactive material	UN2908	Empty	173.427				1,2	1,2	
	Radioactive material, fissile, n.o.s.	Radioactive material	UN2918	Radioactive	173.453	173.417			1,2	1,2	
	Radioactive material, instruments and articles	Radioactive material	UN2911	None	173.422 173.424				1,2	1,2	
	Radioactive material, limited quantity, n.o.s.	Radioactive material	UN2910	None	173.421				1,2	1,2	
	Radioactive material, low specific activity or LSA, n.o.s.	Radioactive material	UN2912	Radioactive	173.421 173.422 173.424	173.425			1,2	1,2	
	Radioactive material, n.o.s.	Radioactive material	UN2982	Radioactive	173.421 173.422 173.424	173.415 173.416			1,2	1,2	
	Radioactive material, special form, n.o.s.	Radioactive material	UN2974	Radioactive	173.421 173.422	173.415 173.416			1,2	1,2	
	Thorium metal, pyrophoric	Radioactive material	UN2975	Radioactive and flammable solid	None	173.418	Forbidden	Forbidden	1,2	1,2	
	Thorium nitrate	Radioactive material	UN1976	Radioactive and oxidizer	None	173.419	Forbidden	25 lb	1,2	1,2	Separate longitudinally by a complete hold or compartment from explosives
	Uranium hexafluoride, fissile (containing more than 0.72% U-235)	Radioactive material	UN2977	Radioactive and corrosive	173.453	173.417			1,2	1,2	
	Uranium hexafluoride, low specific activity	Radioactive material	UN1978	Radioactive and corrosive	173.421	173.425			1,2	1,2	
	Uranium metal pyrophoric	Radioactive material	UN2979	Radioactive and flammable solid	None	173.418	Forbidden	Forbidden	1,2	1,2	
	Uranyl acetate (RQ-5000/2270)	Radioactive material	NA9180	Radioactive	173.421 173.425	173.415 173.416			1,2	1,2	
	Uranyl nitrate hexahydrate solution (RQ-5000/2270)	Radioactive material	UN2980	Radioactive and corrosive	173.421 173.425	173.415 173.416 173.417			1,2	1,2	

Uranyl nitrate, solid (RQ-5000/2270)	Radioactive material	UN2981	Radioactive and oxidizer	None	173.419	Forbidden	25 lb	1,2	1,2	Separate longitudinally by an intervening hold or compartment from explosives

§172.403 Radioactive material

(b) The proper label to affix to a package of radioactive material is based on the radiation level at the surface of the package, the transport index (§173.403 of this subchapter) and, if appropriate, the fissile characteristics of the package. The proper category of label shall be determined in accordance with paragraph (c) of this section. The label to be applied shall be the highest category required for any of the three determining conditions for the package. Radioactive White-I is the lowest category and Radioactive Yellow-III is the highest. For example: a package with a transport index of 0.8 and a maximum surface radiation level of 60 mrem/hr which contains no fissile material must bear a Radioactive Yellow-III label.

(c) Category of label to be applied to radioactive materials packages:

Transport index (T.I.)	Radiation level at package surface (RL)	Fissile criteria	Label[a] category
T.I. = 0	RL <0.5 mrem/hr	Fissile class I only, no fissile class II or III	White-I
T.I. <1.0	0.5 mrem/h < RL < 50/ mrem/h	Fissile class I, fissile class II, with T.I. <1.0, no fissile class III	Yellow-II
1.0 <T.I.	50 mrem/h < RL	Fissile class II with 1.0 < T.I., fissile class III	Yellow-III

[a] Any package containing a ''highway route controlled quantity'' (§173.403 of this subchapter) must be labeled as Radioactive Yellow-III.

(d)[Reserved]

§172.504 [Amended]

10. In §172.504, footnote 5 to Table 1 is amended by removing section reference ''§§173.389(c) and 173.389(o)'' and inserting in its place ''§173.403'', and by removing section reference ''§173.392(b)'' and inserting in its place ''§173.425(b)''.

10a. Section 172.507 is revised to read as follows:

§172.507 Special placarding provisions: Highway

Each motor vehicle used to transport a package of highway route controlled quantity radioactive materials (see §173.403(l) of this subchapter) must have the required RADIOACTIVE warning placard placed on a square background as described in §172.527.

§172.510 [Amended]

10b. In §172.510, paragraph (d) is amended by removing section reference ''173.426'' and inserting, in its place, ''173.9''.

§172.527 [Amended]

10c. In §172.527, paragraph (a) is amended by removing the term ''large quantity'' and inserting in its place ''highway route controlled quantity''.

Part 173 — Shippers — General Requirements for Shipments and Packagings

§173.7 [Amended]

10d. In §173.7, paragraph (d) is amended by removing section reference ''§§173.393a and 173.394 through 173.396'' and inserting in its place, ''§§173.416 and 173.417''.

§173.22 [Amended]

10e. In §173.22, paragraph (c) is amended by removing the phrase ''large quantity packages of radioactive material (see §173.389 of this subchapter)'' and inserting in its place ''highway route controlled quantity packages of radioactive materials (see §173.403)''; and paragraph (d) is amended by removing the phrase ''large quantity of radioactive material (see §173.389(b))'' and inserting in its place ''highway route controlled quantity of radioactive material (see §173.403(1))''.

§173.29 [Amended]

11. In §173.29, paragraph (b) is removed and reserved.

§173.121 [Amended]

11a. In §173.121, paragraph (a)(6) is amended by removing section reference ''173.432'' and inserting in its place ''173.10.''

§173.123 [Amended]

11b. In §173.123, paragraph (a)(5) is amended by removing section reference ''173.432'' and inserting in its place ''173.10''.

§173.226 [Reserved]

12. Section 173.226 is removed and reserved.

§173.389 through 173.398 [Reserved]

13. Sections 173.389 through 173.398 are removed and reserved.

§173.9 [Redesignated from §173.426]

13a. Section 173.426 is transferred to Subpart A and redesignated as §173.9

§173.10 [Redesignated from §173.432]

13b. Section 173.432 is transferred to Subpart A and redesignated as §173.10.

14. Subpart I is revised to read as follows:

Subpart 1 — Radioactive Materials

Sec.

173.401 Scope.
173.403 Definitions.
173.411 General design requirements.
173.412 Additional design requirements for Type A packages.
173.413 Requirements for Type B packages.
173.415 Authorized Type A packages.
173.416 Authorized Type B packages.
173.417 Authorized packaging — fissile materials.
173.418 Authorized packaging — pyrophoric radioactive materials.
173.419 Authorized packaging — oxidizing radioactive materials.
173.421 Limited quantities of radioactive materials.
173.422 Exceptions for instruments and articles.
173.423 Table of activity limits — excepted quantities and devices.

§173.401 Scope

(a) This subpart sets forth requirements for the transportation of radioactive materials by carriers and shippers subject to this subchapter. The requirements prescribed in this subpart are in addition to, but not in lieu of, other requirements set forth in this subchapter and in

10 CFR Part 71 for the packaging and transportation of radioactive materials.
(b) This subpart does not apply to

(1) Radioactive materials produced, used, transported, or stored within an establishment other than during the course of transportation.
(2) Radioactive materials contained in a medical device, such as a heart pacemaker, which is implanted in a human being or live animal.
(3) Radiopharmaceuticals that have been injected into, or ingested by, and are still in human beings or live animals.

§173.403 Definitions
In this subpart:

(a) "A_1" means the maximum activity of special form radioactive material permitted in a Type A package.
(b) "A_2" means the maximum activity of radioactive material, other than special form or low specific activity radioactive material, permitted in a Type A package. These values are either listed in §173.435 or may be derived in accordance with the procedure prescribed in §173.433.
(c) "Closed transport vehicle" means a vehicle equipped with a securely attached exterior enclosure that during normal transportation restricts the access of authorized persons to the cargo space containing the radioactive materials. The enclosure may be either temporary or permanent, and in the case of packaged materials may be of the "see-through" type, and must limit access from top, sides, and ends.
(d) "Containment system" means the components of the packaging intended to retain the radioactive contents during transportation.
(e) "Conveyance" means any vehicle, aircraft, vessel, freight container, or hold, compartment or defined deck area of an inland waterway craft or seagoing vessel.
(f) "Depleted uranium" means uranium containing less uranium-235 than the naturally occurring distribution of uranium isotopes.
(g) "Design" means the description of a special form material, a package, or a packaging, that enables those items to be fully identified. The description may include specifications, engineering drawings, reports showing compliance with regulatory requirements, and other relevent documentation.
(h) "Enriched uranium" means uranium containing more uranium-235 than the naturally occurring distribution of uranium isotopes.
(i) "Exclusive use" (also referred to in other regulations as "sole use" or "full load") means the sole use of a conveyance by a single consignor and for which all initial, intermediate, and final loading and unloading are carried out in accordance with the direction of the consignor or consignee.
(j) "Fissile material" means any material consisting of or containing one or more fissile radionuclides. Fissile radionuclides are plutonium-238, plutonium-239, plutonium-241, uranium-233, and uranium-235. Neither natural nor depleted uranium are fissile material. Fissile materials are classified according to the controls needed to provide nuclear criticality safety during transportation, as provided in §173.455. Certain exclusions are provided in §173.453.
(k) "Freight container" means a reusable container having a volume of 1.81 m^3 (64 ft^3) or more, designed and constructed to permit being lifted with its contents intact and intended primarily for containment of packages in unit form during transportation. A small freight container is one which has either one outer dimension less than 1.5 m (4.9 ft) or an internal volume of not more than 3.0 m^3 (106 ft^3). All other are designated as "large freight containers."

(l) ''Highway route controlled quantity'' means a quantity within a single package which exceeds:

1. 3000 times the A_1 value of the radionuclides as specified in §173.433 for special form radioactive material,
2. 3000 times the A_2 value of the radionuclides as specified in §173.433 for normal form radioactive material, or
3. 30,000 Ci, whichever is least.

(m) ''Limited quantity of radioactive materials'' means a quantity of radioactive material not exceeding the limits given in §173.423.

(n) ''Low specific activity material (LSA)'' means any of the following:

(1) Uranium or thorium ores and physical or chemical concentrates of those ores.
(2) Unirradiated natural or depleted uranium or unirradiated natural thorium.
(3) Tritium oxide in aqueous solutions provided the concentration does not exceed 5.0 mCi/mℓ.
(4) Material in which the radioactivity is essentially uniformly distributed and in which the estimated average concentration per gram of contents does not exceed:

(i) 0.0001 mCi of radionuclides for which the A_2 quantity is not more than 0.05 Ci,
(ii) 0.005 mCi of radionuclides for which the A_2 quantity is more than 0.05 Ci, but not more than 1 Ci, or
(iii) 0.3 mCi of radionuclides for which the A_2 quantity is more than 1 Ci.

(5) Objects of nonradioactive material externally contaminated with radioactive material, provided that the radioactive material is not readily dispersible and the surface contamination, when averaged over an area of 1 m^2, does not exceed 0.0001 millicurie (220,000 disintegrations/min)/cm^2 of radionuclides for which the A_2 quantity is not more than 0.05 Ci, or 0.001 mCi (2,200,000 disintegrations/min)/cm^2 for other radionuclides.

(o) ''Multilateral approval'' means approval by both the appropriate competent authority of the country of origin and of each country through or into which the shipment is to be transported. This definition does not imply approval from countries over which radioactive materials are carried in aircraft, if there is no scheduled stop in that country.

(p) ''Natural thorium'' means thorium with the naturally occuring distribution of thorium isotopes (essentially 100 weight percent thorium-232).

(q) ''Natural uranium'' means uranium with the naturally occuring distribution of uranium isotopes (approximately 0.711 weight percent uranium-235 and the remainder essentially uranium-238).

(r) ''Nonfixed radioactive contamination'' means radioactive contamination that can be readily removed from a surface by wiping with an absorbent material. Nonfixed (removable) radioactive contamination is not significant if it does not exceed the limits specified in §173.443.

(s) ''Normal form radioactive material'' means radioactive material which has not been demonstrated to qualify as ''special form radioactive material.''

(t) ''Package'' means, for radioactive materials, the packaging together with its radioactive contents as presented for transport.

(w) ''Packaging'' means, for radioactive materials, the assembly of components necessary to ensure compliance with the packaging requirements of this subpart. It may consist of one or more receptacles, absorbent materials, spacing structures, thermal insulation, radiation shielding, and devices for cooling or absorbing mechanical shocks. The vehicle, tie-down system, and auxiliary equipment may sometimes be designated as part of the packaging.

(v) ''Radiation level'' means the radiation dose-equivalent rate expressed in millirem per hour (mrem/hr). Neutron flux densities may be converted into radiation levels according to the following table:

Neutron Flux Densities to be Regarded as Equivalent to a Radiation Level of 1 mrem/hr[a]

Energy of neutron	Flux density equivalent to 1 mrem/hr (neutrons per square centimeter per second) (n/cm^2sec)
Thermal	268.0
5 keV	228.0
20keV	112.0
100 keV	32.0
500 keV	12.0
1 MeV	7.2
5 MeV	7.2
10 Mev	6.8

[a] Flux densities equivalent for energies between those listed above may be obtained by linear interpolation.

(w) ''Radioactive article'' means any manufactured device such as an instrument, clock, electronic tube or apparatus, or similar device having radioactive material as a component part.

(x) ''Radioactive contents'' means the radioactive material, together with any contaminated liquids or gases, within the package.

(y) ''Radioactive material'' means any material having a specific activity greater than 0.002 microcuries per gram (μCi/g)(see definition of ''specific activity'').

(z) ''Special form radioactive material'' means radioactive material which satisfies the following conditions:

(1) It is either a single solid piece or is contained in a sealed capsule that can be opened only by destroying the capsule,

(2) The piece or capsule has at least one dimension not less than 5 mm (0.197 in.), and

(3) It satisfies the test requirements of §173.469. Special form encapsulations designed in accordance with the requirements of §173.389(g) in effect on June 30, 1983, and constructed prior to July 1, 1985 may continue to be used. Special form encapsulations either designed or constructed after June 30, 1985 must meet the requirements of this paragraph.

(aa) ''Specific activity'' of a radionuclide, means the activity of the radionuclide per unit mass of that nuclide. The specific activity of a material in which the radionuclide is essentially uniformly distributed is the activity per unit mass of the material.

(bb) ''Transport index'' means the dimensionless number (rounded up to the first decimal place) placed on the label of a package to designate the degree of control to be exercised by the carrier during transportation. The transport index is determined as follows:

(1) The number expressing the maximum radiation level in millirem per hour at 1 m (3.3 ft) from the external surface of the package; or
(2) For Fissile Class II packages or packages in a Fissile Class III shipment, the number expressing the maximum radiation level at 1 m (3.3 ft) from the external surface of the package, or the number obtained by dividing 50 by the allowable number of packages which may be transported together, whichever is larger.

(cc) "Type A package" means a Type A packaging together with its limited radioactive contents. A Type A package does not require competent authority approval, since its contents are limited to A_1 or A_2.
(dd) "Type B package" means a Type B packaging together with its radioactive contents.
(ee) "Type B(M)" means a Type B packaging, together with its radioactive contents, that for international shipments requires multilateral approval of the package design, and may require approval of the conditions of shipment. Type B(M) packages are those Type B package designs which have a maximum normal operating pressure of more than 7 kg/cm^2 (100 lb/in^2) gauge or a relief device which would allow the release of radioactive material to the environment under the hypothetical accident conditions specified in 10 CFR Part 71.
(ff) "Type B(U) package" means a Type B packaging, together with its radioactive contents, that for international shipments, requires unilateral approval only of the package design and of any stowage provisions that may be necessary for heat dissipation.
(gg) "Type A packaging" means a packaging designed to retain the integrity of containment and shielding required by this part under normal conditions of transport as demonstrated by the tests set forth in §§173.465 or 173.466, as appropriate.
(hh) "Type B packaging" means a packaging designed to retain the integrity of containment and shielding required by this part when subjected to the normal conditions of transport and hypothetical accident test conditions set forth in 10 CFR Part 71.
(ii) "Uncompressed gas" means, for the purposes of this subpart, gas at a pressure not exceeding the ambient atmospheric pressure at the time and location the containment system is closed. All other radioactive gases are considered to be compressed.
(jj) "Unilateral approval" means approval by the competent authority of the country of origin only.
(kk) "Unirradiated thorium" means thorium containing not more than 10^{-7}g uranium-233/g of thorium-232.
(ll) "Unirradiated uranium" means uranium containing not more than 10^{-6}g plutonium/g of uranium-235 and a fission product activity of not more than 0.25 mCi of fission products/g of uranium-235.

§173.411 General design requirements

Except for a package that contains a limited quantity or excepted device under §§173.421 through 173.424, each package used for shipment of radioactive materials shall be designed so that

(a) The package can be easily handled and properly secured in or on a conveyance during transport.
(b) A package with a gross weight exceeding 10 kg (22 lb) and up to 50 kg (110 lb) has a means for manual handling.
(c) A package with a gross weight of 50 kg (110 lb) or more can be safely handled by mechanical means,
(d) Each lifting attachment on the package, when used in the intended manner, with a minimum safety factor of three, does not impose an unsafe stress on the structure of the package. In addition, the lifting attachment shall be so designed that failure under excessive load would not impair the ability of the package to meet all other requirements of this subpart. Each attachment or other feature on the outer surface of the packaging that could be used to lift the package must be removable or otherwise capable of being made inoperable for transport, or shall be designed with strength equivalent to that required for lifting attachments,
(e) The external surface, as far as practicable, may be easily decontaminated,
(f) The outer layer of packaging will avoid, as far as practicable, pockets or crevices where water might collect, and
(g) Each feature that is added to the package at the time of transport, and that is not a part of the package, will not reduce the safety of the package.

§173.412 Additional design requirements for Type A packages

In addition to meeting the general design requirements prescribed in §173.411, each Type A packaging shall be designed so that:

(a) The smallest overall external dimension of the package is not less than 10 cm (4 in.),
(b) The outside of the packaging incorporates a feature, such as a seal, that is not readily breakable, and that, while intact, is evidence that the package has not been opened. In the case of packages shipped in exclusive use closed transport vehicles, the cargo compartment may be sealed instead of the individual packages,
(c) As far as practicable, the external surfaces are free from protrusions and are designed and finished so that they can be easily decontaminated,
(d) Containment and shielding would be maintained during transportation and storage in a temperature range of −40°C (−40°F) to 70°C (158°F) with account being taken of the possibility of brittle fracture,
(e) It is able to withstand the effects of any acceleration, vibration, or vibration resonance that may arise during normal transportation, without any deterioration of the effectiveness of closing devices or of the integrity of the package as a whole and without loosening or unintentional release of nuts, bolts, or other securing devices even after repeated use,
(f) It includes a containment system securely closed by a positive fastening device that cannot be opened unintentionally or by pressure that may arise within the package during normal transport. Special form, as demonstrated in accordance with §173.469 may be considered as a component of the containment system,
(g) The materials of the packaging and any components or structures are physically and chemically compatible with each other and with the contents, taking into account the behavior of each under irradiation,
(h) For each component of the containment system account is taken, where applicable, of radiolytic decomposition of materials and the generation of gas by chemical reaction and radiolysis,
(i) The containment system will retain its radioactive contents under the reduction of ambient pressure to 0.25 kg/cm^2 (3,5 lb/in.^{2}),
(j) Each valve through which the radioactive contents could otherwise escape is protected

against damage and unauthorized operation and, except for a pressure relief device, has an enclosure to retain any leakage,

(k) Any radiation shield that encloses a component of the packaging specified as part of the containment system will prevent the unintentional escape of that component from the shield,

(l) Failure of any tie down attachment on the packaging under excessive load will not impair the ability of the package to meet other requirements of this subpart,

(m) When subjected to the tests specified in §173.465 or evaluated against these tests by any of the methods authorized by §173.461(a), the packaging will prevent

 (1) Loss or dispersal of the radioactive contents, and
 (2) Any significant increase in the maximum radiation level recorded or calculated at the external surface for the condition before the test,

(n) Each packaging designed for liquids will

 (1) Meet the conditions prescribed in paragraph (m) of this section when subjected to the tests specified in §173.466 or evaluated against these tests by any of the methods authorized by §173.461(a),
 (2) For any package with a liquid volume not exceeding 50 cm^3 (1.7 fluid oz), have sufficient suitable absorbent material to absorb twice the volume of the liquid contents. The absorbent material shall be compatible with the package contents and suitably positioned to contact the liquid in the event of leakage, and
 (3) For any package with a liquid volume exceeding 50 cm^3 (1.7 fluid oz), either,

  (i) Have sufficient absorbent material as prescribed in paragraph (n)(2) of this section, or
  (ii) Have a containment system composed of primary inner and secondary outer containment components designed to assure retention of the liquid contents within the secondary outer components in the event that the primary inner components leak, and

(o) Each package designed for compressed or uncompressed gases other than tritium or argon-37 not exceeding 200 Ci will be able to prevent loss of contents when the package is subjected to the tests prescribed in §173.466 or evaluated against these tests by any of the methods authorized by §173.461(a).

§173.413 Requirements for Type B packages

Each Type B(U) or Type B(M) package must be designed and constructed to meet the applicable requirements in 10 CFR Part 71.

§173.415 Authorized Type A packages

The following packages are authorized for shipment, if they do not contain quantities exceeding A_1 or A_2 as appropriate:

(a) U.S. Department of Transportation (DOT) Specification 7A (§178.350 of this subchapter) Type A general packaging. Each shipper of a Specification 7A package must maintain on file for at least 1 year after the latest shipment, and shall provide to DOT on request, a complete documentation of tests and an engineering evaluation or comparative data showing that the construction methods, packaging design, and materials of construction comply with that specification. Specification 7A packagings designed in accordance with the requirements of §178.350 in effect on June 30, 1983, and constructed prior to July 1, 1985, may continue to be used. Packagings either designed or constructed after June 30, 1985, must meet the requirements of §178.350 applicable at the time of their design or construction.

(b) DOT Specification 55 metal-encased shielded packaging constructed before April 1, 1975. Such packaging constructed after March 31, 1975 is not authorized unless it is requalified under DOT Specification 7A. Each packaging designed for liquids must also meet the requirements of §173.412 (m) and (n). Use of this package as DOT Specification 55 is not authorized after June 30, 1985.

(c) Any Type B(U) or B(M) packaging, pursuant to §173.416.

(d) Any foreign-made packaging that bears the marking "Type A" and complies with the regulations of the country of origin applicable to Type A packages.

§173.416 Authorized Type B packages

Each of the following packages is authorized for shipment of quantities exceeding A_1 or A_2, as appropriate:

(a) DOT Specification 55 metal-encased shielded packaging constructed before April 1, 1975, for domestic shipments only of special form radioactive materials of 300 Ci or less. Such packaging constructed after March 31, 1975 may not be designated as DOT Specification 55. Use of this packaging is not authorized after June 30, 1985 unless approved in accordance with paragraph (b) of this section.

(b) Any Type B(U) or Type B(M) packaging that meets the applicable requirements in the regulations of the U.S. Nuclear Regulatory Commission (10 CFR Part 71) and that has been approved by that Commission may be shipped pursuant to §173.471.

(c) Any type B(U) or B(M) packaging that meets the applicable requirements of the regulations of the International Atomic Energy Agency (IAEA) in its "Regulations for the Safe Transport of Radioactive Materials, Safety Series No. 6, 1973 Revised Edition (as amended)" and for which the foreign competent authority certificate has been revalidated by DOT pursuant to §173.472. Authorized only for export and import shipments.

(d) DOT Specification 6M (§178.104 of this subchapter) metal packaging, only for solid or gaseous radioactive materials that will not undergo pressure generating decomposition at temperatures up to 121°C (250°F) and that do not generate more than 10 W of radioactive decay heat.

(e) For contents in other than special form; DOT Specification 20 WC (§178.194 of this subchapter), wooden protective jacket, when used with a single, snug-fitting inner DOT Specification 2R (§178.34 of this subchapter), or a DOT Specification 55 container constructed prior to April 1, 1975. Such packagings constructed after March 31, 1975, may not be designated as DOT Specification 55. For liquid contents, the inner packaging must comply with §173.412 (m) and (n).

(f) For contents in special form only; DOT Specification 20WC (§178.194 of this subchapter), wooden protective jacket, with a single snug-fitting inner Type A packaging that has a metal outer wall and conforms to §178.350 of this subchapter, or an inner DOT Specification 55 packaging constructed prior to April 1, 1975. Such packagings constructed after March 31, 1975, may not be designated as DOT Specification 55. Radioactive decay heat may not exceed 100 W.

(g) For contents in special form only; DOT Specification 21 WC (§178.195 of this subchapter), wooden protective overpack, with a single inner DOT Specification 2R (§178.34 of this subchapter) or an inner DOT Specification 55 container constructed prior to April 1, 1975. Such packagings constructed after March 31, 1975, may not be designated as DOT Specification 55. Contents shall be loaded within the inner packaging in such a manner as to prevent loose movement during transportation. The inner packaging shall be securely positioned and centered within the overpack so that there will be no significant displacement of the inner packaging if subjected to the 9 m (30 ft) drop test described in 10 CFR Part 71.

§173.417 Authorized packaging — Fissile materials
(a) Except as provided in §173.453, fissile materials containing not more than A_1 or A_2 as appropriate, shall be packaged in one of the following packagings:

(1) DOT Specification 6L (§178.103 of this subchapter), metal packaging, for materials prescribed in paragraph (b)(1) of this section.
(2) DOT Specification 6M (§178.104 of this subchapter), metal packaging, for materials prescribed in paragraph (b)(2) of this section.
(3) Any packaging listed in §173.415, limited to the following radioactive materials:

 (i) 500 g of uranium-235 in a single shipment as Fissile Class III or not more than 40 g of uranium-235 per package as Fissile Class II. For Fissile Class II shipments, the transport index assigned to each package shall not be less than 0.4 for each gram of uranium-235 above 15 g up to the maximum of 40 g (transport index of 10).
 (ii) 320 g of plutonium-239 as plutonium-beryllium neutron sources in special form. Total radioactivity content may not exceed 20 Ci. The transport index to be assigned to each package must be 0.5 of each 20 g, or fraction thereof, of fissile plutonium.

(4) Any other Type A or Type B packaging for fissile radioactive materials that also meets the applicable standards for fissile materials in the regulations of the U.S. Nuclear Regulatory Commission (10 CFR Part 71), and is used in accordance with §173.471.
(5) Any other Type A or Type B packaging that also meets the applicable requirements for fissile material packaging in Section VI of the International Atomic Energy Agency "Regulations for the Safe Transport of Radioactive Materials, Safety Series No. 6, 1973 Revised Edition (as amended)", and for which the foreign competent authority certificate has been revalidated by the Associate Director for HMR, in accordance with §173.472. Authorized only for export and import shipments.
(6) A DOT Specification 6J (§178.100 of this subchapter) or 17H (§178.118 of this subchapter) 55-gal steel drum, subject to the following conditions:

 (i) The quantity may not exceed 350 g of uranium-235 in any nonpyrophoric form, enriched to any degree in the uranium-235 isotope.
 (ii) Each drum must have a minimum 18-gauge body and bottom head and 16-gauge removable top head with one or more corrugations in the cover near the periphery.
 (iii) Closure must conform to §178.103-5(a) of this subchapter.
 (iv) At least four equally spaced 12 mm (0.5 in.) diameter vent holes shall be provided on the sides of the drum near the top, each covered with weatherproof tape or equivalent device.
 (v) Appropriate primary inner containment of the contents and sufficient packaging material, such as plastic or metal jars or cans shall be provided such that Specification 7A (§173.350 of this subchapter) provisions are satisfied by the inner packaging.
 (vi) Each inner container shall be capable of venting if subjected to the thermal test described in 10 CFR Part 71.
 (vii) Liquid contents shall be packaged in accordance with §173.412(m) and (n).
 (viii) The maximum weight of contents including internal packaging may not exceed 91 kg (200 lb) with fissile material content limited as shown in the table below.

Fissile Material Content and Transport Index for Specification 6J or 17H Packages

Maximum U-235 per package (g)	Minimum transport index per package as Fissile Class II	Maximum packages per transport vehicle as Fissile Class III
350	1.8	72
300	1.0	129
250	0.5	256
200	0.3	500
150	0.1	500
100	0.1	500
50	[a]	[a]

[a] Fissile Class I.

(7) Any metal cylinder that meets the performance requirements of §§173.415 and 178.350 of this subchapter for Specification 7A Type A packaging may be used as a Fissile Class I package for the transport of residual ''heels'' of enriched solid uranium hexafluoride without a protective overpack in accordance with the table below.

Allowable Content of Uranium Hexafluoride (UF_6) ''Heels'' in a Specification 7A Cylinder

Maximum cylinder diameter		Cylinder volume		Maximum uranium-235 enrichment	Maximum ''heel'' weight per cylinder			
					UF_6		Uranium-235	
Inches	Centimeters	Cubic feet	Liters	(weight percent)	kg	lb	kg	lb
5	12.7	0.311	8.8	100.0	0.045	0.1	0.031	0.07
8	20.3	1.359	39	12.5	0.227	0.5	.019	0.04
12	30.5	2.410	68	5.0	0.454	1.0	.015	0.03
30	76	25.64	725	5.0	11.3	25.0	.383	0.84
48	122	108.9 (10 ton)	3084	4.5	22.7	50	.690	1.52
		142.7 (14 ton)	4041					

(8) DOT Specifications 20PF-1, 20PF-2, or 20PF-3 (§178.120 of this subchapter) or Specifications 21PF-1 or 21PF-2 (§178.121 of this subchapter) phenolic-foam insulated overpack with snug fitting inner metal cylinders, for materials prescribed in paragraph (b)(5) of this section.

(b) Fissile radioactive materials with radioactive content exceeding A_1 or A_2 shall be packaged in one of the following packagings:

(1) DOT Specification 6L (§178.103 of this subchapter), metal packaging. Authorized only for uranium-235, plutonium-239 or plutonium-241, as metal, oxide, or compounds that do not decompose at temperatures up to 149°C (300°F). Radioactive decay heat output may not exceed 5 W. Radioactive materials in normal form shall be packaged in one or more tightly sealed metal cans or polyethylene bottles within a DOT Specification 2R (§178.34 of this subchapter) containment vessel. Packages are authorized as Fissile Class II and III with materials limited in accordance with the table below

Authorized Contents in Kilograms (kg) and Conditions for Specification 6L Packages

Uranium-235		Plutonium[a]		Fissile Class II Transport index	Fissile Class III maximum number of packages per transport vehicle
H/X ≤3[b]	3 ≤H/X≤10	H/X≤10	10 < H/X ≤20		
14	3.6[c]	—	—	1.3	80
—	—	2.5	2.4	1.8	50

[a] Plutonium solutions are not authorized.
[b] H/X is the ratio of hydrogen to fissile atoms in the inner containment with all sources of hydrogen in the containment considered.
[c] Volume not to exceed 3.6 ℓ.

(2) DOT Specification 6M (§178.104 of this subchapter), metal packaging. Authorized only for solid radioactive materials that will not decompose at temperatures up to 121°C (250°F). Radioactive decay heat output may not exceed 10 W. Radioactive materials in other than special form shall be packaged in one or more tightly sealed metal cans or polyethylene bottles within a DOT Specification 2R (§178.34 of this subchapter) containment vessel.
For fissile materials:

(i) Fissile Class I packages are limited to the following amounts of fissile radioactive materials: 1.6 kg of uranium-235; 0.9 kg of plutonium (except that due to the 10-W thermal decay heat limitation, the limit for plutonium-238 is 0.02 kg; and 0.5 kg of uranium-233. The maximum ratio of hydrogen to fissile material must not exceed three, including all of the sources of hydrogen within the DOT Specification 2R containment vessel.

(ii) Maximum quantities of fissile material for Fissile Class II and Fissile Class III, and other restrictions are given in the table below. For a Fissile Class II package, the minimum transport index to be assigned is shown in the table below and for a Fissile Class III shipment, the allowable number of similar packages per transport vehicle is shown. Each Fissile Class III shipment is also subject to the requirements in §173.457. Where a maximum ratio of hydrogen to fissile material is specified in the table below, only the hydrogen interspersed with the fissile material need be considered. For a uranium-233 shipment, the maximum inside diameter of the inner containment vessel must not exceed 12.1 cm (4.75 in.). Where necessary, a tight fitting steel insert shall be used to reduce a larger diameter inner containment vessel specified in §178.104-3(b) of this subchapter to the 12 cm (4.75 in.) limit.

(3) Type B(U) or B(M) packaging that meets the standards for packaging of fissile materials in 10 CFR Part 71, and is approved by the U.S. Nuclear Regulatory Commission in accordance with §173.471.

(4) Type B(U) or B(M) packaging that meets the applicable requirements for fissile radioactive materials in Section VI of the IAEA "Regulations for the Safe Transport of Radioactive Materials, Safety Series No. 6, 1973 Revised Edition (as amended)" and for which the foreign competent authority certificate has been revalidated by the Associate Director for HMR in accordance with §173.472. Authorized only for import and export shipments.

(5) DOT Specification 20PF-1, 20PF-2, or 20PF-3 (§178.120 of this subchapter) or Specification 21PF-1 or 21PF-2 (§178.121 of this subchapter) phenolic-foam insulated protective overpacks, with snugfitting inner metal cylinders meeting all of the appli-

AUTHORIZED CONTENTS FOR SPECIFICATION 6M PACKAGES[a]

Uranium-233[e]			Uranium-235			Plutonium[b,c,d]				
Metal or alloy	Compounds		Metal or alloy	Compounds		Metal or alloy	Compounds			Fissile Class III maximum number of packages per transport vehicle
H/X = 0[h]	H/X = 0	H/X < 3	H/X = 0	H/X = 0	H/X < 3	H/X = 0	H/X = 0	H/X < 3	Fissile Class II transport index	
3.6	4.4	2.9	7.2	7.6	5.3	3.1	4.1	3.4	0.1	1250
4.2[f]	5.2	3.5	8.7	9.6	6.4	3.4	4.5	4.1	0.2	625
5.2[f]	6.8	4.5	11.2	13.9	8.3	4.2	—	4.5	0.5	250
—	—	—	13.5	16.0	10.1	4.5	—	—	1.0	125
—	—	—	—	26.0	16.1	—	—	—	5.0	25
—	—	—	—	32.0	19.5	—	—	—	10.0	12

[a] Quantity in kilograms.
[b] Minimum percentage of plutonium-240 is 5 weight percent.
[c] 4.5 kg limitation of plutonium due to 10 W decay heat limitation.
[d] For a mixture of uranium-235 and plutonium an equal amount of uranium-235 may be substituted for any portion of plutonium authorized.
[e] Maximum inside diameter of Specification 2R containment vessel not to exceed 12 cm (4.75 in.) (see par. (b)(2)(ii) of this section).
[f] Granulated or powdered metal with any particle less than 8 mm (0.25 in.) in the smallest dimension is not authorized.
[g] Maximum permitted uranium-235 enrichment is 93.5%.
[h] H/X is the ratio of hydrogen to fissile atoms in the inner containment with all sources of hydrogen in the containment considered.

cable requirements of §§173.24, 173.411, and 173.412. Handling procedures and packaging criteria shall be in accordance with U.S. Department of Energy Report No. ORO-651 or ANSI Standard N-14.1-1971. Quantities of uranium; hexafluoride are authorized as shown in the table below, with each package to be shipped as Fissile Class II, and assigned a minimum transport index as also shown:

Authorized Quantities of Uranium Hexafluoride (UF_6) as Fissile Class II

Protective over-pack specification number	Maximum inner cylinder diameter		Maximum weight of UF_6 contents		Maximum U-235 enrichment (weight percent)	Fissile Class II transport index
	Centimeter	Inch	Kilograms	Pounds		
PF-1	12.7	5	25	55	100.0	0.1
20PF-2	20.3	8	116	255	12.5	4.0
20PF-3	30.5	12	209	460	5.0	1.1
21PF-1[a]	76[b]	30[b]	2,247	4,950	5.0	6.0
	76[c]	30[c]	2,279	5,020	5.0	5.0
21PF-2[a]	76[b]	30[b]	2,247	4,950	5.0	6.0
	76[c]	30[c]	2,279	5,020	5.0	5.0

[a] For 76-cm cylinders, the maximum permitted H/U atomic ratio is 0.066.
[b] Model 30A inner cylinder (Reference: ORO-651).
[c] Model 30B inner cylinder (Reference: ORO-651).

§173.418 Authorized packaging-pyrophoric radioactive materials

(a) Pyrophoric radioactive materials, as referenced in §172.101 of this subchapter, in quantities not exceeding A_2 per package shall be packaged in Type A packagings which are constructed of materials which will not react nor be decomposed by the contents. Contents must be:

(1) In solid form and must not be fissile unless excepted by §173.453,
(2) Contained in sealed and corrosion resistant receptacles with positive closures (friction or slip-fit covers or stoppers are not authorized),
(3) Free of water and any contaminants which would increase the reactivity of the material, and
(4) Made inert to prevent self-ignition during transport by either:

(i) Mixing with large volumes of inerting materials such as graphite or dry sand, or other suitable inerting material, or blended into a matrix of hardened concrete, or
(ii) By filling the innermost receptacle with an appropriate inert gas.

(b) In addition to the applicable requirements of §173.24 each package must be capable of passing the test conditions of §173.465 without leakage of contents.

§173.419 Authorized packaging-oxidizing radioactive materials

Certain oxidizing radioactive materials, as referenced in §172.101 of this subchapter, and which are not fissile materials and not in quantities exceeding A_2, shall be packed in suitable inside packagings of glass, metal or compatible plastic and suitably cushioned with a material which will not react with the contents. Inner packaging and cushioning shall be enclosed within an outside packaging of wood, metal, or plastic. The package shall be capable of meeting the applicable test requirements of §173.465 without leakage of contents. For shipment by air, the maximum quantity in any package may not exceed 11.3 kg (25 lb).

§173.421 Limited quantities of radioactive materials

Radioactive materials whose activity per package does not exceed the limits specified in §173.423 are excepted from the specification packaging, marking, and labeling requirements of this subchapter and requirements of this subpart if

(a) The materials are packaged in strong, tight packages that will not leak any of the radioactive materials during conditions normally incident to transportation,
(b) The radiation level at any point on the external surface of the package does not exceed 0.5 mrem/hr,
(c) The nonfixed (removable) radioactive surface contamination on the external surface of the package does not exceed the limits specified in §173.443(a),
(d) The outside of the inner packaging or if there is no inner packaging, the outside of the packaging itself bears the marking "Radioactive", and
(e) Except as provided in §173.424, the package does not contain more than 15 g of uranium-235.

§173.422 Exceptions for Instruments and articles

Instruments and manufactured articles (including clocks, electronic tubes or apparatus) or similar devices having radioactive materials in gaseous or nondispersible solid form as a component part are excepted from the specification packaging, marking and labeling requirements of this subchapter and requirements of this subpart, if

(a) The activity of the instrument or device does not exceed the relevant limit listed in the table in §173.423;
(b) The total activity per package does not exceed the relevant limit listed in the table in §173.423;
(c) The radiation level at 10 cm (4 in.) from any point on the external surface of any unpackaged instrument or device does not exceed 10 mrem/hr,
(d) The radiation level at any point on the external surface of a package bearing the device or instrument does not exceed 0.5 mrem/hr, or, for exclusive use domestic shipments, 2 mrem/hr,
(e) The nonfixed (removable) radioactive surface contamination on the external surface of the package does not exceed the limits specified in §173.443(a);
(f) Except as provided in §173.424, the package does not contain more than 15 g of uranium-235, and
(g) At least one external dimension of the package is not less than 10 cm (4 in.).

§173.423 Table of activity limits — excepted quantities and devices

The limits applicable to instruments, devices, and limited quantities Subject to exceptions under §§173.421 and 173.422 are shown in the table below

Activity Limits for Limited Quantities, Instruments, and Devices

Nature of contents	Instruments and devices: Instrument and article limits[a]	Instruments and devices: Package limits	Materials package limits
Solids			
Special form			
Other forms	$10^{-2}A_1$	A_1	$10^{-3}A_1$
	$10^{-2}A_2$	A_2	$10^{-3}A_2$
Liquids			
Tritiated water			
<0.1 Ci/ℓ	—	—	1000 Ci
0.1 to Ci to 1.0 Ci/ℓ	—	—	100 Ci
>1.0 Ci/ℓ	—	—	1 Ci
Other liquids	$10^{-3}A_2$	$10^{-1}A_2$	$10^{-4}A_2$
Gases			
Tritium[b]	20 Ci	200 Ci	20 Ci
Special form	$10^{-3}A_1$	$10^{-2}A_1$	$10^{-3}A_1$
Other forms	$10^{-3}A_2$	$10^{-2}A_2$	$10^{-3}A_2$

[a] For mixture of radionuclides see §173.433(b).

[b] These values also apply to tritium in activated luminous paint and tritium absorbed on solid carriers.

§173.424 Excepted articles containing natural uranium or thorium

Manufactured articles in which the sole radioactive material content is natural or depleted uranium or natural thorium are excepted from the specification packaging, marking and labeling requirements of this subchapter and requirements of this subpart if

(a) The outer surface of the uranium or thorium is enclosed in an inactive sheath made of metal or other protective material, and
(b) The conditions specified in §173.421(b), (c), and (d) are met.

§173.425 Transport requirements for low specific activity (LSA) radioactive materials

In addition to other applicable requirements specified in this subchapter, low specific activity (LSA) materials shall be transported in accordance with paragraph (a) of this section, or if transported as exclusive-use may be transported in accordance with paragraph (b) or (c) of this section.

(a) DOT Specification 7A (§178.350 of this subchapter) Type A package. The requirements of §173.412(a), (b), (d), and (n) do not apply.

(b) Packaged shipments of LSA material consigned as exclusive use shall either be in accordance with paragraph (a) of this section or shall comply with the following in which case they are excepted from specification packaging, marking and labeling:

(1) Materials must be packaged in strong, tight packages so that there will be no leakage of radioactive material under conditions normally incident to transportation.
(2) Packages must not have any significant removable surface contamination (see §173.443).
(3) External radiation levels must comply with §173.441.
(4) Shipments must be loaded by consignor and unloaded by consignee from the transport vehicle in which originally loaded.
(5) There must be no loose radioactive material in the car or vehicle.
(6) Shipment must be braced so as to prevent shifting of lading under conditions normally incident to transportation.
(7) Except for shipments of unconcentrated uranium or thorium ores, the transport vehicle

must be placarded with the placards prescribed in accordance with Subpart F of Part 172 of this subchapter, as appropriate.

(8) The exterior of each outside package must be stenciled or otherwise marked ''Radioactive — LSA''.

(9) Specific instructions for maintenance of exclusive use shipment controls must be provided by the shipper to the carrier. Such instructions must be included with the shipping paper information.

(10) Transportation by aircraft is prohibited.

(c) Unpackaged (bulk) shipments of LSA materials shall be transported only in exclusive use closed transport vehicles and shall comply with the following:

(1) Authorized materials are limited to the following:

(i) Uranium or thorium ores and physical or chemical concentrates of those ores.

(ii) Uranium metal or natural thorium metal, or alloys of these materials.

(iii) Materials of low radioactive concentration, if the average estimated radioactivity concentration does not exceed 0.001 mCi/g and the contribution from materials with an A_2 value (see §173.435) of less than 0.05 Ci does not exceed 1% of the total radioactivity.

(iv) Objects of nonradioactive material externally contaminated with radioactive material, if the radioactive material is not readily dispersible and the surface contamination, when averaged over $1m^2$, does not exceed 0.0001 mCi/cm^2 of radionuclides for which the A_2 value is less than 0.05 or 0.0001 mCi/cm^2 of other radionuclides. Such objects must be suitably wrapped or enclosed.

(2) Bulk liquids must be transported in the following:

(i) Specification 103CW, 111A60W7 (§§179.200, 179.201, 179.202 of this subchapter) tank cars. Bottom openings in tanks prohibited.

(ii) Specification MC310, MC311, MC312, or MC331 (§§178.343 or 178.337 of this subchapter) cargo tanks. Authorized only where the radioactivity concentration does not exceed 10% of the specified low specific activity levels (see §173.403(n)). The requirements of §173.412(n) do not apply to these cargo tanks. Bottom fittings and valves are not authorized. Trailer-on-flat-car service is not authorized.

(3) External radiation levels must comply with §173.441(b).

(4) Shipments must be loaded by the consignor, and unloaded by the consignee from the transport vehicle in which originally loaded.

(5) Except for shipments of unconcentrated uranium or thorium ores, the transport vehicle must be placarded with the placards prescribed in Subpart F of Part 172 of this subchapter, as appropriate.

(6) There must be no leakage of radioactive materials from the vehicle.

(7) Specific instructions for maintenance of exclusive use shipment controls must be provided by the shipper to the carrier. Such instructions must be included with the shipping paper information.

(8) Transportation by aircraft is prohibited.

§173.427 Empty radioactive materials packaging

Any packaging which previously contained radioactive materials and has been emptied of contents as far as practical, is excepted from marking and labeling requirements of this subchapter and from requirements of this subpart, provided that:

(a) It complies with the requirements of §173.421(b), (c), and (e).
(b) The packaging is in unimpaired condition and is securely closed so that there will be no leakage of radioactive material under conditions normally incident to transportation,
(c) Internal contamination does not exceed 1000 times the limits specified in the table in §173.443, and
(d) Any labels previously applied in conformance with Subpart E of Part 172 of this subchapter are removed, obliterated or covered and the ''Empty'' label prescribed in §172.450 is affixed to the packaging.

§173.431 Activity limits for Type A and Type B packages

(a) A Type A package shall not contain radioactive contents with an activity greater than the following, as listed in §173.435, or for other materials as determined under §173.433:

(1) For special form radioactive materials, A_1, or
(2) For all other radioactive materials, A_2.

(b) The limits on activity contained in a Type B(U) and Type B(M) package are those prescribed in §173.416 or in the applicable approval recertificate under §§173.471 and 173.472.

§173.433 Requirements for determination of A_1 and A_2 values for radionuclides

(a) Single radionuclides

(1) For single radionuclides of known identity, the values of A_1 and A_2 are those given in the table in §173.435. The values of A_1 and A_2 are also applicable for radionuclides contained in (α,n) or (γ,n) neutron sources.

(2) For any single radionuclide of known identity, which is not listed in §173.435, the values of A_1 and A_2 shall be determined in accordance with the following:

(i) If the radionuclide emits only one type of radiation, A_1 is determined in accordance with paragraphs (A), (B), (C), and (D) of this subparagraphs. For radionuclides emitting different kinds of radiation, A_1 is the most restrictive value of those determined for each kind of radiation. However, in both cases, A_1 is restricted to a maximum of 1000 Ci. If a parent nuclide decays into a shorter lived daughter, of a half-life not greater than 10 days, A_1 is calculated for both the parent and the daughter, and the more limiting of the two values is assigned to the parent nuclide.

(A) For gamma emitters, A_1 is determined by the expression: $A_1 = 9\,\Gamma$ Ci where Γ is the gamma-ray constant, corresponding to the dose in roentgens per hour at 1 m/Ci; the number 9 results from the choice of 1 rem/hr at a distance of 3 m as the reference dose-equivalent rate.

(B) For X-ray emitters, A_1 is determined by the atomic number (Z) of the nuclide:

$$Z < 55 \qquad A_1 = 1000 \text{ Ci}$$
$$\text{for } Z > 55 \qquad A_1 = 200 \text{ Ci}$$

(C) For beta emitters, A_1 is determined by the maximum beta energy (E_{max}) according to the following table:

A_1 for Beta Emitters

E_{max}(MeV)	A_1(Ci)
<0.5	1000
0.5 — <1.0	300
1.0 — <1.5	100
1.5 — <2.0	30
≥2.0	10

(D) For alpha emitters, A_1 is determined by the expression:

$$A_1 = 1000\ A_3$$

where A_3 is the value listed in the following table

A_3 for Alpha Emitters

Atomic number	Half-life less than 1000 days	Half-life 1000 days to 10^6 years	Half-life greater than 10^6 years
1 to 81	3 Ci	50 mCi	3 Ci
82 and above	2 mCi	2 mCi	3 Ci

(ii) For assignment of A_2 values, A_2 is the more restrictive of the following values:
(A) The corresponding A_1.
(B) The value A_3 obtained from the above table.

(3) For any single radionuclide whose identity is unknown, the value of A_1 is 2 Ci and the value of A_2 is 0.002 Ci. However, if the atomic number of the radionuclide is less than 82, the value of A_1 is 10 Ci and the value of A_2 is 0.4 Ci.

(b) Mixture of radionuclides, including radioactive decay chains

(1) For mixed fission products, where a detailed analysis of the mixture is not carried out, the following activity limits apply:

(i) $A_1 = 10$ Ci
(ii) $A_2 = 0.4$ Ci

(2) A single radioactive decay chain is considered to be a single radionuclide when the radionuclides are present in their naturally occurring portions and no daughter nuclide has a half-life either longer than 10 days or longer than that of the parent nuclide. The activity to be taken into account and the A_1 or A_2 value to be applied are those corresponding to the parent nuclide of that chain. When calculating A_1 or A_2 values, radiation emitted by daughters must be taken into account. However, in the case of radioactive decay chains in which any daughter nuclide has a half-life either longer than 10 days or greater than that of the parent nuclide, the parent and daughter nuclides are considered to be mixtures of different nuclides.

(3) In the case of a mixture of different radionuclides, where the identity and activity of each radionuclide is known, the permissible activity of each radionuclide $R_1, R_2, \ldots R_n$ must be such that $F_1 + F_2 + \ldots F_n$ is not greater than unity, when

$$F_1 = \frac{\text{Total activity of } R_1}{A_1(R_1)}$$

$$F_2 = \frac{\text{Total activity of } R_2}{A_1(R_2)}$$

$$F_n = \frac{\text{Total activity of } R_n}{A_1 R_n}$$

Where A_1 (R_1R_2 . . . R_n) is the value of A_1 or A_2 as appropriate for the nuclide R_1,R_2 . . . R_n.

(4) When the identity of each radionuclide is known but the individual activities of some of the radionuclides are not known, the formula given in subparagraph (3) of this paragraph must be applied to establish the values of A_1 or A_2 as appropriate. All the radionuclides whose individual activities are not known (but whose total activity is known) must be classed in a single group and the most restrictive value of A_1 or A_2 applicable to any one of them shall be used as the value of A_1 and A_2 in the denominator of the fraction.

(5) Where the identity of each radionuclide is known but the individual activity of the radionuclides is not known, the most restrictive value of A_1 or A_2 applicable to any one of the radionuclides present is the applicable value.

(6) When the identity of the radionuclides is not known, the value of A_1 is 2 Ci and the value of A_2 is 0.002 Ci. However, if alpha emitters are known to be absent, the value of A_2 is 0.4 Ci.

§173.434 Activity-mass relationships for uranium and natural thorium

Radioactive material	Ci/g	g/Ci
Uranium — (Wt% ^{235}U present)[a]		
0.45	5.0×10^{-7}	2.0×10^{6}
0.72 (natural)	7.06×10^{-7}	1.42×10^{6}
1.0	7.6×10^{-7}	1.3×10^{6}
1.5	1.0×10^{-6}	1.0×10^{6}
5.0	2.7×10^{-6}	3.7×10^{5}
10.0	4.8×10^{-6}	2.1×10^{5}
20.0	1.0×10^{-5}	1.0×10^{5}
35.0	2.0×10^{-5}	5.0×10^{4}
50.0	2.5×10^{-5}	4.0×10^{4}
90.0	5.8×10^{-5}	1.7×10^{4}
93.0	7.0×10^{-5}	1.4×10^{4}
95.0	9.1×10^{-5}	1.1×10^{4}
Natural thorium	2.2×10^{-7}	4.6×10^{6}

[a] The figures for uranium include representative values for the activity of uranium-234 which is concentrated during the enrichment process. The activity for thorium includes the equilibrium concentration of thorium-228.

§173.435 Table of A_1 and A_2 values for radionuclides

Symbol of radionuclide	Element and atomic number	A_1(Ci)	A_2(Ci)	Specific activity (CI/g)
227_{Ac}	Actinum (89)	1000	0.003	7.2×10
228_{Ac}		10	4	2.2×10^{6}
105_{Ag}	Silver (47)	40	40	3.1×10^{4}
$110m_{Ag}$		7	7	4.7×10^{3}
111_{Ag}		100	20	1.6×10^{5}
241_{Am}	Americum (95)[a]	8	0.008	3.2
243_{Am}		8	0.008	1.9×10^{-2}

Symbol of radionuclide	Element and atomic number	A_1(Ci)	A_2(Ci)	Specific activity (CI/g)
37_{Ar} (compressed or uncompressed)	Argon (18)	1000	1000	1.0×10^5
41_{Ar} (uncompressed)		20	20	4.3×10^7
41_{Ar} (compressed)		1	1	4.3×10^7
73_{As}	Arsenic (33)	1000	400	2.4×10^4
74_{As}		20	20	1.0×10^5
76_{As}		10	10	1.6×10^6
77_{As}		300	20	1.1×10^6
211_{At}	Astatine (85)	200	7	2.1×10^6
193_{Au}	Gold (79)	200	200	9.3×10^5
196_{Au}		30	30	1.2×20^5
198_{Au}		40	20	2.5×10^5
199_{Au}		200	25	2.1×10^5
131_{Ba}	Barium (56)	40	40	8.7×10^4
133_{Ba}		40	10	4.0×10^2
140_{Ba}		20	20	7.3×10^4
7_{Be}	Beryllium (4)	300	300	3.5×10^5
206_{Bi}	Bismuth (83)	5	5	9.9×10^4
207_{Bi}		10	10	2.2×10^2
$201_{Bi(RaE)}$		100	4	1.2×10^5
212_{Bi}		6	6	1.5×10^7
249_{Bk}	Berkelium (97)	1000	1	1.8×10^3
77_{Br}	Bromine (35)	70	25	7.1×10^5
82_{Br}		6	6	1.1×10^6
11_{c}	Carbon (6)	20	20	8.4×10^8
14_{c}		1000	60	4.6
45_{Ca}	Calcium (20)	1000	25	1.9×10^4
47_{Ca}		20	20	5.9×10^5
109_{Cd}	Cadmium (48)	1000	70	2.6×10^3
$115m_{Cd}$		30	30	2.6×10^4
115_{Cd}		80	20	5.1×10^5
139_{Ce}	Cerium (58)	100	100	6.5×10^3
141_{Ce}		300	25	2.8×10^4
143_{Ce}		60	20	6.6×10^5
144_{Ce}		10	7	3.2×10^3
249_{Cf}	Californium (98)	2	0.002	3.1
250_{Cf}		7	0.007	1.3×10^2
252_{Cf}		2	0.009	6.5×10^2
36_{Cl}	Chlorine (17)	300	10	3.2×10^{-2}
38_{Cl}		10	10	1.3×10^8
242_{Cm}	Curium (96)	200	0.2	3.3×10^3
243_{Cm}		9	0.009	4.2×10
244_{Cm}		10	0.01	8.2×10
245_{Cm}		6	0.006	1.0×10^{-1}
246_{Cm}		6	0.006	3.6×10^{-1}
56_{Co}	Cobalt (27)	5	5	3.0×10^4
57_{Co}		90	90	8.5×10^3
$58m_{Co}$		000	1000	5.9×10^6
58_{Co}		20	20	3.1×10^4
60_{Co}		7	7	1.1×10^3
51_{Cr}	Chromium (24)	600	600	9.2×10^4
129_{Cs}	Cesium (55)	40	40	7.6×10^5
131_{Cs}		1000	1000	1.0×10^5
$134m_{Cs}$		1000	10	7.4×10^6
134_{Cs}		10	10	1.2×10^3
135_{Cs}		1000	25	8.8×10^{-4}
136_{Cs}		7	7	7.4×10^4
137_{Cs}		30	10	9.8×10
64_{Cu}	Copper (29)	80	25	3.8×10^5

Symbol of radionuclide	Element and atomic number	A_1(Ci)	A_2(Ci)	Specific activity (CI/g)
67_{Cu}		200	25	7.9×10^5
165_{Dy}	Dysprosium (66)	100	20	8.2×10^6
166_{Dy}		1000	200	2.3×10^5
169_{Er}	Erbium (68)	1000	25	8.2×10^4
171_{Er}		50	20	2.4×10^6
$152m_{Eu}$	Europium (63)	30	30	2.2×20^6
152_{Eu}		20	10	1.9×10^2
154_{Eu}		10	5	1.5×10^2
155_{Eu}		400	60	1.4×10^3
18_F	Fluorine (9)	20	20	9.3×10^7
52_{Fe}	Iron (26)	5	5	7.3×10^6
55_{Fe}		1000	1000	2.2×10^3
59_{Fe}		10	10	4.9×10^4
67_{Ga}	Gallium (31)	100	100	6.0×10^5
68_{Ga}		20	20	4.0×10^7
72_{Ga}		7	7	3.1×10^6
153_{Gd}	Gadolinium (64)	200	100	3.6×10^3
159_{Gd}		300	20	1.1×10^4
68_{Ge}	Germanium (32)	20	10	7.0×10^2
71_{Ge}		1000	1000	1.6×10^5
3_H	Hydrogen (1)(see T-Tritium)	—	—	—
181_{Hf}	Hafnium (72)	30	25	1.6×10^4
$197m_{Hg}$	Mercury (80)	200	200	6.6×10^5
197_{Hg}		200	200	2.5×10^5
203_{Hg}		80	25	1.4×10^4
166_{Ho}	Holmium (67)	30	30	6.9×10^5
123_I	Iodine (53)	50	50	1.9×10^6
125_I		1000	70	1.7×10^4
126_I		40	10	7.8×10^4
129_I		1000	2	1.6×10^{-4}
131_I		40	10	1.2×10^5
132_I		7	7	1.1×10^7
133_I		30	10	1.1×10^6
134_I		8	8	2.7×10^7
135_I		10	10	3.5×10^6
111_{In}	Indium (49)	30	25	4.2×10^5
$113m_{In}$		60	60	1.6×10^7
$114m_{In}$		30	20	2.3×10^4
$115m_{In}$		100	20	6.1×10^6
190_{Ir}	Iridium (77)	10	10	6.2×10^4
192_{Ir}		20	10	9.1×10^3
194_{Ir}		10	10	8.5×10^5
42_K	Potassium (19)	10	10	6.0×10^6
43_K		20	10	3.3×10^6
$85m_{Kr}$ (uncompressed)	Krypton (36)	100	100	8.4×10^6
$85m_{Kr}$ (compressed)		3	3	8.4×10^6
85_{Kr} (uncompressed)		1000	1000	4.0×10^2
85_{Kr} (compressed)		5	5	4.0×10^2
87_{Kr} (uncompressed)		20	20	2.8×10^7
87_{Kr} (compressed)		0.6	0.6	2.8×10^7
140_{La}	Lanthanum (57)	30	30	5.6×10^5
LSA	Low specific activity material (see × 173.403)	—	—	—
177_{Lu}	Lutetium (71)	300	25	1.1×10^5
MFP	Mixed fission products	10	0.4	—
28_{Mg}	Magnesium (12)	6	6	5.2×10^6
52_{Mn}	Manganese (25)	5	5	4.4×10^5
54_{Mn}		20	20	8.3×10^3
56_{Mn}		5	5	2.2×10^7

Symbol of radionuclide	Element and atomic number	A_1(Ci)	A_2(Ci)	Specific activity (CI/g)
99_{Mo}	Molybdenum (42)	100	20	4.7×10^{5}
13_{N}	Nitrogen (7)	20	10	1.5×10^{9}
22_{Na}	Sodium (11)	8	8	6.3×10^{3}
24_{Na}		5	5	8.7×10^{6}
$93m_{Nb}$	Niobium (41)	1000	200	1.1×10^{3}
95_{Nb}		20	20	3.9×10^{4}
97_{Nb}		20	20	2.6×10^{7}
147_{Nd}	Neodymium (60)	100	20	8.0×10^{4}
149_{Nd}		30	20	1.1×10^{7}
59_{Ni}	Nickel (28)	1000	900	8.1×10^{-2}
63_{Ni}		1000	100	4.6×10
65_{Ni}		10	10	1.9×10^{7}
237_{Np}	Neptunium (93)	5	0.005	6.9×10^{-4}
239_{Np}		200	25	2.3×10^{5}
185_{Os}	Osmium (76)	20	20	7.3×10^{3}
191_{Os}		600	200	4.6×10^{4}
$191m_{Os}$		200	200	1.2×10^{6}
193_{Os}		100	20	5.3×10^{5}
32_{P}	Phosphorus (15)	30	30	2.9×10^{6}
230_{Pa}	Protoactinium (91)	20	0.8	3.2×10^{4}
231_{Pa}		2	0.002	4.5×10^{-2}
233_{Pa}		100	100	2.1×10^{4}
201_{Pb}	Lead (82)	20	20	1.7×10^{6}
210_{Pb}		100	0.2	8.8×10
212_{Pb}		6	5	1.4×10^{6}
103_{Pd}	Palladium (46)	1000	700	7.5×10^{4}
109_{Pd}		100	20	2.1×10^{6}
147_{Pm}	Promethium (61)	1000	25	9.4×10^{2}
149_{Pm}		100	20	4.2×10^{6}
210_{Po}	Polonium (84)	200	0.2	4.5×10^{3}
142_{Pr}	Praseodymium (59)	10	10	1.2×10^{6}
143_{Pr}		300	20	6.6×10^{4}
191^{Pt}	Platinum (78)	100	100	2.3×10^{5}
$193m^{Pt}$		200	200	2.0×10^{5}
$197m^{Pt}$		300	20	1.2×10^{7}
197^{Pt}		300	20	8.8×10^{5}
238^{Pu}	Plutonium (94)[a]	3	0.003	1.7×10
239^{Pu}		2	0.002	6.2×10^{-2}
240^{Pu}		2	0.002	2.3×10^{-1}
241^{Pu}		1000	0.1	1.1×10^{2}
242^{Pu}		3	0.003	3.9×10^{-3}
223^{Ra}	Radium (88)	50	0.2	5.0×10^{4}
224^{Ra}		6	0.5	1.6×10^{5}
226^{Ra}		10	0.005	1.0
228^{Ra}		10	0.05	2.3×10^{2}
81^{Rb}	Rubidium (37)	30	25	8.2×10^{6}
86^{Rb}		30	30	8.1×10^{4}
87^{Rb}		Unlimited	Unlimited	6.6×10 [illegible]
Rb (natural)		Unlimited	Unlimited	1.8×10^{-8}
186^{Re}	Rhenium (75)	100	20	1.9×10^{-5}
187^{Re}		Unlimited	Unlimited	3.8×10^{-8}
188^{Re}		10	10	1.0×10^{-6}
Re (natural)		Unlimited	Unlimited	2.4×10^{-8}
$103m^{Rh}$	Rhodium (45)	1000	1000	3.2×10^{7}
105^{Rh}		200	25	8.2×10^{5}
222^{Rn}	Radon (86)	10	2	1.5×18^{3}
97^{Ru}	Ruthenium (44)	80	80	5.5×10^{5}
103^{Ru}		30	25	3.2×10^{4}
105^{Ru}		20	20	6.6×10^{6}

Symbol of radionuclide	Element and atomic number	A_1(Ci)	A_2(Ci)	Specific activity (CI/g)
106^{Ru}		10	7	3.4×10^{3}
35^{S}	Sulphur (16)	1000	60	4.3×10^{4}
122^{Sb}	Antimony (51)	30	30	3.9×10^{5}
124^{Sb}		5	5	1.8×10^{4}
125^{Sb}		40	25	1.4×10^{3}
46^{Sc}	Scandium (21)	8	8	3.4×10^{4}
47^{Sc}		200	20	8.2×10^{5}
48^{Sc}		5	5	1.5×10^{6}
75^{Sc}	Selenium (34)	40	40	1.4×10^{4}
31^{Si}	Silicon (14)	100	20	3.9×10^{7}
147^{Sm}	Samarium (62)	Unlimited	Unlimited	2.0×10^{-8}
151^{Sm}		1000	90	2.6×10
153^{Sm}		300	20	4.4×10^{5}
113^{Sn}	Tin (50)	60	60	1.0×10^{4}
$119m^{Sn}$		100	100	4.4×10^{3}
125^{Sn}		10	10	1.1×10^{5}
$85m^{Sr}$	Strontium (38)	80	80	3.2×10^{7}
85^{Sr}		30	30	2.4×10^{4}
$87m^{Sr}$		50	50	1.2×10^{7}
89^{Sr}		100	10	2.9×10^{4}
90^{Sr}		10	0.4	1.5×10^{2}
91^{Sr}		10	10	3.6×10^{6}
92^{Sr}		10	10	1.3×10^{7}
T (uncompressed)	Tritium (1)	1000	1000	9.7×10^{3}
T (compressed)		1000	1000	9.7×10^{3}
T (activated luminous paint)		1000	1000	9.7×10^{3}
T (adsorbed on solid carrier)		1000	1000	9.7×10^{3}
T (tritialed water)		1000	1000	9.7×10^{3}
T (other forms)		20	20	9.7×10^{3}
182^{Ta}	Tantalum (73)	20	20	6.2×10^{3}
160^{Tb}	Terbium (65)	20	10	1.1×10^{4}
$96m^{Tc}$	Technetium (43)	1000	1000	3.8×10^{7}
96^{Tc}		6	6	3.2×10^{5}
$97m^{Tc}$		1000	200	1.5×10^{4}
97^{Tc}		1000	400	1.4×10^{-4}
$99m^{Tc}$		100	100	5.2×10^{6}
99^{Tc}		1000	25	1.7×10^{-2}
$125m^{Te}$	Tellurium (52)	1000	100	1.8×10^{4}
$127m^{Te}$		300	20	4.0×10^{4}
127^{Te}		300	20	2.6×10^{6}
$129m^{Te}$		30	10	2.5×10^{4}
129^{Te}		100	20	2.0×10^{7}
$131m^{Te}$		10	10	8.0×10^{5}
132^{Te}		7	7	3.1×10^{5}
227^{Th}	Thorium (90)	200	0.2	3.2×10^{4}
228^{Th}		6	0.008	8.3×10^{2}
230^{Th}		3	0.003	1.9×10^{-2}
231^{Th}		1000	25	5.3×10^{5}
232^{Th}		Unlimited	Unlimited	1.1×10^{-7}
234^{Th}		10	10	2.3×10^{4}
Th (natural)		Unlimited	Unlimited	2.2×10^{-7}
Th (irradiated)[b]		—	—	—
200^{Tl}	Thallium (81)	20	20	5.8×10^{5}
201^{Tl}		200	200	2.2×10^{5}
202^{Tl}		40	40	5.4×10^{4}
204^{Tl}		300	10	4.3×10^{2}
170^{Tm}	Thulium (69)	300	40	6.0×10^{3}
171^{Tm}		1000	10	1.1×10^{3}
230^{U}	Uranium (92)	100	0.1	2.7×10^{4}

Symbol of radionuclide	Element and atomic number	A_1(Ci)	A_2(Ci)	Specific activity (CI/g)
232^{U}		30	0.03	2.1×10
233^{U}		100	0.1	9.5×10^{-3}
234^{U}		100	0.1	6.2×10^{-3}
235^{U}		100	0.2	2.1×10^{-6}
236^{U}		200	0.2	6.3×10^{-5}
238^{U}		Unlimited	Umlimited	3.3×10^{-7}
U (natural)		Unlimited	Unlimited	(see §173.434)
U (enriched) <20%		Unlimited	Unlimited	(see §173.434)
20% or greater		100	0.1	(see §173.434)
U (depleted)		Unlimited	Unlimited	(see §173.434
U (irradiated)[c]		—	—	—
48^{V}	Vanadium (23)	6	6	1.7×10^{5}
181^{W}	Tungsten (74)	200	100	5.0×10^{3}
185^{W}		1000	25	9.7×10^{-3}
187^{W}		40	20	7.0×10^{5}
127^{Xe} (uncompressed)	Xenon (54)	70	70	2.8×10^{4}
127^{Xe} (compressed)		5	5	2.8×10^{4}
$131m^{Xe}$ (compressed)		10	10	1.0×10^{5}
$131m^{Xe}$ (uncompressed)		100	100	1.0×10^{5}
133^{Xe} (uncompressed)		1000	1000	1.9×10^{5}
133^{Xe} (compressed)		5	5	1.9×10^{5}
135^{Xe} (uncompressed)		70	70	2.5×10^{5}
135^{Xe} (compressed)		2	2	2.5×10^{5}
87^{Y}	Yttrium (39)	20	20	4.5×10
90^{Y}		10	10	2.5×10^{5}
$91m^{Y}$		30	30	4.1×10^{7}
91^{Y}		30	30	2.5×10^{4}
92^{Y}		10	10	9.5×10^{6}
93^{Y}		10	10	3.2×10^{6}
169^{Yb}	Ytterbium (70)	80	80	2.3×10^{5}
175^{Yb}		400	25	1.8×10^{5}
65^{Zn}	Zinc (30)	30	30	8.0×10^{3}
$69m^{Zn}$		40	20	3.3×10^{6}
69^{Zn}		300	20	5.3×10^{7}
93^{Zr}	Zirconium (40)	1000	200	3.5×10^{-3}
95^{Zr}		20	20	2.1×10^{4}
97^{Zr}		20	20	2.0×10^{6}

[a] For shipments solely within the U.S. the A^1 value is 20 Ci for americium and plutonium contained in Am-Be or Pu-Be neutron sources or in nuclear-powdered pacemakers.

[b] The values of A_1 and A_2 must be calculated in accordance with the procedure specified in §173.433 of this subchapter, taking into account the activity of the fission products and of the uranium-233 in addition to that of the thorium.

[c] The values of A_1 and A_2 must be calculated in accordance with the procedure specified in §173.433 of this subchapter, taking into account the activity of the fission products and plutonium isotopes in addition to that of the uranium.

§173.441 Radiation level limitations

(a) Except as provided in paragraph (b) of this section, each package of radioactive materials offered for transportation shall be designed and prepared for shipment so that under conditions normally incident to transportation the radiation level does not exceed 200 mrem/hr at any point on the external surface of the package, and the transport index does not exceed 10.

(b) Except for shipments by air, a shipment which exceeds the radiation level limits specified in paragraph (a) of this section, may be transported as an exclusive-use shipment if the radiation level does not exceed any of the following at any time during transportation:

(1) 200 mrem/hr on the accessible external surface of the package unless the following conditions are met, in which case the limit is 1000 mrem/hr:

   (i) The shipment is made in a closed transport vehicle,
   (ii) Provisions are made to secure the package so that its position within the vehicle remains fixed during transportation, and
   (iii) There are no loading or unloading operations between the beginning and end of the transportation.

(2) 200 mrem/hr at any point on the outer surface of the vehicle, including the upper and lower surfaces, or, in the case of an open vehicle, at any point on the vertical planes projected from the outer edges of the vehicle, on the upper surface of the load, and on the lower external surface of the vehicle,
(3) 10 mrem/hr at any point 2 m (6.6 ft) from the vertical planes represented by the outer lateral surfaces of the vehicle, or, in the case of an open vehicle, at any point 2 m from the vertical planes projected from the outer edges of the conveyance, and
(4) 2 mrem/hr in any normally occupied position in the car or vehicle, except that this provision does not apply to private motor carriers when the personnel are operating under a radiation protection program and wear radiation exposure monitoring devices.

(c) For shipments made under the provisions of paragraph (b) of this section, the shipper shall provide specific written instructions for maintenance of the exclusive use shipment controls to the carrier. The instructions shall be included with the shipping paper information.

§173.442 Thermal limitations

Each package of radioactive material shall be designed, constructed, and loaded so that

(a) The heat generated within the package because of the radioactive contents will not, at any time during transportation, affect the integrity of the package under conditions normally incident to transportation, and
(b) The temperature of the accessible external surfaces of the loaded package will not, assuming still air in the shade at an ambient temperature of 38°C (100°F), exceed either

   (1) 50°C (122°F) in other than an exclusive use shipment, or
   (2) 82°C (180°F) in an exclusive use shipment.

§173.443 Contamination control

(a) The level of nonfixed (removable), radioactive contamination on the external surfaces of each package offered for shipment shall be kept as low as practicable. The level of nonfixed radioactive contamination may be determined by wiping an area of 300 cm^2 of the surface concerned with an absorbent material, using moderate pressure, and measuring the activity on the wiping material. Sufficient measurements shall be taken in the most appropriate locations to yield a representative assessment of the nonfixed contamination levels. Except as provided in paragraph (b) of this section, the amount of radioactivity measured on any single wiping material when averaged over the surface wiped shall not exceed the limits given in the table below at any time during transport. Other methods of assessment of equal or greater efficiency may be used. When other methods are used the detection efficiency of the method used shall be taken into account and in no case shall the nonfixed contamination on the external surfaces of the package exceed ten times the limits listed in the following table.

REMOVABLE EXTERNAL RADIOACTIVE CONTAMINATION LIMITS

Contaminant	Maximum permissible limits	
	μCi/cm²	dpm/cm²
Beta-gamma emitting radionuclides; all radionuclides with half-lives less than 10 days, natural uranium, natural thorium, uranium-235, uranium-238, thorium-232, thorium-228, and thorium-230 when contained in ores or physical concentrates	10^{-5}	22
All other alpha emitting radionuclides	10^{-6}	2.2

(b) Except as provided in paragraph (d) of this section, in the case of packages transported as exclusive use shipments by rail or highway only, the removable (nonfixed) radioactive contamination at any time during transport shall not exceed 10 times the levels prescribed in paragraph (a) of this section.

(c) Except as provided in paragraph (d) of this section, each transport vehicle used for transporting radioactive materials as an exclusive use shipment which utilizes the provisions of paragraph (b) of this section shall be surveyed with appropriate radiation detection instruments after each use. A vehicle shall not be returned to service until the radiation dose rate at each accessible surface is 0.5 mrem/hr or less, and there is no significant removable (nonfixed) radioactive surface contamination as specified in paragraph (a) of this section.

(d) Paragraph (b) and (c) of this section do not apply to any closed transport vehicle used solely for the transportation of radioactive material packages with contamination levels that do not exceed 10 times the levels prescribed in paragraph (a) of this section if

(1) A survey of the interior surfaces of the empty vehicle shows that the radiation dose rate at any point does not exceed 10 mrem/hr at the surface or 2 mrem/hr at 1 m (3.3 ft) from the surface,
(2) Each vehicle is stenciled with the words "For Radioactive Materials Use Only" in letters at least 76 mm (3 in.) high in a conspicuous place on both sides of the exterior of the vehicle, and
(3) Each vehicle is kept closed the except for loading or unloading.

§173.444 Labeling requirements

Each package of radioactive materials, unless excepted by §§173.421, 173.422, 173.424, 173.425(b), or 173.427 shall be labeled as provided in Subpart E of Part 172 of this subchapter.

§173.446 Placarding requirements

See Subpart F of Part 172 of this subchapter.

§173.447 Storage Incident to transportation-general requirements

The following requirements apply to temporary storage during the course of transportation but not to Nuclear Regulatory Commission or Agreement State licensed facilities or U.S. Government owned or contracted facilities.

(a) The number of packages bearing Radioactive Yellow II or Radioactive Yellow III labels stored in any one storage area, such as a transit area, terminal building, store-room, or assembly yard, shall be limited so that the sum of the transport indexes in any individual group of packages does not exceed 50. Groups of these packages must be stored so as to maintain a spacing of at least 6 m (20 ft) from other groups of packages containing radioactive materials.

(b) Mixing of different kinds of packages, including Fissile Class I packages with Fissile Class II packages, is authorized in accordance with §173.459 of this subchapter.

§173.448 General transportation requirements

(a) Each shipment of radioactive materials shall be secured in order to prevent shifting during normal transportation conditions.

(b) Except as may be specifically required by the competent authority in the applicable certificate, a package of radioactive materials may be carried among packaged general cargo without special stowage provisions, if:

(1) The heat output in watts does not exceed 0.1 times the minimum package dimension in centimeters, or
(2) The average surface heat flux of the package does not exceed 15 W/m^2 and the immediately surrounding cargo is not in sacks or bags or otherwise in a form that would seriously impede air circulation for heat removal.

(c) Packages bearing labels prescribed in §172.403 of this subchapter may not be carried in compartments occupied by passengers, except in those compartments exclusively reserved for couriers accompanying those packages.

(d) Mixing of different kinds of packages, including Fissile Class I packages with Fissile Class II packages, is authorized in accordance with §173.459.

(e) No person shall offer for transportation aboard a passenger-carrying aircraft any single package with a transport index greater than 3.0 or an overpack with a transport index greater than 3.0.

(f) No person shall offer for transportation aboard a passenger-carrying aircraft any radioactive material unless that material is intended for use in, or incident to, research, or medical diagnosis or treatment, or is excepted under the provisions of §175.10 of this subchapter.

(g) If an overpack is used to consolidate individual packages of radioactive materials, the packages shall comply with the packaging, marking, and labeling requirements of this subchapter, and the following:

(1) The overpack shall be labeled as prescribed in §172.403 of this subchapter except as follows:

   (i) the "contents" entry on the label may state "mixed" unless each inside package contains the same radionuclide(s).
   (ii) The "number of curies" entry on the label must be determined by adding together the number of curies of the radioactive materials packages contained therein.
   (iii) For a nonrigid overpack, the required label together with required package markings shall be affixed to the overpack by means of a securely attached, durable tag. The transport index shall be determined by adding together the transport indexes of the radioactive materials packages contained therein.
   (iv) For a rigid overpack, the transport index shall be determined by

      (A) Adding together the transport indexes of the radioactive materials packages contained in the overpack, or
      (B) Except for fissile radioactive materials, direct measurements as prescribed in §173.403(bb) which have been taken by the person initially offering the packages contained within the overpack for shipment.

(2) The overpack shall be marked as prescribed in Subpart D of Part 172 of this subchapter and §173.25(a).
(3) The transport index of the overpack shall not exceed 3.0 for passenger-carrying aircraft shipments, or 10.0 for cargo-only aircraft shipments.

§173.451 Fissile materials — general requirements

(a) Except as provided in §173.453, each package containing fissile radioactive materials must comply with §§173.451 through 173.459.

§173.453 Fissile materials — exceptions

The requirements of §§173.451 through 173.459 do not apply to

(a) A package containing not more than 15 g of fissile radionuclides. If the material is transported in bulk, the quantity limitation applies to the conveyance,
(b) A package containing irradiated natural or depleted uranium including the products of irradiation if the irradiation has taken place only in the thermal reactor,
(c) A package containing homogeneous solutions or mixtures where:

    (1) The minimum ratio of the number of hydrogen atoms to the number of atoms of fissile radionuclides (H/X) is 5200;
    (2) The maximum concentration of fissile radionuclides is 5 g/ℓ, and
    (3) The maximum mass of fissile radionuclides in the package is 500 g, except for a mixture where the total mass of plutonium and uranium-233 does not exceed 1% of the mass of uranium-235 the limit is 800 g. If the material is transported in bulk, the quantity limitations apply to the conveyance;

(d) A package containing uranium enriched in uranium-235 to a maximum of 1% by weight, and with a total plutonium and uranium-233 content of up to 1% of the mass of uranium-235, if the fissile radionuclides are distributed homogeneously throughout the package contents, and do not form a lattice arrangement within the package,
(e) A package containing any fissile material if it does not contain more than 5 g of fissile radionuclides in any 10-ℓ volume, and if the material is packaged so as to maintain this limit of fissile radionuclide concentration during normal transport,
(f) A package containing not more than 1 kg of plutonium of which not more than 20% by mass may consist of plutonium-239, plutonium-241, or any combination of those radionuclides,
(g) A package containing liquid solutions of uranyl nitrate enriched in uranium-235 to a maximum of 2% by weight, with total plutonium and uranium-233 not more than 0.1% of the mass of uranium-235, or
(h) A package containing thorium or uranium with not more than 0.72% by weight of fissile material used for shipment solely within the U.S.

§173.455 Classification of fissile materials packages

(a) Except as provided in §173.453, each package of fissile materials shall be classified as follows:

(1) Fissile Class I. Packages that may be transported in unlimited number, and in any arrangement, and that require no nuclear criticality safety controls during transportation. A transport index is not assigned to Fissile Class I packages for the purposes of nuclear criticality safety control, although, the external radiation levels may require a transport index number.

(2) Fissile Class II. Packages that may be transported together in any arrangement but in numbers that do not exceed an aggregate transport index of 50. For the purposes of nuclear criticality safety control, individual packages may have a transport index of not less than 0.1 and not more than 10. However, the external radiation levels may require a higher transport index number. These shipments require no nuclear criticality safety control by the shipper during transportation.

(3) Fissile Class III. Shipments of packages of fissile materials that do not meet the requirements of Fissile Class I or Fissile Class II and that are controlled in transportation as prescribed in §173.457 by appropriate arrangements between the shipper and the carrier.

(b) The numerical values for package assignments as Fissile Class I, the transport indexes for Fissile Class II packages, and the vehicle limitations for Fissile Class III shipments shall be determined in accordance with 10 CFR Part 71.

§173.457 Transportation of Fissile Class III shipments-specific requirements

(a) Fissile Class III shipments shall incorporate transportation controls which are performed by the shipper or carrier, as appropriate, and which:

(1) Provide nuclear criticality safety,
(2) Protect against loading, storing, or transporting that shipment with any other fissile material, and
(3) Include in the shipping papers the description required by §172.203(d) of this subchapter.

(b) Fissile Class III shipments shall be transported:

(1) In a transport vehicle assigned to the exclusive use of the shipper with a specific restriction for the exclusive use to be provided in the appropriate arrangements between shipper and carrier and with instructions to that effect issued with the shipping papers,
(2) Except for shipments by aircraft, with an escort in a vehicle having the capability, equipment, authority, and instructions to provide administrative controls necessary to assure compliance with this section,
(3) In a transport vehicle containing no other packages of radioactive material that are required to bear one of the labels prescribed in §172.403 of this subchapter. Specific arrangements must be made between the shipper and the carrier, with instructions to that effect issued with the shipping papers, or
(4) Under any other procedure specifically authorized by the Associate Director for HMR in accordance with Part 107 of this subchapter.

§173.459 Mixing of fissile material packages

Shipments of fissile materials packages and the commingling of fissile materials packages with other radioactive materials packages shall be in accordance with the provisions of this section.

(a) Mixing of fissile material packages with other types of radioactive materials, including Fissile Class I with Fissile Class II packages is authorized if the total transport index in any transport vehicle or storage location does not exceed 50.

(b) For Fissile Class II packages shipped under the exclusive use provisions of §173.441(b), the transport index number which is calculated for nuclear criticality control purposes shall not exceed 10 for any single package nor a total of 50 for the load.

(c) Fissile Class II packages may be shipped with an external radiation level greater than 10 mrem/hr at 1 m (3.3 ft), and combined with other packages of the same or different designs in a Fissile Class III shipment, under the conditions prescribed in §173.457, if:

(1) Each package in the shipment has been assigned a transport index for criticality control purposes in accordance with the Fissile Class II criteria,
(2) The transport index which has been assigned in the package approval for nuclear criticality control purposes does not exceed 10 for any single package,
(3) The total transport index for nuclear criticality control purposes does not exceed 100 for all packages in the shipment,
(4) The shipment complies with §173.441(b), and
(5) The shipment is not transported by vessel.

(d) A Fissile Class III shipment of packages may be combined with other packages of the same or different design when each package has been assigned a transport index for nuclear criticality control purposes in accordance with Fissile Class II criteria, and may be combined with Fissile Class II packages into a Fissile Class III shipment under the conditions prescribed in §173.457, if:

(1) The transport index which has been assigned in the package approval for nuclear criticality control purposes does not exceed 50 for any single package,
(2) The total transport index for nuclear criticality control purposes for all packages in the shipment does not exceed 100.
(3) The shipment satisfies the provisions of §173.441(b) if any package has a radiation level exceeding 10 mrem/hr at 1 m (3.3 ft) from any accessible external surface of the package, and
(4) The shipment is not transported by vessel.

§173.461 Demonstration of compliance with tests

(a) Compliance with the test requirements in §§173.463 through 173.469 shall be shown by any of the methods prescribed in this paragraph, or by a combination of these methods appropriate for the particular feature being evaluated:

(1) By performance of tests with prototypes or samples of the packaging as normally presented for transportation, in which case the contents of the packaging for the test shall simulate as closely as practicable the expected normal radioactive contents,
(2) By reference to a previous, satisfactory demonstration of compliance of a sufficiently similar nature,
(3) By performance of tests with models of appropriate scale incorporating those features that are significant with respect to the item under investigation, when engineering experience has shown results of those tests to be suitable for design purposes. When a scale model is used, the need for adjusting certain test parameters, such as the penetrator diameter or the compressive load, must be taken into account, or
(4) By engineering evaluation or comparative data.

(b) With respect to the initial conditions for the tests under §§173.463 through 173.469, except for the water immersion tests, compliance shall be based upon the assumption that the package is in equilibrium at an ambient temperature of 38°C (100°F).

§173.462 Preparation of specimens for testing

(a) Each specimen (i.e., sample, prototype or scale model) shall be examined before testing to identify and record faults or damage, including:

(1) Divergence from the specifications or drawings,
(2) Defects in construction,
(3) Corrosion or other deterioration, and
(4) Distortion of features.

(b) Any deviation found under paragraph (a) of this section from the specified design shall be corrected or suitably taken into account in the subsequent evaluation.

(c) The containment system of the packaging shall be clearly specified.

(d) The external features of the specimen shall be clearly identified so that reference may be made to any part of it.

§173.463 Packaging and shielding — testing for integrity

After each of the applicable tests specified in §173.465 and §173.466, the integrity of the packaging, or of the packaging and its shielding, shall be retained to the extent required by §173.412(m) for the packaging being tested.

§173.465 Tests for proposed packagings designed for normal conditions of transportation

(a) The proposed packaging must be capable of withstanding the tests prescribed in this section. One prototype may be used for all tests if the requirements of paragraph (b) of this section are complied with.

(b) *Water spray test.* The water spray test must precede each test or test sequence prescribed in this section. The water spray test shall simulate exposure to rainfall of approximately 5 cm (2 in.)/hr for at least 1 hr. The time interval between the end of the water spray test and the beginning of the next test shall be such that the water has soaked in to the maximum extent without appreciable drying of the exterior of the specimen. In the absence of evidence to the contrary, this interval may be assumed to be 2 hr if the water spray is applied from four different directions simultaneously. However, no time interval may elapse if the water spray is applied from each of the four directions consecutively.

(c) *Free drop test.* The free drop test consists of a fall onto the target in a manner that causes maximum damage to the safety features being tested, and:

(1) For packages weighing 5000 kg (11,000 lb) or less, the distance of the fall measured from the lowest point of the packaging to the upper surface of the target shall not be less than 1.2 (4 ft).

(2) For packages weighing more than 5000 kg (11,000 lb), the distance of the fall shall not be less than the distance specified in the table below for the applicable packaging weight:

Free-Fall Distance for Packagings Weighing More than 5000 kg

Packaging weight		Free-fall distance	
Kilograms	**Pounds**	**Feet**	**Meters**
5,000 to 100,000	11,000 to 22,000	3	0.9
10,000 to 15,000	22,000 to 33,000	2	0.6
More than 15,000	More than 33,000	1	0.3

(3) For Fissile Class II packagings, the free drop specified in subparagraph (1) or (2) of this paragraph shall be preceded by a free drop from a height of 0.3 m (1 ft) on each corner. For cylindrical packagings, the 0.3 m (1 ft) drop shall be onto each of the quarters of each rim.

(4) For fiberboard or wood rectangular packages not exceeding 50 kg (110 lb) in weight, a separate specimen of the proposed packaging shall be subjected to a free drop onto each corner from a height of 0.3 m (1 ft).

(5) For fiberboard cylindrical packages weighing not more than 100 kg (220 lb) a separate

specimen of the proposed packaging shall be subjected to a free drop onto each of the quarters of each rim from a height of 0.3 m (1 ft).

(6) The target shall have a flat, horizontal surface of such mass and rigidity that any increase in its resistance to displacement or deformation upon impact by the specimen would not significantly increase the damage to the specimen.

(d) *Compression test.* The compression test shall last for a period of at least 24 hr and consists of a compressive load equivalent to the greater of the following:

(1) Five times the weight of the actual package, or

(2) 1300 kg/m^2 (225 lb/ft^2), multiplied by the vertically projected area of the package. The compressive load shall be applied uniformly to two opposite sides of the packaging specimen, one of which must be the base on which the package would normally stand.

(e) *Penetration test.* For the penetration test the packaging specimen shall be placed on a rigid, flat, horizontal surface that will not move while the test is being performed. The test shall consist of:

(1) A bar of 3.2 cm (1.25 in.) in diameter with a hemispherical end, weighing 6 kg (13.2 lb) being dropped with its longitudinal axis vertical, onto the center of the weakest part of the packaging specimen, so that, if it penetrates far enough, it will hit the containment system. The bar must not be deformed by the test, and

(2) The distance of the fall of the bar measured from its lower end to the upper surface of the packaging specimen shall not be less than 1 m (3.3 ft).

§173.466 Additional tests for Type A packagings designed for liquids and gases

(a) In addition to the tests prescribed in §173.465, Type A packagings designed for liquids and gases shall be capable of withstanding the following tests:

(1) *Free drop test.* The packaging specimen shall fall onto the target in a manner which will cause it to suffer the maximum damage to its containment. The distance of the fall measured from the lowest part of the packaging specimen to the upper surface of the target shall be not less than 9 m (30 ft).

(2) *Penetration test.* The specimen must be subjected to the test specified in §173.465(e) except that the distance of the fall shall be 1.7 m (5.5 ft).

§173.467 Tests for demonstrating the ability of Type B and fissile radioactive materials packagings to withstand accident conditions in transportation

Each Type B packaging or packaging for fissile material shall meet the test requirements prescribed in 10 CFR Part 71 for ability to withstand accident conditions in transportation.

§173.469 Tests for special form radioactive materials

(a) Special form radioactive materials must meet the test requirements of paragraph (b) of this section. Each solid radioactive material or capsule specimen to be tested shall be manufactured or fabricated so that it is representative of the actual solid material or capsule which will be transported with the proposed radioactive content duplicated as closely as practicable. Any differences between the material to be transported and the test material shall be taken into account. In addition:

(1) A different specimen may be used for each of the tests,

(2) The specimen must not break or shatter when subjected to the impact, percussion, or bending tests,

(3) The specimen must not melt or disperse when subjected to the heat test, and
(4) After each test, leaktightness or indispersibility of the specimen shall be determined by a method no less sensitive than the leaching assessment prescribed in paragraph (c) of this section. For a capsule resistant to corrosion by water, and which has an internal void volume greater than 0.1 mm, an alternative to the leaching assessment is a demonstration of leaktightness of 10^{-4} torr-1/s (1.3×10^{-4} atm-cm^3/s) based on air at 25°C (77°F) and 1 atm differential pressure for solid radioactive content, or 10^{-6} torr-1/s (1.3×10^{-6} atm-cm^3/s) for liquid or gaseous radioactive content.

(b) *Test methods:*

(1) *Impact Test.* The specimen must fall onto the target from a height of not less than 9 m (30 ft). The target must be as specified in §173.465(c)(6);

(2) *Percussion Test.*

(i) The specimen shall be placed on a sheet of lead that is supported by a smooth solid surface, and be struck by the flat face of a steel billet so as to produce an impact equivalent to that resulting from a free fall of 1.4 kg (3 lb) through 1 m (3.3 ft);
(ii) The flat face of the billet shall be 25 mm (1 in.) in diameter with the edges rounded off to a radius of 3 mm ± 0.3 mm (0.12 in. 0.012 in.),
(iii) The lead shall be of a hardness within 3.5 to 4.5 on the Vickers scale, and not more than 25 mm (1 in.) thick, and shall cover an area greater than that covered by the specimen,
(iv) A fresh surface to lead shall be used for each impact, and
(v) The billet must strike the specimen in a manner that causes maximum damage.

(3) *Bending test.*

(i) This test applies only to long slender sources with a length of 10 cm (4 in.) or more and with a length at least 10 times the minimum width,
(ii) The specimen must be securely clamped in a horizontal position so that one half of its length protrudes from the face of the clamp,
(iii) The position of the specimen must be such that it will suffer maximum damage when its free end is struck by the flat face of a steel billet,
(iv) The billet must strike the specimen in a manner that produces an impact equivalent to that resulting from a free vertical fall of 1.4 kg (3 lb) through 1 m (3.3 ft), and
(v) The flat face of the billet must be 25 mm (1 in.) in diameter with the edges rounded off to a radius of 3 mm (0.12 in. ± 0.3 mm (0.012 in.).

(4) *Heat test.* The specimen shall be heated in air to a temperature of not less than 800°C (1472°F), held at that temperature for a period of 10 min, and then allowed to cool.

(c) *Leaching assessment methods.*

(1) For indispersible solid material

(i) The specimen shall be immersed for 7 days in water at ambient temperature. The water must have a pH of 6 to 8 and a maximum conductivity of 10 μΩ/cm at 20°C (68°F),
(ii) The water and specimen shall then be heated to a temperature of 50°C ± 5° (122°F ± 9°) and maintained at this temperature for 4 hr,
(iii) The activity of the water shall then be determined,

(iv) The specimen shall then be stored for at least 7 days in still air with humidity not less than 90% at 30°C (86°F),

(v) The specimen shall then be immersed in water with the same pH and maximum conductivity specifications as in subparagraph (1)(i) of this paragraph. The water and specimen must be heated to 50°C ± 5° (122°F ± 9°) and maintained at that temperature for 4 hr,

(vi) The activity of the water shall then be determined. The activities determined in subparagraph (1)(iii) and this subparagraph shall not exceed 0.05 μCi.

(2) For encapsulated material

(i) The specimen shall be immersed in water at ambient temperature. The water must have a pH of 6 to 8 and a maximum conductivity of 10 μΩ/cm. The water and specimen shall be heated to a temperature of 50°C ± 5° (122°F ± 9°) and maintained at this temperature for 4 hr,

(ii) The activity of the water shall then be determined.

(iii) The specimen shall then be stored for at least 7 days in still air at a temperature not less than 30°C (86°F),

(iv) Step (i) shall be repeated, and

(v) The activity of the water shall be determined. The activities determined in paragraph (c)(2)(ii) and this paragraph (c)(2)(v) shall not exceed 0.05 μCi.

§173.471 Requirements for U.S. Nuclear Regulatory Commission approved packages

In addition to the applicable requirements of the U.S. Nuclear Regulatory Commission (USNRC) and Parts 171 to 177 of this subchapter, any shipper of a Type B or fissile material package that has been approved by the USNRC in accordance with 10 CFR Part 71 shall also comply with the following requirements:

(a) The shipper shall be registered with the USNRC as a party to the approval, and the shipment must be made in compliance with the terms of the approval (approved by the Office of Management and Budget under OMB control number 2137-0512),

(b) The outside of each package shall be durably and legibly marked with the package identification marking indicated in the USNRC approval,

(c) Each shipping paper related to the shipment of the package shall bear the package identification marking indicated in the USNRC approval,

(d) Before the first export shipment of the package, the shipper shall obtain a U.S. Competent Authority Certificate for that package design or if one has already been issued, the shipper shall register with the U.S. Competent Authority as a user of the certificate. Upon registration as a user of the certificate the shipper will be furnished with a copy of it. The shipper shall then submit a copy of the U.S. Competent Authority Certificate applying to that package design to the national competent authority of each country into or through which the package will be transported, unless a copy has already been furnished (approved by the Office of Management and Budget under OMB control numbers 2137-0514 and 2137-0515),

(e) The U.S. Competent Authority responsible for administering the requirements of Section VIII of the IAEA "Regulations for the Safe Transport of Radioactive Materials, Safety Series No. 6, 1973 Revised Edition (as amended)," is the Materials Transportation Bureau, Office of Hazardous Materials Regulation (OHMR), U.S. Department of Transportation, Washington, D.C. 20590,

(f) Each request for a U.S. Competent Authority Certificate as required by the IAEA regulations shall be submitted in writing to the address set forth in paragraph (e) of this section. The request shall be in duplicate and include copies of the applicable

USNRC approval and a reproducible drawing showing the make-up of the package. Each request is considered in the order in which it is received. To allow sufficient consideration by OHMR, requests should be received at least 45 days before the requested effective date (approved by the Office of Management and Budget under OMB control number 2137-0514), and

(g) Import and export shipments may be made in accordance with §171.12 of this subchapter.

§173.472 Requirements for exporting DOT specification Type B and fissile packages

(a) Any shipper who exports a DOT specification Type B of fissile material package authorized by §§173.416 or 173.417 shall comply with paragraphs (b) through (f) of this section.

(b) The shipper shall register with the U.S. Competent Authority as a user of the appropriate U.S. Competent Authority Certificate and the shipment shall be made in accordance with the certificate (approved by the Office of Management and Budget under OMB control number 2137-0515),

(c) The outside of each package must be durably and legibly marked with the package identification marking indicated in the U.S. Competent Authority Certificate,

(d) Each shipping paper related to the shipment of the package must bear the package identification marking indicated in the U.S. Competent Authority Certificate,

(e) Before the first export shipment of the package, the shipper must submit a copy of the U.S. Competent Authority Certificate applying to that package design to the national competent authority of each country into or through which the package will be transported, unless a copy has already been furnished (approved by the Office of Management and Budget under OMB control number 2137-1515), and

(f) import and export shipments may be made in accordance with §171.12 of this subchapter.

§173.473 Requirements for foreign-made packages

In addition to the applicable requirements of Parts 171 through 177 of this subchapter, each shipper of a foreign-made Type B or fissile material package for which a competent authority certificate is required by the IAEA ''Regulations for the Safe Transport of Radioactive Materials, Safety Series No. 6, 1973 Revised Edition (as amended)'' shall also comply with the following requirements:

(a) Prior to the first shipment of such a package of radioactive materials into or from the U.S., the shipper shall:

(1) Have the foreign competent authority certificate revalidated by the U.S. Competent Authority, unless this has been done previously. The request must be in duplicate and contain all the information required by Section VIII of the IAEA regulations. Each request is considered in the order in which it is received. To allow sufficient consideration by OHMR, requests should be received at least 45 days before the requested effective date,

(2) Submit a copy in English of the foreign competent authority certificate with the request for revalidation,

(3) Register its identity in writing with the U.S. Competent Authority as a user of the package covered by the foreign competent authority certificate and its revalidation. If the shipper is requesting the revalidation, this is automatically done by OHMR, and

(4) Supply to the carrier, upon request, the applicable competent authority certificates. However, the competent authority certificates are not required to accompany the packages to which they apply (approved by the Office of Management and Budget under OMB control number 2137-0517.)

(b) The outside of each package shall be durably and legibly marked with the same competent authority identification marking indicated on the competent authority certificate and revalidation,
(c) Each shipping paper for a shipment of radioactive materials shall bear a notation of the package identification marking indicated on the competent authority certificate or revalidation, and
(d) Import and export shipments may be made in accordance with §171.12 of this subchapter.

§173.474 Quality control for construction of packaging
(a) Prior to the first use of any packaging for the shipment of radioactive material, the shipper shall determine, that

(1) The packaging meets the quality of design and construction requirements as specified in this subchapter, and
(2) The effectiveness of the shielding, containment, and, when required, the heat transfer characteristics of the package, are within the limits specified for the package design.

§173.475 Quality control requirements prior to each shipment of radioactive materials
Before each shipment of any radioactive materials package, the shipper shall ensure by examination or appropriate tests, that

(a) The packaging is proper for the contents to be shipped,
(b) The packaging is in unimpaired physical condition, except for superficial marks,
(c) Each closure device of the packaging, including any required gasket, is properly installed, secured, and free of defects,
(d) For fissile material, each moderator and neutron absorber, if required, is present and in proper condition,
(e) Each special instruction for filling, closing, and preparation of the packaging for shipment has been followed,
(f) Each closure, valve, or other opening of the containment system through which the radioactive content might escape is improperly closed and sealed,
(g) Each packaging containing liquid in excess of an A_2 quantity and intended for air shipment has been tested to show that it will not leak under an ambient atmospheric pressure of not more than 0.25 atm, absolute, (0.25 kg/cm^2 or 3.6 psia). The test must be conducted on the entire containment system, or on any receptacle or vessel within the containment system, to determine compliance with this requirement,
(h) The internal pressure of the containment system will not exceed the design pressure during transportation, and
(i) External radiation and contamination levels are within the allowable limits specified in this subchapter.

§173.476 Approval of special form radioactive materials
(a) Each shipper of special form radioactive materials shall maintain on file for at least 1 year after the latest shipment, and provide to the MTB on request, a complete safety analysis, including documentation of any tests, demonstrating that the special form material meets the requirements of §173.469 (approved by the Office of Management and Budget under OMB control number 2137-0516.)
(b) Prior to the first export shipment of a special form radioactive material from the U.S., each shipper shall obtain a U.S. Competent Authority Certificate for the specific material. Each petition shall be submitted in accordance with §173.471(e) and must include the following information:

(1) A detailed description of the material or if a capsule, a detailed description of the contents. Particular reference must be made to both physical and chemical states,
(2) If a capsule is to be used, a detailed statement of its design and dimensions, including complete engineering drawings and schedules of material, and methods of construction, and
(3) A statement of the tests that have been made and their results; evidence based on calculative methods to show that the material is able to pass the tests; or other evidence that the special form radioactive material complies with §173.469 (approved by the Office of Management and Budget under OMB control number 2137-0518).

(c) Paragraphs (a) and (b) of this section do not apply in those cases where A_1 equals A_2 and the material is not described on the shipping papers as "Radioactive Material Special Form, n.o.s."

§173.477 Approval for export shipments

(a) Each export shipment of a package for which an IAEA certificate of competent authority has been issued or revalidated in accordance with §§173.471, 173.472, or 173.473 shall have multilateral approval, if the shipment includes

(1) A vented Type B(M) package,
(2) A Type B(M) packaging containing radioactive materials with an activity greater than $3 \times 10^3\ A_1$, or $3 \times 10^3 A_2$, as appropriate, or 3×10^4 Ci, whichever is less,
(3) A Fissile Class III shipment, or
(4) Transportation by special arrangement.

(b) Each application for shipment approval shall contain

(1) The period of time for which the approval is sought,
(2) A description of the contents, the expected modes of transportation, the type of vehicle to be used, and the proposed route, and
(3) An explanation of how the special precautions and special administrative and operational controls referred to in the package design certificates are to be put into effect.

(c) The packaging and shipment approvals may be combined into a single approval issued in accordance with §§173.471, 173.472, or 173.473.

(d) Approval by competent authorities is not required for packagings designed for materials covered by §§173.421 through 173.427 nor for Type A packagings designed for nonfissile radioactive materials.

§173.478 Notification to competent authorities for export shipments

(a) Before the first export shipment of any packaging with contents exceeding A_1 or A_2, the shipper shall ensure that copies of each applicable competent authority certificate issued in accordance with §§173.471, 173.472, or 173.473 have been submitted to the competent authority of each country through which or into which it is to be transported. The shipper is not required to await an acknowledgment from the competent authority prior to shipping the radioactive material, nor is the competent authority required to acknowledge receipt of the certificate. (approved by the Office of Management and Budget under OMB control number 2137-0515.)

(b) For each of the shipments described in this paragraph, the shipper shall notify the competent authority of each country through which or into which the shipment is to be transported. This notification must be received by each competent authority at least 15 days before the shipment starts for the following:

(1) Type B(U) packagings containing radioactive materials with an activity greater than 3×10^3 A_1, 3×10^3 A_2, as appropriate, or 3×10^4 Ci, whichever is the least,
(2) Type B(M) packages,
(3) Fissile Class III shipments under Section VIII of the IAEA "Regulations for the Safe Transport of Radioactive Materials, Safety Series No. 6, 1973 Revised Edition (as amended)", or
(4) Transportation by special arrangements.

(c) The shipper notification must include

(1) Sufficient information to enable the packaging to be identified, including all applicable certificate numbers and identification marks, and
(2) Information as to the date of shipment, the expected date of arrival, and the proposed routing.

(d) The shipper is not required to send a separate notification if the required information has been included in the application for shipment approval.

Part 174 — Carriage by Rail

§174.208 [Amended]

14a. In §174.208, paragraph (b) is amended by removing section reference "173.426" and inserting, in its place, "173.9".

15. In §174.700, paragraph (a) is amended by removing section reference "§173.389(c) and §173.392" and inserting in their respective places "§§173.403 and 173.425"; paragraph (b) is amended by removing section reference "§173.389(i)" and inserting in its place "§173.403(bb)"; and by removing section references "§§173.389(o) and 173.392, 173.393(j), or 173.396(f)" and inserting in their respective places "§§173.403, 173.425, 173.441, and 173.457"; paragraph (d) is amended by removing section references "§173.389(a)(3) and §173.396(g)" and inserting in their respective places "§173.455(a)(3) and §173.457"; and a new paragraph (g) is added to read as follows:

§174.700 Special handling requirements for radioactive materials

(g) In the case of packages shipped under the exclusive use provisions of §173.441(b) for packages with external radiation levels in excess of 200 mrem/hr at the package surface:

(1) The rail car shall meet the requirements for a closed transport vehicle (§173.403 of this subchapter), and
(2) Provisions must be made to secure the packages so that their position within the vehicle remains fixed under conditions normally incident to transportation.

§174.715 [Amended]

16. In §174.715, paragraph (a) is amended by removing section reference "§173.389(o)" and inserting in its place "§173.403"; and by removing section reference "§173.397(a)" and inserting in its place "§173.443".

§174.750 [Amended]

17. In §174.750, paragraph (a) is amended by removing section reference "§173.397" and inserting in its place "§173.443."

Part 175 — Carriage by Aircraft

§175.710 [Amended]

18. In §175.10, paragraph (a)(6) is amended by removing section reference "§173.391(a),

(b), or (c)'' and inserting in its place ''§§173.421, 173.422, or 173.424.''

19. In §175.700, the section heading is revised; paragraph (b) is amended by removing section reference ''§173.397'' and inserting in its place ''§173.443''; paragraph (c) is amended by removing section reference ''§173.391(a), (b), or (c)'' and inserting in its place ''§§173.421, 173.422, or 173.424''; and a new paragraph (d) is added to read as follows:

§175.700 Special limitations and requirements for radioactive materials

(d) Type B(M) packages may not be offered or accepted for transportation, nor transported, on passenger-carrying aircraft.

20. In §175.703, paragraph (b) is amended by removing section reference ''§173.393(r)'' and inserting in its place ''§173.448(g)''; paragraph (c) is amended by removing section reference ''§173.389(a)(3)'' and inserting in its place ''§173.455(a)(3)''; and paragraphs (d) and (e) are added to read as follows:

§175.703 Other special requirements for the acceptance and carriage of packages containing radioactive materials

(d) No person may offer or accept for transportation, nor transport, by air:

(1) Any Type B(U) or Type B(M) package with an accessible surface temperature in excess of 50°C (122°F),
(2) Continuously vented Type B(M) packages, packages which require external cooling by an ancillary cooling system or packages subject to operational controls during transport, or
(3) Liquid pyrophoric radioactive materials.

(e) Exclusive use shipments of packages having a surface radiation level in excess of 200 mrem/hr may not be transported by air except by special arrangement approved by MTB.

Part 176 — Carriage by Vessel

21. In Part 176, Subpart M is revised to read as follows:

Subpart M — Detailed Requirements for Radioactive Materials

Sec.

- 176.700 General stowage requirements.
- 176.704 Requirements relating to transport.
- 176.708 Segregation distance table.
- 176.710 Care following leakage or sifting of radioactive materials.
- 176.715 Contamination control.

Subpart M — Detailed Requirements for Radioactive Materials

§176.700 General stowage requirements

(a) Radioactive materials must not be stowed in the same hold with mail bags.

(b) A package of radioactive materials which in still air has a surface temperature more than 5°C (9°F) above the ambient air may not be overstowed with any other cargo. If the package is stowed under deck, the hold or compartment in which it is stowed must be ventilated.

(c) Each Fissile Class III shipment must be stowed in a separate hold, compartment, or defined deck area and be separated by a distance of at least 6 m (20 ft) from all other Radioactive Category II or III-Yellow labeled packages. For a shipment of radioactive materials requiring supplemental operational procedures, the shipper must furnish the master or person in charge of the vessel a copy of the necessary operational instructions (paperwork requirement excepted from Office of Management and Budget approval)

(d) A person may not remain unnecessarily in a hold or compartment or in the immediate vicinity of any package on deck containing radioactive materials.

§176.704 Requirements relating to transport indexes

(a) The sum of the transport indexes for all packages of radioactive materials not in a freight container on board a vessel, may not exceed 200.

(b) Except as provided in paragraph (e) of this section, the sum of transport indexes for packages not in a freight container may not exceed 50 in any hold, compartment, or defined deck area. Each group of radioactive material packages must be separated by a distance of at least 6 m (20 ft) at all times.

(c) Except as provided in paragraph (e) of this section, the number of freight containers with packages of radioactive materials contained therein must be limited so that the total sum of the transport indexes in the containers in any hold or defined deck area does not exceed 200, and:

(1) The sum of transport indexes for any individual freight container, or group of freight containers, does not exceed 50, and
(2) Each freight container or group of freight containers is handled and stowed in such a manner that groups are separated from each other by a distance of at least 6 m (20 ft).

(d) The limitations specified in paragraphs (a), (b), and (c) of this section do not apply to consignments of low specific activity materials if the packages are marked "RADIO-ACTIVE LSA" and no Fissile Class II or Fissile Class III radioactive materials are included in the shipment.

(e) For exclusive use shipments, the limitations specified in paragraphs (b) and (c) of this section do not apply if

(1) For packages not in freight containers, the sum of the transport indexes of Fissile Class II packages does not exceed 50 in each hold,
(2) For packages in freight containers, the radiation level does not exceed 200 mrem/hr at any point on the surface and 10 mrem at 2 m (6 ft) from the outside surface of the freight container and the sum of transport indexes of Fissile Class II packages does not exceed 50 in each freight container and 200 in each hold or defined deck area, and
(3) Each group of Fissile Class II packages is separated from other redioactive material by a distance of at least 6 m (20 ft) at all times.

(f) The limitations specified in paragraphs (a) through (e) of this section do not apply when the entire vessel is reserved or chartered for use by a single shipper under exclusive use conditions if the number of Fissile Class II and Fissile Class III packages of radioactive materials aboard the vessel does not exceed the amount authorized in §§173.451 through 173.459 of this subchapter. The entire shipment operation must be approved by the Office of Hazardous Materials Regulation (OHMR) in advance.

§176.708 Segregation distance table

(a) The table below applies to the stowage of packages of radioactive materials on board a vessel with regard to transport index numbers which are shown on the labels of individual packages. Radioactive Category II or III-Yellow labeled packages may not be stowed any closer to living accommodations, regularly occupied working spaces, spaces that may be continually occupied by any person (except those spaces exclusively reserved for couriers

Minimum distance in feet from undeveloped film and plates

Sum of transport indexes of the packages	Minimum distance in feet from living accommodation or regularly occupied working space		1 day voyage			2 day voyage			4 day voyage			10 day voyage			20 day voyage			30 day voyage			40 day voyage			50 day voyage		
	Cargo thickness in feet (unit density)																									
	Nil	3	Nil	3	6	Nil	3	6	Nil	3	6	Nil	3	6	Nil	3	6	Nil	3	6	Nil	3	6	Nil	3	6
0.1 to 0.5	5	X	6	X	X	8	X	X	11	X	X	17	4	X	25	6	X	30	7	X	35	8	X	39	9	X
0.6 to 1	6	X	8	X	X	11	X	X	16	4	X	25	6	X	35	8	X	42	10	X	50	12	X	55	13	X
1.1 to 2	9	X	11	X	X	16	4	X	22	5	X	35	8	X	50	12	X	61	14	X	70	17	X	78	19	X
2.1 to 3	10	X	14	X	X	19	5	X	27	6	X	42	10	X	61	14	X	74	18	X	86	20	X	96	23	X
3.1 to 5	13	X	17	4	X	25	6	X	35	8	X	55	13	X	78	19	X	96	23	X	110	26	X	124	29	7
5.1 to 10	19	4	25	6	X	35	8	X	50	12	X	78	19	X	110	26	X	135	33	8	155	37	9	175	42	10
10.1 to 20	26	6	35	8	X	50	12	X	69	17	X	110	26	X	155	37	9	190	46	11	220	53	13	250	59	14
20.1 to 30	32	8	43	10	X	61	14	X	85	20	X	135	32	8	190	45	11	235	56	13	270	65	16	305	72	17
30.1 to 50	42	10	55	13	X	78	19	X	110	26	X	175	42	10	245	58	14	300	73	17	350	84	20	390	94	22
50.1 to 100	59	14	78	19	X	110	26	X	155	37	9	245	59	14	350	82	20	430	105	24	515	118	28	550	130	32
100.1 to 150	72	17	96	23	X	135	32	8	190	46	11	300	72	17	425	100	24	525	125	30	600	145	34	[a]	165	39
150.1 to 200	84	20	110	26	X	155	37	9	200	53	13	350	84	20	490	115	28	600	140	35	[a]	165	40		190	45
200.1 to 300	105	24	135	32	X	190	46	11	270	64	15	425	105	25	600	145	35	[a]	180	42	[a]	205	49	[a]	230	55
300.1 to 400	120	28	160	37	9	220	53	13	310	75	18	500	120	28	[a]	165	40	[a]	205	49	[a]	235	57	[a]	265	63
0.1 to 0.5	2	X	2	X	X	3	X	X	4	X	X	6	2	X	8	2	X	10	3	X	11	3	X	12	3	X
0.6 to 1.0	2	X	3	X	X	4	X	X	5	2	X	8	2	X	11	3	X	13	4	X	15	4	X	17	4	X
1.1 to 2.0	3	X	4	X	X	5	2	X	7	2	X	11	3	X	15	4	X	19	5	X	22	5	X	24	6	X
2.1 to 3.0	4	X	5	X	X	6	2	X	9	2	X	13	4	X	19	5	X	23	6	X	27	7	X	30	7	X
3.1 to 5.0	4	X	6	2	X	8	2	X	11	3	X	17	4	X	24	6	X	30	7	X	34	8	X	38	9	3
5.1 to 10.0	6	2	8	2	X	11	3	X	15	4	X	24	6	X	34	8	X	42	10	3	48	12	3	54	13	3
10.1 to 20.0	8	2	11	3	X	15	4	X	22	5	X	34	8	X	48	12	3	59	14	4	68	16	4	76	18	5
20.1 to 30.0	10	3	13	4	X	19	5	X	26	7	X	42	10	3	59	14	4	72	17	4	83	20	5	93	22	6

30.1 to 50.0	13	3	17	4	X	24	6	X	34	8	X	54	13	3	76	18	5	92	23	6	110	26	7	120	29	7
50.1 to 100.0	18	5	24	6	X	34	8	X	48	12	3	76	18	5	110	25	6	130	32	8	150	36	9	170	40	10
100.1 to 150.0	22	6	30	7	X	42	10	3	59	14	4	93	22	6	130	31	8	160	39	10	185	45	11	[a]	50	12
150.1 to 200.0	26	6	34	8	X	48	12	3	68	16	4	110	26	7	150	36	9	185	43	11	[a]	51	13	[a]	58	14
200.1 to 300.0	32	8	42	10	3	59	14	4	83	20	5	130	32	8	185	44	11	[a]	55	13	[a]	63	15	[a]	70	17
300.1 to 400.0	36	9	48	12	3	68	16	4	95	23	6	150	36	9	[a]	50	13	[a]	63	15	[a]	73	18	[a]	81	20

Note: X — indicates that thickness of screening cargo is sufficient without any additional segregation distance. By using 2 m of intervening unit density cargo for persons and 3 m for film and plates, no distance shielding is necessary for any length of voyage specified. Using 1 steel bulkhead or steel deck, multiply segregation distance by 0.8. Using 2 steel bulkheads or steel decks, multiply segregation distance by 0.64. ''Cargo of Unit Density'' means cargo stowed at a density of 1 ton (metric) per cubic meter; where the density is less than this the depth cargo specified must be increased in proportion. ''Minimum distance'' means the least in any direction whether vertical or horizontal from the outer surface of the nearest package. The total consignment on board at any time must not exceed transport indexes totalling 200 unless if carried under the provisions of §176.704(f). The figures below the double line of the table should be used in such a contingency.

[a] Not to be carried unless screening by other cargo and bulkheads can be arranged in accordance with the other columns.

specifically authorized to accompany such packages), and undeveloped film than the distance specified to the table below. Where only one consignment of a radioactive substance is to be loaded on board a vessel under exclusive use conditions, the appropriate segregation distance may be established by demonstrating that the direct measurement of the radiation level at regularly occupied working spaces and living quarters is less than 0.75 mrem/hr. More than one consignment may be loaded onboard vessel with the appropriate segregation distance established by demonstrating that direct measurement of the radiation level at regularly occupied working spaces and living quarters is less than 0.75 mrem/hr, provided that the vessel has been chartered for the exclusive use of a competent person specialized in the carriage of radioactive material. Stowage arrangements shall be predetermined for the entire voyage, including any radioactive substances to be loaded at ports of call enroute. The radiation level shall be measured by a responsible person skilled in the use of monitoring instruments.

§176.710 Care following leakage or sifting of radioactive materials

(a) In case of fire, collision, or breakage involving any shipment of radioactive materials, other than materials of low specific activity, the radioactive materials must be segregated from unnecessary contact with personnel. In case of obvious leakage, or if the inside container appears to be damaged, the stowage area (hold, compartment, or deck area) containing this cargo must be isolated as much as possible to prevent radioactive material from entering any person's body through contact, inhalation, or ingestion. No person may handle the material or remain in the vicinity unless supervised by a qualified person.

(b) A hold or compartment in which leakage of radioactive materials has occurred may not be used for other cargo until it is decontaminated in accordance with the requirements of §176.715.

(c) For reporting requirements, see §171.15 of this subchapter.

§176.15 Contamination control

(a) Each hold, compartment, or deck area used for the transportation of low specific activity radioactive materials under exclusive use conditions shall be surveyed with appropriate radiation detection instruments after each use. Such holds, compartments, and deck areas may not be used again until the radiation dose rate at any accessible surface is less than 0.5 mrem/hr, and the removable (nonfixed) radioactive surface contamination is not greater than the limits prescribed in §173.443 of this subchapter.

Part 177—Carriage by Public Highway

§177.825 [Amended]

21a. In §177.825, paragraphs (b), (c), and (d) are amended by removing the phrase "large quantity radioactive material as defined in §173.389(b)" and inserting in its place "highway route controlled quantity radioactive materials as defined in §173.403(l)"; and paragraphs (b)(2)(iii) and (d)(2)(iv) are amended by removing the term "large quantity" and inserting in its place "highway route controlled quantity."

22. In §177.842, paragraph (a) is amended by removing section references "§173.389(i), §173.393(j), §173.396(f), and §173.392", and inserting in their respective places "§§173.403, §173.441(b), §173.457, and §173.425"; paragraph (c) is amended by removing section references "§173.389(c) and §173.392", and inserting in their respective places §§173.403 and §173.425"; paragraph (f) is amended by removing section references "§173.389(a)(3) and §173.396(g)", and inserting in their respective places "§§173.455(a)(3) and 173.457"; and paragraph (g) is added to read as follows:

§177.842 Radioactive material

(g) For shipments transported under exclusive use conditions the radiation dose rate must not exceed 2 mrem/hr in any position normally occupied in the vehicle. For shipments transported as exclusive use under the provisions of §173.441(b) for packages with external radiation levels in excess of 200 mrem/hr at the package surface, the vehicle must meet the requirements of a closed transport vehicle (§173.403 of this subchapter).

23. In §177.843, paragraph (a) is revised to read as follows:

§177.843 Contamination of vehicles

(a) Each motor vehicle used for transporting radioactive materials under exclusive use conditions in accordance with §§173.425(c) or 173.443(c) shall be surveyed with radiation detection instruments after each use. A vehicle may not be returned to service until the radiation dose rate at each accessible surface is 0.5 mrem/hr or less and the removable (nonfixed) radioactive surface contamination is not greater than the level prescribed in §173.443(a).

§177.861 [Amended]

24. In §177.861, paragraph (a) is amended by removing section reference §173.397 and inserting in its place §173.443.

Appendix A—[Amended]

24a. In Appendix A, all references to ''large quantity'' throughout Appendix A are changed to read ''highway route controlled quantity''.

Part 178—Shipping Container Specifications

§178.350-2 [Amended]

25. In §178.350-2, paragraph (a) is amended by removing section references ''§173.389(j) and §173.398(b)'', and inserting in their respective places §§173.403, and §173.465''.

(49 U.S.C. 1803, 1804, 1808; 49 CFR 1.53, App. A. to Part 1)

Issued in Washington, D.C., on February 24, 1983.

L. D. Santman, Director, Materials Transportation Bureau.

(FR Doc. 83-5215 Filed 3-9-84; 8:45 am)

BILLING CODE 4910-60-M

APPENDIX A
HAZARDOUS MATERIALS REGULATIONS*

PART 171—GENERAL INFORMATION, REGULATIONS, AND DEFINITIONS

§171.1 Purpose and scope

This subchapter prescribes the requirements of the Department of Transportation governing the transportation of hazardous materials in commerce.

[Amdt. 171-32, 41 FR 15993, Apr. 15, 1976].

§171.2 General transportation requirements

(a) Except as provided in §171.12, no person may offer or accept a hazardous material for transportation in commerce within the U.S. unless that material is properly classed, described, packaged, marked, labeled, and in the condition for shipment as required by this subchapter.

(b) Except as provided in §171.12, no person may transport a hazardous material in commerce within the U.S. unless that material is handled and transported in accordance with this subchapter.

(c) No person may represent, mark, certify, or sell a packaging or container as meeting the requirements of this subchapter governing the use of that packaging or container in the transportation in commerce of a hazardous material unless the packaging or container is manufactured, fabricated, marked, maintained, reconditioned, or repaired, as the case may be, in accordance with this subchapter.

[Amdt. 171-32, 41 FR 15993, Apr. 15, 1976, as amended by Amdt. 171-34, 41 FR 38179, Sept. 9, 1976].

§171.3 [Reserved]

§171.4 Changes in specifications for tank cars

(a) See §179.4 of this subchapter.

[31 FR 9068, July 1, 1966. Redesignated at 32 FR 5606, Apr. 5, 1967, and amended by Amdt. 171-42, 43 FR 48643, Oct. 19, 1978]

§171.5 Procedure covering tank car construction

(a) See §179.3 of this subchapter.

[Order 71.31 FR 9068, July 1, 1966. Redesignated at 32 FR 5606, Apr. 5, 1967, and amended by Amdt. 171-42, 43 FR 48643, Oct. 19, 1978]

§171.6 [Reserved]

§171.7 Matter incorporated by reference

(a) There is incorporated by reference in Parts 170 to 189 of this subchapter all matter referred to that is not specifically set forth. These materials are hereby made a part of the regulations in Parts 170 to 189 of this subchapter. Unless the reference provides otherwise, matter subject to change is incorporated only as it is in effect on the date of issuance of the regulation referring to that matter.

(b) All incorporated matter is available for inspection in the Dockets Branch, Room 6500 of the Trans Point Building, 2100 Second Street SW., Washington, D.C. 20590.

(c) Matter incorporated by reference is available for distribution as follows:

* From *Fed. Reg.*, June 30, 1977.

(1) ASME: American Society of Mechanical Engineers, United Engineering Center, 345 East 47th Street, New York, N.Y. 10017.
(2) American National Standard: American National Standards Institute, Inc., 1430 Broadway, New York, N.Y. 10018.
(3) CGA: Compressed Gas Association, Inc., 500 Fifth Avenue, New York, N.Y. 10036.
(4) Bureau of Explosives: Bureau of Explosives, Association of American Railroads, American Railroads Building, 1920 L Street NW., Washington, D.C. 20036.
(5) AAR: Association of American Railroads, 59 East Van Buren Street, Chicago, Ill. 60605.
(6) ASTM: American Society for Testing and Materials, 1916 Race Street, Philadelphia, Pa. 19103.
(7) API: American Petroleum Institute, 1801 K Street NW., Washington, D.C. 20006.
(8) AISI: American Iron and Steel Institute, 1000 16th Street NW., Washington, D.C. 20036.
(9) The Chlorine Institute, 342 Madison Avenue, New York, N.Y. 10017.
(10) MCA: Manufacturing Chemists' Association, Inc., 1825 Connecticut Avenue, NW., Washington, D.C. 20009.
(11) NFPA: National Fire Protection Association, 60 Batterymarch Street, Boston, Mass. 02110.
(12) Aluminum Association: The Aluminum Association, 420 Lexington Avenue, New York, N.Y. 10017.
(13) NACE: National Association of Corrosion Engineers, 2400 West Loop South, Houston, TX 77027.
(14) IME: Institute of Makers of Explosives, 420 Lexington Avenue, New York, NY 10017.
(15) IAEA: International Atomic Energy Agency, Karnter Ring 11, Post Office Box 590, A-1011, Vienna, Austria (IAEA publications may be purchased in the U.S. from: Unipub, Inc., Post Office Box 433, New York, NY 10016).
(16) USDOE: United States Department of Energy, Washington, D.C. 20545. Regulations of the USDOE are available from the Superintendent of Documents, U.S. Government Printing Office, Washington, D.C. 20402. Other publications by the USDOE may be obtained from the National Technical Information Center, U.S. Department of Commerce, Springfield, Virginia 22151.
(17) Superintendent of Documents, U.S. Government Printing Office, Washington, D.C. 20402.
(18) National Wooden Box Association, Post Office Box 1010, Cumberland, Md. 21502.
(19) TFI: The Fertilizer Institute, 1015 18th Street NW., Washington, D.C. 20036.
(20) AWWA: American Water Works Association, 2 Park Avenue, New York, NY 10016.
(21) AWS: American Welding Society, 345 East 47th Street, New York, NY 10016.
(22) USDC: U.S. Department of Commerce, National Technical Information Service, 5285 Port Royal Road, Springfield, Va. 22151.
(23) Inter-governmental Maritime Consultative Organization, 101-104 Piccadilly, London, WIV OAE, England.
(24) Uniform Classification Committee, 222 South Riverside Plaza, Chicago, Ill. 60606.
(25) USERDA: United States Energy Research and Development Administration, Washington, D.C. 20545.
(26) USNRC: United States Nuclear Regulatory Commission, Washington, D.C. 20555.

(d) The full title and application of the matter incorporated by reference in Parts 170—189 of this chapter are as follows:

(1) ASME Code means section VIII (Division I) and IX of the 1977 edition of the "American Society of Mechanical Engineers Boiler and Pressure Vessel Code," and

addenda thereto through December 31, 1978, except paragraph UW-11(a)(7) of the code does not apply.

(2) AAR Specifications for Tank Cars means the 1970 edition of the ''Association of American Railroads Specification for Tank Cars''.

(3) Compressed Gas Association:

(i) CGA Pamphlet C-3 is titled, ''Standards for Welding and Brazing

Note: For amendments to §171.8 see the List of CFR Sections Affected appearing in the Finding Aids section of this volume.

§171.9 Rules of construction

(a) In this subchapter, unless the context requires otherwise

(1) Words imparting the singular include the plural;
(2) Words imparting the plural include the singular; and
(3) Words imparting the masculine gender include the feminine;

(b) In this subchapter, the word:

(1) ''Shall'' is used in an imperative sense;
(2) ''Must'' is used in an imperative sense;
(3) ''Should'' is used in a recommendatory sense;
(4) ''May'' is used in a permissive sense to state authority or permission to do the act described, and the words ''no person may ***'' or ''a person may not***'' means that no person is required, authorized, or permitted to the act described; and
(5) ''Includes'' is used as a word of inclusion not limitation.

[Amdt. 171-32, 41 FR 15996, Apr. 15, 1976, as amended by Amdt. 171-32A, 41 FR 40630, Sept. 20, 1976]

§171.10 Flammable or combustible liquids in bulk on board vessels

(a) Nothing in Parts 170 to 189 of this subchapter shall be construed as affecting the transportation of flammable or combustible liquids in bulk on board vessels which transportation is governed by the rules and regulations promulgated under R.S. 4417a; 46 U.S.C. 391a (46 CFR Part 146).

[29 FR 18653, Dec. 29, 1964. Redesignated at 32 FR 5606, Apr. 5, 1967, and amended by Amdt. 171-42, 43 FR 48643, Oct. 19, 1978]

§171.11 [Reserved]

§171.12 Import and export shipments

(a) Except in the case of a shipment from Canada conforming to §173.8, each person importing a hazardous material into the U.S. shall provide the shipper and the forwarding agent at the place of entry into the U.S. timely and complete information as to the requirements of this subchapter that will apply to the shipment of the material within the U.S. The shipper, directly or through the forwarding agent at the place of entry, shall provide the initial carrier in the U.S. the certificate of compliance required by §172.204. The carrier may not accept the material for transportation unless the required certification is provided.

(b) The requirements of §171.2 with respect to classification and labeling notwithstanding, a hazardous material (other than Class A or B explosives or radioactive materials) which is classed and labeled in accordance with the IMCO Code and being imported into or exported from the U.S. or passing through the U.S. in the course of being shipped between places outside the U.S., may be offered and accepted for transportation and transported within the

U.S. if it is otherwise offered, accepted, and transported in accordance with this subchapter. When a material is transported within the U.S. by air, highway, or rail under an IMCO class, the entry on the shipping paper required by §172.202(a)(2) must include a class set forth in this subchapter that most appropriately corresponds to the IMCO class. For example, according to IMCO, the description and class for ethylene oxide is ''Ethylene Oxide, 2'' or ''Ethylene Oxide, Gas 2''. While ethylene oxide in domestic transportation would be classed a flammable liquid, the class in this subchapter that most appropriately corresponds to the IMCO class is ''flammable gas''. The proper entry would therefore be ''Ethylene Oxide, Flammable Gas'' or ''Ethylene Oxide, 2 Flammable Gas''.

(c) The requirements of §171.2 with respect to specification identification markings on packages notwithstanding, a package of hazardous materials (other than a compressed gas cylinder or a package of more than 110 gal capacity) being imported into or exported from the U.S. or passing through the U.S. in the course of being shipped between places outside the U.S. may be offered and accepted for transportation and transported within the U.S. if the package specification identification markings required by Part 178 are clearly and legibly displayed on the surface of the package or on decals or tags securely affixed to the package, and the package is otherwise offered, accepted, and transported in accordance with this subchapter.

(d) Section 171.2 notwithstanding, a hazardous material (other than Class A or B explosives or radioactive materials) being imported into or exported from the U.S. or passing through the U.S. in the course of being shipped between places outside the U.S. may be offered and accepted for transportation and transported by motor vehicle within a single port area (including contiguous harbors) when packaged, marked, classed and labeled in accordance with the IMCO Code, if the hazardous material is offered and accepted in accordance with the requirements of Subparts C and F of Part 172 of this subchapter pertaining to shipping papers and placarding. (See §176.11 of this subchapter for exceptions applicable to vessels.

(e) Not withstanding the quantity limitations of §173.389 (c) and (1) of this subchapter, any package of radioactive materials (except for fissile radioactive materials or Type B quantities under §173.393b of this subchapter) which otherwise conform to the requirements of this subchapter applicable to Type A quantities or low specific activity materials may be offered and accepted for transportation and transported within the U.S. if

(1) The package is being imported into the U.S., or is passing through in the course of being shipped between places outside the U. S.;
(2) The country of origin has adopted the Type A quantity limitations and low specific activity materials definition set forth in the IAEA Regulations for the Safe Transport of Radioactive Materials, 1973 Revised Edition; and
(3) The contents of the package have been limited as a Type A quantity or a low specific activity material in accordance with the IAEA Type A quantity limitations and low specific activity materials definition adopted by the originating country.

(49 U.S.C. 1803, 1804, 1808; 49 CFR 1.53 and App. A to Part 1)

[Amdt. 171-32, 41 FR 15996, Apr. 15, 1976, as amended by Amdt. 171-32A, 41 FR 40630, Sept. 20, 1976]

Note: For amendments to §171.12 see the List of CFR Sections Affected appearing in the Finding Aids section of this volume.

§171.14 Specification markings

(a) Notwithstanding any other requirements of Parts 170-189 of this subchapter, the letters ''ICC'' may continue to be placed on any packaging requiring specification markings until January 1, 1970.

(b) Packagings with the specification markings ''ICC'' placed thereon before January 1, 1970, may be continued in service as marked.

[Amdt. 171-2, 33 FR 17918, Dec. 3, 1968, as amended by Amdt. 171-42, 43 FR 48643, Oct. 19, 1978]

§171.15 Immediate notice of certain hazardous materials incidents

(a) At the earliest practicable moment, each carrier who transports hazardous materials shall give notice in accordance with paragraph (b) of this section after each incident that occurs during the course of transportation (including loading, unloading and temporary storage) in which as a direct result of hazardous materials

(1) A person is killed;
(2) A person receives injuries requiring his hospitalization;
(3) Estimated carrier or other property damage exceeds $50,000;
(4) Fire, breakage, spillage, or suspected radioactive contamination occurs involving shipment of radioactive material. (See also §§174.45, 175.45, 176.48, and 177.807 of this subchapter.); or
(5) Fire, breakage, spillage, or suspected contamination occurs involving shipment of etiologic agents; or
(6) A situation exists of such a nature that, in the judgment of the carrier, it should be reported in accordance with paragraph (b) of this section even though it does not meet the criteria of paragraph (a)(1), (2), or (3) of this section; e.g., a continuing danger of life exists at the scene of the incident.

(b) Each notice required by paragraph (a) of this section shall be given to the Department by telephone (toll-free) on 800-424-8802. Notice involving etiologic agents may be given the Director, Center for Disease Control, U.S. Public Health Service, Atlanta, Ga., Area Code (404) 633-5313, in place of the notice to the Department. Each notice must include the following information:

(1) Name of reporter.
(2) Name and address of carrier represented by reporter.
(3) Phone number where reporter can be contacted.
(4) Date, time, and location of incident.
(5) The extent of injuries, if any.
(6) Classification, name, and quantity of hazardous materials involved, if such information is available.
(7) Type of incident and nature of hazardous material involvement and whether a continuing danger to life exists at the scene.

(c) Each carrier making a report under this section shall also make the report required by §171.16.

(49 U.S.C. 1803, 1804, 1808; 49 CFR 1.53 and App. A to Part 1)

[Amdt. 171-7, 35 FR 16837, Oct. 3, 1970, as amended by Amdt. 171-13, 36 FR 21201, Nov. 4, 1971]

Note: For amendments to §171.15 see the List of CFR Sections Affected appearing in the Finding Aids section of this volume.

§171.16 Detailed hazardous materials incident reports

(a) Each carrier who transports hazardous materials shall report in writing in duplicate on DOT Form F 5800.1* to the Department within 15 days of the date of discovery, each incident that occurs during the course of transportation (including loading, unloading, or

* Filed as part of the original document.

temporary storage) in which, as a direct result of the hazardous materials, any of the circumstances set forth in §171.15(a) occurs or there has been an unintentional release of hazardous materials from a package (including a tank).

(b) Each carrier making a report under this section shall send that report to the Associate Director for Hazardous Materials Regulation, Department of Transportation, Washington, D.C. 20590.

[Amdt. 171-7, 35 FR 16837, Oct. 3, 1970, as amended by Amdt. 171-42, 43 FR 48643, Oct. 19, 1978]

§171.17 [Reserved]

§171.18 Continuation of effectiveness of existing Bureau of Explosives registrations

A registration filed with the Bureau of Explosives in compliance with a requirement of the subchapter, which is valid at the time that registration function is assumed by MTB remains valid to the same extent as if it had been filed originally with MTB.

(49 U.S.C. 1803, 1804, 1808; 49 CFR 1.53 and App; A to Part 1)

[Amdt. 171-50, 44 FR 55577, Sept. 27, 1979]

§171.19 Approvals or authorizations issued by the Bureau of Explosives

Unless otherwise specifically restricted by other requirements of this subchapter, an approval or authorization issued by the Bureau of Explosives, which is valid at the time that approval or authorizing function is abolished or is assumed by the Associate Director for OE, remains valid under the conditions and for the period of time for which it was issued by the Bureau of Explosives. However, no such approval or authorization remains valid beyond December 31, 1984 unless reissued by the Associate Director for OE. The Associate Director for OE may amend or extend any approval or authorization issued by the Bureau of Explosives.

(49 U.S.C. 1803, 1804, 1808; 49 CFR 1.53)

[Amdt. 171-45, 44 FR 18027, Mar. 26, 1979]

APPENDIX B
Title 49, Part 172*

PART 172—HAZARDOUS MATERIALS TABLE AND HAZARDOUS MATERIALS COMMUNICATIONS REGULATIONS

SUBPART A—GENERAL

§172.1 Purpose and scope

This part lists and classifies those materials which the Department of Transportation has designated as hazardous materials for purposes of transportation and prescribes the requirements for shipping papers, package marking, labeling, and transport vehicle placarding applicable to the shipment and transportation of those hazardous materials.
[Amdt. 172-29, 41 FR 15997, Apr. 15, 1976]

§172.3 Applicability

(a) This part applies to

(1) Each person who offers a hazardous material for transportation, and
(2) Each carrier by air, highway, rail or water who transports a hazardous material.

(b) When a person, other than one of those provided for in paragraph (a) of this section, performs a packaging labeling or marking function required by this part, that person shall perform the function in accordance with this part.
[Amdt. 172-29, 41 FR 15996, Apr. 15, 1976, as amended by Amdt. 172-32, 41 FR38179, Sept. 9, 1976]

SUBPART B—TABLE OF HAZARDOUS MATERIALS, THEIR DESCRIPTION, PROPER SHIPPING NAME, CLASS, LABEL, PACKAGING, AND OTHER REQUIREMENTS

§172.100 Purpose and use of the table

(a) The table set forth in §172.101 constitutes a designation of the materials listed therein as hazardous materials for purposes of the transportation of those materials in commerce. In addition, it classifies and specifies requirements and references other requirements set forth elsewhere in this subchapter pertaining to the labeling, packaging, and transportation of those materials.

(b) Column 1 contains three symbols:*, A, and W.

(1) * An asterisk before a proper shipping name means that the material described in column 2 may or may not be regulated under the class shown depending on whether or not the commodity meets the definition of the hazard class listed for that entry. If the commodity does not meet the definition of the class stated, the shipper shall determine whether or not the material meets the definition of any other hazard class, and shall prepare the material for shipment in compliance with the requirements of that class. A material meeting the description of an asterisk entry is not subject to the requirements of this subchapter if the material does not meet the definition of a hazardous material.
(2) A: The symbol "A" before the shipping name means that the material described in column 2 is subject to the requirements of this subchapter only for transportation by aircraft.

* From *Fed. Reg.*, June 30, 1977.

(3) W: The symbol "W" before the shipping name means that the material described in column 2 is subject to the requirements of this subchapter only for transportation by vessel.

(c) Column 2 lists the proper shipping name of those materials which are designated as hazardous materials. Proper shipping names are limited to those shown in Roman type (not italics). In the selection of a proper shipping name to describe a particular material, if the correct technical name of that material is not shown, or is not appropriate, selection must be made from the general descriptions or n.o.s. entries corresponding to the specific hazard class of the material being shipped. The name that more appropriately describes the commodity must be used, i.e., an alcohol must be shipped as an alochol n.o.s. rather than a flammable liquid n.o.s. unless the technical name of the alcohol is listed (methyl alcohol). Some mixtures may be more aptly described by their application such as: "Compound, cleaning liquid" or "Compound, rust removing," rather than "Corrosive liquid n.o.s." For materials that meet the definition of more than one hazard class, the hazard class must be determined by using the precedence given in §173.2 of this subchapter. If it is believed that an adequate description of a material is not given in §172.101, the Office of Hazardous Materials Regulation should be contacted for clarification.

(1) Shipping names may be used in the singular or plural in either capital or lower case letters.

(2) The words in italics are not part of the proper shipping name but may be used in addition to the proper shipping name. The word "or" in italics indicates that any terms in the sequence may be used as the proper shipping name as appropriate.

(3) The abbreviation "n.o.i." which means "not otherwise indexed" or "n.o.i.b.n." which means "not otherwise indexed by name" may be used interchangeably with "n.o.s."

(4) When qualifying words are used as part of the proper shipping name, their sequence on package markings and shipping paper descriptions is optional.

(5) When one entry references another entry by use of a "*see*", if both names are in Roman type, either name may be used as a proper shipping name (e.g. Isopropanol *see* Alcohol, n.o.s.).

(6) When a shipping name includes a concentration range as part of the shipping description, the actual concentration being shipped, if it is within the range stated, may be used in place of the concentration range. For example: Hydrogen peroxide solution (8% to 40% peroxide) may be shipped described as "Hydrogen peroxide solution, 30% peroxide." or "30% Hydrogen peroxide solution."

(7) The use of the prefix "mono" is optional in any shipping name when appropriate. Thus, monoethanolamine may be used interchangeably with ethanolamine. In the "trichloromonofluoromethane" the term "mono" is considered as a prefix to the term "fluoromethane."

(d) Column 3 contains a designation of the hazard class corresponding to each proper shipping name or the word "Forbidden". A material for which the class entry is "Forbidden" must not be offered or accepted for transportation. When re-evaluation of test data or new test data indicates a need to modify the hazard class or labels specified for a material specifically identified in §172.101, these data should be reported to the Office of Hazardous Materials Regulation.

(e) Column 4 specifies the labels required to be applied to each outside packaging, subject to the additional labeling requirements in §172.402.

(f) Column 5 references the applicable packaging section of Part 173. Exceptions from some of the requirements of this subchapter are noted in column 5(a). References to specific packaging requirements and exceptions other than those specified in 5(a) are noted in column 5(b).

(g) Column 6 indicates the maximum net quantity in one package for air transportation or passenger railcar;

(1) Column 6(a) specifies the maximum net quantity permitted in one package for passenger-carrying aircraft or passenger railcar. For air transportation, any material forbidden on passenger-carrying aircraft but permitted on cargo aircraft, or which exceeds the maximum quantity authorized on passenger-carrying aircraft, must be shipped by cargo-only aircraft and bear the CARGO AIRCRAFT ONLY label as described in §172.448.

(2) Column 6(b) lists the maximum net quantity for one outside package on cargo aircraft. Packaging must bear the CARGO AIRCRAFT ONLY label when the quantity of hazardous material exceeds that authorized on passenger-carrying aircraft, or is forbidden on passenger-carrying aircraft.

(3) For flammable liquids, the net quantity limitation for carriage aboard a passenger-carrying aircraft or railcar is 1 gal/package, and for cargo-only aircraft is 55 gal/package, if:

(i) The material has a flash point of 73°F. or higher;

(ii) The material does not meet the definition of any other hazard class as defined in this part; and

(iii) The flash point, or an indication that the flash point is 73°F. or higher, is marked on the outside package.

(h) Column 7 specifies each of the authorized locations on board cargo vessels and passenger vessels and certain additional requirements for shipments of each listed hazardous material. Section 176.63 of this subchapter sets forth the physical requirements for each of the authorized locations listed in Column 7. (For bulk shipments by water see 46 CFR Parts 30 to 40, 48, 64, 70, 98, 148, 151, and 154.)

(1) ''1'' means the material may be stowed ''on deck'' subject to the requirements of §176.63(b) of this subchapter. When both ''on deck'' and ''under deck'' are authorized, ''under deck'' should be used if it is available.

(2) ''2'' means the material may be stowed ''under deck'' in a compartment or hold subject to the requirements of §176.63(c). When both ''on deck'' and ''under deck'' are authorized, ''under deck'' should be used if it is available.

(3) ''3'' means the material may be stowed ''under deck away from heat'' in a ventilated compartment or hold subject to the requirements of §176.63(d) of this subchapter.

(4) ''4'' means the material is authorized to be transported in only the limited quantities specified in the CFR section listed in Column 5 and is subject to the stowage requirements specified for a cargo vessel for the same material.

(5) ''5'' means the material is forbidden and may not be offered or accepted for transportation.

(6) ''6'' means the material is authorized to be transported in a magazine subject to the requirements of §§176.135 through 176.144 of this subchapter.

(49 U.S.C. 1803, 1804, 1808; 49 CFR 1.53(e))
[Amdt. 172-29, 41 FR 15996, Apr. 15, 1976, as amended by mdt. 172-29-A. 41 FR 40630, Sept. 20, 1976]

Note: For amendments to §172.100 see the List of CFR Sections Affected appearing in the Finding Aids section of this volume.

172.101 HAZARDOUS MATERIALS TABLE

(1) */ W/ A	(2) Hazardous materials descriptions and proper shipping names	(3) Hazard class	(4) Label(s) required (if not excepted)	(5) Packaging (a) Exceptions	(5) Packaging (b) Specific requirements	(6) Maximum net quantity in one package (a) Passenger carrying aircraft or railcar	(6) Maximum net quantity in one package (b) Cargo only aircraft	(7) Water shipments (a) Cargo vessel	(7) Water shipments (b) Passenger vessel	(7) Water shipments (c) Other requirements
*	Plutonium nitrate solution	Radioactive material	Radioactive (see Sec. 172.403)	173.393	173.396			1.2	1.2	
	Radioactive device, n.o.s.	Radioactive material	None	173.391				1.2	1.2	
*	Radioactive material, fissile, n.o.s.	Radioactive material	Radioactive	173.393	173.396			1.2	1.2	
*	Radioactive material, low specific activity or L.S.A. n.o.s.	Radioactive material	Radioactive	173.392	173.393			1.2	1.2	
*	Radioactive material, n.o.s.	Radioactive material	Radioactive	173.393	173.395			1.2	1.2	
*	Radioactive material, limited quantity, n.o.s.	Radioactive material	None	173.391				1.2	1.2	
*	Radioactive material, special form, n.o.s.	Radioactive material	Radioactive	173.393	173.394			1.2	1.2	
	Thorium metal, pyrophoric	Radioactive material	Radioactive and flammable solid	173.226	173.226			1.2	1.2	
	Thorium nitrate	Radioactive material	Radioactive and oxidizer	173.392	173.393			1.2	1.2	Separate longitudinally by a complete hold or compartment from explosives
	Uranium hexafluoride, fissile (containing more than 0.7% U-235)	Radioactive material	Radioactive and corrosive	173.393	173.396			1.2	1.2	
	Uranium hexafluoride, low specific activity (containing 0.7% or less U-235)	Radioactive material	Radioactive and corrosive	173.392	173.393			1.2	1.2	
	Uranium metal, pyrophoric	Radioactive material	Radioactive and flammable solid	173.392	173.393 173.396			1.2	1.2	
	Uranyl nitrate hexahydrate solution	Radioactive material	Radioactive and corrosive	173.392	173.393 173.395 173.396			1.2	1.2	
	Uranyl nitrate, solid	Radioactive material	Radioactive and oxidizer	173.392	173.393 173.396			1.2	1.2	Separate longitudinally by an intervening hold or compartment from explosives

[Amdt. 172-29, 41 FR 15996, Apr. 15, 1976, as amended by Amdt. 172-29A, 41 FR 40678, Sept. 20, 1976]

§ 172.304 Marking requirements

(a) The marking required in this subpart

(1) Must be durable, in English, and printed on or affixed to the surface of a package or on a label, tag, or sign.
(2) Must be displayed on a background of sharply contrasting color;
(3) Must be unobscured by labels or attachments; and
(4) Must be located away from any other marking (such as advertising) that could substantially reduce its effectiveness.

[Amdt. 172-29, 41 FR 15996, Apr. 15, 1976, as amended by Amdt. 172-29B, 41 FR 57067, Dec. 30, 1976]

§ 172.306 Consignee's or consignor's name and address

(a) Each package containing a hazardous material offered for transportation must be marked with the name and address of the consignee or consignor except when the package is

(1) Transported by highway and will not be transferred from one motor carrier to another, or

(2) Part of a carload lot, truckload lot, or freight container load, and the entire contents of the rail car, truck, or freight container are tendered from one consignor to one consignee, or
(3) A portable tank, cargo tank, or tank car.

[Amdt. 172-29, 41 FR 15996, Apr. 15, 1976, as amended by Amdt. 172-29A, 41 FR 40678, Sept. 20, 1976; Amdt. 172-29B, 41 FR 57067, Dec. 30, 1976]

§172.308 Authorized abbreviations

(a) Abbreviations may not be used except in the following instances

(1) For marking descriptions on ammunition, such as ammunition for cannon without projectiles, etc., the words ''with'' or ''without'' may be abbreviated as ''W'' or ''W/O'' for example: ''Ammunition for cannon W/O projectiles''
(2) The abbreviation ''ORM''maybe used in place of the words ''Other Regulated Materials.''

§172.310 Radioactive materials

(a) In addition to any other markings required by this subpart, each package containing radioactive materials must be marked as follows:

(1) Each package of radioactive materials in excess of 110 lb (50 kg) must have its gross weight plainly and durably marked on the outside of the package.
(2) Each package of radioactive materials which conforms to the requirements for Type A or Type B packaging (§§ 173.389 (j) and (k) and 173.398 (b) and (c) of this subchapter) must be plainly and durably marked on the outside of the package in letters at least $^{1}/_{2}$-in. (13 mm) high, with the words ''TYPE A'' or ''TYPE B'' as appropriate. A packaging which is not in compliance with these requirements may not be so marked.
(3) Each package of radioactive material destined for export shipment must also be marked ''USA'' in conjunction with the specification marking, or other package certificate identification. (See §§ 173.393a and 173.393b of this subchapter.)

§172.312 Liquid hazardous materials

(a) Except as provided in this section and for limited quantities of flammable liquids packed in inside packagings of 1 qt or less, each package having an inside packaging containing liquid hazardous materials must be

(1) Packed with closures upward, and
(2) Legibly marked ''THIS SIDE UP'' or ''THIS END UP'' as appropriate, to indicate the upward position of the inside packaging.

(b) Except as otherwise prescribed in Part 173 of this subchapter cylinders of liquefied compressed gas and specification containers 6D, 37M, 37P, and 21P are not required to be marked ''THIS SIDE UP'' or ''THIS END UP''.

(c) Arrows for purposes other than indicating proper package orientation may not be displayed on a package containing a hazardous material that is a liquid.

(1) An arrow symbol indicating ''This Way Up'' as specified in ANSI MH6.11968 entitled ''Pictorial Marking for Handling of Goods'' should be used in addition to the marking required by this section and §173.25 of this subchapter.

§172.403 Radioactive material

(a) Unless excepted from labeling by 173.391 or §173.392 of this subchapter, each package of radioactive material must be labeled as provided in this section.

(b) A RADIOACTIVE WHITE-I label must be affixed to each package measuring 0.5 mrem or less per hour at each point on the external surface of the package, provided the package

(1) Is not a Fissile Class II or III, or
(2) Does not contain a "large quantity" of radioactive material, as defined in § 173.389 of this subchapter.

(c) A RADIOACTIVE YELLOW-II label must be affixed to each

(1) Package measuring more than 0.5 but not more than 50 mrem/hr at each point and not exceeding one (1.0) mrem/hr at 3 ft from each point on the external surface of the package.
(2) Fissile Class II package having a transport index of one (1.0) or less.

(d) A RADIOACTIVE YELLOW-III label must be affixed to each package which

(1) Measures more than 50 mrem/hr at each point or exceeds one (1.0) mrem/hr at 3 ft from each point on the external surface;
(2) Is a Fissile Class III; or
(3) Contains a "large quantity" of radioactive material as defined in § 173.389 of this subchapter.

(e) Each package containing a radioactive material that also meets the definition of one or more additional hazards must be labeled as a radioactive material as required by this section and for each additional hazard. For example:

(1) Packages containing the solid nitrates of uranium or thorium must be labeled RADIOACTIVE and OXIDIZER.
(2) Packages containing nitric acid solutions of radioactive material must be labeled RADIOACTIVE and CORROSIVE.

(f) Each package required by this section to be labeled with a RADIOACTIVE label must have two of these labels, affixed to opposite sides of the package. (See § 172.406(e)(3) for freight container label requirements).

(g) The following applicable items of information must be entered in the blank spaces on the RADIOACTIVE label by legible printing (manual or mechanical), using a durable weather resistant means of marking:

(1) "Contents." The name of the radionuclides as taken from the listing of radionuclides in § 173.390 (symbols which conform to established radiation protection terminology are authorized, i.e., ^{99}Mo, ^{60}Co, etc.). For mixtures of radionuclides, the most restrictive radionuclides on the basis of radiotoxicity must be listed as space on the label allows.
(2) "Number of curies." Units shall be expressed in appropriate curie units, i.e., curies (Ci), millicuries (mCi), or microcuries (μCi) (abbreviations are authorized). For a fissile material, the weight in grams or kilograms of the fissile radioisotope also may be inserted.
(3) "Transportation index." (See § 173.389(i).)

[Amdt. 172-29, 41 FR 15996, Apr. 15, 1976, as amended by Amdt. 172-29A, 41 FR 40679, Sept. 20, 1976]

§ 172.404 Labels for mixed and consolidated packaging

(a) *Mixed packaging.* When hazardous materials having different hazard classes are packed within the same packaging, or within the same outside container or overpack as described in § 173.25 and authorized by §173.21 of this subchapter, the packaging, outside container or overpack must be labeled as required for each class of hazardous material contained therein.

(b) *Consolidated packaging.* When two or more packages containing compatible hazardous material (see §173.21) are placed within the same outside container or overpack, the outside container or overpack must be labeled as required for each class of hazardous material contained therein.

§172.406 Placement of labels

(a) *General.* Except as provided in paragraphs (b) and (e) of this section, each label required by this subpart must be printed on or affixed to the surface of the package near the marked proper shipping name required by Subpart D of this part.

(b) *Exceptions.* Labels may be printed on or placed on a securely affixed tag, or may be affixed by other suitable means to

(1) A package that contains no radioactive material and which has dimensions less than those of the required label;
(2) A compressed gas cylinder; and
(3) A package which has such an irregular surface that a label cannot be satisfactorily affixed.

(c) *Placement of multiple labels.* When two or more different labels are required, they must be displayed or affixed next to each other.

(d) *Label border.* Each label must be affixed to a background of contrasting color, or must have a dotted or solid line outer border.

(e) *Additional labeling.* When labeling is required, the labels must be displayed on at least two sides or two ends (excluding the bottom) of

(1) Each package containing a radioactive material;
(2) Each package having a volume of 64 ft^3 or more; and
(3) Each freight container having a volume of 64 ft^3 or more, but less than 640 ft^3 except when placarded in accordance with §172.512(b).
    (i) Placarding may not be used instead of labeling on a package containing radioactive material.
    (ii) When labeled, one of each of the appropriate labels must be displayed on or near the closure.
(4) Each portable tank having a rated capacity of less than 1000 gal, except when placarded in accordance with §172.514(a).

(f) *Obscured labels.* A label must not be obscured by markings or attachments.

[Amdt. 172-29, 41 FR 15996, Apr. 15, 1976, as amended by Amdt. 172-29A, 41 FR 40679, Sept. 20, 1976; Amdt. 172-29B, 41 FR 57067, Dec. 30, 1976]

§172.407 Label specifications

(a) Each label, affixed to or printed on a package must be durable and weather resistant. Black and any color on a label must be able to withstand, without substantial change

(1) A 72-hr fadeometer test (for a description of equipment designed for this purpose, see ASTM G 23-69 (1975), or ASTM G 26-70); and

(2) A 30-day exposure to conditions incident to transportation that reasonably could be expected to be encountered by the labeled package.

(b) Each diamond (square-on-point) label prescribed in this part must be at least 4 in. (101 mm) on each side with each side having a black solid line border $^1/_4$ in. (6.3 mm) from the edge.

(c) Except for size and color, the printing, inner border, and symbol on each label must be as shown for each label.

§172.436 RADIOACTIVE WHITE-I label

(a) Except for size and color, the RADIOACTIVE WHITE-I label, must be as follows:

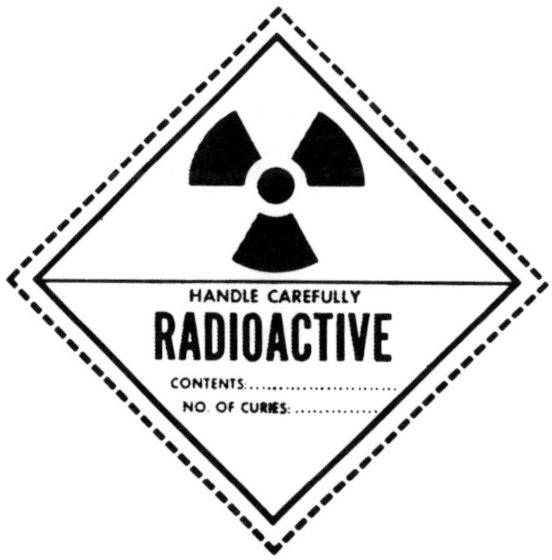

(b) In addition to complying with §172.407, the RADIOACTIVE WHITE-I label must be white. The printing and symbol must be black except for the "I" which must be red.

§172.438 RADIOACTIVE YELLOW-II label

(a) Except for size and color, the RADIOACTIVE YELLOW-II label, must be as follows:

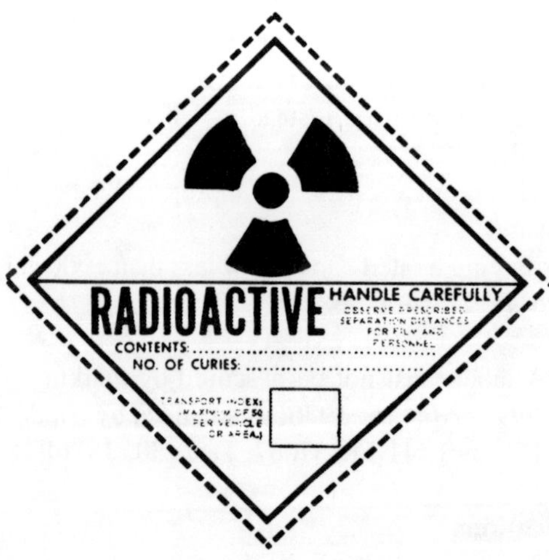

(b) In addition to complying with §172.407, the RADIOACTIVE YELLOW-II label must be yellow in the top half and white in the lower half. The printing and symbol must be black, except for the "II" which must be red.

§172.440 RADIOACTIVE YELLOW-III label

(a) Except for the size and color, the RADIOACTIVE YELLOW-III label must be as follows:

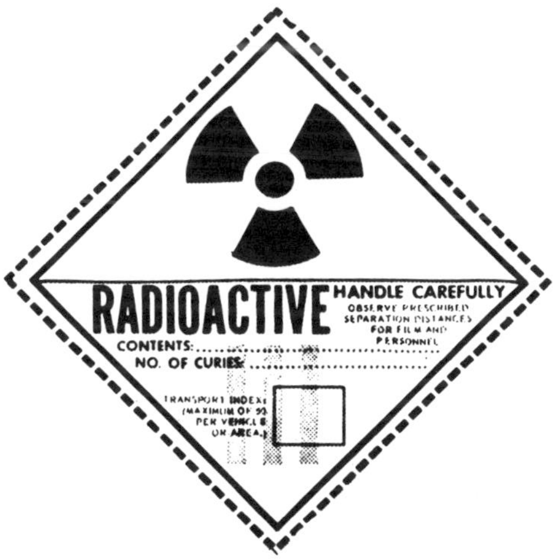

(b) In addition to complying with §172.407, the RADIOACTIVE YELLOW-III label must be yellow in the top half and white in the lower half. The printing and symbol must be black, except for the "III" which must be red.

§172.448 CARGO AIRCRAFT ONLY label

(a) Except for size and color, the CARGO AIRCRAFT ONLY (DANGER—PELIGRO) label including the label name in the lower border must be as follows:

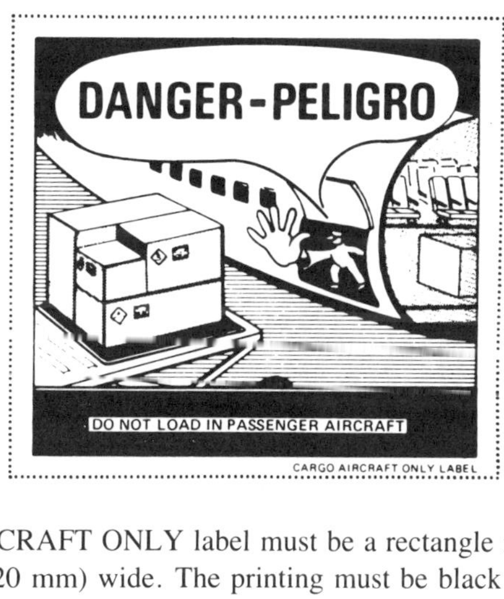

(b) The CARGO AIRCRAFT ONLY label must be a rectangle measuring 4 $^5/_{16}$ in. (110 mm) high by $4^3/_4$ in. (120 mm) wide. The printing must be black and the symbol must be black and orange.

SUBPART F—PLACARDING

§172.500 Applicability of placarding requirements

(a) Each person who offers for transportation or transports any hazardous material subject to this subchapter shall comply with the applicable placarding requirements of this subpart.

(b) This subpart does not apply to

(1) Etiologic agents,
(2) Hazardous materials classed as ORM-A, B, C, or D, or
(3) Hazardous materials authorized by this subchapter to be offered for transportation as Limited Quantities when identified as such on shipping papers in accordance with §172.203(b).

[Amdt. 172-29, 41 FR 15996, Apr. 15, 1976, as amended by Amdt. 172-29A, 41 FR 40679, Sept. 20, 1976]

§172.502 Prohibited placarding

(a) No person may affix or display on a portable tank, freight container, motor vehicle, or rail car any placard described in this subpart unless

(1) The material being offered or transported is a hazardous material, and
(2) The placard represents a hazard of the hazardous material being offered or transported.

(b) No person may affix or display any sign or other device on a motor vehicle, rail car, portable tank, or freight container, that by its color, design, shape, or content could be confused with any placard prescribed in this subpart.

§172.504 General placarding requirements

(a) Except as otherwise provided in this subchapter, each motor vehicle, rail car, and freight container containing any quantity of a hazardous material must be placarded on each end and each side with the type of placards specified in the following tables and other placarding requirements of this subpart, including the specifications for the placards named in the tables and described in detail in §§172.519 through 172.558.

(b) A freight container, motor vehicle, or rail car containing two or more classes of materials requiring different placards specified in Table 2 may be placarded DANGEROUS in place of the separate placarding specified for each of those classes of material specified in Table 2. However, when 5000 lb or more of one class of material is loaded therein at one loading facility, the placard specified for that class in Table 2 must be applied. This paragraph does not apply to a portable tank, cargo tank, or tank car.

(c) No placard is required on a

(1) Motor vehicle, or a freight container if transported by highway only, containing less than 1000 lb (aggregate gross weight) of one or more materials covered by Table 2, or
(2) Rail car loaded with freight containers or motor vehicles when each freight container or motor vehicle contains less than 1000 lb (aggregate gross weight) of one or more materials, covered by Table (2). This paragraph does not apply to portable tanks, cargo tanks, or tank cars or to transportation by air or water.

Table 1

If the motor vehicle, rail car, or freight container contains a material classed (described) as	The motor vehicle, rail car, or freight container must be placarded on each side and each end
Class A explosives	EXPLOSIVES A[a]
Class B explosives	EXPLOSIVES B[b]
Poison A	POISON GAS[a]
Flammable solid (DANGEROUS WHEN WET label only)	FLAMMABLE SOLID W[c]
Radioactive material	
Uranium hexafluoride, fissile (containing more than 0.7% U^{235})	RADIOACTIVE[d,e] AND CORROSIVE[f]
Uranium hexafluoride, low specific activity (containing 0.7% or less U^{235})	RADIOACTIVE[d,e] AND CORROSIVE[f]

[a] See §172.510(a).

[b] EXPLOSIVES B placard not required if the freight container, motor vehicle, or rail car contains class A explosives and is placarded EXPLOSIVES A as required.

[c] FLAMMABLE SOLID "W" placard is required only when the DANGEROUS WHEN WET label is specified in § 172.101 for a material classed as a Flammable solid.

[d] Applies only to any quantity of packages bearing the RADIOACTIVE YELLOW III label. (See § 172.403.)

[e] See §§ 173.389(c) and 173.389(o), for full-load shipments of radioactive materials meeting the definition of low specific activity when transported pursuant to § 173.392(b).

[f] CORROSIVE placard not required for shipments of less than 1000 lb gross weight.

Table 2

If the motor vehicle, rail car, or freight container contains a material classed (described) as	The motor vehicle, rail car, or freight container must be placarded on each side and each end
Class C explosives	FLAMMABLE[a]
Blasting agents	BLASTING AGENT
Nonflammable gas	NONFLAMMABLE GAS
Nonflammable gas (chlorine)	CHLORINE[a]
Nonflammable gas (fluorine)	POISON
Nonflammable gas (oxygen, pressurized liquid)	OXYGEN[b]
Flammable gas	FLAMMABLE GAS
Combustible liquid	COMBUSTIBLE[c,d]
Flammable liquid	FLAMMABLE
Flammable solid	FLAMMABLE SOLID[e]
Oxidizer	OXIDIZER
Organic peroxide	ORGANIC PEROXIDE
Poison B	POISON
Corrosive material	CORROSIVE[f]
Irritating material	DANGEROUS

[a] Applies only to a class C explosive required to be labeled with an EXPLOSIVE C label.

[b] OXYGEN placards may be used to identify liquefied pressurized oxygen contained in a manner so it does not meet the definition in sec. 173.300 of this subchapter.

[c] COMBUSTIBLE placard required only when a material classed as a combustible liquid is transported in a packaging having a rated capacity of more than 110 gal, a cargo tank, or a tank car.

[d] A FLAMMABLE placard may be used on a cargo tank and a portable tank during transportation by highway and water.

[e] Except when offered for transportation by water, a FLAMMABLE placard may be displayed in place of a FLAMMABLE SOLID placard except when a DANGEROUS WHEN WET label is specified for the material in sec. 172.101. (See Table 1. this section.)

[f] See §173.245(b) of this subchapter for authorized exemptions.

[g] CHLORINE placard required only for a packaging having a rated capacity of more than 110 gal; the NONFLAMMABLE GAS placard for packagings having a rated capacity of 110 gal or less.

[Amdt. 172-29, 41 FR 15996, Apr. 15, 1976, as amended by Amdt. 172-29A, 41 FR 40679, Sept. 20, 1976; Amdt. 172-29B, 41 FR 57067, Dec. 30, 1976; Amdt. 172-48, 44 FR 31182, May 31, 1979]

§ 172.506 Providing and affixing placards: Highway

(a) Each person offering a motor carrier a hazardous material for transportation by highway shall provide to the motor carrier the required placards for the material being offered prior to or at the same time the material is offered for transportation, unless the carrier's motor vehicle is already placarded for the material as required by this subpart.

(1) No motor carrier may transport a hazardous material in a motor vehicle, unless the placards required for the hazardous material are affixed thereto as required by this subpart.

[Amdt. 172-29, 41 FR 15996, Apr. 15, 1976, as amended by Amdt. 172-29A, 41 FR 40679, Sept. 20, 1976]

§ 172.508 Placarding and affixing placards: Rail

(a) Each person offering a hazardous material for transportation by rail shall affix to the rail car containing the material, the placards specified by this subpart for the material unless the placards already displayed on motor vehicles, transport containers, or portable tanks that are on a rail car comply with §§ 172.502 and 172.504 as these sections pertain to placarding the rail car.

(b) No rail carrier may accept a rail car containing a hazardous material for transportation unless the placards for the hazardous material are affixed thereto as required by this subpart.

[Amdt. 172-29, 41 FR 15996, Apr. 15, 1976, as amended by Amdt. 172-29B, 41 FR 57068, Dec. 30, 1976]

§ 172.510 Special placarding provisions: Rail

(a) *Square background required.* Each Explosive A placard, Poison Gas placard and POISON GAS—EMPTY, placard affixed to a rail car must be placed on a square background as described in § 172.527.

(b) *DOME placard.* Each domed tank car containing a flammable liquid having a vapor pressure exceeding 16 p.s.i. at 100°F. (37.8°C.) must have a DOME placard affixed thereto as specified in § 173.119(h) of this subchapter.

(c) *EMPTY placard.* Each empty tank car must be placarded with an EMPTY placard as required and described in § 172.525 or paragraph (a) of this section, as appropriate, that corresponds to the placard that was required for the material the tank car last contained unless the tank car last contained a Combustible liquid or has been

(1) Reloaded with a material not subject to this subchapter; or
(2) Sufficiently cleaned of residue and purged of vapor to remove any potential hazard.

(d) *FUMIGATION placard.* Each freight container, motor vehicle, and rail car containing lading that has been fumigated or treated with poisonous liquid, solid, or gas, and that is offered for transportation by rail must have the placard specified in § 173.426 of this subchapter affixed on or near each door.

[Amdt. 172-29, 41 FR 15996, Apr. 15, 1976, as amended by Amdt. 172-29A, 41 FR 40680, Sept. 20, 1976]

§ 172.512 Freight container

(a) *Capacity of 640 ft^3 or more.* Each person who offers for transportation a hazardous material in a freight container having a capacity of 640 ft^3 or more shall affix to the freight container the placards specified for the material in accordance with § 172.504. However,

(1) The placarding exception provided in § 172.504(c)(1) applies, and

(2) The placarding exception provided by paragraphs (c)(1) and (c)(2) of § 172.504 applies to each freight container being transported for delivery to a consignee immediately following an air or water shipment.

(b) *Capacity less than 640 ft³*. Each person who offers for transportation by air a hazardous material in a freight container having a capacity of less than 640 ft^3 shall affix one placard of the type specified by paragraph (a) of this section unless the freight container is labeled in accordance with § 172.406(e)(3) or contains radioactive materials requiring the RADIOACTIVE YELLOW III label and is placarded with one RADIOACTIVE placard and is labeled in accordance with § 172.406(e). When hazardous materials are offered for transportation, not involving air transportation, in a freight container having a capacity of less than 640 ft^3, the freight container need not be placarded. However, it must be labeled in accordance with Subpart E of this part.

(c) Notwithstanding paragraphs (a) and (b) of this section, packages containing hazardous materials, other than ORM-D, offered for transportation by air in freight containers are subject to the inspection requirements of § 175.30 of this chapter.

[Amdt. 172-29, 41 FR 15996, Apr. 15, 1976, as amended by Amdt. 172-29A, 41 FR 40680, Sept. 20, 1976; Amdt. 172-29B, 41 FR 57068, Dec. 30, 1976]

§ 172.514 Cargo tanks and portable tanks

(a) Each person who offers for transportation a cargo tank or a portable tank containing a hazardous material shall affix the placards specified for the material in accordance with § 172.504(a). However, if placarded instead of labeled as provided in § 172.406(e)(4), a portable tank having a rated capacity of less than 1000 gal need be placarded on only two opposite sides.

(b) Each cargo tank and portable tank that is required to be placarded when it contains a hazardous material must remain placarded when it is emptied unless it is

(1) Reloaded with a material not subject to this subchapter; or
(2) Sufficiently cleaned and purged of vapors to remove any potential hazard.

[Amdt. 172-29, 41 FR 15996, Apr. 15, 1976, as amended by Amdt. 172-29A 41 FR 40680, Sept. 20, 1976; Amdt. 172-29B, 41 FR 57068, Dec. 30, 1976]

§ 172.516 Visibility and display of placards

(a) Each placard on a motor vehicle and each placard on a rail car must be readily visible from the direction it faces except from the direction of another motor vehicle or rail car to which the motor vehicle or rail car is coupled. This requirement may be met by the placards displayed on the freight containers or portable tanks loaded on a motor vehicle or rail car.

(b) The required placarding of the front of a motor vehicle may be on the front of a truck-tractor instead of or in addition to the placarding on the front of the cargo body to which a truck-tractor is attached.

(c) Each placard on a transport vehicle, portable tank or freight container must

(1) Be securely attached or affixed thereto or placed in a holder thereon. (See Appendix C to this part.);

(2) Be located clear of appurtenances and devices such as ladders, pipes, doors, and tarpaulins;

(3) So far as practicable, be located so that dirt or water is not directed to it from the wheels of the transport vehicle;

(4) Be located away from any marking (such as advertising) that could substantially reduce its effectiveness, and in any case at least 3 in. (76.0 mm) away from such marking;

(5) Have the words printed on it displayed horizontally, reading from left to right;

(6) Be maintained by the carrier in a condition so that the format, legibility, color, and visibility of the placard will not be substantially reduced due to damage, deterioration, or obscurement by dirt or other matter.

(d) Recommended specifications for a placard holder are set forth in Appendix C of this part. Except for a placard holder similar to that contained in Appendix C to this part, the means used to attach a placard may not obscure any part of its surface other than the borders.

(e) A placard or placard holder may be hinged provided the required format, color, and legibility of the placard are maintained.

§ 172.519 General specifications for placards

(a) A placard may be made of any plastic, metal, or other material that is equal to or better in strength and durability than the tagboard specified in paragraph (b) of this section. Also, reflective or retroreflective materials may be used on a placard providing the prescribed colors, strength and durability are maintained.

(b) A placard made of tagboard must be of material that has

(1) A quality at least equal to that designated commercially as white tagboard;
(2) A weight of 125 lb/ream of 24 by 36-in. sheets;
(3) The ability to pass a 60 p.s.i. Mullen test; and
(4) The ability to withstand open weather exposure for 30 days without a substantial reduction in effectiveness.

(c) A placard may contain form identification information, including the name of its maker if that information is printed in the outer $^1/_2$-in. (12.7 mm) border in no larger than 10-point type.

(d) The hazard class and division number prescribed for dangerous goods in the United Nations Recommendations entitled "Transport of Dangerous Goods (1970)" may be entered on each placard in the lower corner of the diamond. The numerals should be approximately 0.75-in. (19.0 mm) in height and black on each placard except the NONFLAMMABLE GAS, FLAMMABLE GAS, and CORROSIVE placards. The numbers on the NONFLAMMABLE GAS, FLAMMABLE GAS, and FLAMMABLE placards may be white, and numbers on the CORROSIVE placards should be white.

(e) Surface pigmentation on a placard must meet the following requirements:

(1) Black and any color must be able to withstand, without substantial change

  (i) A 72-hr fadeometer test (for a description of equipment designed for this purpose, see ASTM G 23-69 (1975), or ASTM G 26-70); and
  (ii) A 30-day exposure to open weather conditions.

(2) A color on a placard, upon visual examination, must fall within the color tolerances displayed on the appropriate Office of Hazardous Materials Label and Placard Color Tolerance Chart (see § 172.407(d)).

(f) Dimensional specifications for placards are prescribed in Appendix B to this part.

(g) The dotted line at the outside of the $^1/_2$-in. (12.7 mm) white border on each placard is not part of the placard specification. However, a dotted or solid line outer border may be used when needed to indicate the full size of a placard that is part of a larger format or is on a background the color of which does not contrast with the placard color.

(49 U.S.C. 1803, 1804, 1808; 49 CFR 1.53(e)) [Amdt. 172-29, 41 FR 15996, Apr. 15,

1976, as amended by Amdt. 172-29A 41 FR 40680, Sept. 20, 1976; Amdt. 172-37, 42 FR 34285, July 5, 1977]

§ 172.556 RADIOACTIVE placard

(a) Except for size and color, the RADIOACTIVE placard must be as follows:

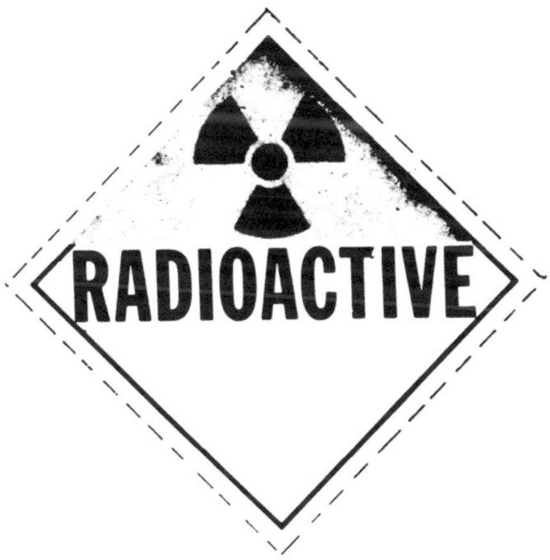

(b) In addition to meeting the requirements of § 172.519, and Appendix B to this part, the RADIOACTIVE placard must have the top portion yellow with the symbol black. The lower portion must be white and the inscription black.

§ 172.558 CORROSIVE placard

(a) Except for size, the CORROSIVE placard must be as follows:

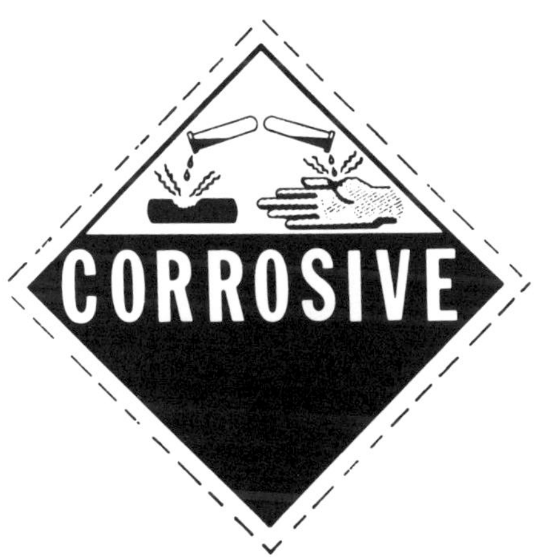

(b) In addition to meeting the requirements of § 172.519, and Appendix B to this part, the CORROSIVE placard must have the center and lower area black except for the letters in the word "CORROSIVE" which must be white. The symbol must be black and white.

(17) *RADIOACTIVE placard.* The word "RADIOACTIVE" must be centered on the placard horizontal center line in letters 2 in. (50.8 mm) with an $^{11}/_{32}$-in. (8.7 mm) stroke. The lower edge of the yellow triangle must be $1^1/_8$ in. (28.6 mm) above the placard horizontal center line. The lower edge of the symbol must be $1^1/_4$ in. (31.7 mm) above the placard horizontal center line. The symbol must be made as shown with the following dimensions:

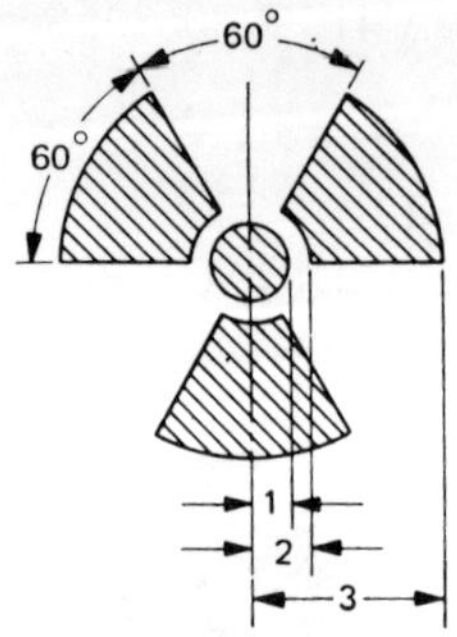

1 = Radius of Circle – 1/2 inch (12.7 mm.)
2 = 1 1/2 Radii
3 = 4 1/2 Radii

(18) The lower white area must have a $^1/_8$-in. (3.2 mm) black solid line border extended from the edge of the yellow area to indicate the outer $^1/_2$-in. (12.7 mm) white placard border. The placard color must be yellow, black, and white.

CORROSIVE placard. The word "CORROSIVE" must be across the center of the placard and made with letters $2^1/_{16}$-in. (52.4 mm) high with a $^{11}/_{32}$-in. (8.7 mm) stroke. The base of the top white triangle must be $1^1/_2$ in. (38.1 mm) above the placard horizontal center line. The lowest part of the symbol must be $1^5/_8$ in. (41.3 mm) above the placard horizontal center line. The height of the symbol measured from a horizontal line extended from the lowest part of the symbol must be $3^1/_4$ in. (82.5 mm) and the width across the widest part must be $7^3/_8$ in. (187.3 mm). The upper white area must have a $^1/_8$-in. (3.2 mm) black solid line border as an extension from the edge of the black area to indicate the outer $^1/_2$-in. (12.7 mm) white placard border. The placard color must be black and white.

APPENDIX C
TITLE 49, PART 173

PART 173—SHIPPERS—GENERAL REQUIREMENTS FOR SHIPMENTS AND PACKAGINGS

SUBPART A—GENERAL

§ 173.1 Purpose and scope

(a) This part defines hazardous materials for transportation purposes and prescribes certain requirements to be observed in preparing them for shipment by air, highway, rail, or water, or any combination thereof.

(b) A shipment that is not prepared for shipment in accordance with this subchapter may not be offered for transportation by air, highway, rail, or water. It is the duty of each person who offers hazardous materials for transportation to instruct each of his officers, agents, and employees having any responsibility for preparing hazardous materials for shipment as to applicable regulations in this subchapter.

(c) When a person other than the person preparing a hazardous material for shipment performs a function required by this part, that person shall perform the function in accordance with this part.

[Amdt. 173-94, 41 FR 16062, Apr. 15, 1976, as amended by Amdt. 173-100, 41 FR 40476, Sept. 20, 1976]

§ 173.2 Classification of a material having more than one hazard as defined in this Part

(a) Except as provided in paragraph (b) of this section, a hazardous material, having more than one hazard as defined in this part must be classed according to the following order of hazards:

(1) Radioactive material.
(2) Poison A.
(3) Flammable gas.
(4) Nonflammable gas.
(5) Flammable liquid.
(6) Oxidizer.
(7) Flammable solid.
(8) Corrosive material (liquid).
(9) Poison B.
(10) Corrosive material (solid).
(11) Irritating materials.
(12) Combustible liquid (in containers having capacities exceeding 110 gal).
(13) ORM-B.
(14) ORM-A.
(15) Combustible liquid (in containers having capacities of 110 gal or less.)

(b) *Exceptions.* Paragraph (a) of this section does not apply to

(1) A material specifically identified in §172.101 of this subchapter;

(2) An explosive required to be classed and approved under § 173.86, or a blasting agent required to be classed and approved under § 173.114a.
(3) An etiologic agent identified in § 173.386 as those materials listed in 42 CFR 72.25(c); or
(4) An organic peroxide. (See § 172.101 and § 173.151a of this subchapter.)

(49 U.S.C. 1803, 1804, 1808; 49 CFR 1.53 and App. A to Part 1)
[Amdt. 173-94, 41 FR 16062, Apr. 15, 1976, as amended by Amdt. 173-94A, 41 FR 40680, Sept. 20, 1976; Amdt. 173-124, 44 FR 31182, May 31, 1979]

§ 173.3 Packaging and exceptions

(a) The packaging of hazardous materials for transportation by air, highway, rail, or water must be as specified in this Part. Methods of manufacture, packing, and storage of hazardous materials, that affect safety in transportation, must be open to inspection by a duly authorized representative of the initial carrier or a representative of the Department. Methods of manufacture and related functions necessary for completion of a DOT specification packaging must be open to inspection by a representative of the Department.

(b) The regulations setting forth packaging requirements for a specific material apply to all modes of transportation unless otherwise stated, or unless exceptions from packaging requirements are authorized. For example, the restriction in § 173.249(b) applicable to cargo-only aircraft applies only to quantities in excess of those allowable under § 173.244. Quantities covered under § 173.244 may also be shipped by cargo-only aircraft.

(c) Packages, other than freight containers, overpacks, portable tanks, cargo tanks and tank cars, that are damaged or leaking and which contain corrosive liquids, corrosive solids, flammable liquids, flammable solids, oxidizers, poison B liquids, poison B solids, or irritating agents may be placed inside a DOT specification drum that is compatible with the lading, provided with adequate closures and, when necessary and appropriate, provided with sufficient cushioning and absorption material to prevent excessive movement of the inner containers and to absorb leaking liquid. Alternatively, a non-DOT specification drum, not exceeding 110-gal capacity, having equal or greater structural integrity than that prescribed in this subchapter for the respective material, may be used as a recovery drum. Either drum is authorized only for the purpose of shipping damaged, or defective packages to a facility for disposal or repackaging.
[Amdt. 173-94, 41 FR 16062, Apr. 15, 1976, as amended by Amdt. 173-94A, 41 FR 40680, Sept. 20, 1976; Amdt. 173-116, 43 FR 17944, Apr. 27, 1978]

§§ 173.4—173.5 [Reserved]

§ 173.6 Shipments by air

(a) *General shipping requirements.* When the regulations indicate a hazardous material is forbidden aboard cargo-only aircraft, the material is also forbidden aboard passenger-carrying aircraft.

(b) *General packaging requirements.*

(1) In addition to the requirements of this part and Parts 175 and 178 of this subchapter, for air shipments each packaging must be designed and constructed to prevent leakage that may be caused by changes in altitude and temperature during air transportation.
(2) Inner containers that are breakable (such as earthenware, glass, or brittle plastic), must be packaged to prevent breakage and leakage under conditions normally incident to transportation. These completed packagings must be capable of withstanding a 4-ft drop on solid concrete in the position most likely to cause damage. Cushioning and absorbent materials must not be capable of reacting dangerously with the contents.

Where any plastic packaging is specified in this part, a plastic bag or pouch is not permitted unless specifically authorized.

(3) For any packaging with a capacity of 110 gal or less containing liquids, sufficient outage (ullage) must be provided to prevent liquid contents from completely filling the packaging at 130°F. The primary packaging (which may include composite packaging), for which retention of the liquid is the basic function, must be capable of withstanding, without leakage, an internal absolute pressure of no less than 26 lb/in.^{2} or no less than the sum of the absolute vapor pressure of the contents at 130°F. (55°C.) and the atmospheric pressure at sea level, whichever is greater.

(4) Stoppers, corks, or other such friction-type closures must be held securely, tightly, and effectively in place with wire, tape, or other positive means. Each screw-type closure on any inside plastic packaging must be secured to prevent the closure from loosening due to vibration or substantial changes in temperature.

(5) Bags permitted by regulations as outside packaging for transportation aboard aircraft must be water resistant.

(6) For any cylinder containing hazardous materials incorporating valves, sufficient protection must be provided to prevent operation and damage to such valves during transportation, by one of the following methods:

(i) By equipping each cylinder with securely attached valve caps or protective headrings, or

(ii) By boxing or crating of the cylinder.

(7) Tank cars and tank motor vehicles containing hazardous materials may not be transported aboard aircraft.

(c) *Special labeling requirements.* see "Magnetized materials" in §§ 172.101 and 173.1020 of this subchapter and see § 172.101 for cargo-only aircraft labeling requirements.
[Amdt. 173-94, 41 FR 16063, Apr. 15, 1976, as amended by Amdt. 173-94B, 41 FR 57068, Dec. 30, 1976]

§ 173.7 U.S. Government material

(a) Shipments of hazardous materials offered by or consigned to the Department of Defense (DOD) of the U.S. Government must be packaged, including limitations of weight, in accordance with the regulations in this subchapter or in containers of equal or greater strength and efficiency as required by DOD regulations. Hazardous materials shipped by DOD under this provision may be reshipped by any shipper to any consignee provided the original packaging has not been damaged or altered in any manner.

(1) Hazardous materials sold by the DOD in packagings that are not marked in accordance with the requirements of this subchapter may be shipped from DOD installations if the DOD certifies in writing that the packagings are equal to or greater in strength and efficiency than the packaging prescribed in this subchapter. The shipper shall obtain such a certification in duplicate for each shipment. He shall give one copy to the originating carrier and retain the other for no less than 1 year.

(b) Shipments of radioactive materials, made by or under the direction or supervision of the U.S. Energy Research and Development Administration or the Department of Defense, and which are escorted by personnel specifically designated by or under the authority of those agencies, for the purpose of national security, are not subject to the regulations in Parts 100—189 of this subchapter.

(c) Shipments of explosive samples, not exceeding 1 g net weight, offered by and consigned to the Bureau of Alcohol, Tobacco and Firearms (ATF) of the Department of the Treasury are not otherwise subject to the relations in Parts 110—189 of this subchapter when placed in a specifically designed multi-unit assembly packed in a strong outside packaging. The packaging must be of a type accepted by ATF as capable of precluding a propagation of any explosion outside the packaging. The second component from the outside of the packaging must be marked or tagged to indicate the presence of an explosive.
(49 U.S.C. 1803, 1804, 1808; 49 CFR 1.53 and App. A to Part 1)
[29 FR 18671, Dec. 29, 1964, as amended by Order 74, 32 FR 5274, Mar. 29, 1967. Redesignated, 32 FR 5606, Apr. 5, 1967]

Note: For amendments to § 173.7 see the List of CFR Sections Affected appearing in the Finding Aids section of this volume.

§ 173.8 Canadian shipments and packagings

(a) Shipments of hazardous materials which conform to the regulations of the Canadian Transport Commission (formerly the Board of Transport Commissioners for Canada), may be transported from the point of entry in the U.S. to their destination in the U.S. or through the U.S. en route to a point in Canada. Empty rail tank cars may be transported in conformity with Canadian Transport Commission regulations from point of origin in the U.S. to point of entry into Canada.

(b) Except as specified in § 173.301(i) specification packagings made and maintained in full compliance with the corresponding specifications prescribed by the Railway Transport Committee of the Canadian Transport Commission (formerly the Board of Transport Commissioners for Canada), in its regulations for the Transportation of Dangerous Commodities by Rail, and marked in accordance therewith (e.g., BTC, CTC, etc.) may be used for the shipment of hazardous materials within the U.S.
[Amdt. 173-11, 34 FR 12589, Aug. 1, 1969, as amended by Amdt. 173-94B, 41 FR 57068, Dec. 30, 1976; Amdt. 173-113, 43 FR 6786, Feb. 16, 1978]

SUBPART B—PREPARATION OF HAZARDOUS MATERIALS FOR TRANSPORTATION

§ 173.21 Prohibited packing

(a) The offering of packages of hazardous materials in the same packaging, freight container, or overpack with other hazardous materials, the mixture of contents of which would be liable to cause a dangerous evolution of heat or gas or produce corrosive materials, is forbidden except as specified in §§ 173.152(a), 173.242(a), (b), and 173.301(a).

(b) The offering for transportation of any package or container of any liquid solid or gaseous material which under conditions incident to transportation may polymerize (combine or react with itself) or decompose so as to cause dangerous evolution of heat or gas is prohibited. Such materials may be offered for transportation when properly stabilized or inhibited. Refrigeration may be used as a means of stabilization only when approved by the Bureau of Explosives.

(c) The offering for transportation of any package or container of any material which will cause a dangerous evolution of heat or gas under conditions normally incident to transportation is forbidden.

(d) The offering for transportation of any package containing a cigarette lighter or other similar ignition device charged with fuel and equipped with an ignition element, or any self-lighting cigarette, is forbidden unless design of the device and its packaging insofar as they affect safety in transportation have been examined by the B or E or another test facility recognized by the MTB and, based on the results of that examination, approved by the Associate Director for OE. (An approval which was issued by the B of E before August

17, 1978, remains valid to the same extent as if it had been issued by MTB.) For lighters containing flammable gases, also see § 173.308.

(49 U.S.C. 1803, 1804, 1808; 49 CFR 1.53 and App. A to Part 1)

[29 FR 18671, Dec. 29, 1964. Redesignated at 32 FR 5606, Apr. 5, 1967]

Note: For amendments to § 173.21 see the List of CFR Sections Affected appearing in the Finding Aids section of this volume.

§ 173.22 SHIPPER'S RESPONSIBILITY

(a) Unless otherwise provided in this part, before offering a hazardous material for shipment in a container the shipper shall determine that the container has been made, assembled with all parts or fittings in their proper place and properly secured, and marked in compliance with applicable specifications prescribed in Parts 178 and 179 of this subchapter or with specifications of the Department in effect at date of manufacture of container. In determining whether a specification container is manufactured in accordance with applicable specifications, the shipper may accept the manufacturer's certification or specification marking. (See §§ 178.0-2 and 179.1 of this subchapter.) For containers supplied by the carrier, the shipper may rely on the manufacturer's identification plate, specification marking, or on certification by the carrier. When a shipper performs a function covered by or having an effect on a specification requirement of Part 178 or Part 179, the shipper must perform that function in accordance with the specification.

(b) Prior to each shipment of fissile radioactive materials, and Type B or large quantities of radioactive materials, the shipper shall notify the consignee of the dates of shipment and of expected arrival. The shipper shall also notify each consignee of any special loading/unloading instructions prior to his first shipment.

[Amdt. 173-3, 33 FR 14921, Oct. 4, 1968; Amdt. 173-14, 34 FR 17523, Oct. 30, 1969; Amdt. 173-94, 41 FR 16063, Apr. 15, 1976; Amdt. 173-100, 42 FR 2689, Jan. 13, 1977]

§ 173.22a Use of packagings authorized under exemptions

(a) Except as provided in paragraph (b) of this section, no person may offer a hazardous material for transportation in a packaging the use of which is dependent upon an exemption issued under Subpart B of Part 107 of this title, unless that person is the holder of or a party to the exemption.

(b) If an exemption authorizes the use of a packaging for the shipment or transportation of a hazardous material by any person or class of persons other than or in addition to the holder of the exemption, that person or a member of that class of persons may use the packaging for the purposes authorized in the exemption subject to the terms specified therein. However, no person may use a packaging under the authority of this paragraph unless he maintains a copy of the exemption at each facility where the packaging is being used in connection with the shipment or transportation of the hazardous material concerned. Copies of exemptions may be obtained from the Office of Hazardous Materials Regulation, U.S. Department of Transportation, Washington, D.C. 20590, Attention: Docket Section

[Amdt. 173-93, 41 FR 3478, Jan. 23, 1976, as amended by Amdt. 173 121, 43 FR 48643, Oct. 19, 1978]

§ 173.23 Previously authorized packaging

(a) Where the regulations require Spec. 6D or 37M (§ 178.102 or § 178.134 of this subchapter) cylindrical steel overpacks, Spec. 5B, 6J, or 37A (single-trip container) (§ 178.82, § 178.100, or § 178.131 of this subchapter) metal drums manufactured before March 18, 1964, having inside Spec. 2S, 2SL, 2T, or 2TL (§ 178.21, § 178.27, § 178.35, or § 178.35a of this subchapter) polyethylene container, may be continued in use for the commodities and gross weights for which they were previously authorized.

(b) Reusable molded polyethylene containers for use without overpack complying with Spec. 34 (§ 178.19 of this subchapter), manufactured before September 5, 1966, may be continued in use, if they are plainly marked "ICC-34," and are embossed with the maker's name or symbol, rated capacity, and the month and year of manufacture.
[Amdt. 173-3, 33 FR 14921, Oct. 4, 1968, as amended by Amdt. 173-90, 39 FR 45240, Dec. 31, 1974; Amdt. 173-94; 41 FR 16063, Apr. 15, 1976]

§ 173.27 Aircraft quantity limitations

(a) The maximum quantity of hazardous material that may be offered for transportation by air in a package that is required for the material by this subchapter may not exceed that quantity prescribed for the material in §172.101 of this subchapter.

(b) When offered for transportation by air, the combined quantity of any one class of materials may not exceed the lowest maximum quantity prescribed in §172.101 of this subchapter for any one of the materials in that class contained in the same package that meets the minimum requirements for the material contained therein.
[Amdt. 173-94, 41 FR 16064, Apr. 15, 1976]

§173.28 Reuse of containers

(a) Containers used more than once (refilled and reshipped after having been previously emptied) must be in such condition, including closure devices and cushioning materials, that they comply in all respects with the prescribed requirements for those containers. Repairs must be made in an efficient manner in accordance with requirements for materials and construction as prescribed in Parts 178 and 179 of this subchapter for new containers, or as otherwise prescribed. Parts that are weak, broken, or otherwise deteriorated must be replaced.

(1) Retest of carboy packages must have been made by or for shippers, or their authorized agents, as required by applicable provisions of the specifications in Part 178 of this subchapter before carboys which are to be offered for transportation are filled.

Note 1: Tests not required by shipper who fills and ships or who reships filled carboys for one shipment only carboy packages which have been properly tested by another shipper or a duly authorized agency.

(b) Markings applied as prescribed by the specifications must be maintained in a legible condition.

(c) If, on account of painting or any other reason, the markings as prescribed for any container cannot be kept plain and legible, a metal plate, brazed or soldered, or otherwise securely fastened to the container, with a reproduction of the prescribed markings plainly stamped thereon, will be permitted.

(d) Containers previously used for the shipment of any hazardous material must have the old markings, including name of contents, addresses, and labels, if any, thoroughly removed or obliterated before being used for the shipment of other articles.

e) Boxes previously used for high explosives containing a liquid explosive ingredient not contained in an inside metal container must not be again used for shipments of any character.

(1) Boxes that have been contaminated by liquid explosive composition must not again be used for shipments of any character.

(f) Kegs previously used for any chlorate must not be again used for shipments of any character.

(g) Metal kegs previously used for black powder not contained in an interior package must not be again used for shipment of any explosive.

Note 1: Because of the present emergency and until further order of the Department, metal kegs, previously used for the shipment of black powder not contained in an interior package, may be used provided the kegs are in good physical condition and are not liable to permit escape of contents during transportation. Empty kegs previously used for shipment of black powder must be entirely free of black powder on the inside and outside before being offered for transportation.

(h) Except as provided in paragraphs (m) and (n) of this section and paragraph (h)(1) of this section, single-trip containers made under specifications prescribed in Part 178 of this subchapter, from which contents have once been removed following use for shipment of any material, must not be used thereafter for shipment of hazardous materials.

(1) Single-trip containers inspected and tested prior to January 1, 1971, that have been approved for reuse by the Bureau of Explosives may be used until July 1, 1971, under the terms and conditions specified.

(i) Containers which are designated as nonreusable containers, marked NRC, and made under specifications prescribed in Part 178 of this subchapter, from which contents have once been removed following use for shipment of any article, must not be again used as shipping containers for explosives, flammable liquids, flammable solids, organic peroxides, oxidizers, corrosive liquids, or poisons, class B or C, as defined in this Part.

(j) Cylinders or other containers which are designated as nonrefillable or for single-trip use under the specifications prescribed in Part 178 of this subchapter, and from which contents have once been removed following use for the shipment of any article, must not be again used as shipping containers for compressed gases.

(k) Containers used for shipments of etching acid liquid, n.o.s. must not be reused for shipment of any commodity.

(l) Cylinders used in anhydrous hydrofluoric acid service must comply with the requirements of §173.264(b)(1) and must not be used in any other service.

(m) Specifications 17C, 17E, and 17H steel drums (§§178.115, 178.116, 178.118 of this subchapter) from which contents have been removed, may be reused as prescribed in this part as packagings for shipment of flammable liquids, flammable solids, organic peroxides, oxidizers, poisons covered by §173.370, radioactive materials, and corrosive liquids covered by §§173.249 and 173.249a, only if the following requirements, in addition to the other requirements of this section, are complied with prior to each reuse:

(1) Each drum must be thoroughly cleaned to remove all residues and foreign matter, inspected for deterioration or defects, and returned to its original shape and contour. All closure devices and parts must be removed (if removable), inspected for defects, and replaced as necessary. Each open head cover gasket must be replaced. Any drum which shows evidence of deterioration (e.g., visible pitting, creases; significant reduction in parent metal thickness from rust, corrosion, or cleaning processes; metal fatigue; or other material defects) or which cannot be returned to its original shape and contour does not qualify for reuse.

(2) The entire surface of each closed-head drum (and after December 31, 1971, each open-head drum, except for its removable head and adjacent chime area) must be tested for leakage by constant internal air pressure. The leakage test must be conducted by submersion under water, by completely covering the surface with soap suds or oil, or by some other method that will be equally sensitive. The air pressure must be maintained for a period of time sufficient to permit a complete inspection for leaks.

The minimum air pressure for the test must be as follows:

Specification No.	Capacity	Minimum test pressure p.s.i.
17C	All	15
17E	Over 12 gal	7
	12 gal or less	5
17H	Over 12 gal	7
	12 gal or less	5

If leaking, the drum does not qualify for reuse.
(3) Marking:

(i) All previous test markings, commodity identification markings, and labels must be removed.
(ii) The outside of each drum qualifying for reuse under this section must be marked on the body within 10 in. of the top head with the following information: ''Tested'' (or ''Inspected'' as appropriate), the month and year of the test (or inspection, if an open-head drum) and the DOT registration number of the reconditioner. For example:

TESTED 2
70
DOT R1001

The registration number required for this marking must be obtained from the Office of Hazardous Materials, Department of Transportation, Washington, D.C. 20590.
(iii) Markings must be in at least $^1/_4$-in. figures and letters on a contrasting background.
(iv) The printed marking of the month and year of test is not required if each is clearly indicated by other means, such as perforations on a decal.

(n) A single-trip packaging (STC) may be reused for the shipment of any corrosive solid, ORM-A, ORM-B, ORM-C, or any material not required by this subchapter to be shipped in a DOT specification packaging and paragraph (m) of this section does not apply to these materials.

(o) Any drum meeting one specification which has been altered to meet another specification must be capable of meeting the new specification in all respects.

(1) Each drum so altered must be inspected, tested, and marked in accordance with paragraph (m) of this section. In addition, the drum must

(i) Bear the specification markings required by the specification under which it was originally manufactured, and
(ii) Bear both the old and the new specification identification in conjunction with the markings required by paragraph (m) of this section with the specification to which the drum is converted shown last, e.g., ''17E/17H''. For example:

17E/17H
TESTED 2
70
DOT R1001

[29 FR 18671, Dec. 29, 1964 Redesignated at 32 FR 5606, Apr. 5, 1967]

Note: For amendments to §173.28 see the List of CFR sections affected in the back of this volume.

§173.29 Empty packagings, portable tanks, cargo tanks, and tank cars

(a) Empty cylinders, barrels, kegs, drums, or other containers, except carboys (see paragraph (b) of this section) previously used for the shipment of any hazardous materials, as defined in this Part, if authorized for reuse must have all openings including removable heads, and filling and vent holes, tightly closed before being offered for transportation. Small quantities of the material with which containers were loaded may remain in "empty" containers. When the vapors remaining therein are unstable, it is permissible to add sufficient inert gas to render the vapors stable. They may be loaded in open or stock cars when desired. Cars should not be placarded but lighted open-flame lanterns or other open-flame lights should be kept away.

(b) Carboys previously used for the shipment of corrosive liquids, when offered to carriers for transportation as "empty" carboys, must have been thoroughly (completely) drained.

(c) Empty bottles, other than carboys previously used for the shipment of corrosive liquids, must be securely stoppered.

(d) Any packaging or accessory which has been used for a shipment of radioactive materials and which contains residual internal radioactive contamination, when shipped as empty, must be securely closed. The external surface must be free of significant removable radioactive contamination as provided in §173.397(a). The radiation at the external surface of the packaging must not exceed 0.5 mrem/hr. The "Empty" label, described in §172.450 of this subchapter, must be affixed to the packaging.

(e) Unless otherwise specifically provided, any empty packaging offered for transportation (see paragraph (a) of this section) bearing labels described in §§172.411 through 172.446 (except §172.450 of this subchapter) must have these labels removed, obliterated, or completely covered. The label described in §172.450 of this subchapter is authorized for the latter purpose. Each packaging which last contained explosives and on which the word "EXPLOSIVES" or the shipping name is printed, stenciled, or otherwise marked or applied, when shipped as empty, must have this marking completely covered or obliterated if shipped in less-than-carload or less-than-truckload lots, or on open-top or flat cars, or on open-top or flat bed motor vehicles or trailers. Covering or obliteration of these labels and markings is not required for carload or truckload shipments made in closed cars or van-type motor vehicles when loaded by the shipper and unloaded by the consignee or their authorized agents.

(f) An empty portable tank, cargo tank, tank car or multi-unit tank car tank may not be offered for transportation unless

(1) Each opening is tightly closed except heater coil inlet and outlet pipes of empty tank cars; and

(2) Except as otherwise specified in this subchapter it is offered for transportation in the same manner as when it previously contained a greater quantity of a hazardous material. This requirement, as well as other provisions in this subchapter, does not apply to any tank that has been cleaned or purged of all hazardous materials residue or when it is reloaded with a material not subject to this subchapter.

[Amdt. 173-94B, 41 FR 57068, Dec. 30, 1976]

§173.30 Loading and unloading of transport vehicles.

A person who loads or unloads hazardous materials into or from a transport vehicle or vessel shall comply with the applicable loading and unloading requirements of Parts 174, 175, 176, and 177 of this subchapter.

[Amdt. 173-94, 41 FR 16064, Apr. 15, 1976]

§173.226 Thorium metal, powdered

Note: Thorium metal, a low specific activity radioactive material, is also subject to the applicable provisions of §§173.389 through 173.399.

(a) Thorium metal, powdered, must be packed in specification containers as follows:

(1) Spec. 15A or 15B (§§178.168 or 178.169 of this subchapter). Wooden boxes with inside metal containers, tightly and securely closed by push-in covers held in place by soldering at least at four points, or in screw-cap type metal cans. Inside containers must not exceed 10 lb net each. Gross weight of outside packages must not exceed 75 lb each.

(b) Limited quantities of thorium metal powder packed in tightly and securely closed metal cans, cushioned with incombustible material in strong outside wooden or fiberboard boxes, and not exceeding 4 oz net weight in one outside packaging, is excepted from labeling (except labeling is required for transportation by air) and the specification packaging requirements of this subchapter. In addition, shipments are not subject to Subpart F of Part 172 of this subchapter, to Part 174 of this subchapter except §174.24 and to Part 177 of this subchapter except §177.817.

[29 FR 18709, Dec. 29, 1964. Redesignated at 32 FR 5606, Apr. 5, 1967]

Note: For amendments to §173.226 see the List of CFR Sections Affected appearing in the Finding Aids section of this volume.

§ 173.386 Etiologic agents; definition and scope

(a) *Definition.* For the purpose of Parts 170—189 of this subchapter:

(1) An ''etiologic agent'' means a viable microorganism, or its toxin, which causes or may cause human disease, and is limited to those agents listed in 42 CFR 72.25(c) of the regulations of the Department of Health, Education, and Welfare.
(2) A ''diagnostic specimen'' means any human or animal material including, but not limited to, excreta, secreta, blood, and its components, tissue, and tissue fluids, being shipped for purposes of diagnosis.
(3) A ''biological product'' means a material prepared and manufactured in accordance with the provisions of 9 CFR Part 102 (Licensed veterinary biological products), 21 CFR Part 601 (Licensing), 21 CFR 312.1 (Conditions for exemption of new drugs for investigational use), 9 CFR Part 103 (Biological products for experimental treatment of animals), or 21 CFR 312.9 (New drugs for investigational use in laboratory research animals or in vitro tests), and which in accordance with these provisions, may be shipped in interstate commerce.

(b) *Applicability.* Except as provided in paragraph (d), no person may ship any material, including a diagnostic specimen or a biological product, containing an etiologic agent unless this material is packaged and prepared for shipment in accordance with § 173.24 and the other applicable regulations of this subchapter.

(c) *General provisions.* The requirements of these regulations (Parts 170—189 of this subchapter) supplement the requirements of the Department of Health, Education, and Welfare's regulations contained in 42 CFR 72.25.

(d) *Exceptions.* The following substances are not subject to any requirements of this subchapter if the items as packaged do not contain any material otherwise subject to the requirements of Parts 170—189 of this subchapter:

(1) Diagnostic specimens; and
(2) Biological products.

(3) Cultures of etiologic agents of 50 mℓ (1.666 fluid oz) or less total quantity in one outside package.

[Amdt. 173-67, 37 FR 20555, Sept. 30, 1972, as amended by Amdt. 173-72, 38 FR 8162, Mar. 29, 1973, Amdt. 173-94B, 41 FR 57070, Dec. 30, 1976; Amdt. 173-121, 43 FR 48644, Oct. 19, 1978]

§ 173.387 Packaging requirements for etiologic agents

(a) Except as provided in § 173.386(d) no person may ship a package containing over 4ℓ gross volume of an etiologic agent.

(b) In addition to the requirements of 42 CFR 72.25(c), each package containing an etiologic agent must be designed and constructed so that, if it were subject to the environment and test conditions prescribed in this section, there would be no release of the contents to the environment, and the effectiveness of the packaging would not be significantly reduced.

(1) *Environmental conditions.*
- (i) Heat — direct sunlight in an ambient temperature of 130°F in still air.
- (ii) Cold — an ambient temperature of −40°F in still air and shade.
- (iii) Reduced pressure — ambient atmospheric pressure of 0.50 atm (7.3 p.s.i.a.).
- (iv) Vibration — vibration normally incident in the mode of transportation the package is to be shipped.

(2) *Test conditions.*
- (i) Water spray — a water spray heavy enough to keep the entire exposed surface of the package (except the bottom) continuously wet during a period of 30 min. Packages for which the outer layer consists of metal, wood, ceramic, or plastic, or combination thereof, are exempt from this test.
- (ii) Freedrop — a freedrop through a distance of 30 ft onto a flat, essentially unyielding horizontal target surface, the package striking the surface in a position for which maximum damage is expected.
- (iii) Penetration — impact of the hemispheric end of a steel cylinder 1.25 in. in diameter and weighing 15 lb dropped from a height of 40 in. on to the exposed surface of the package expected to be most vulnerable to puncture. The long axis of the cylinder must be perpendicular to the impacted surface. This test is not required for a package subject to paragraph (b)(2)(iv) of this section.
- (iv) Penetration (required for packages exceeding 15 lb gross weight only) — a freedrop of the package through a distance of 40 in. striking the top end of a vertical cylindrical mild steel solid bar on an essentially unyielding surface, in a position for which maximum damage is expected. The bar must be 1.5 in. in diameter. The top of the bar must be horizontal, with its edge rounded to a radius not exceeding $^1/_4$ in. The bar must be of such length as to cause maximum damage to the package, but not less than 8 in. long. The long axis of the bar must be vertical to the unyielding horizontal impact surface of the package.

(3) *Testing procedure.*
- (i) At least one sample of each type package (maximum size and gross weight), filled with water, must be subjected to the water spray test unless exempted by paragraph (b)(2)(i) of this section.
- (ii) This sample package then must be given the freedrop and one of the penetration tests, as applicable. Separate wetted sample packages may be used for the freedrop and the penetration test.
- (iii) If the sample package is exempted from the water spray test by paragraph (b)(2)(i) of

this section, at least one sample of each type package (maximum size and gross weight), filled with water, must be subjected consecutively to the freedrop and the penetration test.

[Amdt. 173-67, 37 FR 20556, Sept. 30, 1972]

§ 173.388 Labeling of packages containing etiologic agents

(a) Each package containing an etiologic agent, except a diagnostic specimen or a biological product, must be labeled as prescribed by the regulations of the Department of Health, Education, and Welfare, 42 CFR 72.25(c)(4). For information, this label is required to be a rectangle measuring 51 mm (2 in.) high and 102.5 mm (4 in.) long, predominantly red printing on a white background, and appears as follows:

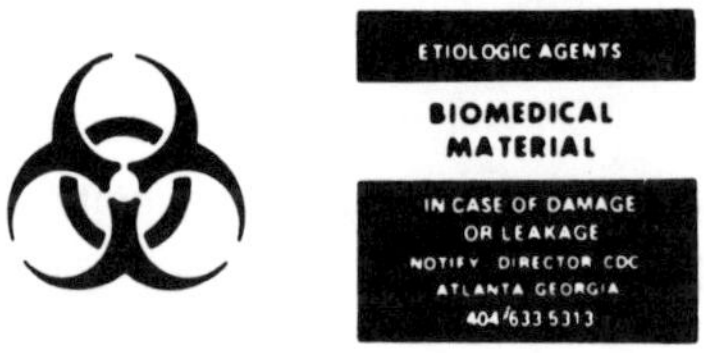

[Amdt. 173-67, 37 FR 20556, Sept. 30, 1972]

§ 173.389 Radioactive materials; definitions

For the purpose of Parts 170—189 of this subchapter:

(a) "Fissile radioactive material" means the following material: Plutonium-238, plutonium-239, plutonium-241, uranium-233, or uranium-235, or any material containing any of the foregoing materials. See § 173.396(a) for exclusions. Fissile radioactive material packages are classified according to the controls needed to provide nuclear criticality safety during transportation as follows:

(1) *Fissile Class I.* Packages which may be transported in unlimited numbers and in any arrangement, and which require no nuclear criticality safety controls during transportation. For purposes of nuclear criticality safety control, a transport index is not assigned to Fissile Class I packages. However, the external radiation levels may require a transport index number.

(2) *Fissile Class II.* Packages which may be transported together in any arrangement but in numbers which do not exceed an aggregate transport index of 50. For purposes of nuclear criticality safety control, individual packages may have a transport index of not less than 0.1 and not more than 10. However, the external radiation levels may require a higher transport index number but not to exceed 10. Such shipments require no nuclear criticality safety control by the shipper during transportation.

(3) *Fissile Class III.* Shipments of packages which do not meet the requirements of Fissile Class I or II and which are controlled to provide nuclear criticality safety in transportation by special arrangements between the shipper and the carrier.

Note 1: Uranium-235 exists only in combination with various percentages of uranium-234 and uranium-238. "Fissile radioactive material" as applied to uranium-235 refers to the amount of uranium-235 actually contained in the total quantity of uranium being transported.

Note 2: Radioactive material may consist of mixtures of fissile and nonfissile radionuclides.

''Fissile radioactive material'' refers to the amount of plutonium-238, plutonium-239, plutonium-241, uranium-233, uranium-235, or any combination thereof actually contained in the mixture. The ''radioactivity'' of the mixture consists of the total activity of both the fissile and nonfissile radionuclides. All mixtures containing ''fissile material'' shall be subject to § 173.396.

(b) ''Large quantity radioactive materials'' means a quantity the aggregate radioactivity of which exceeds that specified as follows:

(1) Groups I or II (see paragraph (h) of this section) radionuclides: 20 Ci.
(2) Groups III or IV radionuclides: 200 Ci.
(3) Group V radionuclides: 5000 Ci.
(4) Groups VI or VII radionuclides: 50,000 Ci.
(5) Special form material: 5000 Ci.

(c) ''Low specific activity material'' means any of the following:

(1) Uranium or thorium ores and physical or chemical concentrates of those ores;
(2) Unirradiated natural or depleted uranium or unirradiated natural thorium;
(3) Tritium oxide in aqueous solutions provided the concentration does not exceed 5 mCi/mℓ;
(4) Material in which the activity is essentially uniformly distributed and in which the estimated average concentration per gram of contents does not exceed:

   (i) 0.0001 mCi of Group I (see § 173.389(h) radionuclides; or
   (ii) 0.005 mCi of Group II radionuclides; or
   (iii) 0.3 mCi of Groups III or IV radionuclides.

Note: This includes, but is not limited to, materials of low radioactivity concentration such as residues or solutions from chemical processing; wastes such as building rubble, metal, wood, and fabric scrap, glassware, paper and cardboard; solid or liquid plant waste, sludges, and ashes.

(5) Objects of nonradioactive material externally contaminated with radioactive material, provided that the radioactive material is not readily dispersible and the surface contamination when averaged over an area of 1 m^2 does not exceed 0.0001 mCi (220,000 disintegrations per minute) per square centimeter of Group I radionuclides or 0.001 mCi (2,200,000 disintegrations per minute) per square centimeter of other radionuclides.

(d) ''Normal form radioactive materials'' means those which are not special form radioactive materials. Normal form radioactive materials are grouped into transport groups (see paragraph (h) of this section).

(e) ''Radioactive material'' means any material or combination of materials, which spontaneously emits ionizing radiation. Materials in which the estimated specific activity is not greater than 0.002 μCi/g of material, and in which the radioactivity is essentially uniformly distributed, are not considered to be radioactive materials.

(f) ''Removable radioactive contamination'' means radioactive contamination which can be readily removed in measurable quantities by wiping the contaminated surface with an absorbent material. The measurable quantities shall be considered as being not significant if they do not exceed the limits specified in § 173.397

(g) ''Special form radioactive materials'' means those which, if released from a package, might present some direct radiation hazard but would present little hazard due to radiotoxicity and little possibility of contamination. This may be the result of inherent properties of the material (such as metals or alloys), or acquired characteristics, as through encapsulation. The criteria for determining whether a material meets the definition of special form are prescribed in § 173.398(a).

(h) ''Transport group'' means any one of seven groups into which normal form radionuclides are classified according to their radiotoxicity and their relative potential hazard in transportation and as listed in §173.390.

(i) ''Transport index'' means the number placed on a package to designate the degree of control to be exercised by the carrier during transportation. The transport index to be assigned to a package of radioactive materials shall be determined by either paragraph (i)(1) or (2) of this section, whichever is larger. The number expressing the transport index shall be rounded up to the next highest tenth; e.g., 1.01 becomes 1.1.

(1) The highest radiation dose rate, in millirem per hour at three feet from any accessible external surface of the package; or

(2) For Fissile Class II packages only the transport index number calculated by dividing the number ''50'' by the number of similar packages which may be transported together (see § 173.396), as determined by the procedures prescribed in the regulations of the U.S. Nuclear Regulatory Commission, Title 10, Code of Federal Regulations, Part 71.

(j) ''Type A packaging'' means packaging which is designed in accordance with the general packaging requirements of §§ 173.24 and 173.393, and which is adequate to prevent the loss or dispersal of the radioactive contents and to retain the efficiency of its radiation shielding properties if the package is subject to the tests prescribed in § 173.398(b).

(k) ''Type B packaging'' means packaging which meets the standards for Type A packaging, and, in addition, meets the standards for hypothetical accident conditions of transportation as prescribed in § 173.398(c).

(l) ''Type A quantity'' and ''Type B quantity'' radioactive materials means a quantity the aggregate radioactivity of which does not exceed that specified as follows:

Transport group (see § 173.389(h))	**Type A quantity (in curies)**	**Type B quantity (in curies)**
I	0.001	20
II	0.05	20
III	3	200
IV	20	200
V	20	5,000
VI and VII	1,000	50,000
Special form	20[a]	5,000

[a] Except that for Californium-252 the Type A quantity limit for special form is 2 Ci.

(m) *Containment system.* Containment system of a radioactive materials package means those components of the packaging including special form encapsulation where used, which have been specified by the package designer as intended to retain the radioactive contents during transport, whether or not individual vessels in the packaging retain their integrity of containment.

(n) *Maximum normal operating pressure.* Maximum normal operating pressure means the maximum pressure above atmospheric pressure at mean sea level that would develop in the containment system in a period of 1 year, under the conditions of temperature and solar radiation corresponding to environmental conditions of transport in the absence of venting, external cooling by an ancillary system, or operational controls during transport.

(o) "Exclusive Use" (also referred to as "sole use" or "Full Load" as used in IAEA regulations) means any shipment:

(1) From a single consignor having the exclusive use of a transport vehicle or of an aircraft, or of a hold or compartment of an inland watercraft, or of a hold, compartment, or defined deck area of a seagoing vessel; and
(2) For which all initial, intermediate, and final loading and unloading is carried out by or under the direction of the consignor, consignee, or his designated agent.

(p) "Radioactive Device" means any manufactured article such as an instrument, clock, electronic tube or apparatus, or similar device having radioactive material (other than liquid) in a nondispersible form as a component part.

(q) "Closed transport vehicle" means a vehicle equipped with a securely attached exterior enclosure, which during normal transport, restricts the access of unauthorized persons to the cargo space containing the radioactive materials. The enclosure may be either temporary or permanent, may be of the "see-through" type, and must limit access from top, sides, and ends.

[Amdt. 173-3, 33 FR 14922, Oct. 4, 1968; 33 FR 19823, Dec. 27, 1968, as amended by Amdt. 173-64, 37 FR 14588, July 21, 1972]

Note: For amendments to § 173.389 see the List of CFR Sections Affected appearing in the Finding Aids section of this volume.

§ 173.390 Transport groups of radio-nuclides

(a) List of radionuclides:

		Transport group						
Element[a]	**Radionuclide**[c]	**I**	**II**	**III**	**IV**	**V**	**VI**	**VII**
Actinium (89)	Ac-227	X						
	Ac-228	X						
Americium (95)	Am-241	X						
	Am-243	X						
Antimony (51)	Sb-122				X			
	Sb-124			X				
	Sb-125			X				
Argon (18)	Ar-37						X	
	Ar-41		X					
	Ar-41 (uncompressed)[b]					X		
Arsenic (33)	As-73				X			
	As-74				X			
	As-76				X			
	As-77				X			
Astatine (85)	At-211			X				
Barium (56)	Ba-131				X			
	Ba-133		X					
	Ba-140			X				
Berkelium (97)	Bk-249	X						
Berylium (4)	Be-7				X			
Bismuth (83)	Bi-206				X			
	Bi-207			X				
	Bi-210		X					
	Bi-212			X				

		Transport group						
Element[a]	**Radionuclide[c]**	**I**	**II**	**III**	**IV**	**V**	**VI**	**VII**
Bromine (35)	Br-82				X			
Cadmium (48)	Cd-109				X			
	Cd-115m			X				
	Cd-115				X			
Calcium (20)	Ca-45				X			
	Ca-47				X			
Californium (98)	Cf-249	X						
	Cf-250	X						
	Cf-252	X						
Carbon (6)	C-14				X			
Cerium (58)	Ce-141				X			
	Ce-143				X			
	Ce-144			X				
Cesium (55)	Cs-131				X			
	Cs-134m			X				
	Cs-134			X				
	Cs-135				X			
	Cs-136				X			
	Cs-137			X				
Chlorine (17)	Cl-36			X				
	Cl-38				X			
Chromium (24)	Cr-51				X			
Cobalt (27)	Co-56			X				
	Co-57				X			
	Co-58m				X			
	Co-58				X			
	Co-60			X				
Copper (29)	Cu-64				X			
Curium (96)	Cm-242	X						
	Cm-243	X						
	Cm-244	X						
	Cm-245	X						
	Cm-246	X						
Dysporsium (66)	Dy-154			X				
	Dy-165				X			
	Dy-166				X			
Erbium (68)	Er-169				X			
	Er-171				X			
Europium (63)	Eu-150			X				
	Eu-152m				X			
	Eu-152			X				
	Eu-154		X					
	Eu-155				X			
Fluorine (9)	F-18				X			
Gadolinium (64)	Gd-153				X			
	Gd-159				X			
Gallium (31)	Ga-67			X				
	Ga-72				X			
Germanium (32)	Ge-71				X			
Gold (79)	Au-193			X				
	Au-194			X				
	Au-195			X				
	Au-196				X			
	Au-198				X			
	Au-199				X			
Hafnium (72)	Hf-181				X			
Holmium (67)	Ho-166				X			
Hydrogen (1)	H-3 (see tritium)							

Element[a]	Radionuclide[c]	Transport group						
		I	II	III	IV	V	VI	VII
Indium (49)	In-113m				X			
	In-114m			X				
	In-115m				X			
	In-115				X			
Iodine (53)	I-124			X				
	I-125			X				
	I-126			X				
	I-129			X				
	I-131			X				
	I-132				X			
	I-133			X				
	I-134				X			
	I-135				X			
Iridium (77)	Ir-190				X			
	Ir-192			X				
	Ir-194				X			
Iron (26)	Fe-55				X			
	Fe-59				X			
Krypton (36)	Kr-85m			X				
	Kr-85m (uncompressed)[b]					X		
	Kr-85			X				
	Kr-85 (uncompressed)[b]						X	
	Kr-87		X					
	Kr-87 (uncompressed)[b]					X		
Lanthanum (57)	La-140				X			
Lead (82)	Pb-203				X			
	Pb-210		X					
	Pb-212		X					
Lutecium (71)	Lu-172			X				
	Lu-177				X			
	Lu-177							
Magnesium (12)	Mg-28			X				
Manganese (25)	Mn-52				X			
	Mn-54				X			
	Mn-56				X			
Mercury (80)	Hg-197m				X			
	Hg-197				X			
	Hg-203				X			
Mixed Fission Products	MF-P		X					
Molybdenum (42)	Mo-99				X			
Neodymium (60)	Nd-147				X			
	Nd-149				X			
Neptunium (93)	Np-237	X						
	Np-239	X						
Nickel (28)	Ni-56			X				
	Ni-59				X			
	Ni-63				X			
	Ni-65				X			
Niobium (41)	Nb-93m				X			
	Nb-95				X			
	Nb-97				X			
Osmium (76)	Os-185				X			
	Os-191m				X			
	Os-191				X			
	Os-193				X			
Palladium (46)	Pd-103				X			
	Pd-109				X			
Phosphorus (15)	P-32				X			

Element[a]	Radionuclide[c]	Transport group I	II	III	IV	V	VI	VII
Platinum (78)	Pt-191					X		
	Pt-193					X		
	Pt-193m					X		
	Pt-197m					X		
	Pt-197					X		
Plutonium (94)	Pu-238[d]		X					
	Pu-239[d]		X					
	Pu-240		X					
	Pu-241[d]		X					
	Pu-242		X					
Polonium (84)	Po-210		X					
Potassium (19)	K-42					X		
	K-43				X			
Praseodymium (59)	Pr-142					X		
	Pr-143					X		
Promethium (61)	Pm-147					X		
	Pm-149					X		
Protactinium (91)	Pa-230		X					
	Pa-231		X					
	Pa-233			X				
Radium (88)	Ra-223			X				
	Ra-224			X				
	Ra-226		X					
	Ra-228		X					
Radon (86)	Rn-220					X		
	Rn-222			X				
Rhenium (75)	Re-183					X		
	Re-186					X		
	Re-187					X		
	Re-188					X		
	Re Natural					X		
Rhodium (45)	Rh-103m					X		
	Rh-105					X		
Rubidium (37)	Rb-86					X		
	Rb-87					X		
	Rb Natural					X		
Ruthenium (44)	Ru-97					X		
	Ru-103					X		
	Ru-105					X		
	Ru-106				X			
Samarium (62)	Sm-145				X			
	Sm-147				X			
	Sm-151					X		
	Sm-153					X		
Scandium (21)	Sc-46				X			
	Sc-47					X		
	Sc-48					X		
Selenium (34)	Se-75					X		
Silicon (14)	Si-31					X		
Silver (47)	Ag-105					X		
	Ag-110m				X			
	Ag-111					X		
Sodium (11)	Na-22				X			
	Na-24					X		

Element[a]	Radionuclide[c]	Transport group I	II	III	IV	V	VI	VII
Strontium (38)	Sr-85m				X			
	Sr-85				X			
	Sr-89			X				
	Sr-90		X					
	Sr-91			X				
	Sr-92				X			
Sulphur (16)	S-35				X			
Tantalum (73)	Ta-182			X				
Technetium (43)	Tc-96m				X			
	Tc-96				X			
	Tc-97m				X			
	Tc-97				X			
	Tc-99m				X			
	Tc-99				X			
					X			
Tellirium (52)	Te-125m				X			
	Te-127m				X			
	Te-127				X			
	Te-129m			X				
	Te-129				X			
	Te-131m			X				
	Te-132				X			
Terbium (65)	Tb-160			X				
Thallium (81)	Tl-200				X			
	Tl-201				X			
	Tl-202				X			
	Tl-204			X				
Thorium (90)	Th-227		X					
	Th-228	X						
	Th-230	X						
	Th-231	X						
	Th-232			X				
	Th-234		X					
	Th Natural			X				
Thulium (69)	Tm-168			X				
	Tm-170			X				
	Tm-171				X			
Tin (50)	Sn-113				X			
	Sn-117m			X				
	Sn-121			X				
	Sn-125				X			
Tritium (1)	H-3				X			
	H-3 (as a gas, as luminous paint, or absorbed on solid material)							X
Tungsten (74)	W-181				X			
	W-185				X			
	W-187				X			
Uranium (92)	U-230		X					
	U-232	X						
	U-233[d]		X					
	U-234		X					
	U-235[d]			X				
	U-236		X					
	U-238			X				
	U Natural			X				
	U Enriched[d]			X				
	U Depleted			X				

Element[a]	Radionuclide[c]	Transport group I	II	III	IV	V	VI	VII
Vanadium (23)	V-48				X			
	V-49			X				
Xenon (54)	Xe-125			X				
	Xe-131m			X				
	Xe-131m (uncompressed)[b]					X		
	Xe-133			X				
	Xe-133 (uncompressed)[b]						X	
	Xe-135		X					
	Xe-135 (uncompressed)[b]					X		
Ytterbium (70)	Yb-175				X			
Yttrium (39)	Y-88			X				
	Y-90				X			
	Y-91m			X				
	Y-91			X				
	Y-92				X			
	Y-93				X			
Zinc (30)	Zn-65				X			
	Zn-69m				X			
	Zn-69				X			
Zirconium (40)	Zr-93				X			
	Zr-95			X				
	Zr-97				X			

[a] Atomic number shown in parentheses.
[b] Uncompressed means at a pressure not exceeding 14.7 p.s.i. (absolute).
[c] Atomic weight shown after the radionuclide symbol.
[d] Fissile radioactive material.

(b) Any radionuclide not listed in the above table shall be assigned to one of the groups in accordance with the following table:

Radionuclide	Radioactive half-life: 0—1000 days	1000 days to 10^6 years	Over 10^6 years
Atomic number 1—81	Group III	Group II	Group III
Atomic number 82 and over	Group I	Group I	Do

Note 1: No unlisted radionuclides shall be assigned to Groups IV, V, VI, or VII.

(c) For mixtures of radionuclides the following shall apply:

(1) If the identity and respective activity of each radionuclide are known, the permissible activity of each radionuclide shall be such that the sum, for all groups present, of the ratio between the total activity for each group to the permissible activity for each group will not be greater than unity.
(2) If the groups of the radionuclides are known but the amount in each group cannot be reasonably determined, the mixture shall be assigned to the most restrictive group present.
(3) If the identity of all or some of the radionuclides cannot be reasonably determined, each of those unidentified radionuclides shall be considered as belonging to the most restrictive group which cannot be positively excluded.
(4) Mixtures consisting of a single radioactive decay chain where the radionuclides are in

the naturally occurring proportions shall be considered as consisting of a single radionuclide. The group and activity shall be that of the first member present in the chain, except if a radionuclide ''x'' has a half-life longer than that of that first member and an activity greater than that of any other member including the first at any time during transportation; in that case, the transport group of the nuclide ''x'' and the activity of the mixture shall be the maximum activity of that nuclide ''x'' during transportation.

[Amdt. 173-3, 33 FR 14923, Oct. 4, 1968]

§ 173.391 Limited quantities of radioactive materials and radioactive devices

(a) Limited quantities of radioactive materials in normal form not exceeding 0.01 mCi of Group I radionuclides; 0.1 mCi of Group II radionuclides; 1 mCi of Groups III, IV, V, or VI radionuclides; 25 Ci of Group VII radionuclides; tritium oxide in aqueous solution with a concentration not exceeding 0.5 mCi/mℓ and with a total activity per package of not more than 3 Ci; or 1 mCi of radioactive material in special form; and not containing more than 15 g of uranium-235 are excepted from specification packaging, marking, and labeling, and are excepted from the provisions of § 173.393, if the following conditions are met:

(1) The materials are packaged in strong tight packages such that there will be no leakage of radioactive materials under conditions normally incident to transportation.

(2) The package must be such that the radiation dose rate at any point on the external surface of the package does not exceed 0.5 mrem/hr.

(3) There must be no significant removable radioactive surface contamination on the exterior of the package (see § 173.397).

(4) The outside of the inner container must bear the marking ''Radioactive.''

(b) Manufactured articles such as instruments, clocks, electronic tubes or apparatus, or other similar devices, having limited quantities of radioactive materials (other than liquids) in a nondispersible form as a component part, are excepted from specification packaging, marking, and labeling, and are excepted from the provisions of § 173.393, if the following conditions are met:

Note 1: For radioactive gases, the requirement for the radioactive material to be in a nondispersible form does not apply.

(1) Radioactive materials are securely contained within the devices, or are securely packaged in strong, tight packages, so that there will be no leakage of radioactive materials under conditions normally incident to transportation.

(2) The radiation dose rate at 4 in. from any unpackaged device does not exceed 10 mrem/hr.

(3) The radiation dose rate at any point on the external surface of the outside of the package may not exceed 0.5 mrem/hr. However, for exclusive use shipments only, the radiation at the external surface of the package or the item may exceed 0.5 mrem/hr, but must not exceed 2 mrem/hr.

(4) There must be no significant removable radioactive surface contamination on the exterior of the package (see § 173.397).

(5) The total radioactivity content of a package containing radioactive devices must not exceed the quantities shown in the following table:

Transport group	Quantity in curies: Per device	Per package
I	0.0001	0.001
II	0.001	0.05
III	0.01	3
IV	0.05	3
V or VI	1	1
VII	25	200
Special form	0.05	20

(6) No package may contain more than 15 g of fissile material.

(c) A manufactured article, other than a reactor fuel element, in which the only radioactive material is metallic natural or depleted uranium or natural thorium or alloys thereof, is excepted from specification packaging, marking, and labeling, and is excepted from the provisions of § 173.393, if the following conditions are met:

(1) The radiation dose rate at any point on the external surface of the outside container does not exceed 0.5 mrem/hr.
(2) There must be no significant radioactive surface contamination on the exterior of the package. To determine whether "significant," the standard in § 173.397 must be used.
(3) The total radioactivity content of each article must not exceed 3 Ci.
(4) The outer surface of the uranium or thorium is enclosed in a nonradioactive, sealed, metallic sheath.

Note: Such articles may be packagings for the transportation of radioactive materials.

(d) Shipments made under this section for transportation are not subject to Subpart F of Part 172 of this subchapter, to Part 174 of this subchapter except § 174.24 and to Part 177 of this subchapter except § 177.817.

[Amdt. 173-3, 33 FR 14925, Oct. 4, 1968, as amended by Amdt. 173-90, 39 FR 45241, Dec. 31, 1974; Amdt. 173-94, 41 FR 16086, Apr. 15, 1976; Amdt. 173-94A, 41 FR 40684, Sept. 20, 1976]

§ 173.392 Low specific activity radioactive material

(a) Low specific activity (LSA) radioactive materials, other than materials consigned as exclusive use, are exempt from the provisions of § 173.393(a) through (e) and (g). However, they must be packaged in accordance with the requirements of § 173.395 and must be marked and labeled as required in §§ 172.300 and 172.400 of this subchapter.

(b) LSA radioactive materials which are transported in a transport vehicle (except aircraft) and consigned as exclusive use are exempt from specification packaging, marking, and labeling, provided the shipment meets the requirements of paragraph (c) or (d) of this section.

(c) Packaged shipments of low specific activity materials transported in transport vehicles (except aircraft) assigned for the sole use of that consignor must comply with the following:

(1) Materials must be packaged in strong, tight packages so that there will be no leakage of radioactive material under conditions normally incident to transportation.
(2) Packages must not have any significant removable surface contamination (see § 173.397).
(3) External radiation levels must comply with § 173.393(j).
(4) Shipments must be loaded by consignor and unloaded by consignee from the transport vehicle in which originally loaded.

(5) There must be no loose radioactive material in the car or vehicle.
(6) Shipment must be braced so as to prevent leakage or shift of lading under conditions normally incident to transportation.
(7) Except for shipments of uranium or thorium ores, unconcentrated, the transport vehicle must be placarded with the placards prescribed in accordance with § 172.500 of this subchapter, as appropriate.
(8) The outside of each outside package must be stencilled or otherwise marked "Radioactive—LSA."
(9) Specific instructions for maintenance of exclusive use (sole use) shipment controls must be provided by the shipper to the carrier. Such instructions must be included with the shipping paper information.

(d) Unpackaged (bulk) shipments of low specific activity materials transported in closed transport vehicles (except aircraft) assigned for the sole use of that consignor must comply with the following:

(1) Authorized materials are limited to the following:

(i) Uranium or thorium ores and physical or chemical concentrates of those ores.
(ii) Uranium metal or natural thorium metal, or alloys of these materials; or
(iii) Materials of low radioactive concentration, if the average estimated radioactivity concentration does not exceed 0.001 mCi/g and the contribution from Group I material does not exceed 1% of the total radioactivity.
(iv) Objects of nonradioactive material externally contaminated with radioactive material, if the radioactive material is not readily dispersible and the surface contamination, when averaged over 1 m^2, does not exceed 0.0001 mCi/cm^2 of Group I radionuclides or 0.001 mCi/cm^2 of other radionuclides. Such objects must be suitably wrapped or enclosed.

(2) Bulk liquids must be transported in the following:

(i) Specification 103CW, 111A60W7 (§§ 179.200, 179.201, 179.202 of this subchapter) tank cars. Bottom openings in tanks prohibited.
(ii) Spec. MC 310, MC 311, MC 312, or MC 331 (§ 178.330, § 178.331, § 178.337, or § 178.343 of this subchapter) cargo tanks. Authorized only where the radioactivity concentration does not exceed 10% of the specified low specific activity levels (see § 173.389(c)). The requirements of § 173.393(g) do not apply to these cargo tanks. Bottom fittings and valves are not authorized. Trailer-on-flatcar service is not authorized.

(3) External radiation levels must comply with paragraphs (2), (3), and (4) of § 173.393(j).
(4) Shipments must be loaded by the consignor, and unloaded by the consignee from the transport vehicles in which originally loaded.
(5) Except for shipments of uranium or thorium ores, unconcentrated, the transport vehicle must be placarded with the placards prescribed in accordance with § 172.500 of this subchapter, as appropriate.
(6) There must be no leakage of radioactive materials from the vehicle.
(7) Specific instructions for maintenance of exclusive use (sole use) shipment controls must be provided by the shipper to the carrier. Such instructions must be included with the shipping paper information.

[Amdt. 173-3, 33 FR 14925, Oct. 4, 1968; 33 FR 19823, Dec. 27, 1968]

Note: For amendments to § 173.392 see the List of CFR Sections Affected appearing in the Finding Aids section of this volume.

§ 173.393 General packaging and shipment requirements

(a) Unless otherwise specified, all shipments of radioactive materials must meet all requirements of this section, and must be packaged as prescribed in §§ 173.391 through 173.396.

(b) The outside of each package must incorporate a feature such as a seal, which is not readily breakable and which, while intact, will be evidence that the package has not been illicitly opened.

(c) The smallest outside dimension of any package must be 4 in. or greater.

(d) Each radioactive material must be packaged in a packaging which has been designed to maintain shielding efficiency and leak tightness, so that, under conditions normally incident to transportation, there will be no release of radioactive material. If necessary, additional suitable inside packaging must be used. Each package must be capable of meeting the standards in §§ 173.398(b) and 173.24.

(1) Internal bracing or cushioning, where used, must be adequate to assure that, under the conditions normally incident to transportation, the distance from the inner container or radioactive material to the outside wall of the package remains within the limits for which the package design was based, and the radiation dose rate external to the package does not exceed the transport index number shown on the label. Inner shield closures must be positively secured to prevent loss of the contents.

(e) The packaging must be designed, constructed, and loaded so that during transport:

(1) The heat generated within the package because of the radioactive materials present will not, at any time during transportation, affect the efficiency of the package under the conditions normally incident to transportation, and
(2) The temperature of the accessible external surfaces of the package will not exceed 122°F. in the shade when fully loaded, assuming still air at ambient temperature. If the package is transported in a transport vehicle consigned for the sole use of the consignor, the maximum accessible external surface temperature shall be 180° F.

(f) Pyrophoric materials, in addition to the packaging prescribed in this subpart, must also meet the packaging requirements of § 173.134 or § 173.154. Pyrophoric radioactive liquids may not be shipped by air.

(g) Liquid radioactive material in Type A quantities must be packaged in or within a leak-resistant and corrosion-resistant inner containment vessel. In addition:

(1) The packaging must be adequate to prevent loss or dispersal of the radioactive contents from the inner containment vessel if the package were subjected to the 9 m (30-ft) drop test prescribed in § 173.398(c)(2)(i); and either
(2) Enough absorbent material must be provided to absorb at least twice the volume of radioactive liquid contents. The absorbent material may be located outside the radiation shield only if it can be shown that if the radioactive liquid contents were taken up by the absorbent material the resultant dose rate at the surface of the package would not exceed 1000 mrem/hr; or
(3) A secondary leak-resistant and corrosion-resistant containment vessel must be provided to retain the radioactive contents under the normal conditions of transport as prescribed in § 173.398(b), assuming the failure of the inner primary containment vessel.

(h) There must be no significant removable radioactive surface contamination on the exterior of the package (see § 173.397).

(i) Except for shipments described in paragraph (j) of this section, all radioactive materials must be packaged in suitable packaging (shielded, if necessary) so that at any time during the normal conditions incident to transportation the radiation dose rate does not exceed 200 mrem/hr at any point on the external surface of the package, and the transport index does not exceed 10.

(j) Packages for which the radiation dose rate exceeds the limits specified in paragraph (i) of this section, but does not exceed at any time during transportation any of the limits specified in paragraphs (j) (1) through (4) of this section may be transported in a transport vehicle which has been consigned as exclusive use (except aircraft). Specific instructions for maintenance of the exclusive use (sole use) shipment controls must be provided by the shipper to the carrier. Such instructions must be included with the shipping paper information:

(1) 1000 mrem/hr at 3 ft from the external surface of the package (closed transport vehicle only);
(2) 200 mrem/hr at any point on the external surface of the car or vehicle (closed transport vehicle only);
(3) 10 mrem/hr at any point 2 m (six ft) from the vertical planes projected by the outer lateral surface of the car or vehicle; or if the load is transported in an open transport vehicle, at any point 2 m (six ft) from the vertical planes projected from the outer edges of the vehicle.
(4) 2 mrem/hr in any normally occupied position in the car or vehicle, except that this provision does not apply to private motor carriers.

(k) [Reserved]

(l) Packages consigned for export are also subject to the regulations of the foreign governments involved in the shipment. See §§ 173.8, 173.9, and 173.393b. (The regulations of the International Atomic Energy Agency (IAEA) are used by most foreign governments.)

(m) Prior to the first shipment of any package, the shipper shall determine by examination or appropriate test that:

(1) The packaging meets the specified quality of design and construction; and
(2) The effectiveness of the shielding and containment, and, where necessary, the heat transfer characteristics of the package are within the limits applicable to or specified for the package design.

(n) Prior to each shipment of any package, the shipper shall insure by examination or appropriate test that:

(1) The package is proper for the contents to be shipped;
(2) The packaging is in unimpaired physical condition except for superficial marks;
(3) Each closure device of the packaging, including any required gasket, is properly installed and secured and free of defects;
(4) For a fissile material, any moderator and neutron absorber, if required, is present in proper condition;
(5) Any special instructions for filling, closing, and preparation of the package for shipment have been followed;
(6) Each closure, valve, and any other opening of the containment system through which the radioactive content might escape is properly closed and sealed;
(7) Each package containing liquid in excess of a Type A quantity and destined for air shipment is tested to demonstrate that it is leak tight under an ambient atmospheric

pressure differential of at least 0.5 atmosphere (absolute) (7.3 p.s.i.a. or 0.5 kgl/cm^2); the test may be conducted on the entire containment system or on any receptacle or vessel within the containment system, as appropriate to determine compliance with the requirement;

(8) If the maximum normal operating pressure of a package is likely to exceed 0.35 kg/cm^2 (gage), the internal pressure of the containment system will not exceed the design pressure during transportation; and

(9) External radiation and contamination levels are within the allowable limits.

(o) No person may offer for transportation a package of radioactive materials until the temperature of the packaging system has reached equilibrium (see also paragraph (e) of this section) unless, for the specific contents, he has ascertained that the maximum applicable surface temperature limits cannot be exceeded.

(p) No person may offer for transportation aboard a passenger carrying aircraft any radioactive material unless that material is intended for use in, or incident to, research, or medical diagnosis or treatment, or is excepted under the provisions of § 175.10 of this subchapter.

[Amdt. 173-3, 33 FR 14926, Oct. 4, 1968, as amended by Amdt. 173-6, 34 FR 7162, May 1, 1969]

Note: For amendments to § 173.393 see the List of CFR Sections Affected appearing in the Finding Aids section of this volume.

§ 173.393a U.S. Atomic Energy Commission approved packages; standard requirements and conditions.

(a) In addition to the applicable requirements of the USAEC approval and Parts 170—189 of this subchapter, each shipper of a package containing radioactive materials, which has been approved by the U.S. Atomic Energy Commission in accordance with § 173.394 (b)(3), (c)(2), § 173.395 (b)(2), (c)(2), § 173.396 (b)(4), or § 173.396 (c)(3), also shall comply with the following:

(1) Before the first shipment in a package approved by the U.S. Atomic Energy Commission for use by another person, each shipper shall register in writing with the USAEC, Division of Materials Licensing, his name and address, the name of the person to whom the USAEC approval was issued, and the approval number assigned to the package. Each shipper shall have a copy of the USAEC approval and the document referred to in the approval in his possession. Each shipment must be made in compliance with the terms and conditions of the approval;

(2) The outside of each package must be durably and legibly marked with the package identification marking indicated in the USAEC approval;

(3) Each shipping paper related to the shipment of this package must bear a notation of the package identification marking indicated in the USAEC approval;

(4) Before the first export shipment of the package, the shipper shall submit a copy of the applicable competent authority certificate applying to that package design to the competent national authority of each country into or through which the package will be transported, unless a copy has already been furnished to this party by another person. (Detailed requirements for the issuance and content of competent authority certificates are provided in marginal C-6 of the IAEA "Regulations for the Safe Transport of Radioactive Materials, safety series No. 6, 1967 edition," hereinafter referred to as the "IAEA Regulations." A list of the national competent authorities of each country is published annually by the IAEA.);

(5) Each package of fissile radioactive material must be marked with the numerical value

for the transport index if the shipment is fissile class II. Any vehicle limitation indicated in the USAEC approval applies if the shipment is fissile class III; and

(6) For a fissile class III shipment the statement prescribed in § 172.203(d)(1)(vi) of this subchapter, must be included with the shipping papers.

[Amdt. 173-69,38 FR 4398, Feb. 14, 1973, as amended by Amdt, 173-121, 43 FR 48644, Oct. 19, 1978]

§ 173.393b International shipments and foreign-made packages; standard requirements and conditions

(a) In addition to the other applicable requirements of Parts 170—189 of this subchapter, each shipper of a package containing radioactive material, for which a foreign competent authority certificate has been issued and revalidated pursuant to the IAEA regulations and § 173.394(b)(4), § 173.394 (c)(3), § 173.395(b)(3), § 173.395(c)(3), § 173,396(b)(5), or § 173.396(c)(4), also shall comply with the following:

(1) Before the first shipment of the package, each shipper shall register in writing his identity and type of package with the Office of Hazardous Materials Regulation, U.S. Department of Transportation, Washington, D.C. 20590, furnishing a copy of the foreign certificate or revalidation thereof which is applicable to that package, unless a copy has already been furnished by another person;

(2) The outside of each package must be durably and legibly marked with the competent authority identification marking indicated on the certificate or revalidation;

(3) Each shipping paper related to the shipment of the package must bear a notation of the package identification marking indicated in the certificate or revalidation;

(4) Before the first export shipment of the package, the shipper shall furnish a copy of the applicable competent authority certificate applying to that package design and any required revalidation, to the competent national authority of each country through or into which the package will be transported, unless a copy has already been furnished by another person;

(5) The applicable competent authority certificates need not accompany the packages to which they relate. However, the shipper shall supply them to the carrier upon request; and

(6) For a fissile class III shipment, the statement prescribed in § 172.203(d)(1)(vi) of this subchapter, must be included with the shipping papers.

(b) The designated competent authority in the USA responsible for administering the requirements (Marginal C-6) of the International Atomic Energy Agency's (IAEA) "Regulations for the Safe Transport of Radioactive Materials," Safety Series No. 6, 1967 Edition, is:

Office of Hazardous Materials Regulation, U.S. Department of Transportation, Washington, D.C. 20590.

(c) Any request for a competent authority certificate required by the IAEA regulations must be submitted in writing to the address given in paragraph (b) of this section. This request should be in duplicate and must contain all the information required by the applicable subsection of Marginal C-6 of the IAEA regulations. Unless there is good reason for priority treatment, each request will be considered in the order in which it is received. To permit timely consideration, requests should be submitted at least 45 days prior to the request effective date.

[Amdt. 173-69, 38 FR 4398, Feb. 14, 1973, as amended by Amdt. 173-121, 43 FR 48644, Oct. 19, 1978]

§ 173.394 Radioactive material in special form

(a) In addition to the applicable requirements of §§ 173.24 and 173.393, a Type A quantity of special form radio-active material must be packaged as follows:

(1) Specification 7A (§ 178.350 of this subchapter) Type A general packaging. Each shipper of a Specification 7A packaging must maintain on file for at least 1 year after the latest shipment, and be prepared to provide the Department, a complete certification and supporting safety analysis demonstrating that the construction methods, packaging design, and materials of construction are in compliance with the specification. This requirement is effective December 31, 1975.
(2) Specification 55 (§ 178.250 of this subchapter) metal encased shielded container. Use of existing container authorized; construction not authorized after March 31, 1975.
(3) Any Type B packaging pursuant to paragraph (b) of this section.
(4) Foreign-made packagings which bear the marking "TYPE A."

(b) Type B quantities of special form radioactive materials must be packaged as follows:

(1) Specification 55 metal encased shielded container. Authorized only for domestic shipments of not more than 300 Ci per package. Use of existing container authorized; construction not authorized after March 31, 1975.
(2) Specification 6M (§ 178.104 of this subchapter) metal packaging.
(3) Any other Type B packaging approved by the U.S. Atomic Energy Commission
(4) Any other Type B packaging which meets the pertinent requirements in the 1967 regulations of the International Atomic Energy Agency and for which the foreign competent authority certificate has been revalidated by the Department.
(5) Specification 20WC (§ 178.194 of this subchapter) wooden outer protective jacket, with a single snug-fitting inner Type A packaging which has a metal outer wall and conforms to § 178.350 of this subchapter or Specification 55. Only use of existing specification 55 container authorized; construction not authorized after March 31, 1975.
(6) Specification 21WC (§ 178.195 of this subchapter) wooden-steel protective overpack, with a single inner specification 2R (§ 178.34 of this subchapter) or specification 55, inner packaging. Only use of existing specification 55 container authorized; construction not authorized after March 31, 1975. Contents must be loaded within the inner packaging to preclude loose movement during transportation. The inner packaging must be securely positioned and centered within the overpack by solid cushioning materials so that there would be no significant displacement of the inner packaging if the packaging were subjected to the 9 m (30-ft) drop test described in § 173.398(c)(1).

(c) Large quantities of radioactive materials in special form must be packaged as follows:

(1) Spec. 6M (§ 178.104 of this subchapter) metal packaging. Radioactive thermal decay energy must not exceed 10 W.
(2) Any other Type B packaging which meets the pertinent requirements for large quantities of radioactive materials in the regulations of the U.S. Atomic Energy Commission (10 CFR Part 71) and is approved by the U.S. Atomic Energy Commission.
(3) Any other Type B packaging which meets the pertinent requirements for large quantities of radioactive materials in the 1967 regulations of the International Atomic Energy Agency, and for which the foreign competent authority certificate has been revalidated by the Department.

(4) Specifications 20WC (§ 178.194 of this subchapter) wooden outer protective jacket, with a single, snug-fitting specification 55 inner packaging. Only use of existing specification 55 container authorized; construction not authorized after March 31, 1975. Radioactive thermal decay energy must not exceed 100.

[Amdt. 173-1, 33 FR 14927, Oct. 4, 1968, as amended by Amdt. 173-34, 35 FR 13836, Sept. 1, 1970]

Note: For amendments to § 173.394 see the list of CFR Sections Affected appearing in the Finding Aids section of this volume.

§ 173.395 Radioactive material in normal form

(a) In addition to the applicable requirements of §§ 173.24 and 173.393, a Type A quantity of normal form radioactive material must be packaged as follows:

(1) Specification 7A (§ 178.350 of this subchapter) Type A general packaging. Each shipper of a specification 7A packaging must maintain on file for at least a year after the latest shipment, and be prepared to provide the Department, a complete certification and supporting safety analysis demonstrating that the construction methods, packaging design, and materials of construction are in compliance with the specification. This requirement is effective December 31, 1975.
(2) Specification 55 metal encased shielded container. Use of existing container authorized; construction not authorized after March 31, 1975. For liquid contents the provisions of § 173.393(g) must also be met.
(3) Any Type B packaging pursuant to paragraph (b) of this section.
(4) Foreign-made packagings which bear the marking "TYPE A."

(b) Type B quantities of radioactive materials in normal form must be packaged as follows:

(1) Spec. 6M (§ 178.104 of this subchapter metal packaging. Authorized only for solid or gaseous radioactive materials which will not decompose at temperatures up to 250°F.
(2) Any other Type B packaging approved by the U.S. Atomic Energy Commission
(3) Any other Type B packaging which meets the pertinent reqirements in the 1967 regulations of the International Atomic Energy Agency, and for which the foreign competent authority certificate has been revalidated by the Department.
(4) Specification 20WC (§ 178.194 of this subchapter) wooden outer protective jacket, when used with a single, snug-fitting inner specification 2R (§ 178.34 of this subchapter) or specification 55 inner packaging. Only use of existing specification 55 container authorized; construction not authorized after March 31, 1975. For liquid contents the provisions of § 173.393(g) must also be met, with respect to the inner packaging.

(c) Large quantities of radioactive materials in normal form must be packaged as follows:

(1) Spec. 6M (§ 178.104) of this chapter) metal packaging. Authorized only for solid or gaseous radioactive materials which will not decompose at temperatures up to 250°F. Radioactive thermal decay energy must not exceed 10 W
(2) Any other Type B packaging for large quantities of radioactive materials which meets the pertinent requirements win the regulations of the U.S. Atomic Energy Commission (10 CFR Part 71) and is approved by the U.S. Atomic Energy Commission.
(3) Any other Type B packaging which meets the pertinent requirements for large quantities of radioactive materials in the 1967 regulations of the International Atomic Energy

Agency, and for which the foreign competent authority certificate has been revalidated by the Department.

[Amdt. 173—3, 33 FR 14927, Oct. 4, 1968, as amended by Amdt. 173—69, 38 FR 4398, Feb. 14, 1973]

Note: For amendments to § 173.395 see the List of CFR Sections Affected appearing in the Finding Aids section of this volume.

§ 173.396 Fissile radioactive material

(a) The following materials are not classified as fissile radioactive materials, are exempted from this section, and must instead be packaged in accordance with the other provisions of this subpart, as appropriate:

(1) Not more than 15 g of fissile material;
(2) Thorium, or uranium containing not more than 0.72 % by weights of fissile material;
(3) Uranium compounds other than metal (e.g., UF_4, UF_6, or uranium oxide in bulk form, not pelleted or fabricated into shapes), and aqueous solutions of uranium, in which the total amount of uranium-233 and plutonium present does not exceed 10% by weight of the uranium-235 content, and the total fissile content does not exceed 1.00% by weight of the total uranium content;
(4) Homogenous hydrogenous solutions or mixtures containing not more than;
    (i) 500 g of any fissile material, provided the atomic ratio of hydrogen to fissile material is greater than 7,600; or
    (ii) 800 g of uranium-235, if the atomic ratio of hydrogen to fissile material is greater than 5200, and the content of other fissile material is not more than 1.0% by weight of the total uranium-235 content; or
    (iii) 500 g of uranium-233 and uranium-235, if the atomic ratio of hydrogen to fissile material is greater than 5200, and the content of plutonium is not more than 1.0% by weight of the total uranium-233 and uranium-235 content.
(5) A package containing less than 350 g of fissile material, if there is not more than 5 g of fissile material in any cubic foot within the package.

(b) Fissile radioactive materials containing not more than Type A quantities of radionuclides, in either normal form or special form, must be packaged as follows:

(1) Specification 6L (§ 178.103 of this subchapter) metal packaging. See paragraph (c)(1) of this section for authorized contents.
(2) Spec. 6M (§ 178.104 of this subchapter) metal packaging. See paragraph (c)(2) of this section for authorized contents.
(3) Any packaging listed in § 173.395(a). Authorized only for not more than the following:
    (i) 500 g of uranium-235 as Fissile Class III, or not more than 40 g of uranium-235 as Fissile Class II. For Fissile Class II shipments, the transport index to be assigned to each package shall be 0.4 for each gram of uranium-235 above 15 g up to a maximum of 40 g (transport index of 10).
    (ii) 320 g of plutonium-239 as plutonium-beryllium neutron sources in special form. Total radioactivity content must not exceed 20 Ci. The transport index to be assigned to each package shall be 0.5 for each 20 g, or fraction thereof, of fissile plutonium.

(4) Any other Type A or B packaging for fissile radioactive materials which also meets the pertinent standards for packaging in the regulations of the U.S. Atomic Energy Commission (10 CFR Part 71), and is approved by the U.S. Atomic Energy Commission.

(5) Any other Type A or B packaging for fissile radioactive materials which also meets the pertinent requirements in the 1967 regulations of the International Atomic Energy Agency, and for which the foreign competent authority certificate has been revalidated by the Department.

(6) Specification 20PF-1, 20PF-2, or 20PF-3 (§ 178.120 of this subchapter) or specification 21PF-1 or 2 (§ 178.121 of this subchapter) phenolic-foam insulated protective over-packs, with snug-fitting inner metal cylinders meeting all of the applicable requirements of §§ 173.24, 173.393, and 173.398(b). Handling procedures and packaging criteria must be in accordance with USAEC Report No. ORO-651 or ANSI Standard N-14.1-1971. Quantities of uranium hexafluoride are authorized as follows, with each package to be shipped as fissile Class II, and assigned a minimum transport index as indicated:

Protective overpack specitication No.	Maximum inner cylinder diameter		Maximum weight of UF_6 contents		Maximum U^{235} enrichment (w/o)	Fissile class II transport index
	Inches	Centimeter	Pounds	Kilograms		
20PF-1	5	12.7	55	25	100	0.1
20PF-2	8	20.3	255	116	12.5	0.4
20PF-3	12	30.5	460	209	5.0	1.1
21PF-1[a]	30[b]	76	4950	2247	5.0	5.0
	30[c]	76	5020	2279	5.0	5.0
21PF-2[a]	30[b]	76	4950	2247	5.0	5.0
	30[c]	76	5020	2279	5.0	5.0

[a] For 30-in cylinders, the maximum H/U automic ratio is 0.088

[b] Model 30A inner cylinder (Reference: ORO-651).

[c] Model 30B inner cylinder (Reference: ORO-651).

(7) Specification 6J (§178.100 of this subchapter) or 17H (§ 178.118 of this subchapter) 55-gal steel drum, for transport of not more than 350 g of uranium-235 in any non-pyrophoric form, enriched to any degree in the U-235 isotope. Each drum must have a minimum 18-gauge body and bottom head and 16-gauge removable top head, with one or more corrugations in the cover near the periphery. Closure must conform to §178.103-5(a) of this subchapter. At least four 1.2 cm (0.5 in.) diameter vent holes must be provided, equally spaced on the sides of the drum near the top, each covered with weatherproof tape, or equivalent device. Appropriate primary inner containment of the contents and any necessary packing material must be provided, such as plastic or metal jars or cans or plastic wrapping, such that Spec. 7A (§ 178.350 of this subchapter) provisions are satisfied. Each inner containment vessel must be capable of venting in the even the package was exposed to the thermal test described in (§ 173.398(c)(2)(iii)). Additionally, liquid contents must be packaged in accordance with § 173.393(g). The maximum weight of contents, including internal packing must not exceed 91 kg (200 lb) with fissile material content limited as follows:

Maximum U^{235} per package (grams)	Minimum transport index per package as fissile class II	Maximum packages per transport vehicle as fissile class III
350	1.8	72
300	1.0	129
250	0.5	256
200	0.3	500
150	0.1	500
100	0.1	500
50	[a]	[a]

[a] Fissile class I.

(8) Any metal cylinder which meets the performance requirements for a specification 7A Type A packaging (see §§ 173.395(a)(1) and 178.350 of this subchapter) for the transport of residual ''heels'' of enriched solid uranium hexafluoride without a protective overpack, are authorized as Fissile Class I packages, in accordance with the following:

Maximum cylinder diameter		Cylinder volume		Maximum U^{235} enrichment (weight percent)	Maximum ''heel'' weight per cylinder UF6 (U^{235})		
Inches	Centimeters	Cubic feet	Liters		Pounds	Kilograms	Kilograms
5	12.7	0.311	8.8	100.0	0.1	0.045	0.031
8	20.3	1.359	39	12.5	0.5	0.227	0.019
12	30.5	2.410	68	5.0	1.0	0.454	0.015
30	76	25.64	725	5.0	25.0	11.35	0.383

(c) Fissile radioactive materials containing Type B quantities of radionuclides, in either normal form or special form, must be packaged as follows:

(1) Specification 6L (§ 178.103 of this subchapter) metal packaging. Authorized only for uranium-235, plutonium-239 or 241, as metal, oxide, or compounds which will not decompose at temperatures up to 149°C (300°F.) Radioactive thermal decay energy output shall not exceed 5 W. Large quantity radioactive materials in normal form must be packaged in one or more sealed and leak tight metal cans or polyethylene bottles within the Spec. 2R containment vessel.

(i) *Fissile Class II and III packages.* The following quantities of fissile radioactive materials are authorized under the Fissile Class II and III conditions listed:

TABLE OF AUTHORIZED CONTENTS[a]

Uranium-235[b]		Plutonium[b,d]			Fissile class III
H/X≤3	3<H/X≤20	H/X≤10	10≤H/X≤20	Fissile class II transport index	maximum number of packages per transport vehicle
14	3.6[c]			1.3	80
		2.5	2.4	1.8	55

[a] Quantity in kilograms.

[b] All sources of hydrogen within the inner containment vessel must be considered in determining the H/X ratio of inner containment vessel.

[c] Volume not to exceed 3.6 ℓ.

[d] Plutonium solutions are not authorized.

(2) Spec. 6M (§ 178.104 of this sub-chapter) metal packaging. Authorized only for solid radioactive materials which will not decompose at temperatures up to 250°F. Radioactive thermal decay energy output shall not exceed 10 W. Large quantity radioactive materials in normal form must be packaged in one or more sealed and leaktight metal cans or polyethylene bottles within the Spec. 2R containment vessels.

(i) *Fissile Class I packages.* The following quantities of fissile radioactive material are authorized for Fissile Class I packages: 1.6 k uranium-235, 0.9 k of plutonium (see Note) 0.5 k of uranium-233. The maximum ratio of hydrogen to fissile material must not exceed three, all sources of hydrogen within the Spec. 2R containment vessel being considered.

Note: Because of the 10-W thermal decay heat limitation, the limit for plutonium 238 is only 0.02 kg.

(ii) *Fissile Class II and III packages.* Quantities of fissile radioactive material as shown in the following table are authorized for a Fissile Class II and Fissile Class III package. Where a maximum ratio of hydrogen to fissile material is specified in the table, only the hydrogen interspersed with the fissile material need be considered. For a Fissile Class II package, the minimum transport index to be assigned is shown in the following table. For a Fissile Class III package, the maximum number of similar packages per transport vehicle is shown. Each Fissile Class III shipment is also subject to a paragraph (g) of this section. For a uranium-233 shipment the maximum inside diameter of the inner containment vessel must not exceed 12 cm (4.75 in.). Where necessary, a tight fitting steel insert must be used to reduce a larger diameter inner containment vessel specified in § 178.104—3(b) of this subchapter to the 12 cm (4.75 in.) limit.

TABLE OF AUTHORIZED CONTENTS[a]

Uranium-233[e]			Uranium-235[d,g]			Plutonium[b,c,d]			Fissile class II transport index	Fissile class III maximum number of packages per transport vehicle
Metal or alloy	Compounds		metalic or alloy	Compounds		Metal or alloy	Compounds			
H/X = O	H/X = O	H/X3	H/X = O	H/X = O	H/X≤3	H/X = O	H/X = O	H/X ≤ 3		
3.6	4.4	2.9	7.2	7.6	5.3	3.1	4.1	3.4	0.1	1250
4.2[f]	5.2	3.5	8.7	9.6	6.4	3.4	4.5	4.1	0.2	625
5.2[f]	6.8	4.5	11.2	13.9	8.3	4.2		4.5	0.5	250
			13.5	16.0	10.1	4.5			1.0	125
				26.0	16.1				5.0	25
				32.0	19.5				10.0	12

[a] Quantity in kilograms.
[b] Minimum percentage of plutonium-240 is 5 weight percent.
[c] 4.5 kg limitation of plutonium due to 10 W decay heat limitation.
[d] For a mixture of uranium-235 and plutonium an equal amount of uranium-235 may be substituted for any portion of plutonium authorized.
[e] Maximum inside diameter not to exceed 12 cm (4.75 in.) (see par. (c)(2)(ii) of this section).
[f] Granulated or powdered metal with any particle less than 8 mm (0.25 in.) in the smallest dimension is not authorized.
[g] Maximum uranium-235 enrichment is 93%.

(3) Any other Type B packaging which also meets the standards for packaging for fissile radioactive materials in the regulations of the U.S. Atomic Energy Commission (10 CFR Part 71), and is approved by the U.S. Atomic Energy Commission.

(4) Any other Type B packaging which also meets the pertinent requirements for fissile radioactive materials in the 1967 regulations of the International Atomic Energy Agency, and for which the foreign competent authority certificate has been revalidated by the Department.

(5) Specification 20PF-1 through 3 (§ 178.120 of this subchapter) or Specification 21PF-1 or 2 (§ 178.121 of this subchapter) phenolic-foam insulated protective overpacks. (See paragraph (b)(6) of this section for authorized use.)

(d) [Reserved]

(e)Mixing of packages of other types of radioactive materials, including Fissile Class I, with Fissile Class II packages is permitted if the total transport index in any one of transport vehicle or storage location does not exceed 50.

(f) For Fissile Class II packages shipped under the exclusive use provisions of § 173.393(j) to provide for package with high radiation dose rates, the transport index number which is calculated for nuclear criticality control purposes must not exceed 10 for any single package or a total of 50 for the full load, unless specifically authorized by the Department for Fissile Class III shipments.

(1) Fissile Class II packages may be shipped with a transport index greater than 10, and combined with other packages of the same or different designs in a Fissile Class III shipment, under the conditions prescribed in paragraph (g) of this section, *provided:*

- (i) The transport index which has been assigned in the package approval for nuclear criticality control purposes does not exceed 10 for any single package;
- (ii) The total transport index for nuclear criticality control purposes for all packages in the shipment does not exceed 100;
- (iii) The shipment satisfies the provisions of § 173.393(j) if any package has radiation dose rates exceeding 10 mrem/hr at 1 m (3ft) from any accessible external surface of the package; and
- (iv) The shipment will not be transported by water.

(2) Fissile Class III packages, which have been assigned a transport index for nuclear criticality control purposes in accordance with Fissile Class II criteria, may be combined

with other Fissile Class III packages of the same or different design for which a transport index has been so assigned for nuclear criticality control purposes, and may be combined with Fissile Class II packages, in a Fissile Class III shipment under the conditions prescribed in paragraph (g) of this section, *provided:*

(i) The transport index which has been assigned in the package approval for nuclear criticality control purposes does not exceed 50 for any single package;
(ii) The total transport index for nuclear criticality control purposes for all packages in the shipment does not exceed 100;
(iii) The shipment satisfies the provisions of § 173.393(j) if any package has radiation dose rates exceeding 10 mrem/hr at 1 m (3 ft) from any accessible external surface of the package; and
(iv) The shipment will not be transported by water.

(g) A fissile class III shipment may be made only in accordance with paragraphs (g) (1), (2), or (3) of this section, or in accordance with other procedures authorized by the Department. The transport controls must provide nuclear criticality safety and must be carried out by the shipper or carrier, as appropriate, to protect against loading, storing, or transporting of that shipment together with any other fissile material.

(1) Transportation in a transport vehicle assigned for the sole use of that consignor, with a specific restriction for such sole use to be provided in the special arrangements, and with instructions to that effect issued with the shipping papers; or
(2) Except for shipments by aircraft, transportation under escort by person in a separate vehicle, with the escort having the capability, equipment, authority, and instructions to provide administrative controls adequate to assure compliance with this paragraph; or
(3) Transportation in a transport vehicle containing no other packages of radioactive material which are required to bear one of the "Radioactive" labels described in § 173.416. Specific arrangements must be effected between shipper and carrier, with instructions to that effect issued with the shipping papers.

(h) The numerical values for package assignments as fissile class I, the transport indices for fissile class II packages, and the vehicle limitations for fissile class III packages must be determined in accordance with §§ 71.36 through 71.40 of Title 10 of the Code of Federal Regulations.
[Amdt. 173—3, 33 FR 14927, Oct. 4, 1968; 33 FR 19823, Dec. 27, 1968, as amended by Amdt. 173-14, 34 FR 17523, Oct. 30, 1969]

Note: For amendments to § 173.396 see the List of CFR Sections Affected appearing in the Finding Aids section of this volume.

§ 173.397 Contamination control

(a) Removable (nonfixed) radioactive contamination is considered significant if the level of contamination, when averaged over any area of 300 cm^2 of any part of the package surface, exceeds any of the following:

Contaminant	Maximum permissible level	
	μCi/Cm^2	dis/min/Cm^2
Natural or depleted uranium and natural thorium		
Beta-gamma	10^{-3}	2200
Alpha	10^{-4}	220
All other beta-gamma emitting radionuclides	10^{-4}	220
All other alpha emitting radionuclides	10^{-5}	22

(1) In assessing the surface contamination of a package, a sufficient number of measurements must be taken in the most appropriate locations so as to yield a representative assessment of the contamination situation. The average amount of removable (nonfixed) radioactive contamination may be determined by wiping the external surface of the package with an absorbent material, using moderate pressure, and then measuring the activity on the wiping material. If the measured activity per square centimeter does not exceed 10% of the levels prescribed above, it may be assumed that those levels have not been exceeded. Other measurement methods of equal or greater efficiency may also be utilized.

(b) When radioactive materials packages are consigned as exclusive use, as defined in § 173.389(o), removable nonfixed radioactive contamination may not exceed 10 times that as specified in paragraph (a)(1) of this section.

(c) Each transport vehicle used for transporting radioactive materials as exclusive use, as defined in § 173.389(o), must be surveyed with appropriate radiation detection instruments after each use. A vehicle may not be returned to service until the radiation dose rate at any accessible surface is 0.5 mrem/hr or less, and there is no significant removable radioactive surface contamination, as defined in paragraphy (a) of this section.
[Amdt. 173-90, 39 FR 45243. Dec. 31, 1974]

§ 173.398 Special tests

(a) Special form material: To qualify as special form material, the radioactive material must either be in massive solid form or encapsulated. Each item in massive solid form or each capsule must either have no overall dimension less than 0.5 mm, or must have at least one dimension greater than 5 mm. Each item, or the capsule material, must not dissolve or convert into dispersible form to the extent of more than 0.005% by weight, by immersion for 1 week in water at pH 6 to 8 and 68°F, and a maximum conductivity of 10 μmho/cm, and by immersion in air at 86°F. If in massive solid form, the radioactive material must not break, crumble, or shatter if subjected to the percussion test prescribed in this section, and must not melt, sublime, or ignite at temperatures below 1000°F. If encapsulated, the capsule must retain its contents when subjected to all of the performance tests prescribed in this section, and must not melt, sublime, or ignite at temperatures below 1475°F.

(1) *Free Drop.* A free drop through a distance of 30 ft on to a flat essentially unyielding horizontal surface, striking the surface in such a position as to suffer maximum damage.
(2) *Percussion.* Impact of the flat circular end of a 1 in. diameter steel rod weighing 3 lb, dropped through a distance of 40 in. The capsule or material shall be placed on a sheet of lead, of hardness number 3.5 to 4.5 on the Vickers scale, and not more than 1 in. thick, supported by a smooth, essentially unyielding surface.
(3) *Heating.* Heating in air to a temperature of 1475° F and remaining at that temperature for a period of 10 min.
(4) Immersion for 24 hr in water at room temperature. The water shall be at pH6 to 8, with a maximum conductivity of 10 μmho/cm.

Note 1: Each shipper of special form radioactive material shall maintain on file for at least 1 year after the last shipment, and be prepared to provide the Department, a complete certification and supporting safety analysis (see Note 2) demonstrating that the special form material meets the requirements of paragraph (a) of this section. This requirement is effective December 31, 1974.

Note 2: Prior to the first shipment of a special form radioactive material outside of the U.S. each shipper shall obtain a Certificate of Competent Authority for the specific material.

Each petition must be submitted in accordance with § 173.393b (b) and (c), and must additionally include the following information:

a. A detailed description of the material, or if a capsule, the contents. Particular reference must be made to both physical and chemical states;
b. A detailed statement of the design of any capsule to be used, including complete engineering drawings and schedules of material, and methods of construction;
c. A statement of the tests which have been done and their results, or evidence based on calculative methods to show that the material is capable of meeting the tests, or other evidence that the special form radioactive material is capable of meeting the tests, or other evidence that the special form radioactive material meets the requirements of paragraphs (a)(1) thru (4) of this section.

(b) Standards for Type A packaging:

(1) Type A packaging must be so designed and constructed that, if it were subject to the environmental and test conditions prescribed in this paragraph:

(i) There would be no release of radioactive material from the package;
(ii) The effectiveness of the packaging would not be substantially reduced; and
(iii) There would be no mixture of gases or vapors in the package which could, through any credible increase of pressure or an explosion, significantly reduce the effectiveness of the package.

(2) Environmental conditions:

(i) *Heat.* Direct sunlight at an ambient temperature of 130° F in still air.
(ii) *Cold.* An ambient temperature of −40° F in still air and shade.
(iii) *Reduced pressure,* Ambient atmospheric pressure of 0.5 atmosphere (absolute) (7.3 p.s.i.a.).
(iv) *Vibration.* Vibration normally incident to transportation.

(3) Test conditions: The packaging shall be subject to all of the following tests unless specifically exempted therefrom, and also to the consecutive application of at least two of the following tests from which it is not specifically exempted:

(i) *Water spray.* A water spray heavy enough to keep the entire exposed surface of the package except the bottom continuously wet during a period of 30 min. Packages for which the outer layer consists entirely of metal, wood, ceramic, or plastic, or combinations thereof, are exempt from the water spray test.
(ii) *Free drop.* Between $1^1/_2$ to $2^1/_2$ hr after the conclusion of the water spray test, a free drop through a distance of 4 ft onto a flat essentially unyielding horizontal surface, striking the surface in a position for which maximum damage is expected.
(iii) *Corner drop.* A free drop onto each corner of the package in succession, or in the case of a cylindrical package onto each quarter of each rim, from a height of 1 ft onto a flat essentially unyielding horizontal surface. This test applies only to packages which are constructed primarily of wood or fiberboard, and do not exceed 110 lb gross weight, and to all Fissile Class II packagings.
(iv) *Penetration.* Impact of the hemispherical end of a vertical steel cylinder $1^1/_4$ in. in diameter and weighing 13 lb, dropped from a height of 40 in. onto the exposed surface of the package which is expected to be most vulnerable to puncture. The long axis of the cylinder shall be perpendicular to the package surface.

(v) *Compression.* For packages not more than 10,000 lb in weight, a compressive load equal to either five times the weight of the package or 2 lb/in.^{2} multiplied by the maximum horizontal cross section of the package, whichever is greater. The load shall be applied during a period of 24 hr, uniformly against the top and bottom of the package in the position in which the package would normally be transported.

(c) Standards for hypothetical accident conditions of transportation for Type B packagings:

(1) Type B packaging must meet the applicable Type A packaging standards and must be designed and constructed and its contents so limited that, if subjected to the hypothetical accident conditions prescribed in this paragraph, it will meet the following conditions:

(i) The reduction of shielding would not be enough to increase the radiation dose rate at 3 ft from the external surface of the package to more than 1000 mrem/hr.

(ii) No radioactive material would be released from packages containing Type B quantities of radioactive material. The allowable release of radioactivity from packages containing large quantities of radioactive material is limited to gases and contaminated coolant containing total radioactivity exceeding neither 0.1% of the total radioactivity of the package contents nor 0.01 Ci of Group I radionuclides, 0.5 Ci of Group I radionuclides, and 10 Ci of Groups III and IV radionuclides, except that for inert gases the limit is 1000 Ci.

(2) Test conditions: The conditions which the package must be capable of withstanding must be applied sequentially, to determine their cumulative effect on a package, in the following order:

(i) *Free drop.* A free drop through a distance of 30 ft onto a flat essentially unyielding horizontal target surface, striking the surface in a position for which maximum damage is expected.

(ii) *Puncture.* A free drop through a distance of 40 in. striking, in a position for which maximum damage is expected, the top end of a vertical cylindrical mild steel bar mounted on an essentially unyielding horizontal surface, the bar shall be 6 in. in diameter, with the top horizontal and its edge rounded to a radius of not more than $^1/_4$ in. and of such a length as to cause maximum damage to the package, but not less than 8 in. long. The long axis of the bar shall be perpendicular to the unyielding horizontal surface.

(iii) *Thermal.* Exposure to a thermal test in which the heat input to the package is no less than that which would result from exposure of the whole package to a radiation environment of 1475°F. for 30 min with an emissivity coefficient of 0.9, assuming the surfaces of the package have an absorption coefficient of 0.8. The package shall not be cooled artificially until 3 hr after the test period unless it can be shown that the temperature on the inside of the package has begun to fall in less than 3 hr.

(iv) *Water immersion (fissile radioactive materials packages only)* Immersion in water to the extent that all portion of the package to be tested are under at least 3 ft of water for a period of not less than 8 hr.

(d) It is not necessary to actually conduct the tests prescribed in this section if it can be clearly shown, through engineering evaluations or comparative data, that the material or item would be capable of performing satisfactorily under the prescribed test conditions. [Amdt. 173-3 33 FR 14929. Oct. 4, 1968; 33 FR 19823, Dec. 27, 1968, as amended by Amdt. 173-90, 39 FR 45244, Dec. 31, 1974; 40 FR 2435, Jan. 13, 1975]

APPENDIX D
TITLE 49, PART 174 *

PART 174 — CARRIAGE BY RAIL

SUBPART A — GENERAL REQUIREMENTS

§ 174.1 Purpose and scope

This part prescribes requirements in addition to those contained in Parts 171, 172, 173, and 179 of this subchapter, to be observed with respect to the transportation of hazardous materials in or on rail cars.

[Amdt. 174-26, 41 FR 16092. Apr. 15, 1976, as amended by Amdt. 174-26A, 41 Fr 40685, Sept. 20, 1976]

§ 174.3 Unacceptable hazardous materials shipments

A shipment of a hazardous material that is not prepared for transportation in accordance with Parts 171,172 and 173 of this subchapter may not be accepted for transportation or transported by rail except as provided in § 174.47(b).

[Amdt. 174-26, 41 FR 16092. Apr. 15, 1976, as amended by Amdt. 174-26A, 41 FR 40685, Sept. 20, 1976]

§ 174.7 Responsibility for Compliance

Unless this subchapter specifically provides that another person is to perform a particular duty, each carrier, including a connecting carrier, shall perform the duties specified and comply with each applicable requirement of this part, and shall instruct its employees in relation thereto.

§ 174.8 Inspection

(a) Methods of manufacture, packing, and storage of hazardous material, insofar as they affect safety in transportation by rail, must be open to inspection by a duly authorized representative of the Department, an initial carrier, and the Bureau of Explosives.

(b) At any point where a train is required to be inspected, each loaded placarded rail car and each rail car immediately adjacent thereto must be inspected. The cars may continue in transit only when the inspection indicates that the cars are in a safe condition for transportation. (See §§ 174.9 and 174.10) The inspection of a rail car other than a tank car or a rail car containing Class A explosives must include a visual inspection for obvious defects of the running gear and any leakage of contents from the car and to determine whether all required placards are in place and conform to the information given on the train consist or other shipping document as required by § 174.26(b).

(c) For inspection requirements applicable to rail cars containing Class A explosives, see §§ 174.10 and 174.104.

[Amdt. 174-26, 41 FR 16092, Apr. 15, 1976, as amended by Amdt. 174-26A, 41 FR 40685, Sept. 20, 1976; Amdt. 174-26B, 41 FR 57071, Dec. 30, 1976]

§ 174.9 Inspection of tank cars

(a) Each loaded placarded tank car must be inspected by the carrier before acceptance at the originating point and when received in interchange to see that it is not leaking and that the air and hand brakes, journal boxes, and trucks are in proper condition for service.

(b) An empty tank car which previously contained a hazardous material and which is

* From *Fed. Reg.*, April 15, 1976.

tendered for movement or received in interchange must have all manhole covers, outlet valve reducers, outlet valve caps, outlet valve cap plugs, end plugs, and plugs or caps or other openings securely in their proper places, except that heater coil inlet and outlet pipes must be left open for drainage.

(c) The safety valves on a tank car may not be tested while the car is loaded. Whenever a test of the safety valves or tank becomes due while a loaded car is in transit, unless the car is leaking or in a manifestly insecure condition, it must be forwarded to its destination, carded on each side with a card exhibiting the following notice:

Safety valves overdue for test:
Tank overdue for test:
Moving under authority of 49 CFR 174.9(c).

A prompt report of each such movement, showing the identifying initials and number of each car, must be made to the Bureau of Explosives by the carrier carding the cars.

§ 174.10 Inspection of cars at interchange

(a) Each rail car containing explosives requiring EXPLOSIVES A placards (see § 174.104) which is offered by a connecting line must be visually inspected externally by the receiving line. If practicable, the receiving carrier should also inspect the lading. The car may not be forwarded until all discovered violations have been corrected.

(b) If the car shows evidence of or if there is any reason to suspect that it has received rough treatment, the lading must be inspected and placed in proper condition before the car is permitted to proceed. When interchange occurs and the inspection is performed after daylight hours, electric flashlights should be used and naked lights may not be used.

(c) A shipment of hazardous materials offered by a connecting carrier must comply with this subchapter, and the revenue waybill, freight bill, manifest of lading, card waybill, switching order, transfer slip ticket, or other billing, must bear the placard notation and endorsement prescribed by § 174.25 of this subpart.

(d) A card containing packages of hazardous materials other than explosives may not be offered in interchange if the packages are in a leaking condition.

(e) In the case of a tank car which has developed small leaks in the course of its movement to an interchange point and which requires a short movement to effect delivery for unloading by the consignee, the movement may be made if it can be made safely adhering to the precautions prescribed by § 174.50.

[Amdt. 174-26, 41 FR 16092, Apr. 15, 1976, as amended by Amdt. 174-26B, 41 FR 57071, Dec. 30, 1976]

§ 174.11 Canadian shipments and packages

A Canadian shipment or package may be transported by rail car within the U.S. if it is in compliance with the requirements of this subchapter or the regulations of the Canadian Transport Commission as provided in § 173.8 of this subchapter.

§ 174.12 Intermediate shippers and carriers

(a) Each origin carrier, including a freight forwarder, must have on file a copy of the shipper's certified shipping paper, as prescribed in Part 172 of this subchapter, for each shipment of hazardous materials it handles. An intermediate shipper or carrier may not forward or transport a shipment of hazardous materials if it does not meet the requirements of this subchapter.

(b) An intermediate carrier offering or delivering for transportation any loaded motor vehicle, trailer, semitrailer, or container containing any hazardous material must show on the shipping paper the information required by §172.201 of this subchapter and a description of the type vehicle or container.

[Amdt. 174-26, 41 FR 16092. Apr. 15, 1976, as amended by Amdt. 174-26B, 41 FR 57071, Dec. 30, 1976]

§ 174.14 Movements to be expedited

(a) A carrier must forward each shipment of hazardous materials promptly and within 48 hr (Saturdays, Sundays, and holidays excluded), after acceptance at the originating point or receipt at any yard, transfer station, or interchange point, except that where biweekly or weekly service only is performed, a shipment of hazardous materials must be forwarded on the first available train.

(b) A tank car loaded with any flammable liquid or gas, or a poison gas, may not be received and held at any point, subject to forwarding orders, so as to defeat the purpose of this section or of § 174.204 of this subchapter.

§ 174.16 Removal and disposition of hazardous materials at destination

(a) *Delivery at nonagency stations.* A shipment of explosives may not be unloaded at nonagency stations unless the consignee is there to receive it or unless properly locked and secure storage facilities are provided at that point for its protection. If delivery cannot be so made, the shipment must be taken to next or nearest agency station for delivery.

(b) *Delivery at agency stations.* A carrier shall require the consignee of each shipment of hazardous materials to remove the shipment from carrier's property within 48 hr (exclusive of Saturdays, Sundays, and holidays) after notice of arrival has been sent or given. If not so removed, the carrier shall immediately dispose of the shipments as follows:

(1) *Class A explosives:* If safe storage is available, by storage at the owner's expense; if safe storage is not available, by return to the shipper, sale, or destruction under supervision of a competent person; or if safety requires, by destruction under supervision of a competent person.

(2) *Hazardous materials, except Class A explosives, in carload shipments:* By storage on the carrier's property; by storage on other than the carrier's property, if safe storage on the carrier's property is not available; or by sale at expiration of 15 calendar days after notice of arrival has been sent or given to the consignee, provided the consignor has been notified of the nondelivery at the expiration of a 48-hr period and orders for disposition have not been received.

(3) *Hazardous materials, except Class A explosives, in less-than-carload shipments:* By return to the shipper if notice of nondelivery was requested and given the consignor prescribed by the carrier's tariff, and orders for return to shipper have been received; by storage on the carrier's property; by storage on other than the carrier's property, if safe storage on carrier's property is not available; or by sale at expiration of 15 calendar days after notice of arrival has been sent or given to the consignee, provided the consignor has been notified of nondelivery at expiration of a 48-hr period and orders for disposition have not been received.

§ 174.18 Astray shipments

An astray package of hazardous materials other than explosives, of known destination and in proper condition for safe transportation, must be forwarded immediately on an "astray bill", showing the information required by Subpart C of Part 172 of this subchapter. When necessary to replace a label and doubt exists as to the kind, the FLAMMABLE LIQUID label must be applied. For astray shipments of explosives, see § 174.103.

§ 174.20 Local or carrier restrictions

(a) When local conditions make the acceptance, transportation, or delivery of hazardous materials unusually hazardous, local restrictions may be imposed by the carrier.

(b) Each carrier must report to the Bureau of Explosives for publication the full information as to any restrictions which it imposes against the acceptance, delivery, or transportation of hazardous materials, over any portion of its lines under this section.

SUBPART B — GENERAL OPERATING REQUIREMENTS

§ 174.24 Shipping papers

(a) Except as provided in paragraph (c) of this section, no person may accept for transportation by rail any hazardous material which is subject to this subchapter unless he has received a shipping paper prepared in the manner specified in Subpart C of Part 172 of this subchapter. In addition, the shipping paper must include a certificate, if required by § 172.204 of this subchapter. However, no member of the train crew of a train transporting the hazardous material is required to have a shipper's certificate on the shipping paper in his possession if the original shipping paper containing the certificate is in the originating carrier's possession.

(b) This subpart does not apply to materials classed as ORM-A, B, C, or D.

[Amdt. 174-26, 41 FR 16092. Apr. 15, 1976, as amended by Amdt. 174-26B, 41 FR 57071, Dec. 30, 1976]

§ 174.25 Additional information on waybills, switching orders and other billings

(a) Each waybill, switching ticket, switching order or other billing used in place thereof, prepared by the carrier from bills-of-lading, shipping orders or other shipping papers, and each shipping order used as a waybill for a rail car required to be placarded by Subpart F of Part 172 of this subchapter must, in addition to containing the information required by §§ 172.202 and 172.203 of this subchapter, be plainly marked by the carrier with

(1) In the case of a flatcar carrying trailers or containers, an indication of which trailers or containers contain the hazardous materials; and

(2) The placard endorsement specified in the following table for the hazardous materials or class concerned near the space on the face of the billing provided for the car number

  (i) In letters not less than $^3/_8$ of an inch, or

  (ii) In bold, uppercase letters not less than $^1/_{10}$ of an inch high inside a rectangle made with any symbol such as asterisk (*), dollar sign ($), capital (X), or the symbol for number (#).

§ 174.69 Removal of placards and car certificates after unloading

When loading requiring placards or car certificates is removed from rail cars other than tank cars, placards and car certificates must be removed by the party unloading the car. For empty tank cars, the placards must be removed, replaced or reversed in accordance with the provisions of § 172.510(c) of this subchapter.

[Amdt. 174-26B, 41 FR 57071, Dec. 30, 1976]

§ 174.81 Segregation and separation requirements for hazardous materials in rail cars

(a) Hazardous materials may not be loaded, transported, or stored together except as provided in the following table:

Low explosives or black powder

High explosives or propellant explosives, class A

Initiating or priming explosives, wet: Diazodinitrophenol, fulminate of mercury, guanyl nitrosamino guanylidene hydrazine, lead azide, lead styphnate, nitro mannite, nitrosoguanidine, pentaerythrite tetranitrate, tetrazene, lead mononitroresorcinate

Blasting caps, with or without safety fuse (including electric blasting caps), detonating primers.

Ammunition for cannon with explosive projectiles, gas projectiles, smoke projectiles, incendiary projectiles, illuminating projectiles or shell; ammunition for small arms with incendiary projectiles; ammunition for small arms with explosive projectiles; rocket ammunition with explosive projectiles, gas projectiles, smoke projectiles, incendiary projectiles, illuminating projectiles; boosters (explosive); bursters (explosive); and supplementary charges (explosive) without detonators[d,e]

Explosive projectiles; bombs; torpedoes; mines; rifle or hand grenades (explosive); jet thrust units (jato), class A; igniters, jet thrust, class A; rocket motors, class A; igniters, rocket motor, class A[e]

Detonating fuzes, class A, with or without radioactive components

Ammunition for cannon with empty, inert-loaded or solid projectiles, or without projectiles; rocket ammunition with empty, inert-loaded or solid projectiles.

Propellant explosives, class B; jet thrust units (jato), class B; igniters, jet thrust, class B; rocket motors, class B; rocket engines (liquid), class B; igniters, rocket motor, class B; starter cartridges, jet engine, class B

Fireworks, special or railway tropedoes

Small arms ammunition, or cartridges, practice ammunition

Primers for cannon or small arms, empty cartridge bags — black powder igniters, empty cartridge cases, primed, empty grenades, primed, combination primers or percussion caps, toy caps, explosive cable cutters, explosive rivets

Percussion fuzes, tracer fuzes or tracers

Time, combination or detonating fuzes, class C

Cordeau detonant fuse, safety squibs, fuse lighters, fuse igniters, delay electric igniters, electric squibs, instantaneous fuse or igniter cord

Fireworks, common

Flammable liquids or flammable gases; Flammable liquid or flammable gas lable

Flammable solids or oxidizing materials; Flammable solid, oxidizer, or organic peroxide label

Corrosive liquids; Corrosive label

Nonflammable gases; Nonflammable gas label

Poisonous gases or liquids, in cylinders, projectiles or bombs, poison gas label

Radioactive materials

[a] Blasting caps or electric blasting caps in quantities not exceeding 1,000 caps may also be loaded and transported with articles named in vertical and horizontal columns 3, 9, 10, 11, 12, and 13. Loading and transportation blasting caps or electric blasting caps in any quantity with articles named in vertical or horizontal columns b, c, e, or f is prohibited.

[b] Unless loaded in opposite ends of car, corrosive liquids must not be loaded with flammable solids, oxidizing materials, ammunition for cannon with or without projectiles, or propellant explosives, except that shippers loading carload shipments of corrosive liquids and flammable solids or oxidizing materials and who have obtained prior approval from the Department may load such materials together when it is known that the mixutre of contents will not cause a dangerous evolution of heat or gas.

[c] Explosives, class A and explosives, class B must not be loaded or stored with chemical ammunition containing incendiary charges or white phosphorus either with or without bursting charges.

[d] Bursters (explosive), boosters (explosive), or supplementary charges (explosive) without detonators when shipped by, to or for the Department of the Army, Navy, and Air Force of the United States Government may be loaded with any of the articles named except those in columns c, d, 3, 9, 10, 11, 12, 13, 14, and 15.

[e] Does not include blasting agent, or ammonium nitrate-fuel oil mixture, ammonium nitrate, fertilizer grade, which may be loaded, transported or stored with high explosive or with blasting caps or electric blasting caps, and detonating primers.

[f] Normal uranium, depleted uranium, and thorium metal in solid form may also be loaded and transported with articles named in vertical and horizontal columns a, b, c, d, e, f, and g.

Note 1: Charged electric storage batteries must not be loaded in the same car nor stored with any class A explosive.

Note 2: Cyanides or cyanide mixtures must not be loaded or stored with acids of corrosive liquids.

Note 3: Gas identification sets may be loaded and transported with all articles named except those in column c.

Note 4: Nitric acid, when loaded in the same car with other acids or other corrosive liquids in carboys, must be separated from the other carboys. A 2 by 6 inch plank set on edge, should be nailed across the car floor at least 12 inches from the nitric acid carboys, and the space between the plank and the carboys of nitric acid should be filled with sand sifted ashes or other incombustible absorbent material.

Note 5: Smokeless powder for small arms in quantities not exceeding 100 pound-net weight in one car shall be classed as a flammable solid for purposes of transportation when approved for such classification by the Bureau of Explosives.

(49 U.S.C. 1803, 1804, 1808; 49 CFR 1.53 and App. A to Part 1)
[Amdt. 174-26, 41 FR 16092, Apr. 15, 1976 as amended by Amdt. 174-26A, 41 FR 40685, Sept. 20, 1976; Amdt. 174-3443 FR 57903, Dec. 11, 1979; Amdt. 174-34, 44 FR 31184, May 31, 1979]

SUBPART D — HANDLING OF PLACARDED CARS

§ 174.83 Switching of cars containing hazardous materials

(a) In switching operations where the use of hand brakes is necessary, a loaded placarded tank car, or a draft which includes a loaded placarded tank car, may not be cut off until the preceding car or cars clear the ladder track and the draft containing the loaded placarded tank car, or a loaded placarded tank car, shall in turn clear the ladder before another car is allowed to follow. In switching operations where hand brakes are used, it must be determined by trial whether a loaded placarded car, or a car occupied by a rider in a draft containing a placarded car, has its hand brakes in proper working condition before it is cut off.

(b) A car placarded ''EXPLOSIVES A'' or ''POISON GAS'' may not be cut off while in motion or coupled into with more force than is necessary to complete the coupling. No car moving under its own momentum shall be allowed to strike any car placarded ''EXPLOSIVES A'' or ''POISON GAS''.

(c) When transporting a car placarded ''EXPLOSIVES A'' in a terminal, yard, or on a side track, or siding, it must be separated from the engine by at least one nonplacarded car.

(d) The doors of each closed car placarded ''EXPLOSIVES A'' must be closed, securely fastened, and the lading securely braced before it is moved.
[Amdt. 174-26, 41 FR 16092, Apr. 15, 1976, as amended by Amdt. 174-26A, 41 FR 40685, Sept. 20, 1976]

§ 174.84 Switching of flatcars carrying placarded trailers or freight containers

(a) A placarded flatcar or a flatcar carrying a placarded trailer or freight container that bears any placard prescribed by Part 172 of this subchapter may not be cut off while in motion.

(b) No rail car moving under its own momentum may be permitted to strike any placarded flatcar or any flatcar carrying a placarded trailer or freight container.

(c) No placarded flatcar or any flatcar carrying a placarded trailer or freight container may be coupled into with more force than is necessary to complete the coupling.
[Amdt. 174-26, 41 FR 16092, Apr. 15, 1976, as amended by Amdt. 174-26B, 41 FR 57071. Dec. 30, 1976]

§ 174.87 Placarded cars prohibited in passenger trains, limited in mixed trains

(a) A placarded rail car may not be transported in a passenger train. However, it may be transported in a mixed train, but only at such times and between such points that freight train service is not in operation and subject to the following limitations:

(1) A placarded car (other than one placarded ''COMBUSTIBLE'') may not be transported

next to an occupied caboose or a car carrying passengers in mixed trains, except as provided in § 174.86.

(2) When a car containing hazardous materials requiring labels is moved in a mixed train and it is not occupied by an employee of the carrier, placards must be applied to the car as required by Subpart F of Part 172 of this subchapter.

§ 174.89 Position in train of cars placarded "RADIOACTIVE"

In a moving or standing train, a car placarded "RADIOACTIVE" may not be placed next to any other loaded placarded car (other than one placarded "COMBUSTIBLE"), an engine, occupied caboose, or carload of undeveloped film. Cars placarded "RADIOACTIVE" may be placed next to each other.

[Amdt. 174-26, 41 FR 16092, Apr. 15, 1976, as amended by Amdt. 174-26A, 41 FR 40685, Sept. 20, 1976; Amdt. 174-26B, 41 FR 57071, Dec. 30, 1976]

SUBPART K — DETAILED REQUIREMENTS FOR RADIOACTIVE MATERIALS

§ 174.700 Special handling requirements for radioactive materials

(a) Each rail shipment of low specific activity materials as defined in § 173.389(c) of this subchapter must be loaded so as to avoid spillage and scattering of loose material. Loading restrictions are prescribed in §173.392 of this subchapter.

(b)The number of packages of radioactive materials that may be transported in any rail car or stored at any single location is limited to that number which does not make a total transport index number (as defined in § 173.389(j) of this subchapter, and determined by adding together the transport index numbers on the labels of the individual packages) of more than 50. This provision does not apply to exclusive use shipments as described in §§ 173.389(o) and 173.392, 173.393(j), or 173.396(f).

(c) Each package of radioactive material bearing RADIOACTIVE YELLOW-II or RADIOACTIVE YELLOW-III labels when being placed in a rail car, depot, or other place may not be placed closer than 3 ft to an area (or dividing partition between areas) which may be continuously occupied by any passenger, rail employee, or shipment of animals, nor closer than 15 ft to any package containing undeveloped film (if so marked). If more than one package of radioactive materials is present, the distance must be computed from the table below on the basis of the total transport index number (determined by adding together the transport index numbers on the labels of the individual packages) of packages in the car or storeroom:

Total transport index	Minimum separation distance in feet to nearest undeveloped film[a]	Minimum distance in feet to area of persons, or minimum distance in feet from dividing partition of a combination car[b]
None	0	0
0.1 to 10.0	15	3
10.1 to 20.0	22	4
20.1 to 30.0	29	5
30.1 to 40.0	33	6
40.1 to 50.0	36	7

[a] In feet to nearest undeveloped filme.

[b] In feet to area of persons, or minimum distance in feet from dividing partition of a combination car.

NOTE: The distance in the table must be measured from the nearest point on the packages of radioactive materials.

(d) Each fissile Class III radioactive material shipment (as defined in § 173.389(a)(3) of this subchapter) must be transported in accordance with one of the methods prescribed in § 173.396(g) of this subchapter. The transport controls must be adequate to assure that no fissile Class III shipment is transported in the same rail car with any other fissile radioactive material shipment. In loading and storage areas each fissile class III shipment must be segregated by a distance of at least 20 ft from other packages required to bear one of the "radioactive" labels described in Part 172 of this subchapter.

(e) A flatcar may be used to transport radioactive materials in a container weighing 15,000 lb or more. A gondola car (other than a drop bottom car) may be used to transport any of the following:

(1) Radioactive materials in containers weighing 5000 lb or more;
(2) Strong wooden boxes with inside containers of solid radioactive material, security braced and cushioned; or
(3) Radioactive material in concrete vaults weighing 700 lb. or more.

(f) A person may not remain unnecessarily in a rail car contining radioactive materials. [Amdt. 174-26, 41 FR 16092, Apr. 15, 1976, as amended by Amdt. 174-26A, 41 FR 40686, Sept. 20, 1976; Amdt. 174032, 43 FR 48645, Oct. 19, 1978]

§ 174.715 Cleanliness of cars after use

(a) Each transport vehicle used for transporting radioactive materials as exclusive use, as defined in § 173.389(e) must be surveyed with appropriate radiation detection instruments after each use. A vehicle may not be returned to service until the radiation dose rate at any accessible surface is 0.5 mrem/hr or less, and there is no significant removable radioactive surface contamination, as defined in paragraph (a) of this section.

(b) This section does not apply to any rail car used solely for transporting radioactive materials if a survey of the interior surface of the car shows that the radiation dose rate does not exceed 10 mrem/hr at the interior surface or 2 mrem/hr at 3 ft from any interior surface. The car must be stenciled with the words "FOR RADIOACTIVE MATERIALS USE ONLY" in lettering at least 3 in. high in a conspicuous place on both sides of the exterior of the car and it must be kept closed at all times other than during loading and unloading. [Amdt. 174-26, 41 FR 16092, Apr. 15, 1976, as amended by Amdt. 174-26A, 41 FR 40686, Sept. 20, 1976]

§ 174.750 Incidents involving leakage

(a) In addition to the incident reporting requirements of §§ 171.15 and 171.16 of this subchapter, the carrier shall also notify the shipper at the earliest practicable moment following any incident in which there has been breakage, spillage, or suspected radioactive contamination involving radioactive materials shipments. Vehicles, buildings, areas, or equipment in which radioactive materials have been spilled may not be again placed in service or routinely occupied until the radiation dose rate at any accessible surface is less than 0.5 mrem/hr and there is no significant removable radioactive surface contamination (see § 173.397 of this subchapter).

(b) The package or materials should be segregated as far as practicable from personnel contact. If radiological advice or assistance is needed, the Energy Research and Development Administration (ERDA) should also be notified. In case of obvious leakage, or if it appears likely that the inside container may have been damaged, care should be taken to avoid inhalation, ingestion, or contact with the radioactive material. Any loose radioactive materials should be left in a segregated area and held pending disposal instructions, from qualified persons. Information involving the handling of radioactive materials in the event of a wreck may be found in Bureau of Explosives Pamphlet No. 1 and No. 2.

APPENDIX E
TITLE 49, PART 175*

PART 175 — CARRIAGE BY AIRCRAFT

SUBPART A — GENERAL INFORMATION AND REGULATIONS

§ 175.1 Purpose and scope

This part prescribes requirements, in addition to those contained in Parts 171, 172, and 173 of this subchapter, to be observed by aircraft operators with respect to the transportation of hazardous materials aboard (including attached to or suspended from) civil aircrafts.

§ 175.3 Unacceptable hazardous materials shipments

A shipment of hazardous materials that is not prepared for shipment in accordance with Parts 172 and 173 of this subchapter may not be accepted for transportation or transported aboard an aircraft.

§ 175.5 Applicability

This part contains regulations pertaining to the acceptance of hazardous materials for transportation of hazardous materials, in any civil aircraft in the U.S. and in civil aircraft of U.S. registry anywhere in air commerce, except aircraft of U.S. registry under lease to and operated solely by foreign nationals outside the U.S.

§ 175.10 Exceptions

(a) This subchapter does not apply to

(1) Aviation fuel and oil in tanks that are in compliance with the installation provisions of 14 CFR, Chapter 1.

(2) Aircraft parts, equipment, and supplies (other than fuel) carried by an aircraft operator if authorized or required aboard his aircraft for their operation including:

- (i) Fire extinguishers;
- (ii) Cylinders containing compressed gases;
- (iii) Aerosol dispensers;
- (iv) Distilled spirits;
- (v) Hydraulic accumulators;
- (vi) Nonspillable batteries;
- (vii) First-aid kits;
- (viii) Signaling devices;
- (ix) Tires; and
- (x) Items of replacement therefore, except that batteries, aerosol dispensers, and signaling devices must be packed in strong outside containers, and tires must be deflated to a pressure not greater than 100 p.s.i.g.

(3) Hazardous materials loaded and carried in hoppers or tanks of aircraft certificated for use in aerial seeding, dusting, spraying, fertilizing, crop improvement, or pest control, to be dispensed during such an operation.

(4) Medicinal and toilet articles carried by a crewmember or passenger in his baggage (including carry-on baggage) when;

* From *Fed. Reg.*, September 20, 1976.

(i) The total capacity of all the containers used by a crewmember or passenger does not exceed 75 oz (net weight ounces and fluid ounces);

(ii) The capacity of each container other than an aerosol container does not exceed 16 fluid oz or 1 lb of material.

(5) Small-arms ammunition for personal use carried by a crewmember or passenger in his baggage (excluding carry-on baggage) if securely packed in fiber, wood, or metal boxes.

(6) Prior to May 3, 1981, radioactive materials which meet the requirements of § 173.391(a), (b), or (c) of this subchapter in effect on May 3, 1979.

(7) Oxygen, or any hazardous material used for the generation of oxygen, carried for medical use by a passenger in accordance with 14 CFR 121.574 or 135.114.

(8) Human beings and animals with an implanted medical device, such as a heart pacemaker, that contains radioactive material or with radio-pharmaceuticals that have been injected or ingested.

(9) Smoke grenades, flares, or similar devices carried only for use during a sport parachute jumping activity.

(10) Personal smoking materials intended for use by any individual when carried on his person except lighters with flammable liquid reservoirs and containers containing lighter fluid for use in refilling lighters.

(11) Smoke grenades, flares, and pyrotechnic devices affixed to aircraft carrying no person other than a required flight crewmember during any flight conducted at and as a part of a scheduled air show or exhibition of aeronautical skill. The affixed installation accommodating the smoke grenades, flares, or pyrotechnic devices on the aircraft must be approved by the FAA for its intended use.

(12) Hazardous materials which are loaded and carried on or in cargo-only aircraft and which are to be dispensed or expended during flight for weather control, forest preservation and protection, or avalanche control purposes when the following requirements are met:

(i) Operations may not be conducted over densely populated areas, in a congested airway, or near any airport where air carrier passenger operations are conducted.

(ii) Each operator shall prepare and keep current a manual containing operational guidelines and handling procedures, for the use and guidance of flight, maintenance, and ground personnel concerned in the dispensing or expending of hazardous materials. The manual must be approved by the FAA District Office having jurisdiction over the operator's certificate, if any, or the FAA Regional Office in the region where the operator is located. Each operation must be conducted in accordance with the manual.

(iii) No person other than a required flight member, FAA inspector, or person necessary for handling or dispensing the hazardous material may be carried on the aircraft.

(iv) The operator of the aircraft must have advance permission from the owner of any airport to be used for the dispensing or expending operation.

(v) When dynamite and blasting caps are carried for avalanche control flights, the explosives must be handled, and, at all times be, under the control of a blaster who is licensed under a state or local authority identified in writing to the FAA district office having jurisdiction over the operator's certificate, if any, or the FAA regional office in the region where the operator is located.

(49 U.S.C. 1803, 1804, 1806, 1808; 49 CFR 1.53 and App. A to Part 1)

[Amdt. 175-1, 41 FR 16106. Apr. 15, 1976, as amended by Amdt. 175-1A, 41 FR 40686, Sept. 20, 1976]

Note: For amendments to § 175.10 see the List of CFR Sections Affected appearing in the Finding Aids section of this volume.

§ 175.20 Compliance

Unless the regulations in this subchapter specifically provided that another person must perform a duty, each operator shall comply with all the regulations in Parts 102, 171, 172, and 175 of this subchapter and shall thoroughly instruct his employees in relation thereto. (See 14 CFR 121.135, 121.401, 121.438a, 135.27 and 135.140.)

§ 175.30 Accepting shipments

(a) No person may accept a hazardous material for transportation aboard an aircraft unless the hazardous material is

(1) Authorized, and is within the quantity limitations specified for carriage aboard aircraft according to § 172.101 of this subchapter;
(2) Described and certified on a shipping paper prepared in duplicate in accordance with Subpart C of Part 172 of this subchapter. The originating aircraft operator must retain one copy of each shipping paper for 90 days;
(3) Labeled and marked, or placarded (when required), in accordance with Subparts D, E and F of Part 172 of this subchapter; and
(4) Labeled with a "CARGO AIRCRAFT ONLY" label (see § 172.448 of this subchapter) if the material as presented is not permitted aboard passenger-carrying aircraft.

(b) Except as provided in paragraph (c) of this section, no person may carry any hazardous material aboard an aircraft unless, prior to placing the material aboard the aircraft, the operator of the aircraft has inspected the package, or the outside container prepared in accordance with § 173.25 of this subchapter which contains the material, and has determined that it has no holes, leakage, or other indications that its integrity has been compromised, and for radioactive materials that the package seal has not been broken.

(c) The requirements of paragraph (b) of this section do not apply to ORM-D materials packed in a freight container and offered for transportation by one consignor.

[Amdt. 175-1, 41 FR 16106. Aprl 15, 1976, as amended by Amdt. 175-1A, 41 FR 40686, Sept. 20, 1976; Amdt. 175-1B, 41 FR 57072, Dec. 30, 1976]

§ 175.33 Notification of pilot-in-command

When materials subject to the provisions of this subchapter are carried in an aircraft, the operator of the aircraft shall give the pilot-in-command the following information in writing before takeoff:

(a) The information required by §§ 172-202 and 172.203 of this subchapter;
(b) The location of the hazardous material in the aircraft; and
(c) The results of the inspection required by § 175.30(b).

[Amdt. 175-1A, 41 FR 40686, Sept. 20, 1976]

§ 175.35 Shipping papers aboard aircraft

(a) A copy of the shipping papers required by § 175.30(a)(2) must accompany the shipment it covers during transportation aboard an aircraft.

(b) The documents required by paragraph (a) of this section and § 175.33 may be combined into one document if it is given to the pilot-in-command before departure of the aircraft.

§ 175.40 Keeping and replacement of labels

(a) Aircraft operators who engage in the transportation of hazardous materials must be kept an adequate supply of the labels specified in Subpart E of Part 172 of this subchapter, on hand at each location where shipments are loaded aboard aircraft.

(b) Lost or detached labels for packages of hazardous materials must be replaced in accordance with the information provided on the shipping papers.

§ 175.45 Reporting hazardous materials incidents

(a) Each operator that transports hazardous materials shall report to the nearest Air Carrier District Office (ACDO), Flight Standards District Office (FSDO), General Aviation District Office (GADO) or other FAA facility, except that in place of reporting to the nearest of those facilities a certificate holder under 15 CFR Part 121, 127, or 135 may report to the FAA District Office holding the carrier's operating certificate and charged with overall inspection of its operations, by telephone at the earliest practicable moment after each incident that occurs during the course of transportation (including loading, unloading or temporary storage) in which as a direct result of any hazardous material

(1) A person is killed;
(2) A person receives injuries requiring his or her hospitalization;
(3) Estimated carrier or other property damage, or both, exceeds $50,000;
(4) Fire, breakage, or spillage or suspected radioactive contamination occurs involving shipment of radioactive materials (see § 175.700(b));
(5) Fire, breakage, spillage, or suspected contamination occurs involving shipment of etiologic agents. In addition to the report required by paragraph (a) of this section, a report on an incident involving etiologic agents should be telephoned directly to the Director, Center for Disease Control, U.S. Public Health, Atlanta, Georgia, area code 404-633-5313; or
(6) A situation exists of such a nature that, in the judgment of the carrier, it should be reported to the Department even though it does not meet the criteria of paragraph (a)(1), (2), or (3) of this section, e.g., a continuing danger to life exists at the scene of the incident.
(7) If the operator conforms to the provisions of this section, the carrier requirements of § 171.15 except § 171.15(c) of this subchapter shall be deemed to have been satisfied.

(b) The following information shall be furnished in each report:

(1) Name of reporting person;
(2) Name and address of carrier represented by reporter;
(3) Phone number where reporter can be contacted;
(4) Date, time, and location of incident;
(5) The extent of the injuries, if any; and
(6) Classification, name and quantity of hazardous material involvement and whether a continuing danger to life exists at the scene.

(c) Each operator who transports hazardous materials shall report in writing, in duplicate, on DOT Form F 5800.1 within 15 days of the date of discovery, each incident that occurs during the course of transportation (including loading, unloading, or temporary storage) in which, as a direct result to hazardous materials, any of the circumstances set forth in paragraph (a) of this section occurs or there has been an unintentional release of hazardous materials from a package. Each operator making a report under this section shall send that report to the Materials Transportation Bureau, Office of Hazardous Materials Regulation, Department

of Transportation, Washington, D.C. 20590, with a separate copy to the FAA facility indicated in paragraph (a) of this section.
[Amdt. 175-1, 41 FR 16106, Aprl 15, 1976, as amended by Amdt. 175-1A, 41 FR 40686, Sept. 20, 1976]

SUBPART B — LOADING, UNLOADING AND HANDLING

§ 175.75 Quantity limitations aboard aircraft

(a) Except as provided in § 175.85(b), no person may carry on an aircraft

(1) A hazardous material except as permitted in Part 172 of this subchapter;
(2) More than 50 lb net weight of hazardous material (and in addition thereto, 150 lb net weight of nonflammable compressed gas) permitted to be carried aboard passenger-carrying aircraft

   (i) In an inaccessible cargo compartment.
   (ii) In any freight container within an accessible cargo compartment, or
   (iii) In any accessible cargo compartment in a cargo-only aircraft in a manner that makes it inaccessible unless in a freight container;

(3) Packages containing radioactive materials when their combined transport indices exceed 50.

(b) No limitation applies to the number of packages of ORM material aboard an aircraft.
[Amdt. 175-1A, 41 FR 40686, Sept. 20, 1976]

§ 175.78 Stowage compatibility of cargo

(a) No person may stow a package of a corrosive material on an aircraft next to or in a position that will allow contact with a package of flammable solids, oxidizing materials, or organic peroxides.

(b) No person may stow a package labeled BLASTING AGENT on an aircraft next to, or in a position that will allow contact with a package of special fireworks or railway torpedoes.
[Amdt. 175-1, FR 16106, Apr. 15, 1976, as amended by Amdt. 175-8, 44 FR 31184, May 31, 1979]

§ 175.79 Orientation of cargo

(a) A package containing hazardous materials marked "THIS SIDE UP", "THIS END UP", or with arrows to indicate the proper orientation of the package, must be stored, loaded aboard an aircraft in accordance with such markings, and secured in a manner that will prevent any movement which would change the orientation of the package.

(b) A package containing liquid hazardous materials not marked as indicated in paragraph (a) of this section must be stored and loaded with closures up.

§ 175.85 Cargo location

(a) No person may carry a hazardous material subject to the requirements of this subchapter in the cabin of a passenger-carrying aircraft.

(b) Each person carrying materials acceptable only for cargo-only aircraft shall carry those materials in location accessible to a crewmember during flight. However, when materials acceptable for cargo-only or passenger carrying aircraft are carried on a small, single pilot, cargo-only aircraft being used where other means of transportation are impracticable or not available, they may be carried without quantity limitation as specified in § 175.75 in a location that is not accessible to the pilot subject to the following conditions.

(1) No person other than the pilot, an FAA inspector, the shipper or consignee of the material or a representative of the shipper or consignee so designated in writing, or a person necessary for handling the material may be carried on the aircraft.
(2) The pilot must be provided with written instructions on characteristics and proper handling of the material.
(3) Whenever a change of pilots occurs while the material is on board, the new pilot must be briefed under a hand-to-hand signature service provided by the operator of the aircraft.

(c) No person may load magnetized material (which might cause an erroneous magnetic compass reading) on an aircraft, in the vicinity of a magnetic compass, or compass master unit, that is a part of the instrument equipment of the aircraft, in a manner that affects its operation. If this requirement cannot be met, a special aircraft swing and compass calibration may be made. No person loading magnetized materials may obscure the warning labels.

(d) No person may carry materials subject to the requirements of this subchapter in an aircraft unless they are suitably safeguarded to prevent their becoming a hazard by shifting. For packages bearing "RADIOACTIVE YELLOW-II" or "RADIOACTIVE YELLOW-III" labels, such safeguarding must prevent movement that would permit the package to be closer to a space that is occupied by a person or an animal than is permitted by § 175.700.

(e) No person may carry a material subject to the requirements of this subchapter that is acceptable for carriage in a passenger-carrying aircraft (other than magnetized materials) unless it is located in the aircraft in a place that is inaccessible to persons other than crewmembers.

[Amdt. 175-1, 41 FR 16106, Apr. 15, 1976, as amended by Amdt. 175-1A, 41 FR 40686, Sept. 20, 1976]

§ 175.90 Damaged shipments

Except as provided for in § 175.700, the operator of an aircraft shall remove from the aircraft any package subject to this subchapter that appears to be damaged or leaking. No person shall place or transport a package that is damaged or appears to be damaged or leaking aboard an aircraft subject to this Part.

[Amdt. 175-1, 41 FR 16106, Apr. 15, 1976, as amended by Amdt. 175-1A, 41 FR 40686, Sept. 20, 1976]

SUBPART C — SPECIFIC REGULATIONS APPLICABLE ACCORDING TO CLASSIFICATION OF MATERIAL

§ 175.700 Special requirements for radioactive materials

(a) No person may place any package of radioactive materials bearing "RADIOACTIVE YELLOW-II" or "RADIOACTIVE YELLOW-III" labels in an aircraft closer than the distances shown in the following table to a space (or dividing partition between spaces) which may be continuously occupied by people, or shipments of animals, or closer than the distances shown in the following table to any package containing undeveloped film (if so marked). If more than one of these packages is present, the distance shall be computed from the following table on the basis of the total transport index numbers shown on labels of the individual packages in the aircraft;

Total transport index	Minimum separation distances in feet to the nearest undeveloped film for various times of transit: Up to 2 hr	2—4 hr	4—8 hr	8—12 hr	Over 12 hr	Minimum distance in feet to area of persons, or minimum distance in feet from dividing partition of cargo compartment
None	0	0	0	0	0	0
0.1 to 1.0	1	2	3	4	5	1
1.1 to 5.0	3	4	6	8	11	2
5.1 to 10.0	4	6	9	11	15	3
10.1 to 20.0	5	8	12	16	22	4
20.1 to 30.0	7	10	15	20	29	5
30.1 to 40.0	8	11	17	22	33	6
40.1 to 50.0	9	12	19	24	36	7

(b) In addition to the reporting requirements of § 175.45, the carrier must also notify the shipper at the earliest practicable moment following any incident in which there has been breakage, spillage, or suspected radioactive contamination involving radioactive materials shipments. Aircraft in which radioactive materials have been spilled may not be again placed in service or routinely occupied until the radiation does rate at any accessible surface is less than 0.5 mrem/hr and there is no significant removable radioactive surface contamination (see § 173.397 of this subchapter). In these instances, the package or materials should be segregated as far as practicable from personnel contact. If radiological advice or assistance is needed, the U.S. Energy Research and Development Administration should also be notified. In case of obvious leakage, or if it appears likely that the inside container may have been damaged, care should be taken to avoid inhalation, ingestion, or contact with the radioactive materials. Any loose radioactive materials should be left in a segregated area pending disposal instructions from qualified persons.

(c) No person may carry aboard a passenger-carrying aircraft any package of radioactive material which contains a large quantity (large radioactive source) of radioactivity (as defined in § 173.389(b) of this subchapter), except as specifically approved by the Director, Office of Hazardous Materials Regulation, Materials Transportation Bureau, Department of Transportation.

(d) Except as provided in this paragraph, no person may carry aboard a passenger-carrying aircraft any radioactive material other than a radioactive material intended for use in, or incident to, research or medical diagnosis or treatment. Prior to May 3, 1981, this prohibition does not apply to materials which meet the requirements of § 173.391(a), (b), or (c) of this subchapter in effect on May 3, 1979.

(49 U.S.C. 1803, 1804, 1806, 1808; 49 CFR 1.53 and App. A to Part 1)

[Amdt. 175-1, 41 FR 16106, Apr. 15, 1976, as amended by Amdt. 175-4, 42 FR 22367, May 3, 1977]

Note: For amendments to § 175.700 see the List of CFR Sections Affected appearing in the Finding Aids section of this volume.

§ 175.710 Special requirements for fissile Class III radioactive materials

(a) No person may carry aboard any aircraft any package of fissile Class III radioactive material (as defined in § 173.389(a)(3) of this subchapter), except as follows:

(1) On a cargo-only aircraft which has been assigned for the sole use of the consignor for the specific shipment of fissile radioactive material. Instructions for such sole use must be provided for in special arrangements between the consignor and carrier, with instructions to that effect issued with shipping papers; or

(2) On any aircraft on which there is no other package of radioactive materials required to bear one of the RADIOACTIVE labels described in §§ 172.436, 172.438, and 172.440 of this subchapter. Specific arrangements must be effected between the shipper and carriers, with instructions to that effect issued with the shipping papers; or

(3) In accordance with any other procedure specifically approved by the Director, Office of Hazardous Materials Regulation, Materials Transportation Bureau.

[Amdt. 175-1, 41 FR 16106, Apr. 15, 1976, as amended by Amdt. 175-6, 43 FR 48645, Oct. 19, 1978]

APPENDIX F
TITLE 49, PART 176*

PART 176 — CARRIAGE BY VESSEL

SUBPART A — GENERAL

§ 176.1 Purpose and scope

This part prescribes requirements in addition to those contained in Parts 171, 172, and 173 of this subchapter to be observed with respect to the transportation of hazardous materials by vessel.

SUBPART D — GENERAL SEGREGATION REQUIREMENTS

§ 176.80 Application

(a) This subpart sets forth segregation requirements in addition to any segregation requirements set forth elsewhere in this subchapter.

(b) Hazardous materials in limited quantities when loaded in transport vehciles and freight containers, are excepted from the segregation requirements of this subpart and any additional segregation specified in this subchapter for transportation by vessel.

[Amdt. 176-1, 41 FR 16110, Apr. 15, 1976, as amended by Amdt. 176-3, 42 FR 57967, Nov. 7, 1977]

§ 176.83 Segregation requirements for cargo vessels and passenger vessels

(a) The following table specifies the categories of explosives which may not be loaded or stowed together within the same hold or compartment. The letter "X" at an intersection of a horizontal and vertical column indicates that these categories may not be stowed together in the same hold or compartment.

(b) The following table (Table 2) specifies the minimum separation requirements that apply when transporting different classes of hazardous materials on board a vessel, other than a ferry vessel. The symbols used in the table below mean the following:

(1) "1" — Away from.
(2) "2" — Separated from.
(3) "3" — Separated by a complete cargo compartment or hold from.
(4) "4" — Separated longitudinally by an intervening complete cargo compartment or hold from.
(5) "0" — No general segregation specified; individual entries in the Hazardous Material Table in § 172.101 of this subchapter should be consulted.
(6) "*" — Consult Table I of this section for segregation requirements between different explosives.

(c) *Definition of terms.*

(1) *Legend.*

(i) Reference package 

* From *Fed. Reg.*, April 15, 1976.

(ii) Incompatible package 

(iii) Deck resistant to liquid and fire 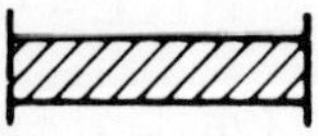

Note: Solid vertical lines represent transverse watertight bulkheads between holds.

(2) *Away from.* ''Away from'' means effectively segregated so that materials may not interact dangerously in the event of an accident. These materials may be stowed in the same cargo compartment, hold, deck area or barge provided a minimum horizontal separation of 10 ft, projected vertically, is provided.

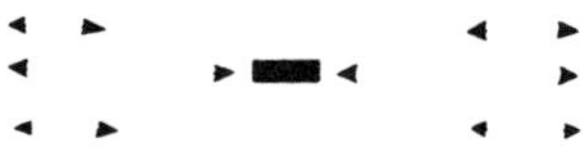

(3) *Separate from*

(i) ''Separate from'' means in separate holds when stowed ''under deck''. If the intervening deck is resistant to fire and liquid, a vertical separation, i.e., in different cargo compartments, is considered equivalent to this requirement. For ''on deck'' stowage, ''away from'' segregation is authorized.

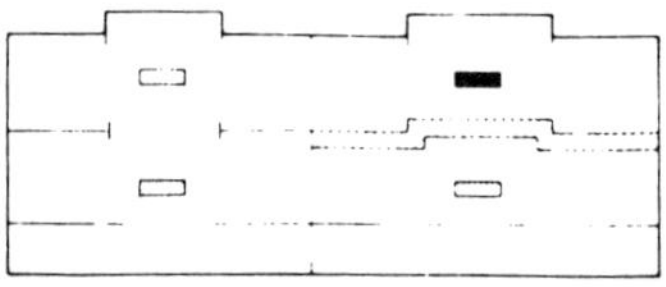

(ii) On barge-carrying vessels, separate barges are required if the barges are constructed of steel. Otherwise separate holds are required.

Table 2

		1(A)	1(B)	1(C)	2(A)	2(B)	3	4(A)	4(B)	4(C)	5(A)	5(B)	6(A)	6(B)	7	8	9
Explosives A	1(a)	·	·	·	4	2	4	4	4	4	4	4	2	2	2	4	0
Explosives B	1(B)	·	·	·	4	2	4	3	3	4	4	4	2	2	2	2	0
Explosives C, blasting agents	1(C)	·	·	·	2	1	2	2	2	2	2	2	1	0	2	2	0
Flammable compressed gases	2(A)	4	4	2	—	0	2	1	2	1	2	4	0	0	2	1	0
Nonflammable compressed bases	2(B)	2	2	1	0	—	2	0	1	0	0	2	0	0	1	0	0
Flammable or combustible liquids	3	4	4	2	2	2	—	2	2	2	2	3	2	0	2	1	0
Flammable solids	4(A)	4	3	2	1	0	2	—	1	1	1	2	0	0	2	1	0
Flammable solids labeled spontaneously combustible	4(B)	4	3	2	2	1	2	1	—	1	2	2	1	0	2	1	0
Flammable solids labeled dangerous when wet	4(C)	4	4	2	1	0	2	1	1	—	2	2	0	0	2	1	0
Oxidizers	5(A)	4	4	2	2	0	2	1	2	2	—	2	0	1	1	2	0
Organic peroxides	5(B)	4	4	2	4	2	3	2	2	2	2	—	2	1	2	2	0
Class A poisons	6(A)	2	2	1	0	0	2	0	1	0	0	2	—	0	1	0	0
Class B poisons or irritating materials	6(B)	2	2	0	0	0	0	0	0	0	1	1	0	—	0	0	0
Radioactive materials	7	2	2	2	2	1	2	2	2	2	1	2	1	0	—	2	0
Corrosive materials	8	4	2	2	1	0	1	1	1	1	2	2	0	0	2	—	0
Other regulated (ORM) materials	9	0	0	0	0	0	0	0	0	0	0	0	0	0	0	0	—

(4) *Separate by a complete cargo compartment or hold from.*

(i) "Separate by a complete cargo compartment or hold from" means either a vertical or horizontal separation. If the decks are not resistant to fire and liquid, a longitudinal separation by an intervening complete cargo compartment is required. For "on deck" stowage this segregation means a separation by a corresponding horizontal distance.

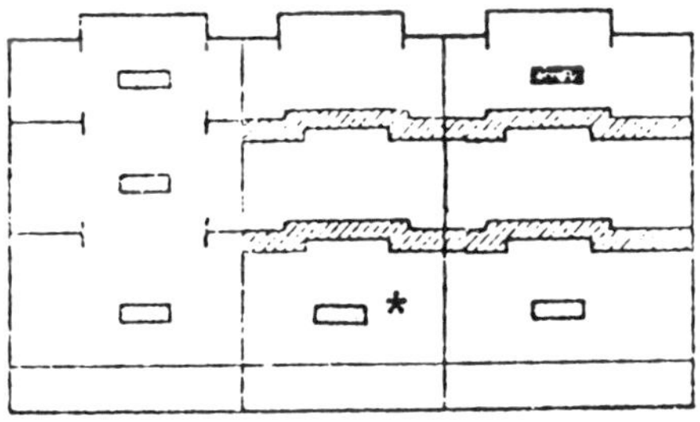

(ii) For barges aboard barge-carrying vessels, the following requirements apply:

(A) For barges loaded on ships having vertical holds, separate barge holds are required.

(B) For barges loaded on ships having horizontal barge levels are required.

(5) *Separate longitudinally by an intervening complete cargo compartment or hold or engine room from*

(i) "Separate longitudinally by an intervening complete cargo compartment or hold or engine room from" means a horizontal separation by a complete intervening hold (two intervening bulkheads) or engine room. Vertical separation alone does not meet this requirement. For "on deck" stowage, this segregation means a separation by the vessel's bridge or superstructure:

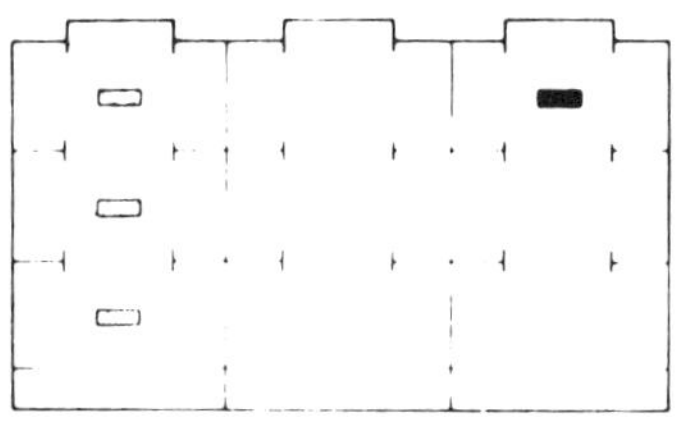

(ii) For barges aboard barge-carrying vessels the following requirements apply:

(A) For barges loaded on ships having vertical holds, separation by an intervening barge hold or engine room is required.

(B) For barges loaded on ships having horizontal barge levels, separate barge levels and a longitudinal separation by at least two intervening barges are required.

(d) In applying the minimum separation requirements specified in Table 2 to freight containers containing hazardous materials, the following additional requirements apply:

* When the stowage location of the incompatible package is in this relation to the reference package, at least one of the intervening decks in the vertical plane must be resistant to fire and liquid.

(1) *Class segregation.* Materials for which any segregation is specified in Table 2 may not be stowed in the same freight container.

(2) *Vertical stowage requirements.* Freight containers either closed or open may not be stowed in the same vertical line when segregation is required unless separated by a deck resistant to fire and liquid. When a solid substance is required to be stowed ''Away from'' another substance, it may be stowed above the other provided a minimum distance of 8 ft intervenes. When ''Separate by a complete cargo compartment or hold from'' is required, freight containers separated by a deck resistant to fire and liquid may not be stowed in the same vertical line unless two such decks intervene.

(3) *Horizontal stowage requirements.*

(i) ''Away from''

- (A) For closed freight containers stowed on or under deck there are no restrictions in regard to freight container location in relation to other freight containers.
- (B) For open containers stowed on or under deck, a minimum separation of 20 ft must be provided in the fore and aft direction unless separated by a bulkhead resistant to fire and water or a minimum athwartships separation of 8 ft must be provided.

(ii) ''Separated from''

- (A) For closed freight containers on or under deck a fore and aft separation of at least 20 ft must be provided unless separated by a bulkhead resistant to fire and water or a minimum athwartships separation of 16 ft must be provided.
- (B) For open freight containers stowed on deck a minimum separation of 20 ft must be provided in the fore and aft direction or a minimum separation of 16 ft must be provided in the athwartships direction.
- (C) Open freight containers stowed under deck must be separated by a bulkhead resistant to fire and water.

(iii) ''Separate by a complete cargo compartment or hold from''

- (A) For closed or open freight containers on deck a minimum separation of 20 ft must be provided in the fore and aft direction or a minimum separation of 24 ft must be provided in the athwartships direction.
- (B) Closed freight containers under deck must be segregated by one bulkhead resistant to fire and water.
- (C) Open freight containers underdeck must be segregated by two bulk-bulkheads resistant to fire and water.

(iv) ''Separated longitudinally by an intervening complete cargo compartment or hold from''

- (A) Closed or open freight containers on deck must be separated by a distance of 80 ft.
- (B) Closed freight containers underdeck must be separated by at least two bulkheads resistant to fire and water or one bulkhead resistant to fire and water and a total distance of at least 80 ft provided the containers are not stowed less than 20 ft from the intervening bulkhead.

(C) Open freight containers under deck must be separated by at least two bulkheads resistant to fire and water.

(e) In applying the minimum separation requirements specified in Table 2 to portable tanks and railroad and highway vehicles containing hazardous materials, paragraph (d) of this section pertaining to freight containers applies.

(f) A ferry vessel (when operating either as a passenger or cargo vessel) which cannot provide the type of separation required in this section may carry incompatible hazardous materials in separate highway or railroad vehicles if they are stowed to give the maximum possible separation.

(49 U.S.C. 1803, 1804, 1808; 49 CFR 1.53 and App. A to Part 1)

[Amdt. 176-1. 41 FR 16110, Apr. 15, 1976, as amended by Amdt. 176-1A, 41 FR 40688. Sept. 20, 1976]

Note: For amendments to § 176.83 see the List of CFR Sections Affected appearing in the Finding Aids section of this volume.

SUBPART E — SPECIAL REQUIREMENTS FOR TRANSPORT VEHICLES LOADED WITH HAZARDOUS MATERIALS AND TRANSPORTED ON BOARD FERRY VESSELS

§ 176.88 Application

The requirements in this subpart are applicable to transport vehicles containing hazardous materials being transported on board ferry vessels and are in addition to any prescribed elsewhere in this subchapter. Vessels in a service similar to a ferry service, but not over a designated ferry route, may be treated as a ferry vessel for the purpose of this subpart if approved in writing by the District Commander.

[Amdt. 176-1, 41 FR 16110, Apr. 15, 1976, as amended by Amdt. 176-1A, 41 FR 40690, Sept. 20, 1976]

176.89 Control of transport vehicles

(a) A transport vehicle containing hazardous materials may be transported on board a ferry vessel, subject to the following conditions:

(1) The operator or person in charge of the vehicle shall deliver to the vessel's representative a copy of the shipping papers and certificate required by § 176.24 and § 176.27;

(2) The vehicle shall be placed at the location indicated by the vessel's representative;

(3) The parking brakes of the vehicle shall be set securely to prevent movement;

(4) The motor of a highway vehicle shall be shut off and not restarted until the vessel has completed its voyage and docked;

(5) All vehicle lights shall be cut off and not relighted until the vessel has completed its voyage and docked;

(6) The operator of a highway vehicle shall remain with the vehicle;

(7) No repairs or adjustments must be made to the vehicle while it is on the vessel;

(8) No hazardous materials are to be released from the vehicle; and

(9) Any instructions given by the vessel's representative during the voyage, and during "roll on" and "roll off" operations must be observed.

(b) Smoking by any person in or around a vehicle is prohibited.

SUBPART M — DETAILED REQUIREMENTS FOR RADIOACTIVE MATERIALS

§ 176.700 General stowage requirements

(a) Each package or container bearing "RADIOACTIVE WHITE" or "RADIOACTIVE YELLOW" labels and being transported on a vessel must be stowed separately from any living accommodations and from any space continuously occupied by any person. Separate stowage is not required from a space occupied by a courier especially authorized to accompany a shipment.

(b) Mail bags may not be stowed in the same hold with radioactive materials.

(c) A package of radioactive materials which is a significant heat source may not be overstowed with any other cargo. If the package is stowed under deck, the hold or compartment in which it is stowed must be ventilated.

(d) Each Fissile Class III shipment must be stowed in a separate hold or compartment and be stowed and handled at least 20 ft from all other packages bearing "RADIOACTIVE YELLOW" labels.

(e) A person may not remain unnecessarily in a hold or compartment or in the immediate vicinity of any package on deck containing radioactive materials. A person may not be exposed to a total of more than 100 mrem in any 7-day period or more than 500 mrem/year whole body dose.

(f) The radiation level in any space or area continuously occupied by passengers, crew, or shipments of animals may not exceed 0.5 mrem/hr.

(g) In the case of a shipment or radioactive materials requiring supplemental operational procedures, the shipper shall furnish the master or person in charge of the vessel a copy of the necessary operational instructions.

(h) The following requirements apply to the stowage of packages of radioactive materials on board a vessel with regard to transport index numbers which are shown on the labels of individual packages:

(1) The sum of the transport indexes of any group of packages may not exceed 50. Each group of packages must be separated by at least 20 ft from all other packages bearing "RADIOACTIVE YELLOW" labels. This separation requirement does not apply to low specific activity or a full load if the consignor has the exclusive use of the entire vessel and the sum of the transport indexes of any group of Fissile Class II packages does not exceed 50.

(2) The sum of the transport indexes of all packages of radioactive materials on board a vessel may not exceed 200.

(3) Packages bearing "RADIOACTIVE YELLOW" labels may not be stowed any closer to persons or undeveloped film than the distances specified in the following table:

Sum of transport indexes of the packages	Minimum distance in feet from living accommodation or regularly occupied working space				Minimum distance[a] in feet from undeveloped films or plates: Less than 24-hr voyage	24 up to 48-hr voyage	Over 2 up 4-day voyage				Over 4 up to 9-day voyage				Over 9 up to 16-day voyage				Over 16 up to 25-day voyage				Over 25 up to 36-day voyage				Over 36 up to 49-day voyage			
	A	B	C	D	A	A	A	B	C	D	A	B	C	D	A	B	C	D	A	B	C	D	A	B	C	D	A	B	C	D
0 through 0.5	10	10	10	10	3	5	10	10	10	10	15	10	10	10	20	10	10	10	20	10	10	10	25	15	10	10	30	15	10	10
Over 0.5 through 1.0	10	10	10	10	5	7	15	10	10	10	20	10	10	10	25	15	10	10	30	15	10	10	35	20	10	10	45	20	10	10
Over 1.0 through 2.0	10	10	10	10	7	12	20	10	10	10	25	15	10	10	35	15	10	10	45	20	10	10	55	25	10	10	65	30	10	10
Over 2.0 through 5.0	10	10	10	10	12	16	35	10	10	10	40	15	10	10	60	20	10	10	70	25	10	10	90	30	10	10	100	35	10	10
Over 5.0 through 10.0	15	10	10	10	16	25	40	15	10	10	55	20	10	10	85	30	10	10	110	35	10	10	135	40	10	10	155	45	10	10
Over 10.0 through 25.0	25	10	10	10	25	35	65	20	10	10	100	30	10	10	140	45	10	10	170	50	10	10	200	60	10	10	230	70	10	10
Over 25.0 through 50.0	40	15	10	10	35	50	90	30	10	10	145	45	10	10	195	60	10	10	240	70	10	10	275	85	15	10	315	105	15	10
Over 50.0 through 100	60	20	10	10	50	70	140	45	10	10	210	65	10	10	270	85	15	10	320	95	15	10	360	115	20	10	400	145	20	10
Over 100 through 200	80	25	10	10	70	100	190	55	10	50	285	85	15	10	325	110	20	10	400	145	20	10	450	180	25	10	520	170	30	10
Over 200 through 300	110	30	10	10	90	125	230	70	10	10	320	105	15	10	400	145	25	10	460	175	25	10	560	230	30	10	[c]	240	35	10
Over 300 through 400[b]	130	35	10	10	100	145	260	80	15	10	360	120	20	10	450	165	30	10	500	200	30	10	[c]	235	35	10	[c]	270	40	10

[a] Column A applies when no intervening cargo or bulkheads screen the radioactive material from the living accommodation or undeveloped photographic film or plane. Column B applies when the radioactive material is to be surrounded by at least 2 ft of cargo of unit density and at least 1 steel bulkhead between the radioactive material and the living accommodation or undeveloped photographic film or plate. Column C applies when the radioactive material is to be surrounded by at least 6 ft of cargo of unit density and at least 2 steel bulkheads between the radioactive material and the living accommodation or undeveloped photographic film or plate. Column D applies when the radioactive material is to be surrounded by at least 14 ft of cargo of unit density and at least 2 steel bulkheads between the radioactive material and the living accommodation or undeveloped photographic film or plate.

"Cargo of unit density" means cargo stowed at a density of 1 ton/36 ft^3 (1 ton metric/m^3). Where the density of the cargo is less than this, the depth of the cargo specified in this note for columns B, C, and D (i.e., 2 feet, 6 feet, and 14 feet) must be increased in proportion.

"Minimum distance" means the least distance in any direction, whether vertical or horizontal.

[b] The total consignment on board at any time must not exceed transport indexes totaling 200 without prior authorization by the Department.

[c] Not to be carried unless screening by other cargo and bulkheads can be arranged in accordance with columns B, C, or D.

§ 176.710 Care following leakage or sifting of radioactive materials

(a) In case of fire, collision, or breakage involving any shipment of radioactive materials, other than materials of low specific activity, the package of material must be segregated from unnecessary contact with personnel. In case of obvious leakage, or if the inside container appears to be damaged, the stowage area (hold, deck area, or compartment) containing this cargo must be isolated as much as possible to prevent radioactive material from entering any person's body through contact, inhalation, or ingestion. No person may handle the material or remain in the vicinity unless supervised by a qualified person.

(b) A hold or compartment in which leakage of radioactive materials has occurred may not be used for other cargo until it is decontaminated in accordance with the requirements of § 176.715.

(c) For reporting requirements, see § 171.15 of this subchapter.

§ 176.715 Contamination control

Each hold, compartment, or deck area used for the transportation of low specific activity radioactive material as a full load must be surveyed with appropriate radiation detection instruments after each use. It may not be used again until the radiation dose rate at any accessible surface is less than 0.5 mrem/hr, and there is no significant removable radioactive surface contamination remaining.

APPENDIX G
TITLE 49, PART 177*

PART 177 — CARRIAGE BY PUBLIC HIGHWAY

SUBPART A — GENERAL INFORMATION AND REGULATIONS

§ 177.800 Purpose of regulations in Parts 170—189 of this chapter

(a) To promote the uniform enforcement of law and to minimize the dangers to life and property incident to the transportation of hazardous materials, by private, common and contract carriers, by motor vehicle engaged in interstate or foreign commerce, the regulations in Parts 170 to 189 of this subchapter are prescribed to define these articles for motor vehicle transportation purposes, and to state the precautions that must be observed by the carrier in handling them while in transit. It is the duty of each such carrier to make the prescribed regulations effective and to thoroughly instruct employees in relation thereto.

[29 FR 18795, Dec. 29, 1964. Redesignated at 32 FR 5606, Apr. 5, 1967]

Note: For amendments to § 177.800 see the List of CFR Sections Affected appearing in the Finding Aids section of this volume.

§ 177.801 Scope of regulations in Parts 170 to 189 of this chapter

(a) Hazardous materials except such as may not be accepted and transported under Parts 170 to 189 of this subchapter, may be accepted and transported by private, common, and contract carriers by motor vehicle engaged in interstate or foreign commerce, provided they are in proper condition for transportation and are certified as being in compliance with Parts 170 to 189 of this subchapter, and provided the method of manufacture, packing, and storage, so far as they affect safety in transportation, are open to inspection by a duly authorized representative of the initial carrier or of the Bureau of Explosives. Shipments of explosives or other dangerous articles not in proper condition for transportation, or loaded or stayed as required, or certified as to proper packing, marking and description as required in Parts 170 to 189 of this subchapter, must not be accepted for transportation or transported.

[29 FR 18795. Dec. 29, 1964. Redesignated at 32 FR 5606. Apr. 5, 1967]

Note: For amendments to § 177.801 see the List of CFR Sections Affected appearing in the Finding Aids section of this volume.

§ 177.802 Application of regulations in Parts 170 to 189 of this chapter

(a) Parts 170 to 189 of this subchapter apply to all private, common, and contract carriers by motor vehicle transporting hazardous materials as defined by Department of Transportation "Regulations for Transportation of Hazardous Materials by Land and Water in Rail Freight, Express, and Baggage Services and by Motor Vehicle (Highway) and Water". When shipments are accepted by motor vehicle for further transportation by rail express (see also paragraph (c) of this section), rail baggage (see also paragraph (d) of this section), rail freight or by water on board vessel, they must, in addition to Parts 170 to 189 of this subchapter, comply with the applicable regulations for the service by which they are to be transported.

[29 FR 18795. Dec. 29, 1964. Redesignated at 32 FR 5606, Apr. 5, 1967, and amended by Amdt. 177-24, 38 FR 5314. Feb. 27, 1973; Amdt. 177-35, 41 FR 16130, Apr. 15, 1976]

§ 177.803 Export and import shipments by domestic carriers by motor vehicles
See § 171.12 of this subchapter.

[Amdt. 177-35, 41 FR 16130, Apr. 15, 1976]

§ 177.804 Compliance with Federal Motor Carrier Safety Regulations
Motor carriers and other persons subject to this part shall comply with 49 CFR Parts 390 through 397 (excluding §§ 397.3 and 397.9) to the extent those rules apply.

[Amdt. 177-39, 43 FR 4859, Feb. 6, 1978]

§ 177.805 Canadian shipments and packagings
(a) Canadian shipments and packagings may be carried under conditions specified in § 173.8 of this subchapter.

[Amdt. 177-7, 34 FR 17524, Oct. 30, 1969, as amended by Amdt. 177-35, 41 FR 16130, Apr. 15, 1976]

§ 177.806 U.S. Government material
(a) Shipments of hazardous materials offered by or consigned to the Department of Defense (DOD) of the U.S. Government must be packaged, including limitations of weight, in accordance with the regulations in this subchapter or in containers of equal or greater strength and efficiency as required by DOD regulations.

(1) Hazardous materials sold by the DOD in packagings that are not marked in accordance with the requirements of this subchapter may be shipped from DOD installations if the DOD certifies in writing that the packagings are equal to or greater in strength and efficiency than the packaging prescribed in this subchapter. The shipper shall obtain such a certification in duplicate for each shipment. He shall give one copy to the originating carrier and retain the other for no less than 1 year.

(b) Shipments of radioactive materials, made by or under the direction or supervision of the U.S. Atomic Energy Commission or the Department of Defense, and which are escorted by personnel specially designated by or under the authority of those agencies, for the purpose of national security, are exempt from the regulations in Parts 170 to 189 of this subchapter.

[29 FR 18795, Dec. 29, 1964. Redesignated at 32 FR 5606. Apr. 5, 1967]

Note: For amendments to § 177.806 see the List of CFR Sections Affected appearing in the Finding Aids section of this volume.

§ 177.807 Reporting hazardous materials incidents
Each carrier shall report incidents involving hazardous materials to the Department as required by §§ 171.15 and 171.16 of this chapter.

[Amdt. 177-14, 35 FR 16838, Oct. 31, 1970; as amended by Amdt. 177-35, 41 FR 16130, Apr. 15, 1976]

§ 177.808 Connecting carrier shipments

Shipments of hazardous materials offered by connecting transportation lines must comply with Parts 170 to 189 of this subchapter.

[29 FR 18795, Dec. 29, 1964. Redesignated at 32 FR 5606. Apr. 5, 1967, and amended by Amdt. 177-35, 41 FR 16130, Apr. 15, 1976]

§ 177.809 Carrier's material and supplies

The regulations in Parts 170 to 189 of this subchapter apply to all shipments of hazardous materials, including carrier's material and supplies.

[29 FR 18795, Dec. 29, 1964. Redesignated at 32 FR 5606. Apr. 5, 1967, and amended by Amdt. 177-35, 41 FR 16130, Apr. 15, 1976]

§ 177.810 Vehicular tunnels

Nothing contained in Parts 170 to 189 of this subchapter shall be so construed as to nullify or supersede regulations established and published under authority of State statute or municipal ordinance regarding the kind, character, or quantity of any hazardous material permitted by such regulations to be transported through any urban vehicular tunnel used for mass transportation.

[29 FR 18795, Dec. 29, 1964. Redesignated at 32 FR 5606. Apr. 5, 1967, and amended by Amdt. 177-35, 41 FR 16130, Apr. 15, 1976]

§ 177.811 Astray shipments

(a) Any carrier in possession of an ashtray shipment of hazardous materials (other than explosives) shall forward it promptly to its destination, if known, after inspection has shown the package to be in proper condition for transportation.

(b) If the package of hazardous materials is not labeled and the exact classification of the contents is not determinable, the carrier shall apply a FLAMMABLE LIQUID label.

[Amdt. 177-35, 41 FR 16130, Apr. 15, 1976, as amended by Admt. 177-35A, 41 FR 40691 Sept. 20, 1976]

§ 177.812 Containers required

Containers required for hazardous materials are prescribed in Part 173 of this subchapter. Regulations Applying to Shippers.

[29 FR 18795, Dec. 29, 1964. Redesignated at 32 FR 5606. Apr. 5, 1967, and amended by Amdt. 177-35, 41 FR 16130, Apr. 15, 1976]

§ 177.813 Inefficient containers

The results of experience gained by examination of broken or leaking containers must be recorded by the Bureau of Explosives to the end that further use of any particular kind of container shown by experience to be inefficient, may be prohibited by the Department.

[29 FR 18795, Dec. 29, 1964. Redesignated at 32 FR 5606, Apr. 5, 1967]

§ 177.814 Retention of manufacturer's certificate and retest reports

(a) Each motor carrier who uses a cargo tank vehicle shall have in his files a certificate or manufacturer's data report signed by a responsible official of the manufacturer or fabricator of the cargo tank, or a competent testing agency, certifying that the cargo tank identified in the certificate was manufactured and tested in accordance with the requirements contained in the specification under which the cargo tank was constructed. The certificate and any other data furnished as required by the specification must be retained at the principal office of the carrier during the time that the cargo tank is used by the carrier and for one year thereafter.

(1) Except for specifications MC 330 and MC 331 cargo tanks, a motor carrier may himself perform the tests and inspections to determine whether the tank meets the requirements of the specification. If the motor carrier performs the tests and inspections and determines that the tank conforms to the specification, he may use the tank if he retains the test data, in place of a certificate, in his files at his principal office for as long as he uses the tank and one year thereafter.
(2) A motor carrier using a specification MC 330 cargo tank for which such carrier is unable to obtain the manufacturer's data report required by the specification may copy the information contained on the cargo tank's identification plate and ASME Code plate and retain such information as required by this section.
(3) Each motor carrier who uses a specification cargo tank which he does not own and has not tested or inspected shall obtain a copy of the manufacturer's certificate or manufacturer's data report and retain it in his files at his principal office during the time he uses the tank and for one year thereafter. A motor carrier using a specification MC 330 cargo tank which he does not own may copy the information contained on the cargo tank's identification plate and ASME Code plate if the manufacturer's data report is not available from the owner of the tank.

(b) Upon a written request to and with the approval of, the Director, Regional Motor Carrier Safety Office, for the region in which a motor carrier has his principal place of business, a motor carrier may retain the certificate and other data specified in paragraph (a) of this section at a regional or terminal office. The address and jurisdictions of the Directors of Regional Motor Carrier Safety Offices are shown in § 390.40 of Chapter III of this title.

(c) *Withdrawal of certification.* See § 177.824(i) of this subchapter.

(d) A copy of retest and inspection reports required by §§ 173.33 and 177.824 of this subchapter and all records of repairs to each cargo tank vessel must be retained in the same file with the manufacturer's certificate or manufacturer's data report for that tank as specified in paragraph (a) of this section. This provision does not apply to a motor carrier leasing a cargo tank for less than 30 days if the lessor has the records required by this section in his files.

[Amdt. 177-31, 39 FR 41742, Dec. 2, 1974, as amended by Amdt. 177-35, 41 FR 17736, Apr. 28, 1976; Amdt. 177-37, 41 FR 40691, Sept. 20, 1976]

§ 177.815 Lost or destroyed labels

Each carrier shall maintain an adequate supply of the labels specified in Subpart E of Part 172 of this subchapter to replace those that become lost or destroyed. The carrier shall replace each lost or destroyed label based on the information on the shipping papers.

[Amdt. 177-35, 41 FR 16130. Apr. 15, 1976]

§ 177.816 [Reserved]

§ 177.817 Shipping papers

(a) *General requirements.* A carrier may not transport a hazardous material unless it is accompanied by a shipping paper that is prepared in accordance with §§ 172.201, 172.202, and 172.203 of this subchapter.

(b) *Shipper certification.* An initial carrier may not accept hazardous material offered for transportation unless the shipping paper describing the material includes a shipper's certification which meets the requirements in § 172.204 of this subchapter. The certification is not required for shipments to be transported entirely by private carriage and for bulk shipments to be transported in a cargo tank supplied by the carrier.

(c) *Requirements when interlining with carriers by rail.* A motor carrier shall mark on the shipping paper required by this section, if it offers or delivers a freight container or transport vehicle to rail carrier for further transportation;

(1) A description of the freight container or transport vehicle; and
(2) The kind of placard affixed to the freight container or transport vehicle.

(d) This section does not apply to materials classed as an ORM-A, B, C, or D.

(e) *Shipping paper accessibility — accident or inspection.* A driver of a motor vehicle containing hazardous material, and each carrier using such a vehicle shall ensure that the shipping paper required by this section is readily avaiable to, and recognizable by authorities in the event of accident or inspection. Specifically, the driver and the carrier shall

(1) Clearly distinguish the shipping paper, if it is carried with other shipping papers or other papers of any kind, by either distinctively tabbing it or by having it appear first; and
(2) Store the shipping paper as follows:
    (i) When the driver is at the vehicle's controls, the shipping paper shall be: (A) Within his immediate reach while he is restrained by the lap belt; and (B) either readily visible to a person entering the driver's compartment or in a holder which is mounted to the inside of the door on the driver's side of the vehicle.
    (ii) When the driver is not at the vehicle's controls, the shipping paper shall be: (A) In a holder which is mounted to the inside of the door on the driver's side of the vehicle; or (B) on the driver's seat in the vehicle.

[Amdt. 177-35, 41 FR 16130, Apr. 15, 1976, as amended by Amdt. 177-35A, 41 FR 40691, Sept. 20, 1976]

§ 177.842 Radioactive material

(a) The number of packages of radioactive materials in any motor vehicle, trailer, or storage location must be limited so that the total transport index number, as defined in § 173.389(i) of this subchapter and determined by adding together the transport index numbers on the labels of the individual packages, does not exceed 50. This provision does not apply to exclusive use shipments described in § 173.393(j), 173,396(f), or 173.392 of this subchapter.

(b) Packages of radioactive material bearing "radioactive yellow-II" or "radioactive yellow-III" labels must not be placed in a motor vehicle or in any other place closer than the distances shown in the following table to any area which may be continuously occupied by passengers, employees, or shipments of animals, nor closer than the distances shown in the table below to any package containing undeveloped film (if so marked). If more than one of these packages is present, the distance shall be computed from the following table on the basis of the total transport index number (determined by adding together the transport index numbers on the labels of the individual packages) or packages in the vehicle or storeroom. Where more than one group of packages is present in any single storage location, a single group may not have a total transport index greater than 50. Each group of packages must be handled and stowed not closer than 6 m (20 ft) (measured edge to edge) to any other group.

(c) Shipments of low specific activity materials, as defined in § 173.391 of this subchapter, must be loaded so as to avoid spillage and scattering of loose materials. Loading restrictions are set forth in § 173.397 of this subchapter.

(d) Packages must be so blocked and braced that they cannot change position during conditions normally incident to transportation.

Total transport index	Minimum separation distances in test to nearest undeveloped film for various times of transit					Minimum distance in feet to area of persons, or minimum distance in feet from dividing partition of cargo compartments
	Up to 2 hr	2—4 hr	4—8 hr	8—12 hr	Over 12 hr	
None	0	0	0	0	0	0
0.1 to 1.0	1	2	3	4	5	1
1.1 to 5.0	3	4	6	8	11	2
5.1 to 10.0	4	6	9	11	15	3
10.1 to 20.0	5	8	12	16	22	4
20.1 to 30.0	7	10	15	20	29	5
30.1 to 40.0	8	11	17	23	33	6
40.1 to 50.0	9	12	19	24	36	7

Note 1: The distance in the table must be measured from the nearest point on the packages of radioactive materials.

(e) Persons should not remain unnecessarily in a vehicle containing radioactive materials.

(f) Each fissile class III radioactive material shipment (as defined in § 173.389(a)(3) of this subchapter) must be transported in accordance with one of the methods prescribed in § 173.396(g) of this subchapter. The transport controls must be adequate to assure that no fissile class III shipment is transported in the same transport vehicle with any other fissile radioactive material shipment. In loading and storage areas each fissile class III shipment must be segregated by a distance of at least 20 ft from other packages required to bear one of the ''Radioactive'' labels described in § 173.416 of this subchapter.

[Amdt. 177-3, 33 FR 14933, Oct. 4, 1968; Amdt. 177-3, 33 FR 19823, Dec. 27, 1968]

Note: For amendments to § 177.842 see the List of CFR Sections Affected appearing in the Finding Aids section of this volume.

§ 177.843 Contamination of vehicles

(a) Each motor vehicle used for transporting low specific activity radioactive materials in truckload lots under the provisions of § 173.392(d) of this subchapter must be surveyed with appropriate radiation detection instruments after each use. Carriers must not return such vehicles to service until the radiation dose rate at any accessible surface is not more than 0.5 mrem/hr and there is no significant removable radioactive surface contamination (see § 173.399 of this subchapter).

(b) This section does not apply to any vehicle used solely for transporting radioactive material if a survey of the interior surface shows that the radiation dose rate does not exceed 10 mrem/hr at the interior surface or 2 mrem/hr at 3 ft from any interior surface. These vehicles must be stenciled with the words ''For Radioactive Materials Use Only'' in lettering at least 3 in high in a conspicuous place, on both sides of the exterior of the vehicle. These vehicles must be kept closed at all times other than loading and unloading.

(c) In case of fire, accident, breakage, or unusual delay involving shipments of radioactive material, see § 177.861.

[Amdt. 177-3, 33 FR 14933. Oct. 4, 1968, as amended by Amdt. 177-35, 41 FR 16131, Apr. 15, 1976]

§ 177.844 Other regulated materials

Asbestos must be loaded, handled, and unloaded, and any asbestos contamination of transport vehicles removed, in a manner that will minimize occupational exposure to airborne asbestos particles released incident to transportation. (See § 173.1090 of this subchapter.)

[Amdt. 177-44, 43 FR 56668, Dec. 4, 1978]

§ 177.848 Loading and Storage Chart of Hazardous Materials

(a) Hazardous materials must not be loaded, transported, or stored together, except as provided in the Loading and Storage Chart of hazardous materials shown in this section.

The following table shows the hazardous materials which must not be loaded or stored together.

Low explosives or black powder.

High explosives or propellant explosives, class A.

Initiating or priming explosives, wet: Diazodinitrophenol, fulminate of mercury, guany, nitrosamino guanylidene hydrazine, lead azide, lead styphnate, nitro mannite. nitrosoguanidine, pentaerythrite tetranitrate, tetrazene, lead mononitroresorcinate.

Detonators, detonating primers.

Ammunition for cannon with explosive projectiles, gas projectiles, smoke projectiles, incendiary projectiles, illuminating projectiles or shell; ammunition for small arms with incendiary projectiles; ammunition for small arms with explosive projectiles, gas projectiles, smoke projectiles, incendiary projectiles, illuminating projectiles; boosters (explosive); bursters (explosive); and supplementary charges (explosive) without detonators[c,d]

Explosive projectiles; bombs; torpedoes; mines; rifle or hand grenades (explosive); jet thrust units (jato), class A; igniters, jet thrust, class A; rocket motors, class A; igniters, rocket motor, class A[c]

Detonating fuzes, class A, with or without radioactive components.

[a] Detonators, Class C Explosives may also be loaded and transported with articles named in vertical and horizontal columns 3, 9, 10, 11, 12 and 13. Loading and transportation of detonating primers or detonators except as prescribed in § 177.835, in any quantity, with articles named in vertical or horizontal columns b, c, e or f is prohibited.

[b] Corrosive liquids must not be loaded above or adjacent to flammable solids, oxidizing materials, ammunition for cannon with or without projectiles, or propellant explosives, except that shippers loading truckload shipments of corrosive liquids and flammable solids or oxidizing materials packages and who have obtained prior approval from the Department may load such materials together when it is known that the mixture of contents would not cause a dangerous evolution of heat or gas.

[c] Explosives, class A and explosives, class B must not be loaded or stored with chemical ammunition containing incendiary charges or white phosphorus either with or without bursting charges.

[d] Bursters (explosive), boosters (explosive), or supplementary charges (explosive) without detonators when shipped by, to or for the Departments of the Army, Navy, and Air Force of the United States Government may be loaded with any of the articles named except those in columns, c, d, 3, 9, 10, 11, 12, 13, 14, and 15.

[e] Does not include blasting agents, Ammonium Nitrate-Fuel oil mixtures or ammonium nitrate, fertilizer grade, which may be loaded, transported or stored with high explosives or with detonators containing not more than 1 gram of explsoive each, excluding ignition and delay charges.

Normal uranium, depleted uranium, and thorium metal in solid form may also be loaded and transported with articles named in vertical and horizontal columns a, b, c, d, e, f, and g.

Note 1: Charged electric storage batteries must not be loaded in the same vehicle with explosives, class A

Note 2: Cyanides or cyanide mixtures must not be loaded or stored with acids or corrosive liquids.

Note 3: Gas identification sets may be loaded and transported with all articles named except those in column c.

Note 4: Nitric acid, when loaded in the same motor vehicles with other acids or other corrosive liquids in carboys, must be separated from the other carboys. A 2 by 6 inch plank, set on edge, should be nailed across the motor vehicle floor at least 12 inches from the nitric acid carboys, and the space between the plank and the carboys of nitric acid should be filled with sand, sifted ashes, or other incombustible absorbent material.

Note 5: Smokeless powder for small arms in quantities not exceeding 100 pounds net weight in one motor vehicle shall be classed as a flammable solid for purposes of transportation when examined for this classification by the Bureau of Explosives and approved by the Associate Director for OE.

SUBPART D — VEHICLES AND SHIPMENTS IN TRANSIT; ACCIDENTS

§ 177.861 Accidents; radioactive materials

(a) In addition to the incident reporting requirements of §§ 171.15 and 171.16 of this subchapter, the carrier must also notify the shipper at the earliest practicable moment following any incident in which there has been breakage, spillage, or suspected radioactive contamination involving radioactive materials shipments. Vehicles, buildings areas, or equipment in which radioactive materials have been spilled may not be again placed in service or routinely occupied until the radiation dose rate at any accessible surface is less than 0.5 mrem/hr and there is not significant removable radioactive surface contamination (see § 173.397 of this subchapter).

Note 1: In these instances, the package or materials should be segregated as far as practicable from personnel contact. If radiological advice or assistance is needed, the U.S. Atomic Energy Commission should also be notified. In case of obvious leakage, or if it appears likely that the inside container may have been damaged, care should be taken to avoid inhalation, ingestion, or contact with the radioactive material. Any loose radioactive material should be left in a segregated area and held pending disposal instructions from qualified persons.

Note 2: Details involving the handling of radioactive materials in the event of an accident can be found in Bureau of Explosives' Pamphlets 1 and 2.

(b) *Cleaning vehicles.* See § 177.843.

[Amdt. 177-3, 33 FR 14934. Oct. 4, 1968, as amended by Amdt. 177-17, 36 FR 18469, Sept. 15, 1971]

Note: For amendments to § 177.861 see the List of CFR Sections Affected appearing in the Finding Aids section of this volume.

SUBPART E — REGULATIONS APPLYING TO HAZARDOUS MATERIAL ON MOTOR VEHICLES CARRYING PASSENGERS FOR HIRE

§ 177.870 Regulations for passenger carrying vehicles

(a) *Vehicles transporting passengers and property.* In addition to the regulations in Parts 170 to 189 of this subchapter the following requirements shall apply to vehicles transporting passengers and property.

(b) *No explosives or other hazardous materials on passenger-carrying vehicles, exceptions.* No hazardous materials except small-arms ammunition, emergency shipments of drugs, chemicals and hospital supplies, and the accompanying munitions of war of the Departments of the Army, Navy, and Air Force of the U.S. Government, are authorized by Parts 170 to 189 of this subchapter to be transported on motor vehicles carrying passengers for hire where other practicable means of transportation is available.

(c) *Explosives in passenger-carrying space forbidden.* No explosive, except small-arms ammunition, may be carried in the passenger-carrying space of any motor vehicle transporting passengers for hire.

(d) *Hazardous materials on passenger-carrying vehicles; quantity.* Where no other practicable means of transportation is available the following articles in the quantities as shown may be transported in motor vehicles carrying passengers for hire in a space other than that provided for passengers: Not to exceed 100 lb gross weight of any or all of the kinds of explosives permitted to be transported by rail express or rail baggage services, may be transported on a motor vehicle transporting passengers: *Provided however,* That samples of explosives for laboratory examination, not exceeding a net weight of $^1/_2$ lb each, and not exceeding 20 samples or not to exceed a total of 100 blasting caps at one time in a single motor vehicle transporting passengers. (See § 172.101 of this subchapter.)

(e) *Articles other than explosives on passenger-carrying vehicles.* The gross weight of any given class of hazardous material other than explosives shall not exceed 100 lb, and the aggregate weight of all such other dangerous articles shall not exceed 500 lb. This provision does not apply to nontoxic, nonflammable refrigerants, when such refrigerant is for servicing operations of a motor carrier on whose motor vehicles the refrigerant is used. A cylinder secured against movement while in transit and not exceeding 250 lb gross weight may be transported.

(f) *Poisons on passenger-carrying vehicles.* No motor carrier may transport any extremely dangerous poison, class A, any tear gas or irritating substance, class C, any less dangerous poison, class B, which is a liquid, or any paranitraniline, in any amount, in or on any bus while engaged in the transportation of passengers; or any less dangerous poison, class B, which is other than a liquid, in any amount exceeding an aggregate of 100 lb gross weight in or on any such bus.

(g) *Radioactive materials.* In addition to the limitations prescribed in paragraphs (b) and (e) of this section, no person may transport any radioactive material requiring labels under §§ 172.436, 172.438, and 172.440 of this subchapter in or on any motor vehicle carrying passengers for hire except where no other practicable means of transportation is available. Packages of radioactive materials must be stored only in the trunk or baggage compartment of the vehicle, and must not be stored in any compartment occupied by persons. Packages of radioactive materials must be handled and placed in the vehicle as prescribed in § 177.842.

[29 FR 18795, Dec. 29, 1964. Redesignated at 32 FR 5606, Apr. 5, 1967]

Note: For amendments to § 177.870 see the list of CFR Sections Affected appearing in the Finding Aids section of this volume.

APPENDIX H
TITLE 49, PART 178

PART 178 — SHIPPING CONTAINER SPECIFICATIONS

§ 178.34 Specification 2R; inside containment vessel

[Amdt. 178-35, 39 FR 45245, Dec. 31, 1974]

§ 178.34-1 General requirements

(a) Each vessel must be made of stainless steel, malleable iron, or brass, or other material having equivalent physical strength and fire resistance.

(b) Each vessel must meet all of the applicable requirements of § 173.24 (c) and (d) of this subchapter. Letters and numerals at least 6 mm ($^{1}/_{4}$-in) in height are authorized for the marking of a vessel not exceeding 5 cm (2 in.) inside diameter.

[Amdt. 178-35, 39 FR 45245, Dec. 31, 1974]

§ 178.34-2 Manufacture

The ends of the vessel must be fitted with screw-type closures or flanges (see § 178.34-4), except that one or both ends of the vessel may be permanently closed by a welded or brazed plate. Welded or brazed side seams are authorized.

[Amdt. 178-35, 39 FR 45245, Dec. 31, 1974]

§ 178.34-3 Dimensions

(a) The inside diameter of the vessel may not exceed 30 centimeters (12 in.) exclusive of flanges for handling or fastening devices and must have wall thickness and length in accordance with the following:

Inside diameter maximum		Threaded closure		Wall thickness minimum	Length maximum	
Inches	**Centimeters**	**Inches**	**Millimeters**	**Flanged closure**	**Inches**	**Centimeters**
2	5	$^{3}/_{32}$	2.5	Not less than that prescribed for schedule 40 pipe.	16	41
6	15	$^{1}/_{8}$	3.2		72	183
12	30	$^{1}/_{4}$	6.5		72	183

[Amdt. 178-35, 39 FR 45245, Dec. 31, 1974]

§ 178.34-4 Closure devices

(a) Each closure device must be as follows:

(1) Screw-type cap or plug; number of threads per inch must not be less than U.S. standard pipe threads and must have sufficient length of thread to engage at least 5 threads when securely tightened. Pipe threads must be luted with an appropriate nonhardening compound which must be capable of withstanding up to 149° C (300° F) without loss

of efficiency. Tightening torque must be adequate to maintain leak tightness with the specific luting compound.

(2) An opening may be closed by a securely bolted flange and leak-tight gasket. Each flange must be welded or brazed to the body of the 2R vessel per (ANSI) Standard B16.5 or (AWWA) Standard C207-55, section 10. A torque wrench must be used in securing the flange with a corresponding torque of no more than twice the force necessary to seal the selected gasket. Gasket material must be capable of withstanding up to 149°C (300° F) without loss of efficiency. The flange, whether of ferrous or nonferrous metal, must be constructed from the same metal as the vessel and must meet the dimensional and fabrication specifications for welded construction as follows:

(i) Pipe flanges described in Tables 13, 14, 16, 17, 19, 20, 22, 23, 25 and 26 of ANSI B16.5

(ii) For nominal pipe sizes, 6, 8, 10, and 12 in. AWWA Standard C207-55, Table 1, class B, may be used in place of the tables prescribed by paragraph (a)(s)(i) of this section.

(iii) Sizes under 6 in. nominal pipe size, the following table with the same configuration as illustrated in AWWA C207-55, Table 1, class B, may be used in place of paragraph (a)(2)(i) of this section.

Nominal pipe size		Flange O.D.			Bolt circle diameter	
Inches	Centimeters	Inches	Centimeters	Number of bolts	Inches	Centimeters
2	5	6	15	4	$4^3/_4$	11.8
$2^1/_2$	6.2	7	17.5	4	$5^1/_2$	13.8
3	7.5	$7^1/_2$	18.8	4	6	15
$3^1/_2$	8.8	$8^1/_2$	21.3	8	7	17.5
4	10	9	22.5	8	$7^1/_2$	18.8
5	12.6	10	25.4	8	$8^1/_2$	21.3

Diameter of bolts		Flange thickness	
Inches	Centimeters	Inches	Centimeters
$^1/_2$	1.2	$^5/_8$	1.6
$^1/_2$	—	$^5/_8$	—
$^1/_2$	—	$^5/_8$	—
$^1/_2$	—	$^5/_8$	—
$^1/_2$	—	$^5/_8$	—
$^1/_2$	—	$^5/_8$	—

(iv) Cast iron flanges prohibited.

[Amdt. 178-35, 39 FR 45245, Dec. 31, 1974; 40 FR 2435, Jan. 13, 1975, as amended at 40 FR 44327, Sept. 26, 1975]

§ 178.103 Specification 6L; metal packaging
[Amdt. 178-35, 39 FR 45246, Dec. 31, 1974]

§ 178.103-1 General requirements
Each packaging must meet the applicable requirements of § 173.24 of this subchapter.
[Amdt. 178-35, 39 FR 45246. Dec. 31, 1974]

§ 178.103-2 Rated capacity

(a) Rated capacity as marked (see § 178.103-6). Not less than 55 gal nor more than 110 gal for the outer steel drum. Not more than 17.74 ℓ for the inner vessel.

(b) The authorized maximum gross weight of the package is 160 kg (350 lb) for sizes not over 210L (55 gal) or 220 k (480 lb) for sizes over 210L (55 gal) but not over 420L (110 gal).

[Amdt. 178-1, 33 FR 14934, Oct. 4, 1968, as amended by Amdt. 178-35, 39 FR 45246, Dec. 31, 1974]

§ 178.103-3 General construction requirements

(a) The outer shell must be of straight sided steel, with welded body seams and at least 18-gauge body and bottom head sheets, and 14-gauge removable head sheets (unless there are one or more corrugations in the cover near the periphery, in which case 16-gauge is authorized). The shell may be either a single sheet of steel or may be fabricated by welding together two appropriate lengths of 210L (55-gal) drums, such as a DOT Specification 6J or 17H, with rolled or swedged in hoops as prescribed for either of those specifications. The head must be convex (crowned), not extending beyond the level of the chime, with a minimum convexity of 1 cm ($^3/_8$-in). The inside diameter of the shell must be at least 57 cm (22.5 in).

(b) Inner containment vessel must conform to specification 2R (except that cast iron is not authorized), with a maximum usable inside dimension of 13.3 cm (5.25 in) maximum height of 127 cm (50 in) (with caps in place) and minimum wall thickness of 6 mm (0.25 in).

(c) Inner containment vessel must be fixed within the outer shell by one of the following types of centering devices:

(1) At least 8 steel rod spacers, of at least 6 mm (0.25-in) diameter (for packages of 210 ℓ (55-gal) capacity) or 1 cm of (0.375-in) diameter (for packages with greater than 210 ℓ (55-gal) capacity) cold rolled steel, welded to the vessel at each end by minimum 5 cm (2-in) continuous weld. Each rod must be welded to the vessel at radial positions not exceeding 45° as not to interfere with closure of the inner vessel. Each spacer rod must extend at least 5.6 cm (2.25 in) beyond the inner vessel at each end, then radially to the wall of the outer drum (to provide a springlike snug fit) and along the entire length of the wall of the outer drum. For a packaging of more than 210 ℓ (55-gal) capacity, each spacer rod must be braced by welding a 6 mm (0.25-in) by 5 cm (2-in.) steel plate to the spacer rod and the pipe with a continuous weld at each joint, the joints being located approximately half way along the length of the drum. For containers manufactured prior to March 31, 1975, this requirement is effective December 31, 1975.

(2) At least three steel "spiders," not more than 24 in. apart, with each spider having at least four legs. Each leg must be constructed of materials having dimensions not less than those listed in this paragraph, welded by continuous weld at each joint to inner and outer steel bands of at least $^1/_4$-in. by 1-in. steel. The inner steel band must be welded to the inner vessel by at least six 2-in welds on both edges of the band. The outer steel band must be welded to the outer drum by at least six 2-in welds on both edges of the top outer band, such that the inner vessel is at least $2^1/_4$ in. from the top and bottom of the drum. Authorized construction materials are:

(i) 2.5 cm (1 in) by 2.5 cm (1 in) by 6 mm($^1/_4$-in) steel angle iron.
(ii) 3 cm ($1^1/_4$ in) by 3 cm ($1^1/_4$in.) by 5 mm ($^3/_{16}$-in) steel angle iron.
(iii) 2.5 cm (1 in.) schedule 40 steel pipe.

(iv) 1$^{1}/_{2}$-in diameter solid steel rods, with only two such spiders required instead of three.

(3) There must not be less than 2 spacer mechanisms for a packaging of 210 ℓ (55-gal) capacity nor less than 3 spacer mechanisms for a packaging greater than 210 ℓ (55-gal) capacity. Each spacer mechanism must consist of not less than 6 steel angles, pipe, or rod radial supports of at least 2.7 cm^2 (0.42 in.^{2}) cross-section. Each radial support must be welded at one end to the containment vessel by a continuous weld or to an inner steel band of at least 6 mm ($^{1}/_{4}$-in) by 2.5 cm (1 in) by a continuous weld at radial positions not exceeding 60° from the center of the package. The inner band, when used, must be welded to the inner containment vessel by at least 6 equally spaced 5 cm (2-in) welds on each edge of the band. The opposite end of the radial support must be welded by a continuous weld to an outer steel band of at least 6 mm ($^{1}/_{4}$-in) by 2.5 cm (1 in.) The outer steel band must be welded to the outer shell by at least 6 equally spaced welds on each edge of the top band, such that the inner vessel is fixed at least 5.7 cm (2.25 in) from the top and bottom of the drum. The spacer mechanism must be welded as specified near each end of the containment vessel so as not to interfere with the vessel closure. For a packaging greater than 210L (55-gal) capacity, the additional spacer mechanism must be located at approximately midpoint along the length of the inner vessel.

(d) The void between the inner containment vessel and the outer shell must be completely filled with bagged or tamped vermiculite (expanded mica), with a density of at least 0.072 g/cc (4.5 lb/ft^3). Loose, untamped vermiculite is not authorized.
[Amdt. 178-1, 33 FR 14934. Oct. 4, 1968, as amended by Amdt. 178-35, 39 FR 45246, Dec. 31, 1974; 40 FR 2435, Jan. 13, 1975; 40 FR 44327, Sept. 26, 1975]

§ 178.103-4 Welding

Welding must be of material having a melting point in excess of 800° C (1475° F) (except that for packages constructed prior to March 31, 1975, this temperature may be 540°C (1000° F), with a joint efficiency of at least 0.85. This requirement applies to welding used in adding spacer rods to comply with 178.103(3)(c)(1).
[Amdt. 178-35, 39 FR 45246, Dec. 31, 1974]

§ 178.103-5 Closure

(a) The outer drum closure must be at least a 12-gauge bolted ring with drop forged lugs, one of which is threaded, and having at least a 1.6 cm ($^{5}/_{8}$-in) diameter steel bolt and a lock nut, or equivalent device.

(b) The closure device must have a means for the attachment of a tamper-proof lock wire and seal, or equivalent.
[Amdt. 178-1, 33 FR 14935, Oct. 4, 1968, as amended by Admt. 178-35, 39 FR 45246, Dec. 31, 1974]

§ 178.103-6 Markings

(a) Markings on each container, by die stamping on a metal plate attached to the outside of the outer container by spot welding, or other equally efficient method, in letters and figures of at least $^{1}/_{4}$ in. in height, as follows:

(1) "DOT-6L".
(2) "FISSILE RADIOACTIVE MATERIAL."
(3) Name or symbol of person making the marks specified in paragraph (a) (1) of this section. Symbol, if used, must br registered with the Associate Director for OE.

(4) Gauge of metal of the outer steel drum in the thinnest part, rated capacity of the outer steel drum in gallons, and the year of manufacture of the assembled package (e.g., 18-110-68). When the gauge of the metal in the drum wall differs from that in the head, both must be indicated with a slanting line between, and with the gauge of the body indicated first (e.g., 18/16-110-68 for 18-gauge body and 16-gauge head).

[Order 70, 30 FR 6496, Apr. 29, 1966. Redesignated at 32 FR 5606, Apr. 5, 1967, and amended by Amdt. 178-1, 33 FR 14935, Oct. 4, 1968; Amdt. 178-40, 41 FR 38181, Sept. 9, 1976]

§ 178.104 Specification 6M; metal packaging
[Amdt. 178-1, 33 FR 14935, Oct. 4, 1968]

§ 178.104-1 General requirements
(a) Each package must meet the applicable requirements of § 173.24 of this chapter.
[Amdt. 178-1, 33 FR 14935, Oct. 4, 1968]

§ 178.104-2 Rated capacity
(a) Rated capacity as marked (see § 178.104-5) Not less than 10 gal nor more than 110 gal for the outer steel drum. Not less than 1.24 ℓ for the inner containment vessel.
[Amdt. 178-1, 33 FR 14935, Oct. 4, 1968]

§ 178.104-3 General construction requirements
(a) The outer shell must be of straight-sided steel, with welded body seams, and may be either a single sheet of steel, or may be fabricated by welding together two appropriate lengths of drums, such as a DOT Specification 6C or 17C, with each length to contain 3 swedged or rolled rolling hoops as prescribed for either of these specifications. A removable head for a packaging of 210 ℓ (55 gal) or larger volume must have one or more corrugations in the cover near the periphery. For a packaging exceeding 57 ℓ (15 gal) volume, the head must be crowned (convexed), not extending beyond the level of the chime, with a minimum convexity of 1 cm ($^3/_8$-in.)

(1) The maximum authorized gross weight, metal thickness, and minimum end insulation thickness for the marked volume is as follows:

Marked capacity	Maximum authorized gross weight			Minimum thickness of un-coated sheets and heads	Minimum thickness of end insulation	
Gallons not over	Liters	Pounds	Kilograms	(gauge)	Inches	Centimeters
15	57	160	73	20	1.98	4.7
30	114	480	219	18	3.75	9.5
55	210	640	292	16	3.75	9.5

(2) Each drum must have at least four 1.2 cm (0.5-in.) diameter vents near the top, each covered with a weatherproof tape or fusible plug; or equivalent device. A layer of porous refractory fiber may be placed behind the pressure-relief vent holes.

(b) Inner containment vessel must conform to specification 2R or equivalent (cast iron or brass are prohibited), with maximum usable inside diameter of 13.3 cm (5.25 in.), minimum usable inside diameter of 10 cm (4 in), and minimum height of 15 cm (6 in.).

(c) Inner containment vessel must be fixed within the outer shell by one of the following types of solid centering media, with the sides of the inner vessel protected by at least 9.5 cm (3.75 in) of insulation media, and the ends with at least the thickness as prescribed in § 178.104-3(a)(1).

(1) Machined discs and rings made of solid industrial cane fiberboard having a density of at least 0.24 g/cc(15 lb/ft^3) fitted such that the radial clearances between the fiberboard, inner vessel, and shell do not exceed 6 mm ($^1/_4$-in.) or
(2) Hardwood or plywood at least 1.2 cm ($^1/_2$-in) thick, having a density of at least 0.45 g/cc (28 lb/ft^3). There must be no gap or direct heat path from the shell to the inner vessel.

(d) Any radiation shielding material used must be placed within the inner containment vessel or must be protected in all directions by at least the thickness of the thermal insulating material prescribed in paragraph (a) of this section.

(e) For a packaging having an authorized gross weight in excess of 219 kg (480 lb), a steel bearing plate, at least 6 mm (0.25-in) thick or a plywood disc, at least 2.5 cm (1-in) thick, and at least 25 cm (10 in.) in diameter must be provided at both ends and adjacent to the specification 2R inner containment vessel, to provide additional load-bearing surface against the insulation-centering medium.
[Amdt. 178-1, 33 FR 14935. Oct. 4, 1968, as amended by Amdt. 178-35, 39 FR 45246, Dec. 31, 1974; 40 FR 44327, Sept. 26, 1975]

§ 178.104-4 Closure

(a) The outer drum closure must be at least 16-gauge bolt-type locking ring having at least a $^5/_{16}$-in steel bolt for drum sizes not over 15 gal. or a 12-gauge bolted ring with drop-forged lugs, one of which is threaded, and a $^5/_8$-in steel bolt for drum sizes over 15 gallons. Each bolt must be provided with a lock nut or equivalent device.

(b) The closure device must have means for the attachment of a tamperproof lock wire and seal, or equivalent.
[Amdt. 178-1, 33 FR 14935, Oct. 4, 1968]

§ 178.104-5 Markings

(a) Marking must be as prescribed in § 173.24 of this chapter.

(b) Marking on the outside of each package must be as follows: ''DOT-6M Type B,'' ''Radioactive Materials,'' or ''Fissile Radioactive Materials,'' as appropriate; and the gauge of metal of the outer drum in the thinnest part, rated capacity of the outer drum in gallons, and year of manufacture (for example, 18-30-69). When the gauge of the metal in the drum wall differs from that in the head, both must be indicated with a slanting line between, and with the gauge of the body indicated first (e.g., 18/16-55-69 for 18-gauge body and 16-gauge head).
[Amdt. 178-1, 33 FR 14395, Oct. 4, 1968]

§ 178.117 Specification 17F; steel drums

Single trip container. Removable head containers not authorized.

§ 178.117-1 Compliance

(a) Required in all details.

§ 178.117-2 Rated capacity

(a) Rated capacity as marked, see § 178.117-11(a)(3). Actual capacity of containers shall be not less than rated (marked) capacity plus 2%, nor greater than rated capacity plus 2% plus 1 qt, except that for containers over 30 gal marked capacity actual capacity shall be not less than rated capacity plus 2% nor greater than rated capacity plus 2% plus 2 qt.

§ 178.117-3 Composition

(a) Sheets for body and heads to be low carbon, open hearth or electric steel. Steel to be as high as practicable in tensile strength, having no loose oxide scale.

§ 178.117-5 Seams

(a) Body seams welded.

(b) Head and chime seams welded or double-seamed.

(c) Flanges for closures welded in place.

§ 178.117-6 Chime reinforcement

(a) Chime reinforcement required to be not less than 12 gauge (see § 178.117-7(b)).

§ 178.117-7 Parts and dimensions

(a) Parts and dimensions as follows:

Marked capacity not over (gallons)	Type of container	Minimum thickness uncoated sheets (gauge)		Rolling hoops		
					Minimum	
		Body sheet	Head sheet	Type	Size	Weight
55	Straight side	16	16	[a]	—	—

[a] Rolled or swedged-in hoops. Use of I-bar hoops authorized.

(b) Steel sheets of specified gauges shall comply with the following:

Gauge No.	Nominal thickness[a] (inch)	Minimum thickness[a] (inch)
12	0.1046	0.0946
16	0.0598	0.0533

[a] Thickness shall be measured at any point on the sheet not less than $^3/_8$ in. from an edge.

§ 178.117-8 Rolling hoops and convex heads

(a) *Rolling hoops.* Rolling hoops to be expanded. Alternate use of I-bar hoops authorized.

(b) *Convex heads.* Convex (crowned) heads; minimum convexity to be $^3/_8$ in., with minimum chime height of $^7/_8$ in.

§ 178.117-9 Closures

(a) Adequate to prevent leakage; gaskets required.

(b) Closing part (plug, cap, plate, etc., see Note 1) must be of metal as thick as prescribed for head of container; this is not required for containers of 12 gal or less when the opening to be closed is not over 2.3 in. in diameter. If unthreaded cap is used it must be provided with outside sealing devices which cannot be removed without destroying the cap or sealing device.

Note 1: This does not apply to cap seal over a closure which complies with all requirements.

(c) Closure must be of screw-thread type or fastened by screw-thread device.

(d) One opening not over 2.3 in. and one opening not over $^{3}/_{4}$ in. allowed; both openings to be welded in one head only. Threads to be standard pipe thread of 11 threads per inch for the larger opening and 14 threads per inch for the $^{3}/_{4}$-in. opening.

§ 178.117-10 Defective containers

(a) Leaks and other defects to be repaired by method used in constructing container, not by soldering.

§ 178.117-11 Marking

(a) Marking on each container by embossing on head with raised marks, or by embossing or die stamping on footring on drums equipped with footrings, or on metal plates securely attached to drum by brazing or welding not less than 20% of the perimeter as follows:

(1) DOT-17F. The letters STC; located near the DOT mark to indicate ''single-trip container.'' In addition, when the container is of stainless steel, the type of steel used in body and head sheets as identified by American Iron and Steel Institute type number, and also the letters HT following steel designation on containers subjected to stress-relieving or heat-treatment during manufacture (for example, DOT-17F-304 or DOT-17F-304 HT as applicable) shall be shown.

(2) Name or symbol of person making the marks specified in paragraph (a)(1) of this section. Symbol, if used, must be registered with the Associate Director for OE.

(3) Gauge of metal in thinnest part, rated capacity in gallons, and year of manufacture (for example, 12-55-50).

[29 FR 18893, Dec. 29, 1964, as amended by Order 66, 30 FR 5755, Apr. 23, 1965. Redesignated at 32 FR 5606, Apr. 5, 1967, and amended by Amdt. 178-40, 41 FR 38181, Sept. 9, 1976]

§ 178.117-12 Size markings

(a) Size of markings (minimum); $^{1}/_{2}$ in. high for 33-gal or less, $^{3}/_{4}$ in. for over 33 and not over 55 gal.

§ 178.117-13 Type tests

(a) Samples taken at random and closed as for use, shall withstand prescribed tests without leakage. Tests to be made of each type and size by each company starting production and to be repeated every 4 months. Samples last tested to be retained until further tests are made for 1 year, whichever period is shorter. The type tests are as follows:

(1) Test by dropping, filled with water to 98% capacity, from height of 6 ft onto solid concrete so as to strike diagonally on chime, or when without chime seam, to strike on other circumferential seam; also additional drop test on any other parts which might be considered weaker than the chime. Closing devices and other parts projecting beyond chime or rolling hoops must also be capable of withstanding this test.

(2) Hydrostatic pressure test of 80 lb/in^2 sustained for 5 min.

[29 FR 18893, Dec. 29, 1964, as amended by Order 66, 30 FR 5755, Apr. 23, 1965. Redesignated at 32 FR 5606, Apr. 5, 1967]

§ 178.117-14 Leakage test

(a) Each container shall be tested, with seams under water or covered with soapsuds or heavy oil, by interior air pressure of at least 15 lb/in.^{2}. Equally efficient means of testing are authorized upon demonstration and proof of satisfactory tests to representative of Bureau of Explosives. Leakers shall be rejected or repaired and retested.

§ 178.118 Specification 17H; steel drums

Single-trip container. Removable head required.

§ 178.118-1 Compliance

(a) Required in all details.

§ 178.118-2 Rated capacity

(a) Rated capacity as marked, see § 178.118-10(a)(3). Minimum actual capacity of containers shall be not less than rated (marked) capacity plus 4% Maximum actual capacity shall not be greater than rated (marked) capacity plus 5% or rated (marked) capacity plus 4% plus 1 qt whichever is the greater.

§ 178.118-3 Composition

(a) Sheets for body and heads to be low carbon, open hearth or electric steel.

§ 178.118-5 Seams

(a) Body seams welded.

§ 178.118-6 Parts and dimensions

(a) Parts and dimensions as follows:

		Minimum thickness, uncoated sheets (gauge)				Rolling hoops	
						Minimum	
Marked capacity not over (gallons)	Type of container	Body sheet	Bottom head sheet	Removable head sheet	Type	Size (gauge or inch)	Weight (pounds per foot)
5	Straight side	24	24	20	None	—	—
30	do	18	18	18	[a]	—	—
55	do	18	18	14[c]	[b]	—	—

[a] Rolled or swedged-in hoops.

[b] Each drum must have three rolled or swedged-in hoops, one to be placed in the body near the top curl.

[c] 16 gauge authorized provided there is at least one corrugation in the removable head near the periphery, 18-gauge authorized provided (1) there are at least two corrugations in the removable head near the periphery, (2) the manufacturer or assembler provides to the Director, OHMO, evidence of satisfactory performance of testing of the complete package design conducted in accordance with this section, and (3) the director issues a registration number which the manufacturer or assembler concerned durably marks on the removable head and its corresponding ring-closure device.

(b) Steel sheets of specified gauge shall comply with the following:

Gauge No.	Nominal thickness[a] (inch)	Minimum thickness[a] (inch)
14	0.0747	0.0677
16	0.0598	0.0533
18	0.0478	0.0428
20	0.0359	0.0324
24	0.0239	0.0209

[a] Thickness shall be measured at any point on the sheet not less than $^3/_8$ in. from an edge.

(49 U.S.C. 1803, 1804, 1808; 49 CFR 1.53(e))
[29 FR 18893, Dec. 29, 1964. Redesignated at 32 FR 5606, Apr. 5, 1967, and amended by Admt. 178-44, 42 FR 61465, Dec. 5, 1977]

§ 178.118-7 Convex heads

(a) Convex (crowned) heads, not extending beyond level of chime, required for drums of 25 gal capacity or over; minimum convexity of $^3/_8$ in. required.

§ 178.118-8 Closures

(a) Adequate to prevent leakage; gaskets required.

(b) Drums over 5 gal capacity must be closed by means of 12 gauge bolted ring with drop forged lugs, one of which is threaded, and having $^3/_8$ in. bolt and nut for drums not over 30 gal capacity and $^5/_8$ in. bolt and nut for drums over 30 gal capacity. Five gallon drums must be of lug type closure with cover having at least 16 lugs. Equally efficient types of closures are authorized upon demonstration and proof of satisfactory tests to representative of Bureau of Explosives.

(c) For closure with threaded plug or cap, the seat (flange, etc.) for plug, or cap, must have 3 or more threads; two drainage holes of not over $^5/_{16}$ in. diameter are allowed. Plug, or cap, must have sufficient length of thread to engage 3 threads when screwed home with gasket in place; *Provided,* That for containers having a capacity of 12 gal and less the seat (flange, etc.) for plug, or cap, must have two or more complete threads and plug, or cap, must have sufficient length of thread to engage two threads when screwed home with gasket in place.

(1) Closures of screw-thread type or closed by other positive means, of any material or design, may be authorized by the Bureau of Explosives for use upon satisfactory proof of efficiency.

[29 FR 18893, Dec. 29, 1964, as amended by Order 67, 30 FR 7425, June 5, 1965. Redesignated at 32 FR 5606, Apr. 5, 1967]

§ 178.118-9 Defective containers

(a) Leaks and other defects to be repaired by method used in constructing container, not by soldering.

§ 178.118-10 Marking

(a) Marking on each container by embossing on head, except that such embossment must be on the permanent head for drums having removable heads, with raised marks, or by embossing or die stamping on footring on drums equipped with footrings, or on metal plates securely attached to drum by brazing or welding not less than 20% of the perimeter, as follows:

(1) DOT-17H. The letters STC; located near the DOT mark to indicate ''single-trip container.'' In addition, when the container is of stainless steel, the type of steel used in body and head sheets as identified by American Iron and Steel Institute type number, and also the letters HT following steel designation on containers subjected to stress-relieving or heat-treatment during manufacture (for example, DOT-17H-304 or DOT-17H-304 HT as applicable) shall be shown.
(2) Name or symbol of person making the marks specified in paragraph (a)(1) of this section. Symbol, if used, must be registered with the Associate Director for OE.
(3) Gauge of metal in thinnest part, rated capacity in gallons, and year of manufacture (for example, 12-55-50). When gauge of metal in body differs from that in head, both must be indicated with slanting line between and with gauge of body indicated first (for example 14/12-55-50 for body 14 gauge and head 12 gauge).

[29 FR 18893, Dec. 29, 1964, as amended by Order 66, 30 FR 5756, Apr. 23, 1965. Redesignated at 32 FR 5606, Apr. 5, 1967, and amended by Amdt. 178-40, 41 FR 38181, Sept. 9, 1976]

§ 178.118-11 Size of markings

(a) Size of markings (minimum): $^1/_2$ in. high for 33-gal or less, $^3/_4$ in. for over 33 and not over 55 gal.

§ 178.118-12 Type tests

(a) Samples taken at random and closed as for use, shall withstand prescribed tests without leakage. Tests to be made of each type and size by each company starting production and to be repeated every 4 months. Samples last tested to be retained until further tests are made or for 1 year, whichever period is shorter. The type tests are as follows:

(1) Test by dropping, filled with water to 98% capacity, from height of 4 ft onto solid concrete so as to strike diagonally on chime, or when without chime seam, to strike on other circumferential seam; also additional drop test on any other parts which might be considered weaker than the chime. Closing devices and other parts projecting beyond chime or rolling hoops must also be capable of withstanding this test.
(2) Hydrostatic pressure test of 15 lb/in.^{2} sustained for 5 min.

[29 FR 18893, Dec. 29, 1964, as amended by Order 66, 30 FR 5756, Apr. 23, 1965, Redesignated at 32 FR 5606, Apr. 5, 1967]

§ 178.118-13 Leakage test

(a) Each container shall be tested, with seams under water or covered with soapsuds or heavy oil, by interior air pressure of at least 7 lb/in.[a] for containers over 12 gal capacity and at least 5 lb for others. Equally efficient means of testing are authorized upon demonstration and proof of satisfactory tests to representative of Bureau of Explosives. Leakers shall be rejected or repaired and retested. Containers not required to be tested with heads in place except that samples taken at random and closed as for use, of each type and size, must be tested at start of production and repeated every four months. Samples so tested must be retained until further tests are made.

§ 178.191 Specification 19B; wooden boxes, glued plywood, nailed

§ 178.191-1 Compliance

(a) Required in all details.

§ 178.191-2 Authorized gross weight.

(a) Authorized gross weight not to exceed 150 lb.

§ 178.191-3 Plywood

(a) Plywood shall be made from veneer which has been rotary cut, sliced or sawed. It shall be well seasoned and commercially dry; free from decay, objectionable knots, that interfere with nailing, splits, gaps, and other defects that materially lessen the strength. Plywood shall be of good commercial box or sheathing grade.

(b) Plywood shall be at least 5 ply; each ply alternately glued with the grain at right angles to the one next.

§ 178.191-4 Nails

(a) Cement coated and of size specified for ''sinkers'' or ''coolers'' as generally known to the trade.

(b) Nail spacing as follows:

Nail (size) in penny	Maximum spacing when driven into end and corner posts	
	Side grain	**End grain**
	Inches	*Inches*
Threepenny	$1^1/_4$	1
Fourpenny	$1^1/_2$	$1^1/_4$
Fivepenny	$1^3/_4$	$1^1/_2$
Sixpenny	2	$1^3/_4$
Sevenpenny	$2^1/_4$	2
Eightpenny	$2^1/_2$	$2^1/_4$
Ninepenny	$2^3/_4$	$2^1/_2$
Tenpenny	3	$2^1/_2$

§ 178.191-5 Corner construction

(a) Boxes exceeding 35 lb gross weight must have 4 vertical corner posts, or other equally suitable devices or fasteners; nailed lap-joint permitted for others.

§ 178.191-6 Assembly

(a) Assemble with grain of outer plywood face in the direction of the longest faces of the box and securely nail or fasten to corner posts or ends as provided in §§ 178.191-4 and 178.191-5.

§ 178.191-7 Special tests

(a) Samples of each type and size manufactured, taken at random, and filled with dummy contents the shape and size of expected contents, or with sand or sawdust, to the gross weight at which container is marked, closed as for use, must be capable of withstanding the following tests without serious rupture or exposure of contents:

(1) 8 drops from height of 1 ft, one on each corner, onto solid concrete.

§ 178.191-8 Closing for shipment

(a) Box to be securely closed. Nails, if used, must be as prescribed in § 178.191-3; hinges and hasps or other equally efficient device authorized.

§ 178.191-9 Marking

(a) Marking on each container with letters and figures at least $^1/_2$ in. high in rectangle as follows.

DOT-19B***

(1) The stars must be replaced by authorized gross weight (for example DOT-19B150).
(2) Name or symbol of person making the mark specified in paragraph (a)(1) of this section and located just above, below, or following that mark. Symbol, if used, must be registered with the Associate Director for OE.

[29 FR 18927, Dec. 29, 1964. Redesignated at 32 FR 5606, Apr. 5, 1967, and amended by Amdt. 178-21, 36 FR 18469, Sept. 15, 1971; Amdt. 178-40, 41 FR 38181, Sept. 9, 1976]

§ 178.194 Specification 20WC wooden protective jacket
[Amdt. 178-35, 39 FR 45252, Dec. 31, 1974]

§ 178.194-1 General requirements
(a) Each jacket must meet the applicable requirements of § 173.24 of this subchapter.
(b) Maximum gross weight of the jacket plus the contents may not exceed the following:

(1) Specification 20WC-1; 225 kg (500 lb.)
(2) Specification 20WC-2; 225 kg (500 lb.)
(3) Specification 20WC-3: 455 kg (1000 lb.)
(4) Specification 20WC-4: 910 kg (2000 lb.)
(5) Specification 20WC-5: 1820 kg (4000 lb).
(6) Specification 20WC-6: 2230 kg (6000 lb.)

[Amdt. 178-35, 39 FR 45252, Dec. 31 1974]

§ 178.194-2 Materials of construction
(a) The general configuration of the wooden protective jacket must be a hollow cylindrical shell constructed of one-piece discs and rings of plywood or solid hardwood reinforced with steel rods.

(1) The specification 20WC-2 must be additionally completely encased, snugly fit, within an 18-gauge steel shell. The steel shell must be provided with at least four 6 mm (0.25-in) diameter vent holes. Each hole must be covered with durable weatherproof tape, or equivalent device.
(2) The specification 20WC-6 jacket must be additionally completely encased, snugly-fit, within a 12-gauge steel shell. The steel shell must be provided with at least twelve 1.2 cm (0.5-in) diameter vent holes, located in 3 rows of 4 holes each, spaced at 90° intervals near the top, middle, and bottom of the drum. Each hole must be covered with durable weatherproof tape, or equivalent device.

(b) Plywood must be exterior-grade, void-free, Douglas fir (or equivalent) not more than 2.5 cm (1 in.) thick. Solid hardwood is authorized for specification 20WC-2 only.
(c) Discs and rings must be glued together with a strong, shock-resistant adhesive, such as either of the following:

(1) A resorcinol-formaldehyde adhesive, which has been bonded under both heat and pressure; or

(2) A polyvinyl-acetate emulsion, which has been reinforced with cement-coated nails. The nails must be randomly spaced and must be at least 2.5 times as long as the minimum thickness of the plywood discs or rings.

(d) Full-length steel rods are required for reinforcement and lid closure.

(1) The minimum number of rods and the minimum rod diameter are as shown in the following table:

Specification	Minimum number or rods	Minimum rod diameter	
		Inches	Millimeters
20WC-1	6	0.25	6.0
20WC-2	6	0.25	6.0
20WC-3	12	0.375	9.5
20WC-4	16	0.375	9.5
20WC-5	16	0.50	12.0
20WC-6	16	0.50	12.0

(2) For specifications 20WC-1 and 20WC-2, steel rods must be equally spaced around the circumference to the rings and discs, midway between the O.D. and I.D. of the rings. For specifications 20WC-3 and 20WC-4, bolts may be staggered alternatvely in two rows, at ±1.2 cm (0.5-in.) from the line midway between the O.D. and I.D. of the rings. For specifications 20WC-5 and 20WC-6, bolts may be staggered alternately in two rows at ±2.5 cm (1 in.) from the line midway between the O.D. and I.D. of the rings.

(3) Rod ends must be threaded and secured with lock nuts and steel washers, or equivalent device, to provide at least a 2.5 cm (1 in.) diameter bearing surface on each end. Ends of the rods must terminate 1.4 cm (0.75-in) below the surface of the plywood for specifications 20WC-1 and 20WC-2. For specifications 20WC-3, 20WC-4, 20WC-5 and 20WC-6, the ends of the rods must terminate 3.7 cm (1.5 in) below the surface of the plywood, and that portion of each end disc which extends beyond the rod ends must be further held in place with lag screws at least 10 cm (4 in) long.

(e) Thickness of wooden shell:

(1) Specification 20WC-1: At least 10 cm (4 in.) thick.

(2) Specification 20WC-2: At least 7.5 cm (3 in.) thick.

(3) Specification 20WC-3: At least 13 cm (5 in.) thick for the jacket wall, and at least 15 cm (6 in.) thick for the end discs. In addition, at least 3 plywood chines, 5 cm (2 in.) wide and protruding 5 cm (2 in.) beyond the outer surfaces, must be located at each end and midway along the length of the jacket.

(4) Specification 20WC-4: At least 15 cm (6 in.) thick for the jacket wall, and at least 15 cm (6 in.) thick for the end discs. In addition, at least 3 plywood chines, 5 cm (2 in.) wide and protruding 5 cm (2 in.) beyond the outer surfaces, must be located at each end and midway along the length of the jacket.

(5) Specifications 20WC-5 and 20WC-6: At least 15 cm (6 in.) thick for the jacket wall, and at least 20 cm (8 in.) thick for the end discs. In addition, at least 5 plywood chines, 5 cm (2 in.) wide and protruding 5 cm (2 in.) beyond the outer surfaces, must be located at each end and equally spaced along the length of the jacket.

[Amdt. 178-35, 39 FR 45252, Dec. 31, 1974]

§ 178.194-3 Closure

(a) Closure for the wooden protective jacket is provided by the steel reinforcing rods. The end cap (lid) must fit tightly to the body of the jacket to prevent a heat path to the inside of the jacket. The lid joint for specifications 20WC-3, 20WC-4, 20WC-5, and 20WC-6, may not be coplanar with the end of the inner containment vessel.

(b) Specifications 20WC-2 and 20WC-6. Locking ring closure, if used, must conform to § 178.104-4. Flanged closure, if used, must have at least 8 steel bolts (at least 6 mm (0.25-in.) diameter for 20WC-2 or 1.2 cm (0.50-in) diameter for 20WC-6) and lock nuts (or equivalent device), spaced not more than 13 cm (5 in) between centers.

[Amdt. 178-35, 39 FR 45252, Dec. 31, 1974]

§ 178.194-4 Tests

Prior to each use, each jacket must be visually inspected for defects such as improper bonding, cracking, corrosion of steel rods, and improperly fitting closure lid, or other manufacturing defects. Particular attention must be given to any separation of the plywood discs and rings which would provide a heat path to the inside of the jacket.

[Amdt. 178-35, 39 FR 45252, Dec. 31, 1974]

§ 178.194-5 Painting

Each jacket (other than 20WC-2 and 20WC-6) must be completely painted with a high quality exterior weather resistant paint.

[Amdt. 178-35, 39 FR 45252, Dec. 31, 1974]

§ 178.194-6 Marking

(a) Each jacket must be marked on the external surface as follows: ''USA-DOT 20WC-( ) TYPE B'' The appropriate numeral must be inserted in the marking to indicate the appropriate specification 20WC category: e.g., ''20WC-2.''

(b) Each jacket must also be marked with the name or symbol of person making the marks specified in paragraph (a) of this section. Symbol, if used, must be registered with the Associate Director for OE.

[Amdt. 178-35, 39 FR 45252, Dec. 31, 1974. as amended by Admt. 178-40, 41 FR 38182, Sept. 9, 1976]

§ 178.194-7 Typical assembly sketches

(a) Spec. 20WC-2.

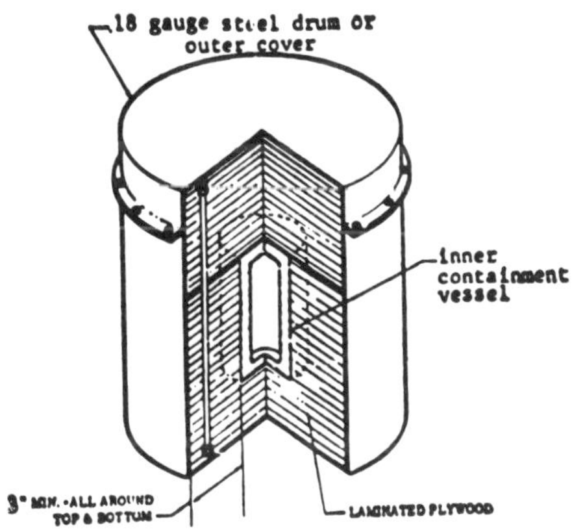

(b) Spec. 20WC-5.

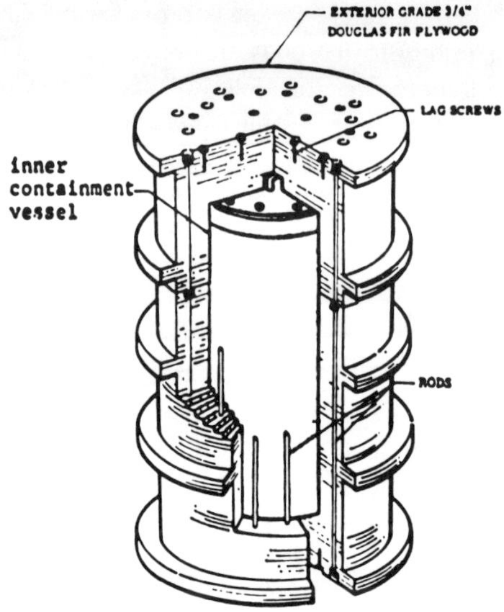

[Amdt. 178-35, 39 FR 45253, Dec. 31, 1974; 40 FR 2435, Jan. 13, 1975]

§ 178.195 Specification 21WC woodensteel protective overpack
[Amdt. 178-35, 39 FR 45253, Dec. 31, 1974]

§ 178.195-1 General requirements

(a) Each jacket must meet all the applicable requirements of § 173.24 of this subchapter.

(b) The maximum authorized gross weight of the overpack, including its inner container and contents may not exceed 1360 kg (3000 lb.)
[Admt. 178-35, 39 FR 45253, Dec. 31, 1974]

§ 178.195-2 Materials of construction and other requirements

(a) The general configuration of the protective overpack must be a combination of two nested plywood boxes, each 2.5 cm (1 in.) thick, nested within a third wooden box of nominal 5 cm (2-in.) thickness solid hardwood. The three nested boxes must be enclosed within a welded framework 10 cement-coated nails spaced on nominally 1 cm ($^3/_8$-in.) thick by 8 to 10 cm (3 to 4 in.) wide. All outer surfaces of each box must be coated with intumescent paint.

(b) Plywood must be exterior-grade, void-free, Douglas fir, or equivalent, at least 2.5 cm (1 in.) thick. Solid hardwood must be maple, or equivalent.

(c) All box joints and interior surfaces must be glued with a strong, shock-resistant adhesive such as polyvinylacetate emulsion, or equivalent.

(d) All hardwood joints must be mitered, or equivalent, reinforced with No. 10 cement-coated nails space on nominal 15 cm (6-in.) centers.

(e) All plywood joints must be butt-type, or equivalent, reinforced with No. 10 cement-coated nails space on nominal 15 cm (6-in.) centers.

(e) All plywood joints must be butt-type, or equivalent, reinforced with No. 10 cement-coated nails spaced on nominal 15 cm (6-in.) centers.

(f) The angles and strapping of the metal frame must be spaced such that separation distances do not exceed 15 cm (6 in.)

(g) The lid must be of the same material as the box and fabricated in such a manner that

closure forms a mitered joint with the hardwood box and 2 stepped-joints with the plywood boxes.
[Amdt. 178-35, 39 FR 45253, Dec. 31, 1974]

§ 178.195-3 Closure

Closure for the protective overpack must be provided by at least 4 mild steel hinges formed from minimum 2.5-cm (1-in.) x 5-mm ($^{3}/_{16}$-in.) bar stock. Hinge pins must be minimum 6-mm ($^{1}/_{4}$-in.) diameter by 13.3 cm ($5^{1}/_{4}$ in.) long mild steel rod drilled at both ends for cotter pins.
[Amdt. 178-35, 39 FR 45253, Dec. 31, 1974]

§ 178.195-4 Tests

Prior to each use, each overpack must be visually inspected for defects such as wood checking or splintering weld cracking, corrosion of steel parts, improper joint bonding, or improperly fitting closure lid.
[Amdt. 178-35, 39 FR 45253, Dec. 31, 1974]

§ 178.195-5 Required marking

(a) Marking must be as prescribed in § 173.24 of this subchapter.

(b) Marking on the outside of each overpack must include the following:

(1) ''USA-DOT 21WC'' and ''TYPE B'' as appropriate.
[Amdt. 178-35, 39 FR 45253, Dec. 31, 1974]

§ 178.195-6 Typical assembly detail.

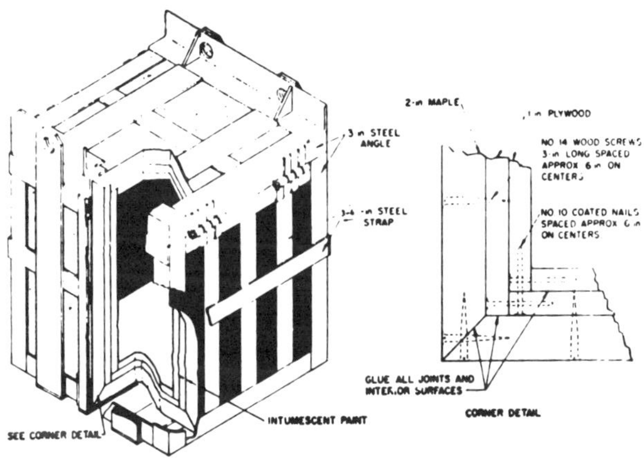

FIGURE 4. Radioisotopes shipping cask fire and impact shield. [Amdt. 178-35, 39 FR 45253, Dec. 31, 1974; 40 FR 2435, Jan. 13, 1975.]

SUBPART K — SPECIFICATIONS FOR GENERAL PACKAGINGS

§ 178.350 Specification 7A; general packaging, Type A
[Amdt. 178-1, 33 FR 14935. Oct. 4, 1968]

§ 178.350-1 General requirements

(a) Each packaging must meet all applicable requirements of § 173.24 of this chapter.
[Amdt. 178-1, 33 FR 14935, Oct. 4, 1968]

§ 178.350-2 Specific requirements

(a) Each packaging must be so designed and constructed that it meets the standards for Type A packaging (see §§ 173.389(j) and 173.398(b) of this chapter).
[Amdt. 178-1, 33 FR 14935, Oct. 4, 1968]

§ 178.350-3 Marking

(a) Marking on the outside of each packaging as follows: "USA DOT 7A Type A" and "Radioactive Material."

(b) The letter and number size and additional marking requirements of § 173.24 of this subchapter must be complied with.
[Amdt. 178-1, 33 FR 14935, Oct. 4, 1968, as amended by Amdt. 178-40, 41 FR 38183, Sept. 9, 1976]

APPENDICES TO PART 178
APPENDIX A — SPECIFICATIONS FOR STEEL

Table 1
OPEN-HEARTH, BASIC OXYGEN, OR ELECTRIC STEEL OF UNIFORM QUALITY. THE FOLLOWING CHEMICAL COMPOSITION ARE BASED ON LADLE ANALYSIS

	Chemical composition, percent-ladle analysis		
Designation	**Grade 1**[a]	**Grade 2**[a,b]	**Grade 3**[c,d,e]
Carbon	0.10/0.20	0.24 maximum	0.22 maximum
Manganese	1.10/1.60	0.50/1.00	1.25 maximum
Phosphorus, maximum	0.04	0.04	0.045[f]
Sulfur, maximum	0.05	0.05	0.05
Silicon	0.15/0.30	0.30 maximum	
Copper, maximum	0.40	—	
Columbium	—	0.01/0.04	
Heat treatment authorized	[c]	[c]	[c]
Maximum stress (p.s.i.)	35,000	35,000	35,000

[a] Addition of other elements to obtain alloying effect is not authorized.
[b] Ferritic grain size 6 or finer according to ASTM E112-63.
[c] Any suitable heat treatment in excess of 1,100°F except that liquid quenching is not permitted.
[d] Other alloying elements may be added and shall be reported.
[e] For compositions with a maximum carbon content of 0.15 % of ladle analysis, the maximum limit for manganese on ladle analysis may be 1.40%.
[f] Rephosphorized Grade 3 steels containing no more than 0.15 % phosphorus are permitted if carbon content does not exceed 0.15% and manganese does not exceed 1%.

CHECK ANALYSIS TOLERANCES
A HEAT OF STEEL MADE UNDER ANY OF THE ABOVE GRADES, THE LADLE ANALYSIS OF WHICH IS SLIGHTLY OUT OF THE SPECIFIED RANGE IS ACCEPTABLE IF THE CHECK ANALYSIS IS WITHIN THE FOLLOWING VARIATIONS

Element	Limit or maximum specified (percent)	Tolerance (percent) over the maximum limit or under the minimum limit	
		Under minimum limit	Over maximum limit
Carbon	To 0.15 inclusive	0.02	0.03
	Over 0.15 to 0.40 inclusive	0.03	0.04
Manganese	To 0.60 inclusive	0.03	0.03
	Over 0.60 to 1.15 inclusive	0.04	0.04
	Over 1.15 to 2.50 inclusive	0.05	0.05
Phosphorus[a]	All ranges	—	0.01
Sulfur	All ranges	—	0.01
Silicon	To 0.30 inclusive	0.02	0.03
Over 0.30 to 1.00	inclusive	0.05	0.05
Copper	To 1.00 inclusive	0.03	0.03
	Over 1.00 to 2.00 inclusive	0.05	0.05
Nickel	To 1.00 inclusive	0.03	0.03
	Over 1.00 to 2.00 inclusive	0.05	0.05
Chromium	To 0.90 inclusive	0.03	0.03
	Over 0.90 to 2.10 inclusive	0.05	0.05
Molybdenum	To 0.20 inclusive	0.01	0.01
	Over 0.20 to 0.40 inclusive	0.02	0.02
Zirconium	All ranges	0.01	0.05
Columbium	To 0.04 inclusive	0.005	0.01
Aluminum	Over 0.10 to 0.20 inclusive	0.04	0.04
	Over 0.20 to 0.30 inclusive	0.05	0.05

[a] Rephosphorized steels not subject to check analysis for phosphorus.

[Amdt. 178-3, 34 FR 12283, July 25, 1969; 34 FR 12593, Aug. 1, 1969]

APPENDIX B — SPECIFICATIONS FOR PLASTICS

Table 1
POLYETHYLENE MUST HAVE THE FOLLOWING PROPERTIES, AS DETERMINED BY THE AMERICAN SOCIETY FOR TESTING MATERIALS (ASTM) METHODS DESIGNATED. TESTS MUST BE PERFORMED ON RESIN WITH ADDITIVES INCLUDED:

Property	Type I	Type II	Type III	ASTM method
Density (g/cc)	0.910 — <0.926	0.926 — <0.941	0.941 — <0.965	D 1505-68.
Melt index (flow rate)	2.0 max	1.0 max	1.0 max	D 1238-65T.
Tensile strength	1500 p.s.i min	1800 p.s.i	3000 p.s.i	D 638-68.
Elongation	400% min	400%	75%	D 638-68.

Note: Other materials may be added to polyethylene resin provided they do not adversely affect the physical properties specified above.

[Amdt. 178-5, 34 FR 12593, Aug. 1, 1969; Amdt. 178-32, 39 FR 12752, Apr. 8, 1974]

APPENDIX I
TITLE 10, PART 20*

§ 20.205 Procedures for Picking Up, Receiving, and Opening Packages

(a)(1) Each licensee who expects to receive a package containing quantities of radioactive material in excess of the Type A quantities specified in paragraph (b) of this section shall:

(i) If the package is to be delivered to the licensee's facility by the carrier, make arrangements to receive the package when it is offered for delivery by the carrier; or
(ii) If the package is to be picked up by the licensee at the carrier's terminal, make arrangements to receive notification from the carrier of the arrival of the package, at the time of arrival.

(2) Each licensee who picks up a package of radioactive material from a carrier's terminal shall pick up the package expeditiously upon receipt of notification from the carrier of its arrival.

(b) (1) Each licensee, upon a receipt of a package of radioactive material, shall monitor the external surfaces of the package for radioactive contamination caused by leakage of the radioactive contents, except:

(i) Packages containing no more than the exempt quantity specified in the table in this paragraph:
(ii) Packages containing no more than 10 mCi of radioactive material consisting solely of tritium, carbon-14 sulfur-35, or iodine-125;
(iii) Packages containing only radioactive material as gases or in special form
(iv) Packages containing only radioactive material in other than liquid form (including Mo-99/Tc-99m generators) and not exceeding the Type A quantity limit specified in the table in this paragraph; and
(v) Packages containing only radionuclides with half-lives of less than 30 days and a total quantity of no more than 100 mCi.

The monitoring shall be performed as soon as practicable after receipt, but no later than 3 hr after the package is received during the licensee's normal working hours, or 18 hr if received after normal working hours.

(2) If removable radioactive contamination in excess of 0.01 μCi (22,000 disintegrations per minute) per 100 square centimeters of package surface is found on the external surfaces of the package, the licensee shall immediately notify the final delivering carrier and, by telephone and telegraph, mailgram, or facsimile, (amended 41 FR 16445), the appropriate Nuclear Regulatory Commission Inspection and Enforcement Regional Office shown in Table 1.

* From *Fed. Reg.*, September 1, 1978.

TABLE OF EXEMPT AND TYPE A QUANTITIES

Transport group[a]	Exempt quantity limit (in millicuries)	Type A quantity limit (in curies)
I	0.01	0.001
II	0.1	0.050
III	1	3
IV	1	20
V	1	20
VI	1	1000
VII	25,000	1000
Special Form	1	20

[a] The definitions of "transport group" and "special form" are specified in § 71.4 of this chapter.

(c) (1) Each licensee, upon receipt of a package containing quantities of radioactive material in excess of the Type A quantities specified in paragraph (b) of this section, other than those transported by exclusive use vehicle, shall monitor the radiation levels external to the package. The package shall be monitored as soon as practicable after receipt, but no later than 3 hr after the package is received at the licensee's facility if received during the licensee's normal working hours, or 18 hr if received after normal working hours.

(2) If radiation levels are found on the external surface of the package in excess of 200 mrem/hr or at 3 ft from the external surface of the package in excess of 10 mrem/hr, the licensee shall immediately notify by telephone and telegraph, maligram, or facsimile, the director of the appropriate NRC Regional Office listed in Appendix D, and the final delivering carrier.

(d) Each licensee shall establish and maintain procedures for safely opening packages in which licensed material is received, and shall assure that such procedures are followed and that due consideration is given to special instructions for the type of package being opened.

§ 20.206 Instruction of personnel

Instructions required for individuals working in or frequenting any portion of a restricted area are specified in § 19.12 of this chapter.

TABLE 1
UNITED STATES NUCLEAR REGULATORY COMISSION INSPECTION AND ENFORCEMENT REGIONAL OFFICES

Region	Address	Telephone	
		Daytime	Nights and holidays
I Connecticut, Delaware, District of Columbia, Maine, Maryland, Massachusetts, New Hampshire, New Jersey, New York, Pennsylvania, Rhode Island, and Vermont	Region I, USNRC Office of Inspection and Enforcement 631 Park Avenue King of Prussia, Pa. 19406	(215) 337-5000	(215) 337-5000
II Alabama, Florida, Georgia, Kentucky, Mississippi, North Carolina, Puerto Rico, South Carolina, Tennessee, Virginia, Virgin Islands, and West Virginia	Region II, USNRC Office of Inspection and Enforcement 101 Marietta Street Suite 3100 Atlanta, Georgia 30303	(404) 221-4503	(404) 221-4503
III Illinois, Indiana, Iowa, Michigan, Minnesota, Missouri, Ohio, and Wisconsin	Region III, USNRC Office of Inspection and Enforcement 799 Roosevelt Road Glen Ellyn, Ill. 60137	(312) 932-2500	(312) 932-2500
IV Arkansas, Colorado, Idaho, Kansas, Louisiana, Montana, Nebraska, New Mexico, North Dakota, Oklahoma, South Dakota, Texas, Utah, and Wyoming	Region IV, USNRC Office of Inspection and Enforcement 611 Ryan Plaza Drive Suite 1000 Arlington, Texas 76012	(817) 334-2841	(817) 334-2841
V Alaska, Arizona, California, Hawaii, Nevada, Oregon, Washington, and U.S. territories and possessions in the Pacific	Region V, USNRC Office of Inspection and Enforcement 1990 N. California Blvd. Suite 202 Walnut Creek, Calif. 94596	(415) 943-3700	(415) 943-3700

APPENDIX J
TITLE 10, PART 20 H-3 AND C-14

WASTE DISPOSAL

§ 20.301 General requirement

No licensee shall dispose of licensed material except:

(a) By transfer to an authorized recipient as provided in the regulations in Parts 30, 40, 60, 70 or 72 of this chapter, whichever may be applicable; or
(b) As authorized pursuant to § 20.302; or
(c) As provided in § 20.303, applicable to the disposal of licensed material by release into sanitary sewerage systems, or in § 20.306 for disposal of specific wastes, or in § 20.106 (Radioactivity in effluents to unrestricted areas).

[25 FR 10914 Nov. 17, 1960, as amended at 46 FR 16234. Mar. 11, 1981; 46 FR 58282, Dec. 1, 1981]

§ 20.302 Method for obtaining approval of proposed disposal procedures

(a) Any licensee or applicant for a license may apply to the Commission for approval of proposed procedures to dispose of licensed material in a manner not otherwise authorized in the regulations in this chapter. Each application should include a description of the licensed material and any other radioactive material involved, including the quantities and kinds of such material and the levels of radioactivity involved, and the proposed manner and conditions of disposal. The application should also include an analysis and evaluation of pertinent information as to the nature of the environment, including topographical, geological, meteorological, and hydrological characteristics; usage of ground and surface waters in the general area; the nature and location of other potentially affected facilities; and procedures to be observed to minimize the risk of unexpected or hazardous exposures.

(b) The Commission will not approve any application for a license to receive licensed material from other persons for disposal on land not owned by the Federal government or by a State government.

(c) The Commission will not approve any application for a license for disposal of licensed material at sea unless the applicant shows that sea disposal offers less harm to a man or the environment than other practical alternative methods of disposal.

[25 FR 10914, Nov. 17, 1960, as amended at 26 FR 352, Jan. 18, 1961; 36 FR 23138, Dec. 4, 1971]

§ 20.303 Disposal by release into sanitary sewerage systems

No licensee shall discharge licensed material into a sanitary sewerage system unless;

(a) It is readily soluble or dispersible in water; and
(b) The quantity of any licensed or other radioactive material released into the system by the licensee in any one day does not exceed the larger of paragraphs (b)(1) or (2) of this section.

    (1) The quantity which, if diluted by the average daily quantity of sewage released into the sewer by the licensee, will result in an average concentration equal to the limits specified in Appendix B, Table I, Column 2 of this part; or
    (2) Ten times the quantity of such material specified in Appendix C of this part; and

(c) The quantity of any licensed or other radioactive material released in any one month, if diluted by the average monthly quantity of water released by the licensee, will not result in an average concentration exceeding the limits specified in Appendix B, Table I, Column 2 of this part; and
(d) The gross quantity of licensed and other radioactive material, excluding hydrogen-3 and carbon-14, released into the sewerage system by the licensee does not exceed 1 Ci/year.

The quantities of hydrogen-3 and carbon-14 released into the sanitary sewerage system may not exceed 5 Ci/year for hydrogen-3 and 1 Ci/year for carbon-14. Excreta from individuals undergoing medical diagnosis or therapy with radioactive material shall be exempt from any limitations contained in this section.
[25 FR 10914, Nov. 17, 1960, as amended at 46 FR 16234, Mar. 11, 1981]

§ 20.305 Treatment or disposal by incineration

No licensee shall treat or dispose of licensed material by incineration except for materials listed under § 20.306 or as specifically approved by the Commission pursuant to §§ 20.106(b) and 20.302.
[46 FR 16234, Mar. 11, 1981]

§ 20.306 Disposal of specific wastes

Any licensee may dispose of the following licensed material without regard to its radioactivity:

(a) 0.05 μCi or less of hydrogen-3 or carbon-14, per gram of medium, used for liquid scintillation counting; and
(b) 0.05 μCi or less of hydrogen-3 or carbon-14, per gram of animal tissue averaged over the weight of the entire animal; provided however, tissue may not be disposed of under this section in a manner that would permit its use either as food for humans or as animal feed.
(c) Nothing in this section, however, relieves the licensee of maintaining records showing the receipt, transfer and disposal of such byproduct material as specified in § 30.51 of this chapter; and
(d) Nothing in this section relieves the licensee from complying with other applicable Federal, State and local regulations governing any other toxic or hazardous property of these materials.

[46 FR 16234, Mar. 11, 1981]

APPENDIX K
TITLE 10, PART 71*

SUBPART A — GENERAL PROVISIONS

§ 71.1 Purpose

(a) This part establishes requirements for transportation and for preparation for shipment of licensed material and prescribes procedures and standards for approval by the Nuclear Regulatory Commission of packaging and shipping procedures for licensed materials and prescribes certain requirements governing such packaging and shipping.

(b) The packaging and transport of these materials are also subject to other parts of this chapter and to the regulations of other agencies having jurisdiction over means of transport. The requirements of this part are in addition to, and not in substitution for, other requirements.

§ 71.2 Scope

The regulations in this part apply to each person authorized by specific license issued by the Commission to receive, possess, use or transfer licensed materials, if he delivers such materials to a carrier for transport or transports such material outside the confines of his plant or other place of use.

§ 71.3 Requirement for license

No licensee subject to the regulations in this part shall (a) deliver any licensed materials to a carrier for transport or (b) transport licensed material except as authorized in a general license or specific license issued by the Commission, or as exempted in this part.

§ 71.4 Definitions

As used in this part:

(a) ''Carrier'' means any person engaged in the transportation of passengers or property, as common, contract, or private carrier, or freight forwarder, as those terms are used in the Interstate Commerce Act, as amended, or the U.S. Post Office:

(b) ''Close reflection by water'' means immediate contract by water of sufficient thickness to reflect a maximum number of neutrons;

(c) ''Containment vessel'' means the receptacle on which principal reliance is placed to retain the radioactive material during transport;

(d) ''Fissile classification'' means classification of a package or shipment of fissile materials according to the controls needed to provide nuclear criticality safety during transportation as follows:

(1) Fissile Class I: Packages which may be transported in unlimited numbers and in any arrangement, and which require no nuclear criticality safety controls during transportation. For purposes of nuclear criticality safety control, a transportation index is not assigned to Fissile Class I packages. However, the external radiation levels may require a transport index number.

(2) Fissile Class II: Packages which may be transported together in any arrangement but in numbers which do not exceed an aggregate transport index of 50. For purposes of nuclear criticality safety control, individual packages may have a transport index of not less than 0.1 and not more than 10. However, the external radiation levels may

* From the United States Nuclear Regulatory Commission Rules and Regulations, Title 10, Chapter 1, Code of Federal Regulations — Energy, September 1, 1982.

require a higher transport index number but not to exceed 10. Such shipments require no nuclear criticality safety control by the shipper during transportation.

(3) Fissile Class III: Shipments of packages which do not meet the requirements of Fissile Classes I and II and which are controlled in transportation by special arrangements between the shipper and the carrier to provide nuclear criticality safety.

(e) "Fissile materials" means uranium-233, uranium-235, plutonium-238, plutonium-239, and plutonium-241;

(f) "Large quantity" means a quantity of radioactive material, the aggregate radioactivity of which exceeds any one of the following:

(1) For transport groups as defined in paragraph (p) of this section:

- (i) Group I or II radionuclides: 20 Ci;
- (ii) Group III or IV radionuclides: 200 Ci;
- (iii) Group V radionuclides: 5000 Ci;
- (iv) Group VI or VII radionuclides: 50,000 Ci; and

(2) For special form material as defined in paragraph (o) of this section: 5,000 Ci.

(g) "Low specific activity material" means any of the following:

(1) Uranium or thorium ores and physical or chemical concentrates of those ores;
(2) Unirradiated natural or depleted uranium or unirraidated natural thorium;
(3) Tritium oxide in aqueous solutions provided the concentration does not exceed 5.0 mCi/μℓ;
(4) Material in which the activity is essentially uniformly distributed and in which the estimated average concentration per gram of contents does not exceed:

- (i) 0.0001 mCi of Group I radionuclides; or
- (ii) 0.005 mCi of Group II radionuclides; or
- (iii) 0.3 mCi of Groups III or IV radionuclides.

Note: This includes but is not limited to, materials of low radioactivity concentration such as residues or solutions from chemical processing; wastes such as building rubble, metal, wood, and fabric scrap, glassware, paper, and cardboard; solid or liquid plant waste, sludges, and ashes.

(5) Objects of nonradioactive material externally contaminated with radioactive material, provided that the radioactive material is not readily dispersible and the surface contamination, when averaged over an area of 1 m^2 does not exceed 0.0001 mCi (220,000 disintegrations per minute) per square centimeter of Group I radionuclides or 0.001 mCi (2,200,000 disintegrations per minute) per square centimeter of other radionuclides.

(h) "Maximum normal operating pressure" means the maximum gauge pressure which is expected to develop in the containment vessel under the normal conditions of transport specified in Appendix A of this part;

(i) "Moderator" means a material used to reduce, by scattering collisions and without appreciable capture, the kinetic energy of neutrons;

(j) "Optimum interspersed hydrogenous moderation" means the occurrence of hydrogenous material between containment vessels to such an extent that the maximum nuclear reactivity results;

(k) "Package" means packaging and its radioactive contents;

(l) "Packaging" means one or more receptacles and wrappers and their contents excluding fissile material and other radioactive material but including absorbent material, spacing structures, thermal insulation, radiation shielding, devices for cooling and for absorbing mechanical shock, external fittings, neutron moderators, nonfissile neutron absorbers, and other supplementary equipment;

(m) "Primary coolant" means a gas, liquid, or solid, or combination of them, in contact with the radioactive material or, if the material is in special form, in contact with its capsule, and used to remove decay heat;

(n) "Sample package" means a package which is fabricated, packed, and closed to fairly represent the proposed package as it would be presented for transport, simulating the material to be transported, as to weight and physical and chemical form;

(o)"Special form" means any of the following physical forms of licensed material of any transport group;

(1) The material is in solid form having no dimension less than 0.5 mm or at least one dimension greater than 5 mm; does not melt, sublime, or ignite in air at a temperature of 1000°F; will not shatter or crumble if subjected to the percussion test described in Appendix D of this part; and is not dissolved or converted into dispersible form to the extent of more than 0.005% by weight by immersion for 1 week in water at 68°F, or in air at 86°F; or

(2) The material is securely contained in a capsule having no dimension less than 0.5 mm or at least one dimension greater than 5 mm, which will retain its contents if subjected to the tests prescribed in Appendix D of this part; and which is constructed of materials which do not melt, sublime, or ignite in air at 1475°F and do not dissolve or convert into dispersible form to the extent of more than 0.005% by weight by immersion for 1 week in water at 68°F, or in air at 86°F.

(p) "Transport group" means any one of seven groups into which radionuclides in normal form are classified, according to their toxicity and their relative potential hazard in transport, in Appendix C of this part.

(1) Any radionuclide not specifically listed in one of the groups in Appendix C shall be assigned to one of the Groups in accordance with the following table:

	Radioactive half-life		
Radionuclide	**0 to 1000 days**	**1000 days to 10^6 years**	**Over 10^6 years**
Atomic number 1—81	Group III	Group II	Group III
Atomic number 82 and over	Group I	Group I	Group III

(2) For mixtures of radionuclides the following shall apply:

(i) If the identity and respective activity of each radionuclide are are known, the permissible activity of each radionuclide shall be such that the sum, for all groups present, of the radio between the total activity for each group to the permissible activity for each group will not be greater than unity.

(ii) If the groups of the radionuclides are known but the amount in each group cannot be reasonably determined, the mixture shall be assigned to the most restrictive group present.

(iii) If the identity of all or some of the radionuclides cannot be reasonably determined, each of those unidentified radionuclides shall be considered as belonging to the most restrictive group which cannot be positively excluded.

(iv) Mixtures consisting of a single radioactive decay chain where the radionuclides are in the naturally occurring proportions shall be considered as consisting of a single radionuclide. The group and activity shall be that of the first member present in the chain, except that if a radionuclide "x" has a half-life longer than that of that first member and an activity greater than that of any other member, including the first, at any time during transportation, the transport group of the nuclide "x" and the activity of the mixture shall be the maximum activity of that nuclide "x" during transportation.

Terms defined in Parts 20, 30 to 35 inclusive, and 70 of this chapter have the same meaning when used in this part.

(q) "Type A quantity" and "type B quantity" means a quantity of radioactive material the aggregate radioactivity of which does not exceed that specified in the following table:

Transport groups see § 71.4(p)	Type A quantity (in curies)	Type B quantity (in curies)
I	0.001	20
II	0.05	20
III	3	200
IV	20	200
V	20	5,000
VI and VII	1000	50,000
Special form	20[a]	5,000

[a] Except that for californium-252, the limit is 2 Ci.

(r) "Nuclear waste" as used in §§ 71.5a-71.5b means:

(1) Any large quantity of source, by-product, or special nuclear material required by this part to be in Type B packaging while transported to, through, or across state boundaries to a disposal site, or to a collection point for transport to a disposal site, or
(2) Any large quantity of irradiated fuel required by this part to be in Type 2 packaging while transported to, through, or across state boundaries irrespective of destination if the quantity of irradiated fuel is less than that subject to advance notification requirements of 10 CFR Part 73.

(s) "State" as used in §§ 71.5a to 71.5b means that several States of the Union, the District of Columbia, the Commonwealth of Puerto Rico, the Virgin Islands, Guam, American Samoa, the Trust Territory of the Pacific Islands, and the Commonwealth of the Northern Mariana Islands.

§ 71.5 Transportation of licensed material

(a) No licensee shall transport any licensed material outside of the confines of his plant or other place of use, or deliver any licensed material to a carrier for transport, unless the licensee complies with the applicable requirements of the regulations appropriate to the mode of transport, of the Department of Transportation in 49 CFR Parts 170 to 189, and the U.S. Postal Service in the Postal Service Manual (Domestic Mail Manual), section 124.3, incorporated by reference, 39 CFR 111.1 (1974), insofar as such regulations relate to the packaging of by-product, source, or special nuclear material, marking and labeling of the packages, loading and storage of packages, placarding of the transportation vehicle, monitoring requirements and accident reporting.

(b) When Department of Transportation regulations are not applicable to shipments of licensed material by rail, highway, or water because the shipment or the transportation of the shipment is not in interstate or foreign commerce, or to shipments of licensed material by air because the shipment is not transported in civil aircraft, the licensee shall conform to the standards and requirements of the Department of Transportation specified in paragraph (a) of this section, to the same extent as if the shipment or transportation were in interstate, or foreign commerce or in civil aircraft. Any requests for modifications, waivers, or exemptions from those requirements, and any notifications referred to in those requirements shall be filed with or made to the Nuclear Regulatory Commission.

(c) Paragraph (a) of this section shall not apply to the transportation of licensed material, or to the delivery of licensed material to a carrier for transport, where such transportation is subject to the regulations of the U.S. Postal Service.

ADVANCE NOTIFICATION TO STATES OF TRANSPORT OF NUCLEAR WASTE

§ 71.5a Transport of nuclear waste — advance notification requirement

Prior to the transport of any nuclear waste outside of the confines of the licensee's plant or other place of use or storage, or prior to the delivery of any nuclear waste to a carrier for transport, each licensee shall comply with the procedures in § 71.5b for advance notification to the governor of a state or the governor's designee for the transport of nuclear waste to, through, or across the boundary of the state.

§ 71.5b Advance notification of shipment of nuclear waste; revision notice; cancellation notice

(a) *Where, when, and how advance notification must be sent.* The notification required by § 71.5a must be made in writing to the office of each appropriate governor or governor's designee and to the Director of the appropriate Nuclear Regulatory Commission Inspection and Enforcement Regional Office listed in Appendix A of Part 73 of this chapter. A notification delivered by mail must be postmarked at least 7 days before the beginning of the 7-day period during which departure of the shipment is estimated to occur. A notification delivered by messenger must reach the office of the governor or of the governor's designee at least 4 days before the beginning of the 7-day period during which departure of the shipment is estimated to occur. A list of the mailing addresses of the governors and governors' designees is available upon request from the Director, Office of State Programs, U.S. Nuclear Regulatory Commission, Washington, D.C. 20555. A copy of the notification shall be retained by the licensee as a record for 1 year.

(b) *Information to be furnished in advance notification of shipment.* Each advance notification of shipment of nuclear waste must contain the following information:

(1) The name, address, and telephone number of the shipper, carrier, and receiver of the nuclear waste shipment.

(2) A description of the nuclear waste contained in the shipment as required by the regulations of the U.S. Department of Transportation in 49 CFR §§ 172.202 and 172.203(d);

(3) The point of origin of the shipment, and the 7-day period during which departure of the shipment is estimated to occur;

(4) The 7-day period during which arrival of the shipment at state boundaries is estimated to occur;

(5) The destination of the shipment, and the 7-day period during which arrival of the shipment is estimated to occur; and
(6) A point of contact with a telephone number for current shipment information.

(c) *Revision notice.* A licensee who finds that schedule information previously furnished to a governor or governor's designee in accordance with § 71.5b(b) will not be met, shall telephone a responsible individual in the office of the governor of the state or of the governor's designee and inform that individual of the extent of the delay relative to the schedule originally reported in writing under the provisions of § 71.5b(b). The licensee shall maintain a record of the name of the individual contact for 1 year.

(d) *Cancellation notice.*

(1) Each licensee who cancels a nuclear waste shipment for which advance notification has been sent as required by § 71.5a shall send a cancellation notice to the governor of each state or the governor's designee previously notified and to the Director of the appropriate Nuclear Regulatory Commission Inspection and Enforcement Regional Office listed in Appendix A of Part 73 of this chapter.
(2) The notice shall state that it is a cancellation and shall identify the advance notification which is being cancelled. A copy of the notice shall be retained by the licensee as a record for 1 year.

EXEMPTIONS

§ 71.6 Specific exemptions

On application of any interested person or on its own initiative, the Commission may grant such exemptions from the requirements of the regulations in this part as it determines are authorized by law and will not endanger life or property or the common defense and security.

§ 71.7 Exemption for no more than type A quantities

(a) A licensee is exempt from all the requirements of this part to the extent that he delivers to a carrier for transport packages each of which contains no licensed material having a specific activity in excess of 0.002 μCi/g.

(b) Except for the requirements specified in §71.5, a licensee is exempt from all the requirements of this part to the extent he delivers to a carrier for transport packages subject to the regulations of the Department of Transportation in 49 CFR Parts 170—189 or the U.S. Postal Service in the Postal Service Manual (Domestic Mail Manual), section 124.3, incorporated by reference, 39 CFR 111.1 (1974), each of which contains no more than a Type A quantity of radioactive materials, as defined in § 71.4(g), which may include one of the following:

(1) Not more than 15 g of fissile material; or
(2) Thorium, or uranium containing not more than 0.72% by weight of fissile material; or
(3) Uranium compounds, other than metal (e.g., UF_4, UF_6, or uranium oxide in bulk form, not pelleted or fabricated into shapes) or aqueous* solutions of uranium, in which the total amount of uranium-233 and plutonium present does not exceed 1.0% by weight of the uranium-235 content, and the total fissile content does not exceed 1.00% by weight of the total uranium content; or

* This applies to light water and does not apply to heavy water.

(4) Homogeneous hydrogenous* solutions or mixtures containing not more than:

   (i) 500 g of any fissile material, provided the atomic ratio of hydrogen to fissile material is greater than 7600; or
   (ii) 800 g of uranium-235; *Provided,* That the atomic ratio of hydrogen to fissile material is greater than 5200, and the content of other fissile material is not more than 1% by weight of the total uranium-235 content; or
   (iii) 500 g of uranium-233 and uranium-235; *Provided* That the atomic ratio of hydrogen to material is greater than 5200, and the content of plutonium is not more than 1% by weight of the total uranium-233 and uranium-235 content; or

(5) Less than 350 g of fissile material: *Provided,* That there is not more than 5 g of fissile material in any cubic foot within the package.

§ 71.8 Exemption of physicians

Physicians, as defined in § 35.3(b) of this chapter, are exempt from the regulations in this part to the extent that they transport licensed material for use in the practice of medicine.

§ 71.9 Exemption for fissile material

A licensee is exempt from requirements in §§71.33, 71.35(b), 71.36(b), 71.37, 71.38, 71.39, and 71.40 to the extent that he delivers to a carrier for transport packages each of which contains one of the following:

(a) Not more than 15 g of fissile material; or
(b) Thorium, or uranium containing not more than 0.72% by weight of fissile material; or
(c) Uranium compounds, other than metal (e.g., UF_4, UF_6, or uranium oxide in bulk form, not pelletted or fabricated into shapes) or aqueous** solutions of uranium, in which the total amount of uranium-233 and plutonium present does not exceed 1.0 percent by weight of the uranium-235 content, and the total fissile content does not exceed 1.00 percent by weight of the total uranium content; or
(d) Homogenous hydrogenous* solutions or mixtures containing not more than:

   (1) 500 g of any fissile material, provided the atomic ratio of hydrogen to fissile material is greater than 7600; or
   (2) 800 g of uranium-235: *Provided,* That the atomic ratio of hydrogen to fissile material is greater than 5200, and the content of other fissile material is not more than 1% by weight of the total uranium-235 content; or
   (3) 500 g of uranium-233 and uranium-235: *Provided,* That the atomic ratio of hydrogen to fissile material is greater than 5200, and the content of plutonium is not more than 1% by weight of the total uranium-233 and uranium-235 content; or

(e) Less than 350 g of fissile material: *Provided,* That there is not more than 5 g of fissile material in any cubic foot within the package.

§ 71.10 Limited exemption for shipment of type B quantities of radioactive material

A person delivering a type B quantity of radioactive material, as defined in § 71.4(q), to a carrier for transport in accordance with the provisions of a special permit, which has been

* This applies to light hydrogen and does not apply to heavy hydrogen (i.e., deuterium or tritium).
** This applies to light water and does not apply to heavy water.

issued by the Department of Transportation and is in effect on June 30, 1973, is exempt from the requirements in this part with respect to such shipments. The exemption granted by this section shall terminate on December 31, 1973, or on the date on which the DOT special permit expires, whichever is later, except as to activities described both in the special permit and in an application for a license which the person has, prior to the termination date of the exemption, filed with the Commission. If the person has filed such an application, the exemption, granted by this section shall continue until the application has been finally determined by the Commission.

GENERAL LICENSES

§ 71.11 General license for shipment of licensed material

A general license is hereby issued, to persons holding specific licenses issued pursuant to this chapter, to deliver licensed material to a carrier for transport, without complying with the package standards of Subpart C of this part, when either:

(a) The material is shipped as a Fissile Class III shipment with the following limitations on its contents:

- (1) No single package contains more than a type A quantity of radioactive material, as defined in § 71.4(q); and
- (2) The fissile material contents of the shipment do not exceed:
  - (i) 500 g of uranium-235; or
  - (ii) 300 g total of uranium-233, plutonium-238, plutonium-239, and plutonium-241; or
  - (iii) Any combination of uranium-233, uranium-235, and plutonium in such quantities that the sum of the ratios of the quantity of each of them to the quantity specified in subdivisions (i) and (ii) of this subparagraph does not exceed unity; or
  - (iv) 2500 g of plutonium-238, plutonium-239, and plutonium-241 encapsulated as plutonium-beryllium neutron sources, with no one package containing in excess of 400 g of plutonium-238, plutonium-239, and plutonium-241; or

(b) The material is shipped as Fissile Class II packages with the following limitations on the contents of each package;

(1) No single package contains more than a type A quantity of radioactive material, as defined in § 71.4(q); and

(2) No package contains fissile material in excess of the amounts specified in the following table, and each package is labeled with the corresponding transport index:

Maximum quantity of fissile material in a single package				
U-235 (grams	U-233 (grams)	Plutonium (grams)	Plutonium as Pu-Be neutron sources (grams)	Corresponding transport index
35—40	27—30	23—25	320—400	10
30—35	24—27	21—23	240—320	8
25—30	21—24	19—21	160—240	6
20—25	18—21	17—19	80—160	4
15—20	15—18	15—17	15—80	2

Note: Combinations of fissile materials are authorized. For combinations of fissile materials, the transport index is the sum of the individual corresponding transport indexes. The total transport index shall not exceed 10.

§ 71.12. General license for shipment in DOT specification containers, in packages approved for use by another person, and in packages approved by a foreign national competent authority

A general license is hereby issued to persons holding a general or specific license issued pursuant to this chapter, to deliver licensed material to a carrier for transport, provided the license has a quality assurance program whose description has been submitted to and approved by the Commission as satisfying the provisions of § 71.51.

(a) In a specification container for fissile material as specified in § 173.396(b) or (c) or for a type B quantity of radioactive material as specified in § 173.394(b) or § 173.395(b), or for a large quantity of radioactive material as specified in § 173.394(c) or § 173.395(c) of the regulations of the Department of Transportation, 49 CFR part 173; or

(b) In a package for which a license, certificate of compliance or other approval has been issued by the Commission's Director of Nuclear Material Safety and Safeguards or the Atomic Energy Commission, provided that:

(1) The person using a package pursuant to the general license provided by this paragraph:

(i) Has a copy of the specific license, certificate of compliance, or other approval authorizing use of the package, and has the drawings and other documents referenced in the approval relating to the use and maintenance of the packaging and to the actions to be taken prior to shipment

(ii) Complies with the terms and conditions of the license, certificate, or other approval, as applicable, and the applicable requirements of this part; and

(iii) Prior to first use of the package submits in writing to the Director of Nuclear Material Safety and Safeguards or the Atomic Energy Commission, his name and license number, the name and license or certificate number of the person to whom the package approval has been issued, and the package identification number specified in the package approval.

(2) The package approval authorizes use of the package under general license provided in this paragraph.

(c) In a package which meets the pertinent requirements in the 1967 regulations of the International Atomic Energy Agency and the use of which has been approved in a foreign national competent authority certificate which has been revalidated by the Department of Transportation: *Provided*, That the person using a package pursuant to the general license provided by this paragraph:

(1) Has and complies with the applicable certificate, the revalidation, and the drawings and other documents referenced in the certificate relating to the use and maintenance of the packaging and to the actions to be taken prior to shipment; and
(2) Complies, with the applicable requirements of this part, and the Department of Transportation regulations in 49 CFR part 173, 14 CFR part 103, and 46 CFR part 146.

§ 71.13 Communications

All communications concerning the regulations in this part should be addressed to the Nuclear Regulatory Commission, Washington, D.C. 20555, Attention: Director of Nuclear Material Safety and Standards, or may be delivered in person at the Commission's offices at 1717 H Street NW., Washington, D.C. or at 7920 Norfolk Avenue, Bethesda, Maryland.

§ 71.14 Interpretations

Except as specifically authorized by the Commission in writing, no interpretation of the meaning of the regulations in this part by an officer or employee of the Commission other than a written interpretation by the General Counsel will be recognized to be binding on the Commission.

§ 71.15 Additional requirements

The Commission may by rule, regulation, or order impose upon any licensee such requirements, in addition to those established in this part, as it deems necessary or appropriate to protect health or to minimize danger to life or property.

§ 71.16 Amendment of existing licenses

(a) Licenses issued pursuant to this part and in effect on October 4, 1968, which authorize Fissile Class II packages are hereby amended by increasing the minimum number of units specified for each Fissile Class II package by a factor of 1.25 The new number shall be rounded up to the first decimal. In addition, the term "radiation units" is changed to "transport index" wherever used in the license.

(b) The reference to § 71.6(b) in licenses issued pursuant to this part prior to March 26, 1972* is changed to § 71.9(b).

(c) The reference to § 71.9(b) in licenses issued pursuant to this part prior to June 30, 1973, is changed to 71.12(b).

SUBPART B — LICENSE APPLICATIONS

§ 71.21 Contents of application

An application for a specific license under this part may be submitted as an application for a license or license amendment under this chapter and shall include, for each proposed packaging design and method of transport, the following information in addition to any otherwise required:

(a) A package description as required by § 71.22;
(b) A package evaluation as required by § 71.23;
(c) An identification of the proposed program of quality assurance as required by § 71.24;
(d) In the case of fissile material, an identification of the proposed fissile class.

§ 71.22 Package description

The application shall include a description of the proposed package in sufficient detail to

* Effective date of this amendment.

identify the package accurately and to provide a sufficient basis for evaluation of the packaging. The description should include:

(a) With respect to the packaging:

(1) Gross weight;
(2) Model number;
(3) Specific materials of construction, weights, dimensions, and fabrication methods of:

(i) Receptacles, identifying the one which is considered to be the containment vessel;
(ii) Materials specifically used as nonfissile neutron absorbers or moderators;
(iii) Internal and external structures supporting or protecting receptacles;
(iv) Valves, sampling ports, lifting devices, and tie-down devices;
(v) Structural and mechanical means for the transfer and dissipation of heat; and

(4) Identification and volumes of any coolants and of receptacles containing coolant.

(b) With respect to the contents of the package:

(1) Identification and maximum radioactivity of radioactive constituents;
(2) Identification and maximum quantities of fissile constituents;
(3) Chemical and physical form;
(4) Extent of reflection, the amount and identity of nonfissile neutron absorbers in the fissile constituents, and the atomic ratio of moderator to fissile constituents;
(5) Maximum weight; and
(6) Maximum amount of decay heat.

§ 71.23 Package evaluation

The applicant shall:

(a) Demonstrate that the package satisfies the standards specified in Subpart C;
(b) For a Fissile Class II package, ascertain and specify the number of similar packages which may be transported together in accordance with § 71.39; and
(c) For a Fissile Class III shipment, describe any proposed special controls and precautions to be exercised during transport, loading, unloading, and handling, and in the event of accident or delay.

§ 71.24 Quality assurance

(a) The applicant shall identify his approved quality assurance program to be applied to the design, fabrication, assembly, testing, maintenance, repair, modification, and use of the proposed packaging.

(b) The applicant shall identify any established codes and standards proposed for use in package design, fabrication, assembly, testing, maintenance, and use. In the absence of such codes and standards, the applicant shall describe the basis and rationale used to formulate the package quality assurance program.

(c) The applicant shall identify any specific provisions to be contained in his quality assurance program which are applicable to the particular package design under consideration.

§ 71.25 Additional information

The Commission may at any time require further information in order to enable it to determine whether a license, certificate of compliance, or other approval should be granted, denied, modified, suspended, or revoked.

SUBPART C — PACKAGE STANDARDS

§ 71.31 General standards for all packaging

(a) Packaging shall be of such materials and construction that there will be no significant chemical, galvanic, or other reaction among the packaging components, or between the packaging components and the package contents.

(b) Packaging shall be equipped with a positive closure which will prevent inadvertent opening.

(c) Lifting devices:

(1) If there is a system of lifting devices which is a structural part of the package, the system shall be capable of supporting three times the weight of the loaded package without generating stress in any material of the packaging in excess of its yield strength.

(2) If there is a system of lifting devices which is a structural part only of the lid, the system shall be capable of supporting three times the weight of the lid and any attachments without generating stress in any material of the lid in excess of its yield strength.

(3) If there is a structural part of the package which could be employed to lift the package and which does not comply with subparagraph (1) of this paragraph, the part shall be securely covered or locked during transport in such a manner as to prevent its use for that purpose.

(4) Each lifting device which is a structural part of the package shall be so designed that failure of the device under excessive load would not impair the containment or shielding properties of the package.

(d) Tie-down devices:

(1) If there is a system of tie-down devices which is a structural part of the package, the system shall be capable of withstanding, without generating stress in any material of the package in excess of its yield strength, a static force applied to the center of gravity of the package having a vertical component of two times the weight of the package with its contents, a horizontal component along the direction in which the vehicle travels of 10 times the weight of the package with its contents, and a horizontal component in the transverse direction of 5 times the weight of the package with its contents.

(2) If there is a structural part of the package which could be employed to tie the package down and which does not comply with subparagraph (1) of this paragraph, the part shall be securely covered or locked during transport in such a manner as to prevent its use for that purpose.

(3) Each tie-down device which is a structural part of the package shall be so designed that failure of the device under excessive load would not impair the ability of the package to meet other requirements of this subpart.

§ 71.32 Structural standards for type B and large quantity packaging

Packaging used to ship a type B or a large quantity of radioactive material, as defined in § 71.4 (q) and (f), shall be designed and constructed in accordance with the structural standards of this section.

Standards different from those specified in this section may be approved by the Commission if the controls proposed to be exercised by the shipper are demonstrated to be adequate to assure the safety of the shipment.

(a) *Load resistance.* Regarded as a simple beam supported at its ends along any major axis, packaging shall be capable of withstanding a static load, normal to and uniformly distributed along its length, equal to 5 times its fully loaded weight, without generating stress in any material of the packaging in excess of its yield strength.
(b) *External pressure.* Packaging shall be adequate to assure that the containment vessel will suffer no loss of contents if subjected to an external pressure of 25 lb/in.^{2} gauge.

§ 71.33 Criticality standards for fissile material packages

(a) A package used for the shipment of fissile material shall be so designed and constructed and its contents so limited that it would be subcritical if it is assumed that water leaks into the containment vessel, and:

(1) Water moderation of the contents occurs to the most reactive credible extent consistent with the chemical and physical form of the contents; and
(2) The containment vessel is fully reflected on all sides by water.

(b) A package used for the shipment of fissile material shall be so designed and constructed and its contents so limited that it would be subcritical if it is assumed that any contents of the package which are liquid during normal transport leak out of the containment vessel, and that the fissile material is then:

(1) In the most reactive credible configuration consistent with the chemical and physical form of the material;
(2) Moderated by water outside of the containment vessel to the most reactive credible extent; and
(3) Fully reflected on all sides by water.

(c) The Commission may approve exceptions to the requirements of this section where the containment vessel incorporates special design features which would preclude leakage of liquids in spite of any single packaging error and appropriate measures are taken before each shipment to verify the leak tightness of each containment vessel.

§ 71.34 Evaluation of a single package

(a) The effect of the transport environment on the safety of any single package of radioactive material shall be evaluated as follows:

(1) The ability of a package to withstand conditions likely to occur in normal transport shall be assessed by subjecting a sample package or scale model, by test or other assessment, to the normal conditions of transport as specified in § 71.35; and
(2) The effect on a package of conditions likely to occur in an accident shall be assessed by subjecting a sample package or scale model, by test or other assessment, to the hypothetical accident conditions as specified in § 71.36.

(b) Taking into account controls to be exercised by the shipper, the Commission may permit the shipment to be evaluated together with or without the transporting vehicle, for the purpose of one or more tests.

(c) Normal conditions of transport and hypothetical accident conditions different from those specified in § 71.35 and § 71.36 may be approved by the Commission if the controls proposed to be exercised by the shipper are demonstrated to be adequate to assure the safety of the shipment.

§ 71.35 Standards for normal conditions of transport for a single package

(a) A package used for the shipment of fissile material or more than a type A quantity of radioactive material, as defined in § 71.4(q), shall be so designed and constructed and its contents so limited that under the normal conditions of transport specified in appendix A of this part:

(1) There will be no release of radioactive material from the containment vessel;
(2) The effectiveness of the packaging will not be substantially reduced;
(3) There will be no mixture of gases or vapors in the package which could, through any credible increase of pressure or an explosion, significantly reduce the effectiveness of the package;
(4) Radioactive contamination of the liquid or gaseous primary coolant will not exceed 10^{-7} Ci of activity of Group I radionuclides per milliliter, 5×10^{-6} Ci of activity of Group II radionuclides per milliliter, 3×10^{-4} Ci of activity of Group III and Group IV radionuclides per milliliter; and
(5) There will be no loss of coolant.

(b) A package used for the shipment of fissile material shall be so designed and constructed and its contents so limited that under the normal conditions of transport specified in Appendix A of this part:

(1) The package will be subcritical;
(2) The geometric form of the package contents would not be substantially altered;
(3) There will be no leakage of water into the containment vessel. This requirement need not be met if, in the evaluation of undamaged packages under § 71.38(a), § 71.39(a)(1), or § 71.40(a), it has been assumed that moderation is present to such an extent as to cause maximum reactivity consistent with the chemical and physical form of the material; and
(4) There will be no substantial reduction in the effectiveness of the packaging, including:

    (i) Reduction by more than 5% in the total effective volume of the packaging on which nuclear safety is assessed;
    (ii) Reduction by more than 5% in the effective spacing on which nuclear safety is assessed, between the center of the containment vessel and the outer surface of the packaging; or
    (iii) Occurrence of any aperture in the outer surface of the packaging large enough to permit the entry of a 4-in. cube.

(c) A package used for the shipment of more than a type A quantity of radioactive material as defined in § 71.4(q), shall be so designed and constructed and its contents so limited that under the normal conditions of transport specified in appendix A of this part, the containment vessel would not be vented directly to the atmosphere.

§ 71.36 Standards for hypothetical accident conditions for a single package

(a) A package used for the shipment of more than a type A quantity of radioactive material, as defined in § 71.4(q), shall be so designed and constructed and its contents so limited that if subjected to the hypothetical accident conditions specified in Appendix B of this part as the free drop, puncture, thermal, and water immersion conditions in the sequence listed in appendix B, it will meet the following conditions:

(1) The reduction of shielding would not be sufficient to increase the external radiation dose rate to more than 1000 mrem/hr at 3 ft from the external surface of the package.
(2) No radioactive material would be released from the package except for gases and contaminated coalant containing total radioactivity exceeding neither:

(i) 0.1% of the total radioactivity of the package contents; nor
(ii) 0.01 Ci of Group I radionuclides, 0.5 Ci of Group II radionuclides, 10 Ci of Group III radionuclides, 10 Ci of Group IV radionuclides, and 1000 Ci of inert gases irrespective of transport group.

A package need not satisfy the requirements of this paragraph if it contains only low specific activity materials, as defined in § 71.4(g), and is transported on a motor vehicle, railroad car, aircraft, inland water craft, or hold or deck of a seagoing vessel assigned for the sole use of the licensee.

(b) A package used for the shipment of fissile material shall be so designed and constructed and its contents to limited that if subjected to the hypothetical accident conditions specified in Appendix B of this part as the Free Drop, Puncture, Thermal, and Water Immersion conditions, in the sequence listed in Appendix B, the package would be subcritical. In determining whether this standard is satisfied, it shall be assumed that:

(1) The fissile materials is in the most reactive credible configuration consistent with the damaged condition of the package and the chemical and physical form of the contents;
(2) Water moderation occurs to the most reactive credible extent consistent with the damaged condition of the package and the chemical and physical form of the contents; and
(3) There is reflection by water on all sides and as close as is consistent with the damaged condition of the package.

§ 71.37 Evaluation of an array of packages of fissile material

(a) The effect of the transport environment on the nuclear safety of any array of packages of fissile material shall be evaluated by subjecting a sample package or a scale model, by test or other assessment, to the hypothetical accident conditions specified in § 71.38, § 71.39, or § 71.40 for the proposed fissile class, and by assuming that each package in the array is damaged to the same extent as the sample package or scale model. In this case of a Fissile Class III shipment, the Commission may, taking into account controls to be exercised by the shipper, permit the shipment to be evaluated as a whole rather than as individual packages, and either with or without the transporting vehicle, for the purpose of one or more tests.

(b) In determining whether the standards of §§ 71.38(b), 71.39(a)(2), and 71.40(b) are satisfied, it shall be assumed that:

(1) The fissile material is in the most reactive credible configuration consistent with the damaged condition of the package, the chemical and physical form of the contents, and controls exercised over the number of packages to be transported together; and
(2) Water moderation occurs to the most reactive credible extent consistent with the damaged condition of the package and the chemical and physical form of the contents.

§ 71.38 Specific standards for a Fissile Class I package

A Fissile Class I package shall be so designed and constructed and its contents so limited that:

(a) Any number of such undamaged packages would be subcritical in any arrangement, and with optimum interspersed hydrogenous moderation unless there is a greater amount of interspersed moderation in the packaging, in which case that greater amount may be considered; and
(b) 250 such packages would be subcritical in any arrangement, if each package were subjected to the hypothetical accident conditions specified in Appendix B of this part as the Free Drop, Thermal, and Water Immersion conditions, in the sequence listed in Appendix B, with close reflection by water on all sides of the array and with optimum interspersed hydrogenous moderation unless there is a greater amount of interspersed moderation in the packaging in which case that greater amount may be considered. The condition of the package shall be assumed to be as described in § 71.37.

§ 71.39 Specific standards for a Fissile Class II package

(a) A Fissile Class II package shall be so designed and constructed and its contents so limited, and the number of such packages which may be transported together so limited, that:

(1) Five times that number of such undamaged packages would be subcritical in any arrangement if closely reflected by water; and
(2) Twice that number of such packages would be subcritical in any arrangement if each package were subjected to the hypothetical accident conditions specified in Appendix B of this part as the Free Drop, Thermal, and Water Immersion conditions, in the sequence listed in Appendix B, with close reflection by water on all sides of the array and with optimum interspersed hydrogenous moderation unless there is a greater amount of interspersed moderation in the packaging, in which case that greater amount may be considered. The condition of the package shall be assumed to be as described in § 71.37.

(b) The transport index for each Fissile Class II package is calculated by dividing the number 50 by the number of such Fissile Class II packages which may be transported together as determined under the limitations of paragraph (a) of this section. The calculated number shall be rounded up to the first decimal place.

§ 71.40 Specific standards for a Fissile Class III shipment

A package for Fissile Class III shipment shall be so designed and constructed and its contents so limited, and the number of packages in a Fissile Class III shipment shall be so limited, that:

(a) The undamaged shipment would be subcritical with an identical shipment in contact with it and with the two shipments closely reflected on all sides by water; and
(b) The shipment would be subcritical if each package were subjected to the hypothetical accident conditions specified in Appendix B of this part as the Free Drop: Thermal, and Water Immersion conditions, in the sequence listed in Appendix B, with close reflection by water on all sides of the array and with the packages in the most reactive arrangement and with the most reactive degree of interspersed hydrogenous moderation which would be credible considering the controls to be exercised over the shipment. The condition of the package shall be assumed to be as described in § 71.37. Hy-

pothetical accident conditions different from those specified, in this paragraph may be approved by the Commission if the controls proposed to be exercised by the shipper are demonstrated to be adequate to assure the safety of the shipment.

§ 71.41 Previously constructed packages for irradiated solid nuclear fuel

(a) Notwithstanding any other provisions of this subpart, a package, the use of which has been authorized by the Atomic Energy Commission for the transport of irradiated solid nuclear fuel on or after September 23, 1961, and which has been completely constructed prior to January 1, 1967, shall be deemed to comply with the package standards of this subpart for that purpose, except as otherwise provided in paragraph (b).

(b) The holder (licensee) of the specific approval providing the authority specified in paragraph (a) shall, within 6 months after October 18, 1977, file a consolidated application for a superseding approval for the use of such packages, demonstrating that the packages satisfy the package standards of this subpart. If the licensee fails to submit such an application, the provisions of paragraph (a) and the authority granted by the approval to deliver the material to a carrier for transport in such packages shall expire at the end of that 6 month period. The Commission may issue a new approval superseding the existing approval, may confirm the existing approval with or without modification, or may deny the application in whole or in part and terminate the existing approval in whole or in part. If modification of the design of a package being used under the authority of this section in effect prior to October 18, 1977, is proposed by a licensee in his application for a superseding approval in accordance with this paragraph, the licensee shall designate in his application the time period needed to modify the package(s) after approval by the Commission.

§ 71.42 Special requirements for plutonium shipments after June 17, 1978

(a) Notwithstanding the exemption in § 71.9, plutonium in excess of twenty (20) curies per package shall be shipped as a solid.

(b) Plutonium in excess of twenty (20) curies per package shall be packaged in a separate inner container placed within outer packaging that meets the requirements of Subpart C for packaging of material in normal form. The separate inner container shall not release plutonium when the entire package is subjected to the normal and accident test conditions specified in Appendices A and B. Solid plutonium in the following forms is exempt from the requirements of this paragraph:

(1) Reactor fuel elements;
(2) Metal or metal alloy; or
(3) Other plutonium bearing solids that the Commission determines should be exempt from the requirements of this section.

(c) Authority in licenses issued pursuant to this part for delivery of plutonium to a carrier for transport under conditions which do not meet the limitations of paragraphs (a) and (b) of this Section shall expire on June 17, 1978.

SUBPART D — OPERATING PROCEDURES

§ 71.51 Establishment and maintenance of a quality assurance program

(a) The licensee shall establish, maintain, and execute a quality assurance program satisfying each of the applicable criteria specified in Appendix E, "Quality Assurance Criteria for Shipping Packages for Radioactive Material," and satisfying any specific provisions which are applicable to the licensee's activities including procurement of packaging. The description of the quality assurance program shall include a discussion of which requirements of Appendix E are applicable and how they will be satisfied.* A description of that program shall be filed, in accordance with this section, by January 1, 1979, with the Director, Office of Nuclear Material Safety and Safeguards, Nuclear Regulatory Commission. Washington, D.C. 20555. If a person has filed such a description, the continued use of his existing quality assurance program is authorized until the acceptability of the program has been finally determined by the Commission.

(b) The provisions of this paragraph deal with packages which have been approved for use in accordance with this part prior to January 1, 1979, and which have been designed in accordance with the provisions of this part in effect at the time of package approval. Notwithstanding the provisions of paragraph (a) of this section, such packages shall be deemed to have been designed in accordance with a quality assurance program which satisfies the provisions of paragraph (a) of this section.

(c) The provisions of this paragraph deal with packages which have been approved for use in accordance with this part prior to January 1, 1979, have been at least partially fabricated prior to that date, and which have been fabricated in accordance with the provisions of this part in effect at the time of package approval. Notwithstanding the provisions of paragraph (a) of this section, such packages shall be deemed to have been fabricated and assembled in accordance with a quality assurance program which satisfies the provisions of paragraph (a) of this section.

(d) A Commission-approved quality assurance program which satisfies the applicable criteria of Appendix B of Part 50, of this chapter and which is established, maintained, and executed with regard to transport packages shall be deemed to satisfy the requirements of paragraph (a) of this section.

§ 71.52 Assumptions as to unknown properties

When the isotopic abundance, mass, concentration, degree of irradiation, degree of moderation, or other pertinent property of fissile material in any package is not known, the licensee shall package the fissile material as if the unknown properties have such credible values as will cause the maximum nuclear reactivity.

§ 71.53 Preliminary determinations

(a) Prior to the first use of any packaging for the shipment of licensed materials, the licensee shall ascertain that there are no cracks, pinholes, uncontrolled voids or other defects which could significantly reduce the effectiveness of the packaging.

(b) Prior to the first use of any packaging for the shipment of licensed materials, where the maximum normal operating pressure will exceed 5 lb/in.^{2} gauge, the licensee shall test the containment vessel to assure that it will not leak at an internal pressure 50% higher than the maximum normal operating pressure.

(c) Packaging shall be conspicuously and durably marked with its model number. Prior to applying the model number, the licensee shall determine that the packaging has been fabricated in accordance with the design approved by the Commission.

§ 71.54 Routine determinations

Prior to each use of a package for shipment of licensed material the licensee shall ascertain that the package with its contents satisfies the applicable requirements of Subpart C of this part and of the license, including determinations that:

(a) The packaging has not been significantly damaged;
(b) Any moderators and nonfissile neutron absorbers, if required, are present and are as authorized by the Commission;

* The pertinent requirements of Appendix E should be applied in a graded approach, i.e., applied to an extent consistent with their importance to safety as described in Section 2 of Appendix E.

(c) The closure of the package and any sealing gaskets are present and are free from defects;
(d) Any valve through which primary coolant can flow is protected against tampering;
(e) The internal gauge pressure of the package will not exceed, during the anticipated period of transport, the maximum normal operating pressure;
(f) Contamination of the primary coolant will not exceed, during the anticipated period of transport, the limits specified in § 71.35(a)(4).
(g) Space provided for contained expansion of liquid coolant or a liquid shielding medium is adequate, and the systems for the liquid coolant and the liquid shielding medium are leaktight.
(h) The pressure relief valve or valves are operable, and set in accordance with written procedures.
(i) The package has been loaded and closed in accordance with written procedures.

The provisions of this section shall not be applicable for packages authorized in the general licenses granted by § 71.6 In such cases the licenseee shall ascertain that the contents of the package are as authorized in the general license.

§ 71.55 Opening instructions

Prior to delivery of a package to a carrier for transport, the licensee shall assure that any special instruction needed to safely open the package are sent to or have been made available to the consignee.

§ 71.61 Reports

The licensee shall report to the Director of Nuclear Material Safety and Safeguards, U.S. Nuclear Regulatory Commission, Washington, D.C. 20555, within 30 days any instance in which there is substantial reduction in the effectiveness of any authorized packaging during use.

§ 71.62 Records

(a) The licensee shall maintain for a period of 2 years after its generation a record of each shipment of fissile material or of more than a type A quantity of radioactive material as defined in §71.4(q), in a single package, showing, where applicable:

(1) Identification of the packaging by model number;
(2) Details of any significant defects in the packaging, with the means employed to repair the defects and prevent their recurrence;
(3) Volume and identification of coolant;
(4) Type and quantity of licensed material in each package, and the total quantity in each shipment;
(5) For each item of irradiated fissile material;

    (i) Identification by model number;
    (ii) Irradiation and decay history to the extent appropriate to demonstrate that its nuclear and thermal characteristics comply with license conditions;
    (iii) Any abnormal or unusual condition relevant to radiation safety.

(6) Date of the shipment;
(7) For Fissile Class III, any special controls exercised;
(8) Name and address of the transferee;
(9) Address to which the shipment was made; and
(10) Results of the determination required by § 71.54.

(b) The licensee shall make available to the Commission for inspection, upon reasonable notice, all records required by this part.

(c) The licensee shall maintain, during the life of the packaging to which they pertain, sufficient quality assurance records to furnish documentary evidence of the quality of packaging components which have safety significance, and of services affecting such quality, including records of the results of the determinations required by § 71.53, and of monitoring, inspection and auditing of work performance during the design, fabrication, assembly, testing, modification, maintenance, and repair of the packaging.

§ 71.63 Inspection and tests

(a) The licensee shall permit the Commission at all reasonable times to inspect the licensed material, packaging, and premises and facilities in which the licensed material or packaging, and premises and facilities in which the licensed material or packaging are used, produced, tested, stored or shipped.

(b) The licensee shall perform and permit the Commission to perform, such tests as the Commission deems necessary or appropriate for the administration of the regulations in this chapter.

(c) The licensee shall notify the Director of Inspection and Enforcement, U.S. Nuclear Regulatory Commission, Washington, D.C., 20555, at least 45 days prior to fabrication of a package to be used for the shipment, in that single package, of radioactive material having a decay heat load in excess of 5 kW or with an operating pressure in excess of 15 psig.

§ 71.64 Violations

An injunction or other court order may be obtained prohibiting any violation of any provision of the Atomic Energy Act of 1954, as amended, or Title II of the Energy Reorganization Act of 1974, or any regulation or order issued thereunder. A court order may be obtained for the payment of a civil penalty imposed pursuant to section 234 of the Act for violation of section 53, 57, 62, 63, 81, 82, 101, 103, 104, 107, or 109 of the Act, or section 206 of the Energy Reorganization Act of 1974, or any rule, regulation, or order issued thereunder, or any term, condition, or limitation of any license issued thereunder, or for any violation for which a license may be revoked under section 186 of the Act. Any person who willfully violates any provision of the Act or any regulation or order issued thereunder may be guilty of a crime and, upon conviction may be punished by fine or imprisonment or both, as provided by law.

Note: The reporting and record keeping requirements contained in this part have been approved by the General Accounting Office und B-180255 (R0056).

APPENDIX A — NORMAL CONDITIONS OF TRANSPORT

Each of the following normal conditions of transport is to be applied separately to determine its effect on a package.

1. *Heat* — Direct sunlight at an ambient temperature of 130°F in still air.
2. *Cold* — An ambient temperature of −40°F in still air and shade.
3. *Pressure* — Atmospheric pressure of 0.5 times standard atmospheric pressure.
4. *Vibration* — Vibration normally incident to transport.
5. *Water Spray* — A water spray sufficiently heavy to keep the entire exposed surface of the package except the bottom continuously wet during a period of 30 min.
6. *Free Drop* — Between 1.5 and 2.5 hr after the conclusion of the water spray test, a free drop through the distance specified below onto a flat essentially unyielding hor-

izontal surface, striking the surface in a position for which maximum damage is expected.

Free fall distance

Package weight (pounds)	Distance (feet)
Less than 10,000	4
10,000 to 20,000	3
20,000 to 30,000	2
More than 30,000	1

7. *Corner Drop* — A free drop onto each corner of the package in succession, or in the case of a cylindrical package onto each quarter of each rim, from a height of 1 ft onto a flat, essentially unyielding horizontal surface. This test applies only to packages which are constructed primarily of wood or fiberboard, and do not exceed 110 lb gross weight, and to all Fissile Class II packagings.
8. *Penetration* — Impact of the hemispherical end of a vertical steel cylinder 1.25 in. in diameter and weighing 13 lb dropped from a height of 40 in. onto the exposed surface of the package which is expected to be most vulnerable to puncture. The long axis of the cylinder shall be perpendicular to the package surface.
9. *Compression.* — For packages not exceeding 10,000 lb in weight, a compressive load equal to either 5 times the weight of the package or 2 lb/in.^{2} multiplied by the maximum horizontal cross section of the package, whichever is greater. The load shall be applied during a period of 24 hr, uniformly against the top and bottom of the package in the position in which the package would normally be transported.

APPENDIX B — HYPOTHETICAL ACCIDENT CONDITIONS

The following hypothetical accident conditions are to be applied sequentially, in the order indicated, to determine their cumulative effect on a package or array of packages.

1. *Free Drop* — A free drop through a distance of 30 ft onto a flat essentially unyielding horizontal surface, striking the surface in a position for which maximum damage is expected.
2. *Puncture* — A free drop through a distance of 40 in. striking, in a position for which maximum damage is expected, the top end of a vertical cylindrical mild steel bar mounted on an essentially unyielding horizontal surface. The bar shall be 6 in. in diameter, with the top horizontal and its edge rounded to a radius of not more than 0.25 in., and of such a length as to cause maximum damage to the package, but not less than 8 in. long. The long axis of the bar shall be perpendicular to the unyielding horizontal surface.
3. *Thermal* — Exposure to a thermal test in which the heat input to the package is not less than that which would result from exposure of the whole package to a radiation environment of 1475°F for 30 min. with an emissivity coefficient of 0.9, assuming the surfaces of the package have an absorption coefficient of 0.8. The package shall not be cooled artificially until 3 hr after the test period unless it can be shown that the temperature on the inside of the package has begun to fall in less than 3 hr.
4. *Water Immersion* (fissile material packages only) — Immersion in water to the extent that all portions of the package to be tested are under at least 3 ft of water for a period of not less than 8 hr.

APPENDIX C — TRANSPORT GROUPING OF RADIONUCLIDES

Element[a]	Radionuclide[c]	Group
Actinium (89)	Ac 227	I
	Ac 228	I
Americium (95)	Am 241	I
	Am 243	I
Antimony (51)	Sb 122	IV
	Sb 124	III
	Sb 125	III
Argon (18)	Ar 37	VI
	Ar 41	II
	Ar 41 (uncompressed)[b]	V
Arsenic (33)	As 73	IV
	As 74	IV
	As 76	IV
	As 77	IV
Astatine (85)	At 211	III
Barium (56)	Ba 131	IV
	Ba 133	II
	Ba 140	III
Berkelium (97)	Bk 249	I
Beryllium (4)	Be 7	IV
Bismuth (83)	Bi 206	IV
	Bi 207	III
	Bi 210	II
	Bi 212	III
Bromine (35)	Br 82	IV
Cadmium (48)	Cd 109	IV
	Cd 115 m	III
	Cd 115	IV
Calcium (20)	Ca 45	IV
	Ca 47	IV
Californium (98)	Cf 249	I
	Cf 250	I
	Cf 252	I
Carbon (6)	C 14	IV
Cerium (58)	Ce 141	IV
	Ce 143	IV
	Ce 144	III
Cesium (55)	Cs 131	IV
	Cs 134 m	III
	Cs 134	III
	CS 135	IV
	Cs 136	IV
	Cs 137	III
Chlorine (17)	Cl 36	III
	Cl 38	IV
Chromium (24)	Cr 51	IV
Cobalt (27)	Co 56	III
	Co 57	IV
	Co 58m	IV
	Co 58	IV
	Co 60	III
Copper (29)	Cu 64	IV
Curium (96)	Cm 242	I
	Cm 243	I
	Cm 244	I
	Cm 245	I
	Cm 246	I
Dysprosium (66)	Dy 154	III
	Dy 165	IV
	Dy 166	IV
Erbium (68)	Er 169	IV
	Er 171	IV
Europium (63)	Eu 150	III
	Eu 152m	IV
	Eu 152	III
	Eu 154	II
	Eu 155	IV
Fluorine (9)	F 18	IV
Gadolinium (64)	Gd 153	IV
	Gd 159	IV
Gallium (31)	Ga 67	III
	Ga 72	IV
Germanium (32)	Ge 71	IV
Gold (79)	Au 193	III
	Au 194	III
	Au 195	III
	Au 196	IV
	Au 198	IV
	Au 199	IV
Hafnium (72)	Hf 181	IV
Holmium (67)	Ho 166	IV
Hydrogen (1)	H 3 (see tritium)	
Indium (49)	In 113 m	IV
	In 114 m	III
	In 115 m	IV
	In 115	IV
Iodine (53)	I 124	III
	I 125	III
	I 126	III
	I 129	III
	I 131	III
	I 132	IV
	I 133	III
	I 134	IV
	I 135	IV
Iridium (77)	Ir 190	IV
	Ir 192	III
	Ir 194	IV
Iron (26)	Fe 55	IV
	Fe 59	IV
Krypton (36)	Kr 85 m	III
	Kr 85 m(uncompressed)	V
	Kr 85	III
	Kr 85 (uncompressed)	VI
	Kr 87	II
	Kr 87 (uncompressed)	V
Lanthanum (57)	La 140	IV
Lead (82)	Pb 203	IV
	Pb 210	II
	Pb 212	II

Element[a]	Radionuclide[c]	Group	Element[a]	Radionuclide[c]	Group
Lutecium (71)	Lu 172	III		Re Natural	IV
	Lu 177	IV	Rhodium (45)	Rh 103 m	IV
Magnesium (12)	Mg 28	III		Rh 105	IV
Manganese (25)	Mn 52	IV	Rubidium (37)	Rb 86	IV
	Mn 54	IV		Rb 87	IV
	Mn 56	IV		Rb Natural	IV
Mercury (80)	Hg 197 m	IV	Ruthenium (44)	Ru 97	IV
	Hg 197	IV		Ru 103	IV
	Hg 203	IV		Ru 105	IV
Mixed fission products MFP		II		Ru 106	III
			Samarium (62)	Sm 145	III
Molybdenum (42)	Mo 99	IV		Sm 147	III
Neodynium (60)	Nd 147	IV		Sm 151	IV
	Nd 149	IV		Sm 153	IV
Neptunium (93)	Np 237	I	Scandium (21)	Sc 46	III
	Np 239	I		Sc 47	IV
Nickel (28)	Ni 56	III		Sc 48	IV
	Ni 59	IV	Selenium (34)	Se 75	IV
	Ni 63	IV	Silicon (14)	Si 31	IV
	Ni 65	IV	Silver (47)	Ag 105	IV
Niobium (41)	Nb 93 m	IV		Ag 110 m	III
	Nb 95	IV		Ag 111	IV
	Nb 97	IV	Sodium (11)	Na 22	III
Osmium (76)	Os 185	IV		Na 24	IV
	Os 191 m	IV	Strontium (38)	Sr 85 m	IV
	Os 191	IV		Sr 85	IV
	Os 193	IV		Sr 89	III
Palladium (46)	Pd 103	IV		Sr 90	II
	Pd 109	IV		Sr 91	III
Phosphorus (15)	P 32	IV		Sr 92	IV
Platinum (78)	Pt 191	IV	Sulfur (16)	S 35	IV
	Pt 193	IV	Tantalum (73)	Ta 182	III
	Pt 193 m	IV	Technetium (43)	Tc 96 m	IV
	Pt 197 m	IV		Tc 96	IV
	Pt 197	IV		Tc 97 m	IV
Plutonium (94)	Pu 238 (F)	I		Tc 97	IV
	Pu 239 (F)	I		Tc 99 m	IV
	Pu 240	I		Tc 99	IV
	Pu 241 (F)	I	Tellurium (52)	Te 125 m	IV
	Pu 242	I		Te 127 m	IV
Polonium (84)	Po 210	I		Te 127	IV
Potassium (19)	K 42	IV		Te 129 m	III
	K 43	III		Te 129	IV
Praseodymium (59)	Pr 142	IV		Te 131 m	III
	Pr 143	IV		Te 132	IV
Promethium (61)	Pm 147	IV	Terbium (65)	Tb 160	III
	Pm 149	IV	Thallium (81)	Tl 200	IV
Protactinium (91)	Pa 230	I		Tl 201	IV
	Pa 231	I		Tl 202	IV
	Pa 233	II		Tl 204	III
Radium (88)	Ra 223	II	Thorium (90)	Th 227	II
	Ra 224	II		Th 228	I
	Ra 226	I		Th 230	I
	Ra 228	I		Th 231	I
Radon (86)	Rn 220	IV		Th 232	III
	Rn 222	II		Th 234	II
Rhenium (75)	Re 183	IV		Th Natural	III
	Re 186	IV	Thulium (69)	Tm 168	III
	Re 187	IV		Tm 170	III
	Re 188	IV		Tm 171	IV

Element[a]	Radionuclide[c]	Group
Tin(50)	Sn 113	IV
	Sn 117 m	III
	Sn 121	III
	Sn 125	IV
Tritium (1)	H 3	IV
	H 3 (as a gas, as luminous paint, or adsorbed on solid material)	VII
Tungsten (74)	W 181	IV
	W 185	IV
	W 187	IV
Uranium (92)	U 230	II
	U 232	I
	U 233(F)	II
	U 234	II
	U 235(F)	III
	U 236	II
	U 238	III
	U Natural	III
	U Enriched (F)	III
	U Depleted	III
Vanadium (23)	V 48	IV
	V 49	III
Xenon (54)	Xe 125	III
	Xe 131 m	III
	Xe 131 m (uncompressed)[b]	V
	Xe 133	III
	Xe 133 (uncompressed)[b]	VI
	Xe 135	II
	Xe 135 (uncompressed)[b]	V
Ytterbium (70)	Yb 175	IV
Yttrium (39)	Y 88	III
	Y 90	IV
	Y 91 m	III
	Y 91	III
	Y 92	IV
	Y 93	IV
Zinc (30)	Zn 65	IV
	Zn 69 m	IV
	Zn 69	IV
Zirconium (40)	Zr 93	IV
	Zr 95	III
	Zr 97	IV

Note: m = Metastable state; (F) = fissile material.

[a] Atomic number shown in parentheses.
[b] Uncompressed means at a pressure not exceeding one atmosphere.
[c] Atomic weight shown after the radionuclide symbol.

APPENDIX D — TESTS FOR SPECIAL FORM LICENSED MATERIAL

1. *Free Drop* — A free drop through a distance of 30 ft onto a flat essentially unyielding horizontal surface, striking the surface in such a position as to suffer maximum damage.

2. *Percussion* — Impact of the flat circular end of a 1 in. diameter steel rod weighing 3 lb, dropped through a distance of 40 in. The capsule or material shall be placed on a sheet of lead, of hardness number 3.5 to 4.5 on the Vickers scale, and not more than 1 in. thick, supported by a smooth essentially unyielding surface.

3. *Heating* — Heating in air to a temperature of of 1475°F and remaining at that temperature for a period of 10 min.

4. *Immersion* — Immersion for 24 hr in water at room temperature. The water shall be at pH 6 to pH 8, with a maximum conductivity of 10 μmhos/cm.

APPENDIX E — QUALITY ASSURANCE CRITERIA FOR SHIPPING PACKAGES FOR RADIOACTIVE MATERIAL

INTRODUCTION

In accordance with § 71.24, every applicant for an approval for use of a shipping package is required to describe his quality assurance program, and every licensee is required by § 71.51 to establish and maintain a quality assurance program for the design, fabrication, assembly, testing, use, and maintenance of each packaging, as defined in § 71.4(1).

This appendix establishes quality assurance requirements which apply to all activities affecting the components of the packaging which are significant to safety. These activities include designing, purchasing, fabricating, handling, shipping, storing, cleaning assembling, inspecting, testing, operating maintaining, repairing and modifying.

As used in this appendix, ''quality assurance'' comprises all those planned and systematic actions necessary to provide adequate confidence that a system or component will perform satisfactorily in service. Quality assurance includes quality control, which comprises those quality assurance actions related to control of the physical characteristics and quality of the material or component to predetermined requirements.

1. ORGANIZATION

The licensee* shall be responsible for the establishment and execution of the quality assurance program. The licensee may delegate to others, such as contractors, agents, or consultants, the work of establishing and executing the quality assurance program, or any part thereof, but shall retain responsibility therefore. The authority and duties of persons and organizations performing activities affecting the safety-related functions of structures, systems, and components shall be clearly established and delineated in writing. These activities include both the performing functions of attaining quality objectives and the quality assurance functions. The quality assurance functions are those of (a) assuring that an appropriate quality assurance program is established and effectively executed and (b) verifying, such as by checking, auditing, and inspection, that activities affecting the safety-related functions have been correctly performed. The persons and organizations performing quality assurance functions shall have sufficient authority and organizational freedom to identify quality problems; to initiate, recommend or provide solutions; and to verify implementation of solutions. Such persons and organizations performing quality assurance functions shall report to a management level such that this required authority and organizational freedom, including sufficient independence from cost and schedule when opposed to safety considerations, are provided. Because of the many variables involved, such as the number of personnel, the type of activity being performed, and the location or locations where activities are performed, the organizational structure for executing the quality assurance program may take various forms provided that the persons and organizations assigned the quality assurance functions have this required authority and organizational freedom. Irrespective of the organizational structure, the individual(s) assigned the responsibility for assuring effective execution of any portion of the quality assurance program at any location where activities subject to this Appendix are being performed shall have direct access to such levels of management as may be necessary to perform this function.

2. QUALITY ASSURANCE PROGRAM

The licensee shall establish at the earliest practicable time, consistent with the schedule, for accomplishing the activities, a quality assurance program which complies with the requirements of this appendix. The quality assurance program shall be documented by written procedures or instructions, and shall be carried out in accordance with those procedures throughout the period during which packaging is used. The licensee shall identify the material and components to be covered by the quality assurance program and the major organizations participating in the program, together with the designated function of these organizations. The quality assurance program shall provide control over activities affecting the quality of the identified materials and components to an extent consistent with their importance to

* While the term ''licensee'' is used in this appendix, the quality assurance requirements are applicable to whatever design, fabrication, assembly and testing of the package is accomplished with respect to a package prior to the time a package approval is issued.

safety, and as necessary to assure conformance to the approved design of each individual package used for the shipment of radioactive material. Activities affecting quality shall be accomplished under suitably controlled conditions. Controlled conditions include the use of appropriate equipment; suitable environmental conditions for accomplishing the activity, such as adequate cleanness; and assurance that all prerequisites for the given activity have been satisfied. The program shall take into account the need for special controls, processes, test equipment, tools and skills to attain the required quality, and the need for verification of quality by inspection and test.

The licensee shall base the requirements and procedures of his quality assurance program on the following considerations concerning the complexity and proposed use of the packaging and its components:

(1) The importance of malfunction or failure of the item to safety;
(2) The design and fabrication complexity or uniqueness of the item;
(3) The need for special controls and surveillance over processes and equipment;
(4) The degree to which functional compliance can be demonstrated by inspection or text; and
(5) The quality history and degree of standardization of the item.

The program shall provide for indoctrination and training of personnel performing activities affecting quality as necessary to assure that suitable proficiency is achieved and maintained. The licensee shall review the status and adequacy of the quality assurance program at established intervals. Management of other organizations participating in the quality assurance program shall regularly review the status and adequacy of that part of the quality assurance program which they are executing.

3. DESIGN CONTROL

Measures shall be established to assure that applicable regulatory requirements and the package design, as specified in the license, for those materials and components to which this appendix applies, are correctly translated into specifications, drawings, procedures, and instructions. These measures shall include provisions to assure that appropriate quality standards are specified and included in design documents and that deviations from such standards are controlled. Measures shall be established for the selection and review for suitability of application of materials, parts, equipment, and processes that are essential to the safety-related functions of the materials, parts, and components of the packaging.

Measures shall be established for the identification and control of design interfaces and for coordination among participating design organizations. These measures shall include the establishment of written procedures among participating design organizations for the review, approval, release, distribution, and revision of documents involving design interfaces. The design control measures shall provide for verifying or checking the adequacy of design, such as by the performance of design reviews, by the use of alternate or simplified calculational methods, or by the performance of a suitable testing program. The verifying or checking process shall be performed by individuals or groups other than those who performed the original design, but who may be from the same organization. Where a test program is used to verify the adequacy of a specific design feature in lieu of other verifying or checking processes, it shall include suitable qualification testing of a prototype or sample unit under the most adverse design conditions. Design control measures shall be applied to items such as the following: criticality physics, radiation shielding, stress, thermal, hydraulic, and accident analyses; compatibility of materials; accessibility for in-service inspection, maintenance and repair; features to facilitate decontamination; and delineation of acceptance criteria for inspections and tests.

Design changes, including field changes, shall be subject to design control measures commensurate with those applied to the original design. Changes in the conditions specified in the package approval require Commission approval.

4. PROCUREMENT DOCUMENT CONTROL

Measures shall be established to assure that applicable requirements of this part which are necessary to assure adequate quality are suitably included or referenced in the documents for procurement of material, equipment, and services, whether purchased by the licensee or by his contractors or subcontractors. To the extent necessary, the licensee shall require contractors or subcontractors to provide a quality assurance program consistent with the pertinent provisions of this part.

5. INSTRUCTIONS, PROCEDURES, AND DRAWINGS

Activities affecting quality shall be prescribed by documented instructions, procedures, or drawings of a type appropriate to the circumstances and shall be accomplished in accordance with these instructions, procedures, or drawings. These shall include appropriate quantitative or qualitative acceptance criteria for determining that important activities have been satisfactorily accomplished.

6. DOCUMENT CONTROL

Measures shall be established to control the issuance of documents, such as instructions, procedures, and drawings, including changes thereto, which prescribe all activities affecting quality. These measures shall assure that documents, including changes, are reviewed for adequacy and approved for release by authorized personnel and are distributed and used at the location where the prescribed activity is performed. Changes to documents shall be reviewed and approved by the same organizations that performed the original review and approval unless the applicant designates another organization.

7. CONTROL OF PURCHASED MATERIAL, EQUIPMENT, AND SERVICES

Measures shall be established to assure that purchased material, equipment, and services, whether purchased directly or through contractors and subcontractors, conform to the procurement documents. These measures shall include provisions, as appropriate, for source evaluation and selection, objective evidence of quality furnished by the contractor or subcontractor, inspection at the contractor or subcontractor, source, and examination of products upon delivery. Documentary evidence that material and equipment conform to the procurement specifications shall be available prior to installation or use of such material and equipment. This documentary evidence shall be retained by or be available to the licensee and shall be sufficient to identify the specific requirements met by the purchased material and equipment. The effectiveness of the control of quality by contractors and subcontractors shall be assessed by the licenseee or designee at intervals consistent with the importance, complexity and quantity of the product or services.

8. IDENTIFICATION AND CONTROL OF MATERIALS, PARTS, AND COMPONENTS

Measures shall be established for the identification and control of materials, parts, and components. These measures shall assure that identification of the item is maintained by heat number, part number, or other appropriate means, either on the item or on records traceable to the item, as required throughout fabrication, installation, and use of the item. These identification and control measures shall be designed to prevent the use of incorrect or defective materials, parts and components.

9. CONTROL OF SPECIAL PROCESSES

Measures shall be established to assure that special processes, including welding, heat treating, and nondestructive testing, are controlled and accomplished by qualified personnel using qualified procedures in accordance with applicable codes, standards, specifications, criteria, and other special requirements.

10. INSPECTION

A program for inspection of activities affecting quality shall be established and executed by or for the organization performing the activity to verify conformance with the documented instructions, procedures, and drawings for accomplishing the activity. Such inspection shall be performed by individuals other than those who performed the activity being inspected. Examination, measurements, or tests of material or products processed shall be performed for each work operation where necessary to assure quality. If inspection of processed material or products is impossible or disadvantageous, indirect control by monitoring processing methods, equipment, and personnel shall be provided. Both inspection and process monitoring shall be provided when quality control is inadequate without both. If mandatory inspection hold points, which require witnessing or inspecting by the licensee's designated representative and beyond which work shall not proceed without the consent of its designated representative, are required, the specifid hold points shall be indicated in appropriate documents.

11. TEST CONTROL

A test program shall be established to assure that all testing required to demonstrate that the packaging components will perform satisfactorily in service is identified and performed in accordance with written test procedures which incorporate the requirements of this part and the requirements and acceptance limits contained in the package approval. The procedures shall include provisions for assuring that all prerequisities for the given test have been met, that adequate test instrumentation is available and used, and that the test is performed under suitable environmental conditions. Test results shall be documented and evaluated to assure that test requirements have been satisfied.

12. CONTROL OF MEASURING AND TEST EQUIPMENT

Measures shall be established to assure that tools, gauges, instruments, and other measuing and testing devices used in activities affecting quality are properly controlled, calibrated, and adjusted at specified times to maintain accuracy within necessary limits.

13. HANDLING, STORAGE, AND SHIPPING

Measures shall be established to control the handling, storage, shipping, cleaning, and preservation of materials and equipment to be used in packaging in accordance with instructions to prevent damage or deterioration. When necessary for particular products, special protective environments, such as inert gas atmosphere, specific moisture content levels and temperature levels shall be specified and provided.

14. INSPECTION, TEST, AND OPERATING STATUS

Measures shall be established to indicate, by the use of markings such as stamps, tags, labels, routing cards, or other suitable means, the status of inspections and tests performed upon individual items of the packaging. These measures shall provide for the identification of items which have satisfactorily passed required inspections and tests, where necessary to preclude inadvertent by-passing of such inspections and tests.

Measures shall also be established for indicating the operating status of components of the packaging, such as tagging valves and switches, to prevent inadvertent operation.

15. NONCONFORMING MATERIALS, PARTS, OR COMPONENTS

Measures shall be established to control materials, parts, or components which do not conform to requirements in order to prevent their inadvertent use or installation. These measures shall include, as appropriate, procedures for identification, documentation, segregation, disposition, and notification to affected organizations. Nonconforming items shall be reviewed and accepted, rejected, repaired or reworked in accordance with documented procedures.

16. CORRECTIVE ACTION

Measures shall be established to assure that conditions adverse to quality, such as deficiencies, deviations, defective material and equipment, and nonconformances, are promptly identified and corrected. In the case of a significant condition adverse to quality, the measures shall assure that the cause of the condition is determined and corrective action taken to preclude repetition. The identification of the significant condition adverse to quality, the cause of the condition, and the corrective action taken shall be documented and reported to appropriate levels of management.

17. QUALITY ASSURANCE RECORDS

Sufficient written records shall be maintained to furnish evidence of activities affecting quality. The records shall include the following: design records, records of use and the results of reviews, inspections, tests, audits, monitoring of work performance, and materials analyses. The records shall also include closely related data such as qualifications of personnel procedures, and equipment. Inspection and test records shall, as a minimum, identify the inspector or data recorder, the type of observation, the results, the acceptability, and the action taken in connection with any deficiencies noted. Records shall be identifiable and retrievable. Consistent with applicable regulatory requirements, the licensee shall establish requirements concerning record retention, such as duration, location, and assigned responsibility.

18. AUDITS

A comprehensive system of planned and periodic audits shall be carried out to verify compliance with all aspects of the quality assurance program and to determine the effectiveness of the program. The audits shall be performed in accordance with the written procedures or check lists by appropriately trained personnel not having direct responsibilities in the areas being audited. Audit results shall be documented and reviewed by management having responsibility in the area audited. Followup action, including reaudit of deficient areas, shall be taken where indicated.

APPENDIX L
TITLE 39, PARTS 21 AND 124

SUBCHAPTER B — INTERNATIONAL MAIL PART 21

21.3 (b)(6) *Radioactive materials.* Radioactive materials are restricted as provided in Part 124 of this chapter and must be mailed by air. Senders of mailable radioactive materials must place on the wrapper of the package a white label bearing the French words Matières radioactives. The label must be supplied by the sender and is to be gummed or taped to the address side of the package. The package must also bear a conspicuous request for return to sender in case of nondelivery.

SUBCHAPTER C — DOMESTIC MAIL PART 124

124.2(e) *Radioactive materials* In addition to special packaging precautions, as prescribed in this part, a package containing radioactive materials must not emit from its exterior any significant alpha, beta, or neutron radiations. The gamma radiation at any surface of the package must be less than 10 mR for 24 hr. The package must not contain more than 0.1 mCi of radium, or polonium, or that amount of strontium-89, strontum-90, or barium-140 which disintegrates at a rate of more than 5 million atoms per second; or that amount of any other radioactive substance which disintegrates at a rate of more than 50 million atoms per second.

[Note — Postal Service Manual Amendment. This amendment has not been published in the *Federal Register* as of August 1, 1974. See editorial note on p. 77 for explanation.

Revise § 124.2(e) to read:

(e) Regulations on radioactive matters are found in Postal Service Publication 6.]

APPENDIX M
SUGGESTED STATE REGULATIONS — RAM TRANSPORT RULE

TRANSPORTATION

Sec. C.100 Preparation of Radioactive Material for Transport

(a) No licensee shall deliver any radioactive material to a carrier* for transport, unless:

(1) the licensee complies with the applicable requirements of the regulations, appropriate to the mode of transport, of the U.S. Department of Transportation insofar as such regulations relate to the packaging of radioactive material, and to the monitoring, marking, and labeling of those packages;

(2) the licensee has established procedures for opening and closing packages in which radioactive material is transported to provide safety and to assure that, prior to the delivery to a carrier for transport, each package is properly closed for transport; and

(3) prior to delivery of a package to a carrier for transport, the licensee shall assure that any special instructions needed to safely open the package are sent to or have been available to the consignee.

(b) C.100(a) shall not apply to the transportation of licensed material, or to the delivery of licensed material to a carrier for transport, where such transportation is subject to the regulations of the U.S. Department of Transportation or the U.S. Postal Service.

* For the purpose of this regulation, a licensee who transports his own licensed material as a private carrier is considered to have delivered such material to a carrier for transport.

APPENDIX N
STATE AND LOCAL RULE SUMMARY (FROM NUREG/CR-1263)

STATE AND LOCAL LAWS AND REGULATIONS GOVERNING THE TRANSPORTATION OF RADIOACTIVE MATERIALS

	Routing	Advance notification	Escorts	Keeping of/ access to records manifests	Qualification of personnel	Accident notification	Accident/ emergency procedures	Loading, packaging, labeling, marking	Regulation, from permits, licensing	Certain shipments prohibited	Financial liability, insurance, bonding	Monitoring, surveillance, inspection	State adoption of federal requirements	Other
Alabama	—	—	—	—	—	As required by DOT in 49 CFR	—	As required by DOT in 49 CFR	Reciprocal with DOT licensing	—	—	—	Dot regulation	—
Alaska	—	—	—	—	—	—	—	As required by DOT in 49 CFR and others	State Dept. of Health and Science registration	—	—	—	DOT and others	—
Arizona	—	—	—	—	—	File with Arizona Atomic Energy Commission	—	As required by DOT in 49 CFR	Reciprocal with DOT licensing	—	—	—	DOT regulations	—
Arkansas	—	Transportation Commission authority (no regs. issued)	Transportation Commission authority (no regs. issued)	Transportation Commission authority (no regs. issued)	—	Notify state police immediately	—	As required by DOT in 49 CFR	Permit required from State Dept. of Pollution Control & Ecology	—	—	State Dept. of Energy Authority	DOT regulations	Enforcement Trans. Commiss. State police, St. Highway Dept.
California	—	—	—	Documents in vehicles describing material	—	Federal requirements	Federal requirements	As required by DOT in 49 CFR and Highway Patrol	Registration $30 fee; Dept. of Health Services	—	—	State Dept. of Industrial Relations	NRC, DOT, regs.	—
Colorado	—	—	—	—	—	As regulated by DOT in 49 CFR	—	As required by DOT in 49 CFR	Reciprocal with DOT licensing	—	—	—	DOT regulations	—
Connecticut	Prescribed by state	1 day	—	—	—	—	—	As required by ICC	Permit required from the State Department of Environmental Protection	—	—	—	IC regulations	No shipments remitted on weekends.
Delaware	—	—		—		As required by DOT in 49 CFR	—	—	Permits for Del. Memorial Bridge	—	—	State police	49 CFR	—
Florida	—	10 days before trip		Inspection of records permitted by Health Dept.		—	—	As required by DOT in 49 CFR	Certificates required for some roads.	—	—	Optional vehicle inspection by Health Dept.	49 CFR	—
Georgia	Prior notice and approval required	Prior notice of route, time of trip, cargo		Annual reports required of nonpermit holders		As required by DOT in 49 CFR	—	As required by DOT, Postal & State Pkg. & Labeling Regs.	Permits, Licenses required. Permits for Talmadge Bridge	—	Liability Insurance required by state DOT	—	Parts of 49 CFR, 14 CFR, and 39 CFR	Restrictions on shipments through Atlanta 5 day limit on trips
Hawaii	—	—		—		—	—	—	—	—	—	—		
Idaho	—	—		—		—	—	—	Reciprocal with DOT licensing	—	—	—	49 CFR, 14 CFR, 39 CFR	—
Illinois	—	—		—		—	Report railroad accidents to Illinois Commerce Comm.	"Radioactive" placed in opening & closing instructions	—	—	$10,000 fine for each civil violation $25,000 criminal	Law enforcement officials enforce on highways	49 CFR, ICC regulations	Radioactive shipments allows on toll highways if NRC, NO & ICC regs followed
Indiana	—	—		—		—	—	—	Permit required for East Indiana Toll road	—	$1 million insurance certificate	—	—	—

	Routing	Advance Notification	Escorts	Keeping of/ Access to Records Manifests	Qualification of Personnel	Accident Notification	Accident/ Emergency Procedures	Loading, Packaging, Labeling, Marking	Registration, Fees, Permits, Licensing	Certain Shipments Prohibited	Financial Liability, Insurance, Bonding	Monitoring, Surveillance, Inspection	State Adoption of Federal Requirements	Other
Iowa	—	—	—	—	—	Iowa Highway Safety Patrol; Dept. of Motor Vehicles	Contact police radio; state safety patrol	—	Permits required for some bridges	—	—	—	—	
Kansas	—	—	—		—	—	—	—	Registration by Sec. of Health and Environ. required	—	—	—	49 CFR 397.1 through 397.21	
Kentucky	—	—	—	—	—	—	—	As required in 49, 46, 39, and 14 CFR	State Dept. of Human Resources, general license to carriers in compliance with DOT	—	—	Inspection by authorized agencies	Parts of 49, 46, 39, and 14 CFR	
Louisiana	—	—	—	Documents in vehicle describing material	Dept. of Public Safety prescribes standards	Dept. of Public Safety and Nuclear Energy Div.; phoned and written reports	—	As required by DOT in 49 CFR	Reciprocal with DOT licensing	Shipment of high level waste prohibited	Liability insurance required; $300,000 public, $100,000 private liability coverage	Monitoring as required by DOT in 49 CFR	DOT, postal serivce inspection	
Maine	—	—	—	Bill of lading describing materials	—	Report to an emergency agency (unnamed)	—	Placard as required by 49 CFR	Permits required for turnpike	—	—	—	49 CFR requirements for placarding	
Maryland	—	Sufficient to allow for inspection and processing permit	—	—	—	—	—	—	Permits required for tall roads, bridges, tunnels	—	—	—	—	
Massachusetts	—	—	—	—	—	—	—	—	Permits required for turnpike	Banned through Callahan-Sumner Tunnels	—	—	49 CFR	
Michigan	—	—	—	—	—	Report "incidents" affecting public health to Dept. of Public Health	—	—	Registration required; permit Saulte Ste. Marie Bridge	Banned on Detroit International Bridge	—	—	Parts of 10, 14, and 49 CFR	
Minnesota	—	—		—		—		As required by 49 CFR	—	—	—	—	Parts of 14 and 49 CFR	—
Mississippi	—	—		—		—		—	Law requires license, no registration issued	—	Liable to state for incidents	—	—	—
Missouri	—	—		—		Accidents reported to state Division of Health		—	—	—	—	—	—	—
Montana	—	—		—		—		—	Law requires license, no regulation issued	—	—	—	—	—
Nebraska	—	—		Quarterly report to Department of Health		—		DOT, Postal Service, plus "Removal Prohibited" warning	Reciprocal with DOT licensing	—	—	As required by DOT	DOT regulations	—

Nevada	—	3 days for out of-state licensee, can be waived		Quarterly reports to Board of Health		—		—	Specific NRC, other licenses granted general state license	—	—	—	Specific parts of 46, 49, and 14 CFR	—
New Hampshire	—	—		—		—		—	—	—	—	—	—	—
New Jersey	Information when applying for certificate	7 days for certificate		—		—		As required by DOT, NRC, Postal Service	Certificate, Dept. Environmental Protection Permit, tall roads	—	—	—	—	—
New Mexico	Authorization in law, no regs	—		—		—		—	—	—	—	—	4/3/74 agreement with AEC	—
New York	—	Yearly permit applications 30 days in advance		Manifest in carrier		—		As in 49 CFR	Permits required	Banned on bridge.	Insurance certificate city thruway	By DOT, FHA, and Div. of State Police	49 CFR, NRC, DOT	See NYC column for special requirements
North Carolina	Notice for spent fuel to Division of Highway Patrol	5 Days spent fuel	—	—	—	—	—	As required by DOT	—	—	—	—	DOT, Coast Guard regulations	Materials not subject to DOT, Special notice
North Dakota	—	—	—	—	—	—	Subject to Health Dept. orders, Health Council hearing in 10 days	As required by DOT	Reciprocal with DOT Licenses	—	—	Health Dept. may Impound	DOT regulation	—
Ohio	—	—	—	—	—	—	—	49 CFR	—	Banned on some bridges	—	—	49 CFR 14 CFR	—
Oklahoma	—	—	—	—	—	—	—	—	—	—	—	—	Board of Health empowered to adopt regs	Compliance with NRC, ICC, and DOT required for turnpike
Oregon	Inform State Health Department	—	—	—	—	As required in 49 CFR	—	As required in 49 CFR	Reciprocal with DOT Licensing	—	—	—	—	Rail transporters advance and incident notice
Pennsylvania	—	30 days prior to transportation to H.S.T.B.[a]	—	—	—	Report accident to H.S.T.B.	—	As required by DOT in 49 CFR	Permits required for turnpike reciprocal with DOT licensing	—	—	Inspection by H.S.T.B. authorized representative	49 CFR	—
Rhode Island	—	48 hr prior to shipment	—	Certificate of compliance with DOT, NRC regulations	—	Immediately notify RI State Police	—	—	Permits required from Public Utilities Carriers	—	Bond may be required from Dir. of Health	—	DOT, NRC regulations	2-way radios required. No shipments between 7—9 a.m. and 4—6 p.m. weekdays
South Carolina	—	—	—	Inspection permitted	—	—	—	As required by DOT in 49 CFR	—	—	—	Inspection by SC Dept. of Health & Environmental Control	For packing, loading, marking, and handling	—
South Dakota	—	2 days prior to entry into state	—	—	—	Notify within 24 hr Dir. of Health Dept.	—	—	State Health Department registration	—	—	—	—	—
Tennessee	—	To Public Service Comm. for spent fuel shipments	—	—	—	—	—	—	PUC has authority to license, no regulation issued	—	—	—	—	—

[a] H.S.T.B. = Hazardous Substance Transportation Board.

	Routing	Advance Notification	Escorts	Keeping of/ Access to Records Manifests	Qualification of Personnel	Accident Notification	Accident/ Emergency Procedures	Loading, Packaging, Labeling, Marking	Registration, Fees, Permits, Licensing	Certain Shipments Prohibited	Financial Liability, Insurance, Bonding	Monitoring, Surveillance, Inspection	State Adoption of Federal Requirements	Other
Texas	—	—	—	—	—	—	—	—	—	Banned through Baytown-La Porte tunnel	—	—	To be consistent with DOT regulations	Fire extinguishers required
Utah	—	—	—	—	—	—	—	—	—	—	—	—	DOT regulations	—
Vermont	Give notice to Director of Occupational Health	2 days	—	—	—	Radiation Control Agency may act, 10 days to hold hearing	—	—	Reciprocal with DOT licensing	—	—	Inspection authorized	Law enables Commission of Health to adopt by reference	Notice of destination date; time of shipment
Virginia	—	—	—	—	—	—	—	—	Permit required for state highways	—	—	Office of Emergency Services monitors	Regulations pending	—
Washington	—	—	—	—	—	Report incidents to Dept. of Social and Health Sciences	—	As required by DOT	Reciprocal with DOT license requirement	—	—	—	—	Physicians exempt
West Virginia	—	—	—	—	—	—	—	As required by DOT and other federal agencies	—	—	—	—	DOT, NRC, and Postal Regulations	—
Wisconsin	—	—	—	—	—	—	—	—	—	—	—	—		
Wyoming	—	—	—	—	—	—	—	—	—	—	—	—	DOT Regulations	—
Chicago	—	—	—	—	—	—	—	—	—	—	—	—	See Illinois	—
Los Angeles	—	—	—	—	—	—	—	—	—	—	—	—	See California	—
New York City	Limited to truck routes	2 weeks	For specific substances	In case of accident, see below	—	Thefts, loss of radiation to notify Dept. of Health	—	Reports to be filed on accident, tests made	Certificates required, permits on thruway, bridges	Banned on Triborough Bridge, Tunnel	$1,000,000 insurance certificate NY thruway	—	—	Weight, load limits for bridges
Philadelphia	—	—	—	—	—	—	—	—	—	—	—	—	See Pennsylvania	—

APPENDIX O
NEW YORK RAM TRANSPORT RULES (NUREG/CR-1263 AND CR38)

NEW YORK

Lead Agencies

- Departments of Transportation/Environmental Conservation

Requirements

- Compliance with U.S. Department of Transportation and Nuclear Regulatory Commission regulations
- Permits required
- Application for permit to be made 30 days in advance
- Manifest in carrier identifying waste

Other restrictions

- Permits required for shipments on facilities of New York State Thruway Authority, and most bridges

New York City — Department of Health requires

- Emergency certificates for certain shipments
- Two weeks advance notice of shipments (include routing)
- Follow designated truck routes
- Escorts
- Vehicles crossing -bridges to comply with weight/size limits
- Reports of thefts of material

Shipments banned on Triborough bridge and tunnel

NEW YORK TRANSPORTATION LAW SEC.

14-F. Transportation of hazardous materials

1. The commissioner of transportation is hereby authorized to promote safety in the transportation of hazardous materials by all modes of transportation, and in connection therewith shall:

(a) Have the power to make rules and regulations governing transportation of hazardous materials, which shall mean a substance or material in a quantity and form which may pose an unreasonable risk to health and safety or property when transported in commerce, by all modes. For purposes of this section, hazardous materials may include, but are not limited to explosives, radioactive materials, etiologic agents, flammable liquids or solids, combustible liquids or solids, poisons, oxidizing or corrosive materials, and compressed gases. Such rules and regulations shall, be no less protective of public safety than the rules and regulations promulgated by the federal government with respect to the transportation of hazardous materials.

(b) Have power to enforce said rules and regulations through the use of department staff or others pursuant to cooperative agreement.
(c) Have power and is hereby authorized to enter into cooperative agreements with agencies of this and other states and of the federal government in relation to enforcement of said rules and regulations.

2. It shall be unlawful for any person to violate any of the rules and regulations promulgated by the commissioner pursuant to this section.

3. Any person found guilty of violating any such rule or regulation shall be subject to a fine of not less than $250 or more than $1000 for the first offense, and upon being found guilty of a second or subsequent offense by a fine of not less than $1000 or more than $2500, or by imprisonment for not more than 90 days. Except as otherwise provided by law, such a violation shall not be a crime and the penalty or punishment imposed therefore shall not be deemed for any purpose a criminal penalty or punishment and shall not impose any disability upon or affect or inpair the credibility as a witness, or otherwise, of a person found guilty thereof.

4. Notwithstanding any other provision of this chapter or other law whether general, special or local, violations of any rules and regulations promulgated hereunder involving the operation of a motor vehicle may be charged through the use of a uniform traffic summons and complaint prescribed by the commissioner of motor vehicles pursuant to section two hundred seven of the vehicle and traffic law.

5. With respect to the transportation of radioactive materials nothing in this section shall be construed to abrogate or effect the provisions of any other federal or state statute or local ordinance, regulation or resolution which are more restrictive than or which supercede* the provisions of this section or regulations adopted pursuant hereto.
Added L.1976, c. 611, & 1.

NEW YORK ENVIRONMENTAL CONSERVATION LAW

C. 27-0905 Manifest system

Not later than 6 months after the promulgation of regulations for hazardous wastes pursuant to paragraph one of section 27-0903 of this title, and after consultation and coordination with the commissioner of transportation, the commissioner shall promulgate in a manner consistent with the state administrative procedure act, regulations establishing a manifest system by which to monitor the transportation, storage, and disposal of hazardous waste and to assure that such acts are performed in a manner consistent with this title. Such manifest systems shall conform to that adopted by the administrator pursuant to RCRA. Where appropriate and consistent with the provisions of RCRA, the commissioner may provide for exemption from the provisions of this section for the transport of hazardous waste by the generator from one facility to another owned and operated by the generator. As a minimum such system shall require that:

1. Hazardous waste generators use a specific form identifying the composition, quantity, and disposition of each shipment of hazardous waste:
2. Copies of manifest be carried during transportation of hazardous waste, and
3. Hazardous waste generators, hazardous waste transporters and owners and operators

* So in original.
Effective Date. Section effective Apr. 1, 1977, pursuant to L.1976, c. 611 & 2.
Library References — Carriers 10, 21(1)
C. J. S. Carriers && 15 et seq., 511 et seq., 568.
United States Code Annotated
Hazardous materials transportation, see section 1501 et seq. of Title 19 Transportation.

of hazardous waste treatment, storage, and disposal facilities maintain copies of manifest for at least 3 years.

Added L. 1978. c. 639 c.7
42 U.S.C.A. c. 6901 et seq.
Effective Date. Section effective Sept. 1, 1978, pursuant to L.1978 c. 639, c. 12.

C. 27-0909. Standards applicable to transporters of hazardous waste

Not later than 18 months after the effective date of this title, and after consultation and coordination with the commissioner of transportation, and after opportunity for public hearings, the commissioner shall promulgate regulations establishing such standards which shall be applicable to transporters of hazardous waste identified or listed under this title, as may be necessary to protect human health and the environment. Such standards shall include but need not be limited to requirements respecting:

1. Recordkeeping practices that accurately identify the hazardous wastes transported, and their sources and delivery points,
2. Transportation and storage of such waste only if properly labeled:
3. Compliance with the manifest system established under section 27-0905 of this title,
4. Transportation of all such hazardous waste only to the hazardous waste treatment, storage, or disposal facility or facilities which are designated on the manifest form, a copy of which shall be presented to the generator prior to transportation, and which either hold operation permits issued under this article, are a permittee under the Federal Resource Conservation and Recovery Act of 1976 or any amendment thereof, or are otherwise duly authorized to accept hazardous waste, and
5. Requirement of a bond to meet all responsibilities in case of release of hazardous wastes causing damage as a condition to the issuance of a certificate of registration to a transporter required by this title.

Effective date same as above.

RULES AND REGULATIONS GOVERNING THE TRANSPORTATION OF HAZARDOUS MATERIALS

Pursuant to Section 14-f of the Transportation Law as added by Chapter 641 of the Laws of 1976, the Commissioner of Transportation hereby adds a new Part 507 to Title 17 of the Official Compilation of Codes, Rules and Regulations to take effect April 1, 1977 and to read as follows:

Part 507
Transportation of Hazardous Materials

Section 507.1 General

(a) Section 14-f of the Transportation Law authorizes the Commissioner of Transportation to make rules and regulations governing transportation of hazardous materials by all modes and provides that these rules shall be no less protective to public safety than the rules and regulations promulgated by the Federal government with respect to the transportation of hazardous materials and that, with respect to the transportation of radioactive materials, these rules shall not be construed to abrogate or effect the provisions of any other Federal or State statute or local ordinance, regulation or resolution which are more restrictive than or which supersede these rules.

(b) Federal law governing the transportation of hazardous materials (section 112 of the Federal Hazardous Materials Transportation Act, title I of Publ. L. 93-633) provides for Federal preemption in the area of hazardous materials transportation. It states that any requirement of the State or political subdivision thereof which is inconsistent with Federal law or regulations in the field is preempted. It affords a procedure whereby State requirements may be determined by the U.S. Secretary of Transportation to be not preempted if the State requirement affords an equal or greater level of protection to the public than the Federal requirements and does not unreasonably burden the commerce.

Section 507.2 Application

(a) Every carrier, whether by highway, by rail, by water or by air, engaged in the transportation of hazardous materials within this State shall be subject to the rules and regulations contained in this Part.

(b) No person shall offer or accept a hazardous material for transportation within this State unless that material is properly classed, described, packaged, clearly marked, clearly labeled, and in the condition for shipment as required by this Part.

(c) No person shall offer or accept a hazardous material for transportation unless that material is handled and transported in accordance with this Part.

Section 507.3 Definitions

For the purposes of this Part, the following definitions shall apply:

(a) *Hazardous materials* shall mean those materials listed in the table of hazardous materials contained in section 172.101 of title 49 of the Code of Federal Regulations, revised as of October 1, 1976, and including any amendments or additions thereto.

(b) *Transports or Transportation* shall mean any movement of property by highway, by rail, by water, and by air and any loading, unloading, or storage incidental thereto.

(c) *Commerce* shall mean trade, traffic, commerce or transportation within the jurisdiction of New York State which affects trade, traffic, commerce or transportation within the State.

(d) *Person* shall mean an individual, firm, copartnership, corporation, company, association, or joint-stock association, and includes any trustee, receiver, assignee, or personal representative thereof.

(e) *Serious harm* shall mean death, serious illness, or severe personal injury.

Section 507.4 Transportation of hazardous materials

(a) To promote the uniform enforcement of law and to minimize the dangers to life and property incident to the transportation of hazardous materials by all modes of transportation, all carriers and persons engaged in the transportation of hazardous materials that are subject to this Part shall classify, describe, package, mark, label and prepare all hazardous materials which are defined and listed in section 172.101 of chapter I of title 49 of the Code of Federal Regulations and any amendments or additions thereto in accordance with the regulations promulgated by the Materials Transportation Bureau of the U.S. Department of Transportation contained in parts 170 to 189 of title 49 of the Code of Federal Regulations, revised as of October 1, 1976, and any amendment or addition thereto, which regulations are hereby adopted in toto, defining these articles and stating the precautions that must be observed by the carrier in handling them while in transit.

(b) All carriers and persons engaged in the transportation of hazardous materials shall afford to authorized employees of the Department of Transportation and the Division of State Police and the Federal Highway Administration reasonable opportunity to enter vehicles or any place where hazardous materials are offered into commerce for the purpose of inspection to determine compliance with the provisions of this Part.

Section 507.5 Cooperative agreements

(a) The cooperative agreement entered into on August 16, 1968 between the New York State Public Service Commission and the Federal Highway Administration accepting the provisions then identified as sections 277c.4, 277c.5, 277c.6, and 277c.7 of title 49 of the Code of Federal Regulations with regard to the exchange of information between the agencies' requests for assistance, joint investigation, inspection and examination, and joint administrative activities relating to the enforcement of safety and hazardous materials laws and regulations shall continue to remain in full force and effect.

(b) The Division of State Police shall refer all violations of this Part to the Department of Transportation, Traffic and Safety Division, 1220 Washington Avenue, Albany, New York 12232 on a form supplied for such purpose by the Department of Transportation.

Section 507.6 Exemptions

With respect to the transportation of radioactive materials nothing in this Part shall be construed to abrogate or effect the provisions of any Federal or State statute or local ordinance, regulation or resolution which are more restrictive than or which supersede the provisions of this Part.

PART 364
SEPTIC TANK CLEANER AND INDUSTRIAL WASTE* COLLECTOR REGISTRATION
(STATUTORY AUTHORITY: ENVIRONMENTAL CONSERVATION LAW, SEC. 9-0101)

Historical Note

Part (secs. 364.1-364.2) added, filed Oct. 15, 1970; renum. Part 458, Title 9, filed Sept., 1971; Part (secs. 364.1-364.4) added, filed June 27, 1972 eff. immediately.

Section 364.1 Definitions

When used in this Part and unless context otherwise requires, the following words and phrases shall mean as follows:

(a) *Department* means the New York State Department of Environmental Conservation.

(b) *Person* means any individual, public or private corporation, political subdivision, municipality, industry, copartnership, association, firm, trust or estate who engages in the business of cleaning septic tanks or cesspools or marina sanitary waste-holding facilities, scavenging or disposing of commercial wastes and industrial process waste products, or otherwise removing or disposing of solid or liquid wastes from domestic sewer systems and treatment facilities.

(c) *Marina sanitary waste-holding facilities* means those tanks and containers which are used for temporary storage of sewage wastes removed from holding tanks in boats.

* Radioactive materials are included in definition of industrial waste.

(d) *Septic tank or cesspool* means the facilities used for the settling of organic or inorganic solids from domestic sewage lines, whether or not the tank is separate from the disposal system or an integral part of it. For the purposes of this definition, septic tank or cesspool shall mean tanks operating under aerobic or anaerobic conditions.

(e) *Commercial wastes and industrial process waste products* mean liquid, solid, or semi-solid wastes generated by industrial or commercial operations which are prohibited by local sewage use ordinances, from discharge into municipal sewage treatment systems and are prohibited from discharge into on-site industrial waste treatment facilities required to be under permit under article 12 of the Public Health Law. Such wastes include, but are not limited to, residue sludges, oils, solvents, spent chemicals, acids, and similar wastes but do not include wood, paper, and packaging materials.

(f) *Waste disposal area* means any land used for disposal.

(g) *Waste receiving station* means a designated location where collected wastes are introduced into a waste treatment system or facility employing mechanical, chemical, biological, or thermal processes.

Historical Note

Secs. added, filed Oct. 15, 1970; renum. 458.1. Title 9, filed Sept., 1971; new added, filed June 27, 1972 eff. immediately.

200.5 CN 6-30-72

Section 364.2 Applications

(a) All applications for disposal permits shall be submitted to the regional office having jurisdiction over the waste disposal area or waste receiving station used by the applicant. If an applicant disposes of collected wastes at multiple locations, the application shall be submitted to the regional office having jurisdiction over the facility receiving the largest portion of collected wastes. Persons utilizing waste disposal areas or waste receiving stations located without the State shall submit initial applications to the department at Albany, 12201.

(b) All persons currently engaged in collecting and transporting such wastes must submit an application for a certificate of registration within 30 days after adoption of this Part. All persons who begin operations to collect and transport such wastes after said adoption shall submit an application for a certificate of registration at least 30 days prior to the anticipated date of initiating operations.

(c) All applications shall be on forms provided by the department. The department may also require such plans, reports, and other data as are necessary to determine whether the disposal facility is suitable and whether the proposed method of operation is acceptable.

(d) Applications for renewal of the certificate of registration shall be submitted at least 30 days in advance of the date of expiration.

(e) Each application for renewal of the certificate of registration shall be accompanied by an annual report on forms provided by the department.

(f) At the discretion of the department, separate applications may be required when a person collects and disposes of more than one type of waste and employs different disposal methods, in which case, one registration fee will cover all applications.

(g) When collected wastes are to be disposed of at a waste disposal area or waste receiving station not owned by the applicant, written permission to discharge at such facility shall accompany the application.

(h) If, within the registration year, the registrant wishes to collect and/or dispose of additional wastes or alter the method or location of disposal, he must so notify the department and receive approval for such modification.

Historical Note

Secs. added, filed Oct. 15, 1970; renum. 458.2, Title 9, filed Sept., 1971; new added, added, filed June 27, 1972 eff. immediately.

Section 364.3 Certificate of registration

(a) The certificate of registration shall be issued for a period not to exceed 1 year and, unless otherwise stated therein, shall expire on March 31.

(b) A copy of the certificate of registration shall be carried in each vehicle provided with cleaning or holding tank equipment or used on public highways for transporting any waste covered by this Part. The certificate of registration shall be presented on demand to any authorized representative of the department or law enforcement officer.

(c) The number of the certificate of registration shall be displayed on all vehicles used on public highways transporting any materials covered by this Part. The registration number shall be displayed in a prominent place on the sides and rear of the vehicle using numerals at least 4 in. high of a color to contrast with the background in order to insure and enhance their visibility at a distance.

Historical Note

Sec. added, filed June 27, 1972 eff. immediately.

Section 364.4 Hearings

(a) A hearing may be held, after 10-day notice to a registrant at a time and location specified by the department to determine whether such person has collected and/or disposed of wastes not specified on the required application(s), or has altered the method or location of disposal as specified on the application(s), or has not complied with conditions imposed by the department, upon the use of a disposal facility, or has not received approval to modifications to the application.

(b) Upon a finding of one or more of the forementioned, the department may suspend or revoke the certificate or assess a fine as provided for by law.

Historical Note

Sec. added, filed June 27, 1972 eff. immediately.

HEALTH SERVICES ADMINISTRATION DEPARTMENT OF HEALTH (RESOLUTIONS ADOPTED)

AT A MEETING OF THE BOARD OF HEALTH OF THE DEPARTMENT OF HEALTH HELD January 15, 1976, the following resolution was adopted:

Resolved, that section 175.111 of the New York City Health Code, as repealed and reenacted by resolution adopted on the fifteenth day of November, nineteen hundred seventy-three and filed with the City Clerk on the twentieth day of November, nineteen hundred seventy-three, be and the same hereby is amended by adding a new subsection (1) thereto, to follow subsection (k) thereof, to be printed together with explanatory notes, to read as follows:

(1) Notwithstanding the foregoing provisions of this section, a Certificate of Emergency Transport issued by the Commissioner or his designated representative shall be required for

each shipment, to be transported through the City or brought into the City, of any of the following materials:

(1) Plutonium isotopes in any quantity and form exceeding 2 g or 20 Ci, whichever is less;
(2) Uranium enriched in the isotope U-235 exceeding 25 atomic % of the total uranium content in quantities where the U-235 content exceeds 1 kg;
(3) Any of the actinides (i.e. elements with atomic number 89 or greater) the activity of which exceeds 20 Ci;
(4) Spent reactor fuel elements or mixed fission products associated with such spent fuel elements the activity of which exceeds 20 Ci; or
(5) Any quantity of radioactive material specified as a ''Large Quantity'' by the Nuclear Regulatory Commission in 10 CFR Part 71, entitled ''Packaging of Radioactive Material for Transport''.

NOTES: Subsection (1) was added by resolution adopted on January 15, 1976 to require the approval of the Commissioner or his designated representative through the issuance of a Certificate of Emergency Transport for the transport or the bringing into this City of specified large quantities of plutonium, enriched uranium, and other actinides and spent reactor fuel elements which would present a great hazard to public health in this densely and highly populated City. It is intended that such Certificate will be issued for the most compelling reasons involving urgent public policy or national security interests transcending public health and safety concerns and that economic consideration alone will not be acceptable as justification for the issuance of such Certificate. Such Certificates are also intended to be issued for hectocurie and kilocurie cobalt-60 and cesium-137 teletherapy sources employed in therapeutic radiology and biomedical research or educational purposes and for medical devices designed for individual human application (e.g., cardiac pacemakers) containing plutonium-238, promethium-147 or other radioactive material. This subsection is not intended to apply to small quantities of specified radioactive materials intended for therapeutic radiology and biomedical research or educational purposes.

Resolved, further, that subsection (c) of section 175.111 of the New York City Health Code, as repealed and reenacted by resolution adopted on the fifteenth day of November, nineteen hundred seventy-three and filed with the City Clerk on the twentieth day of November, nineteen hundred seventy-three, be and the same hereby is amended, to be printed together with explanatory notes, to read as follows:

(c) This section shall not apply to radiation sources shipped by or for the United States Government for military or national security purposes or which are related to national defense. Nothing herein shall be construed as requiring the disclosure of any defense information or restricted data as defined in the Atomic Energy Act of 1954 and the Energy Reorganization Act of 1974, as amended.

NOTES: Subsection (c) was amended by resolution adopted on January 15, 1976 to conform its provisions with subsection (1) adopted by the same resolution.

Resolved, further, that this resolution shall take effect immediately.

A true copy.

PATRICIA J. CARUSO, Acting Secretary

ARTICLE 175 RADIATION CONTROL

Section 175.111 Transportation

(a) The person responsible for the transportation of a radiation source outside of an installation shall take all necessary precautions so that no individual is exposed to ionizing radiation exceeding in amount the maximum permissible dose rate specified in section 175.05 of this Article. Sources shall be containerized and packaged, warning labels shall be affixed to the outer container holding the radiation source, and the airplane, ship, vehicle, or rail carrier concerned placarded in conformity with the regulations of the U.S. Department of Transportation, U.S. Atomic Energy Commission or other related federal or state agencies, regardless of whether the shipment is being made intracity, intrastate or interstate.

(b) When a radiation source which may involve a high degree of hazard in the event of an accident is to be transported into, within, through or out of the City, the shipper shall first notify the Department of the date of shipment, type and quantity of radiation source involved, method of transportation, route, starting point, destination, and such other information as the Department may require. So much of such information as is then available shall be furnished at least 2 weeks prior to such shipment. The unsupplied information shall be furnished no later than 2 hr prior to arrival of the radiation source in the City or in the case of a shipment originating in the City no later than the time of its departure from the point of origin. The radiation source shall be transported through the City over such route or routes, or at such time or times of the day, consistent with the public health and safety and the convenience of the shipper, as the Department may direct.

(c) This section does not apply to radiation sources shipped by or for the United States Government. Nothing herein shall be construed as requiring the disclosure of any defense information or restricted data as defined in the Atomic Energy Act of 1954, as amended.

(d) The following radiation sources may involve a high degree of hazard in the event of accident:

(1) Any quantity of radioactive material specified as a ''Large Quantity'' by the United States Atomic Energy Commission in 10 CFR Part 71, ''packaging of Radioactive Material for Transport'';

(2) Any quantity arrangement and packaging combination of fissle material specified by the United States Atomic Commission as a ''Fissile Class 111'' shipment in 10 CFR Part 71, ''Packaging of Radioactive Material for Transport'', or

(3) Any shipment of radioactive material that is required by the appropriate regulating agency to be accompanied by an escort for safety reasons.

(e) Motor vehicles transporting the radiation sources designated in subsection (b) shall follow the ''Truck Routes'' listed in Article 16 of the Traffic Regulations adopted by the Commissioner of Traffic of the City of New York except that any such motor vehicle may be operated on a street not so listed for the purpose of delivery, loading or servicing, provided it leaves and returns to a listed street by the most direct route.

(f) In addition, in the case of shipments of radiation sources in the following categories the provisions of subsections (g) and (h) below shall be complied with:

(1) More than ten times the quantity specified as a ''Large Quantity'' of:

   (i) Mixed fission products, including that contained in, but not limited to, a shipment of spent nuclear fuel, or

   (ii) Liquid or gaseous radioactive material;

(2) Fissile Class III;

(3) Required to be escorted for safety reasons; or
(4) Any intrastate (New York) or intracity (New York City) ''Large Quantity'' shipment of radioactive material which does not meet the U.S. Department of Transportation packaging, labeling and placarding requirements in all respects.

(g) The shipper shall notify the Department and shall arrange with the Department for an escort through this City at a time to be designated by the Department. He shall report the point of entry into the City or point of origin with the City and such other information as is required by this Code.

(h) If the destination is within this City to a pier, airport, or there delivery point and facilities are not available during the night or unloading upon arrival, the motor vehicle shall be parked out-of-doors and not close to any building. The driver shall remain with the vehicle until the materials are unloaded.

(i) The following exemptions, subject to the specified conditions, will not result in undue danger to life and health:

(1) All shippers of ''Large Quantity'' radiation sources may be exempt from the requirement of reporting their proposed route, provided they follow the ''Truck Routes'' specified in subsection (e) above.
(2) All shippers of ''Large Quantity'' radiation sources ten times or less than the designated quantity may be exempt from supplying the Department with the information prescribed by this section, provided they follow the ''Truck Routes'' specified in subsection (e) above and leave the city without making a delivery and without any loading, servicing, or layover within the City.

(j) Vehicles passing over any bridge under the jurisdiction of the Department of Highways shall meet the provisions of Local Law p. 49 of 1954, section 683a2-1.0 of the Administration Code of the City of New York governing the maximum dimensions and weights for vehicles.

(k) Transport of radioactive material within the City by a physician for use in the practice of medicine is exempt from the requirement of this section, provided that such material is not transported via mass transit facilities.

Section 75.112 Radiation accidents, contaminations, thefts, losses, and reports thereof

(a) When an accident or other situation involving a radiation source occurs which results or may result in contamination or the over-exposure of persons to ionizing radiation, or any level of radiation from, or release of a concentration of, radioactive material in any area which is not a controlled area or which may cause any installation to be rendered inoperative for at least one full working day, the owner, person in charge, or radiation safety officer of the installation concerned or, if the accident occurs outside of an installation the owner or the person responsible for the radiation source involved shall immediately notify the Department by telephone. Such report shall not relieve such owner, person, or radiation safety officer of the responsibility for instituting and performing such corrective and preventive measures as are necessary to reduce the hazards. Upon request of the Department, a written report shall be filed containing such information as may be required by the Department.

(b) If a theft or loss of a radiation source occurs, the owner, person in charge, or radiation safety officer of the installation concerned or, if the theft or loss occurs outside of an installation, the owner or the person responsible for the radiation source shall immediately notify the Department by telephone. Upon request of the Department, a written report shall be filed containing such information as may be required by the Department.

(c) Any written report filed with the Department pursuant to this section shall describe the extent of exposure of individuals to radiation or radioactive material levels of radiation and concentrations of radioactive material involved; the cause of the exposure, levels, or concentrations; and corrective steps taken or planned to assure against a recurrence. Such reports shall be prepared in such a manner that the name, the social security number, and the date of birth of each individual who has received exposure to radiation will be stated in a part of the report separate from the information regarding the exposure.

(d) When necessary or desirable in order to aid in determining the extent of any individual's exposure to radiation subsequent to any radiation accident, contamination, theft or loss, the owner or person in charge of such radiation source shall comply with orders of the Department directing him to make available to such individual appropriate medical evaluation services or appropriate tests and to furnish to the Department a copy of the reports of such evaluation or tests.

Buffalo and Fort Erie Public Bridge Authority
Peace Bridge Plaza
Buffalo, New York 14213*

Radioactive shipments are allowed to travel under permit on the Peace Bridge, provided they conform to the applicable regulations of the Atomic Energy Commission, the United States Department of Transportation, and the Interstate Commerce Commission. The permit is issued by the Authority. A minimum of 2 days is required for processing the permit. Authority regulations, however, exclude weapons of war employing atomic fission or radioactive force.

New York State Thruway Authority
P.O. Box 189
Albany, New York 12201

The Gov. Thomas E. Dewey Thruway
New York State Bridge Authority
P.O. Box 590
Poughkeepsie, New York 12602*

Radioactive shipments are allowed to travel, under permit, on the facilities of the New York State Thruway Authority, provided they comply with the applicable regulations of the Atomic Energy Commission, the United States Department of Transportation and the Interstate Commerce Commission. The permits are issued by the Department of Operations. A special $1,000,000 insurance certificate is required to satisfy financial responsibility for the Authority. Sufficient time must be allowed prior to the shipment for processing paper work related to the permit.

Radioactive shipments are allowed to travel, under permit, on the facilities of the New York State Bridge Authority, provided they conform to the applicable regulations of the Atomic Energy Commission, the United States Department of Transportation and the Interstate Commerce Commission. The permits are issued by the individual Bridge Managers and 1 day is required for processing of the permit.

The Port Authority of New York and New Jersey
One World Trade Center, 56N
New York, New York 10048*

Radioactive shipments are allowed to travel on the Bridges and through the Tunnels of

* From Compendium of Regulations — Shipments of Radioactive Materials over Toll Roads, Bridges and Tunnels — February 1974. Compiled by International Bridge, Tunnel & Turnpike Association, Inc.

The Port Authority of New York and New Jersey, under permit, provided they conform to the application regulations of the Atomic Energy Commission, the United States Department of Transportation and the Interstate Commerce Commission. The permits are issued by the individual Bridge Managers and a minimum of 2 days is necessary to process the permit. Authority regulations exclude weapons of war employing atomic fission or radioactive force.

SECTION 38.39 TRANSPORTATION*

(a) The transportation of radioactive materials is subject to other State and Federal requirements, particularly the following:

(1) *New York State requirements.* Department of Transportation, Department of Motor Vehicles, certain public authorities, and commissions as provided in the Vehicle and Traffic Law and the requirements of cities having populations in excess of one million.
(2) *Federal requirements.* United States Department of Transportation, the Interstate Commerce Commission, the Federal Aviation Agency, the United States Coast Guard, and where the mails are used the United States Postal Service.

(b) When the regulations of the New York State Department of Transportation, the United States Department of Transportation, or the Interstate Commerce Commission are not applicable to the shipment by land of radioactive materials by persons subject to the provisions of this Part (rule), such transportation shall, nevertheless, be in accordance with the requirements relating to the transportation of radioactive materials set forth in the regulations of the United States Department of Transportation, the Interstate Commerce Commission and the New York State Department of Transportation. Any requests for modifications or exceptions to such requirements, any requests for special approvals referred to in such regulations, and any notifications referred to in such requirements shall be filed with, or made to, the commissioner.

(c) No person shall deliver radioactive material to a carrier or accept radioactive material from a carrier for transport unless:

(1) The person has established procedures, prior to delivery of radioactive material to a carrier for transport, to ensure that the radioactive material is packaged and the package monitored in accordance with applicable NYS and U.S. Departments of Transportation regulations and has included on the package for the consignee, instructions to safely open the package when such instructions are appropriate.
(2) The person has established procedures, prior to receipt of radioactive material, to ensure that the receipt and opening of the packages is done in a safe manner.
(3) The person has established procedures to ensure loading and unloading and monitoring of radioactive materials on a carrier's vehicle is done in compliance with applicable NYS and U.S. Departments of Transportation regulations.

(d) The transportation of radioactive materials by persons subject to the provisions of this Part (rule) shall also be subject to such additional requirements as the commissioner may order as reasonably appropriate and necessary to enforce the provisions of this Part (rule) relating to the general duty to protect health and safety.

* Industrial Code, Rule 38 (12NYCRR38); effective July 10, 1978.

APPENDIX P
NEW JERSEY RAM TRANSPORT RULES
NEW JERSEY ADMINISTRATIVE CODE

SUBCHAPTER 12. TRANSPORTATION

7:28-12.1 Purpose and scope

(a) This subchapter establishes requirements for transportation of radioactive material and for approval by the Department of shipping procedures for certain quantities of radioactive materials as defined in N.J.A.C. 7:28-12.3.

(b) The provisions of this subchapter shall apply to the transportation of certain quantities of radioactive materials into, through or within the State of New Jersey and to any storage of such materials during or pending such transportation notwithstanding the applicability of other provisions of this chapter or compliance with other applicable law or regulations.

7:28-12.2 Definitions

The following words and terms, when used in this subchapter, shall have the following meanings, unless the context clearly indicates otherwise.

Certificate of handling means a written document issued by the Department approving the use of certain specified New Jersey routes for the transport of specified quantities of radioactive materials.

Certificate of handling for intransit storage means a written document issued by the Department approving the use of a specifically designated location for the temporary storage of specified quantities of radioactive materials.

Certification number means the number associated with the written document issued by the Department.

Certified shipment means a shipment which meets the certification requirements as set forth in this subchapter.

Intransit storage means the storing, holding, or otherwise detaining of radioactive material during shipment at a location other than its ultimate delivery point or point where material is to be used, processed, disposed of or otherwise utilized.

Irradiated reactor fuel means materials used as a source of fuel in a nuclear reactor and which have been subjected to neutron bombardment.

Radiopharmaceutical means a radionuclide or radioactive compound designed and prepared for organ or body system administration.

7:28-12.3 General requirements

(a) No person shall cause, suffer, allow, or permit the transportation, intransit storage, or detention pending transportation of any of the following materials without first having obtained a certificate of handling or a certification number in advance of such certificate from the Department:

1. Plutonium isotopes in any quantity and form exceeding 2 g or 20 Ci, whichever is less;
2. Uranium enriched in the isotope U-235 exceeding 25 atomic percent of the total uranium content in quantities where the U-235 content exceeds 1 kg;
3. Any quantity of radioactive material which, when combined with any other quantity of such material, exceeds 20 Ci including, but not limited to, any of the actinides, spent reactor fuel elements or mixed fission product associated with such spent fuel elements.

(b) In the case of intrastate shipments, no person shall cause, suffer, allow or permit the transportation or intransit storage of any amount of radioactive material outside the confines of the location authorized for its use unless there is compliance with all relevant rules and regulations, as amended, of the United States Department of Transportation, United States Nuclear Regulatory Commission, and the United States Postal Service to the same extent as if the transportation were subject to the rules and regulations of that agency directly.

7:28-12.4 Application for certificate of handling for the transportation of radioactive material

(a) No person shall cause suffer, allow or permit the transportation of radioactive material in quantities specified in N.J.A.C. 7:28-12.3(a) without having first obtained a certificate of handling or a certification number in advance of such certificate from the Department.

(b) All shipments of radioactive material shall be accompanied by either a certificate of handling or a certification number issued by the Department.

1. In those cases where a certificate of handling is issued by the Department, the certificate of handling shall be included with the shipping documents accompanying the certified shipment;
2. In those cases where a certification number is issued by the Department the certification number and a 24-hr emergency telephone number will be supplied by the Department for notifying the State Police in the event of a public safety accident. Both the certification number and 24-hr emergency telephone number shall appear on all shipping documents accompanying the certified shipment;
3. All documents accompanying a certified shipment shall be available for inspection by authorized enforcement personnel.

(c) All applications for a certificate of handling or certification number shall be made to the Department not less than seven business days prior to shipment and shall include the following information:

1. Name of shipper;
2. Name of carrier and name of driver;
3. Type and quantity of radioactive material;
4. Date and time of shipment;
5. Starting point, scheduled route and destination;
6. Year, make, color, State of Registration, and plate number of vehicle, if applicable;
7. Names and phone numbers of individuals with knowledge as to the type and quantity of material, who will be available on a 24-hr basis to assist in radiological assessment in the event of a public safety accident;
8. An affidavit of insurance which complies with the requirements of subsection(j) of this Section;
9. Any additional information required by the Department.

(d) The Department may require changes in dates, routes, or time of transporting such material, if necessary, to maximize protection to public health and safety.

(e) The Department, upon receipt of the information specified in N.J.A.C. 7:28-12.4(c) and after consultation with the Superintendent of State Police, may approve an application for a certificate of handling or a certification number, if it determines that the shipment of such material shall be accomplished in a manner which does not jeopardize the public health and safety.

(f) Where the applicant supplies a shipping schedule for a number of shipments along with the information specified in N.J.A.C. 7:28-12.4(c) for each shipment, the Department, after consultation with the Superintendent of State Police, may issue certificates of handling or certification numbers for the specified shipments for a period not exceeding 1 year in advance of any shipment.

(g) The Department may issue yearly certificates of handling or yearly certification numbers for the routine shipment of radioactive materials.

(h) In the case of certain shipments, the Department may require an escort and special handling and may prohibit any shipment until the applicant has satisfactorily demonstrated that he has arranged, at his own expense, such escort or other special handling.

1. Where an escort or other special handling is required, the applicant shall submit the plans or specification for review and approval by the Department and by the Superintendent of State Police.
2. The Superintendent of State Police reserves the right to disapprove such specifications and to require such modifications as deemed appropriate or in certain extraordinary cases to direct that any shipment be prohibited until a State Police escort or other action can be arranged. Any condition stipulated by the State Police will be imposed by the Department as a condition of the certificate handling.

(i) All certified shipments which do not require placarding on the outside of the shipping vehicle shall have a placard conspicuously posted in the cab to be readily visible from outside the cab of the vehicle bearing the conventional radiation symbol and the words:

CAUTION: THIS VEHICLE CONTAINS RADIOACTIVE MATERIAL

(j) The applicant shall have adequate insurance coverage in order to indemnify all parties against injury, loss, or damage resulting from accidents.

(k) The Department may amend or revoke any certificate of handling issued pursuant to this subchapter whenever it has cause to believe that the information upon which the certificate is issued is in anyway inaccurate, incomplete or otherwise invalid.

7:28-12.5 Application for a certificate of handling for the transportation of irradiated reactor fuel (spent fuel)

(a) No person shall cause, suffer, allow, or permit the transportation of irradiated reactor fuel without first having obtained a certificate of handling from the Department.

(b) All shipments of irradiated reactor fuel shall be accompanied by a certificate of handling issued by the Department.

(c)The certificate of handling shall be included with the shipping documents accompanying the certified shipment. All such documents shall be available for inspection by authorized enforcement personnel.

(d) In order to obtain a certificate of handling for the shipment of irradiated reactor fuel, the applicant shall satisfy the following requirements in addition to any other regulations applicable to irradiated reactor fuel shipments.

(e) All applications for a certificate of handling shall be made to the Department in writing not less than 30 days prior to the planned shipment date and shall include the following information:

1. Name of shipper;
2. Name of carrier;
3. Type and quantity of radioactive material, including the number of fuel assemblies and activity in curies;
4. Date of shipment;

5. Starting point, scheduled route, and destination including mileage and estimated elapsed time for each distinct segment of the route within New Jersey. The scheduled shipment shall comply with the requirements of N.J.A.C. 7:28-12.5(i),(j),(k), and (m);
6. Type of transport vehicle, cask identification, and loaded weight of the transport vehicle;
7. A written safeguard plan which shall include procedures for the physical protection of the irradiated reactor fuel shipment which complies with, but is not limited to, the requirements of N.J.A.C. 7:28-12.5(h) and (l);
8. Any unusual characteristics of the shipment that would require special preparations or countermeasures in the event of a transportation emergency;
9. Names and phone numbers of available personnel responsible for emergency control and cleanup;
10. The names and phone numbers of individuals with knowledge of the type and quantity of material who will be available on a 24-hr basis to assist in radiological assessment in the event of a public safety accident;
11. An affidavit of insurance which complies with the requirements of N.J.A.C. 7:28-12.5(g); and
12. Any additional information required by the Department.

(f) Upon approval, all applicants shall update and verify information given to the Department on the original application, and shall provide the Department with the following additional information in writing not less than seven (7) days prior to the approved shipment date:

1. Time of shipment, including starting time, and if applicable, estimated time of entry into and departure from the State of New Jersey;
2. Names of personnel accompanying shipment;
3. Year, make, color, State of Registration, and plate number of vehicles escorting the shipment, if applicable; and
4. Means by which the Department can contact the transport and escort vehicles while enroute in New Jersey.

(g) The applicant shall have adequate insurance coverage in order to indemnify all parties against injury, loss, or damage resulting from accident.

(h) The applicant shall provide a statement setting forth arrangements made with law enforcement agencies along the route of the shipment for their response to an emergency or call for assistance.

(i) The proposed route shall utilize railways, roadways, or other transport modalities deemed safe by the Department and State Police. For road shipments, the applicant shall use major highways in all routing except where the Department judges such routing would place a greater threat to the public health and safety than alternate routing, or where secondary roadways must be used for a minimum distance for egress from the point of origin or ingress to the final destination.

(j) In addition to compliance with all applicable standards the applicant shall not transport in any county in New Jersey which has a population density exceeding 1000 persons/square mile as measured in the most recent decennial census. The Department may waive this requirement only when it is shown to the satisfaction of the Department that routing excluding densely populated areas would place a greater threat to the public health and safety than routing tranversing these areas.

(k) If, in accordance with N.J.A.C. 7:28-12.5(j), movement through a densely populated area is unavoidable, the following additional measures shall be taken;

1. Transit of the irradiated reactor fuel shall be nonstop. Provisions shall be made in advance so that refueling will be unnecessary in densely populated areas.
2. Primary roads shall be used for road shipments.
3. Protection by an armed escort force consisting of local police or trained armed private guards shall be provided by the shipper. At least two armed guards in a separate vehicle shall accompany the transport vehicle for road shipments.
4. No movement of irradiated reactor fuel shall occur through densely populated areas between 7:00 a.m. and 9:00 a.m. and 4:00 p.m. and 6:00 p.m.

(l) Each shipment of irradiated reactor fuel shall be accompanied by an armed escort; the plans and specifications for which shall be submitted at the time of application for review by the Department and Superintendent of State Police.

(m) The shipment of irradiated reactor fuel shall be scheduled wherever practicable without any intermediate stops within New Jersey except for refueling and obtaining provisions, and at all stops, at least one individual shall maintain constant surveillance of the transport vehicle. Irradiated reactor fuel is specifically excluded from the provision of N.J.A.C.7:28-12.7.

(n) The Superintendent of State Police reserves the right to disapprove escort or special handling specifications and to require such modifications as deemed appropriate or, in certain extraordinary cases, to direct that any shipment be prohibited until a State Police escort or other action can be arranged. Any conditions stipulated by the State Police will be imposed by the Department as a condition of the certificate of handling.

(o) The Department may require changes in dates, routes, or times of transporting irradiated reactor fuel if necessary to maximize protection of the public health and safety.

(p) The Department will issue certificates of handling for individual shipments only. Irradiated reactor fuel is specifically excluded from the provisions of N.J.A.C.7:28:12.4(f) and (g).

(q) The Department, upon review of the information specified in N.J.A.C. 7:28-5(e), and after consultation with the Superintendent of State Police, may approve the application for a certificate of handling if it determines that the shipment shall be accomplished in a manner which does not jeopardize the public health and safety.

(r) The Department may amend or revoke any certificate of handling issued pursuant to this Section whenever it has cause to believe that the information upon which the certificate is issued is in any way inaccurate, incomplete, or otherwise invalid or has not been verified pursuant to N.J.A.C.7:28-12.5(f).

7:28-12.6 Application for certificate of handling for the transportation of radiopharmaceuticals or radiographic exposure devices

(a) No person shall transport or cause, suffer, allow, or permit the shipment of radiopharmaceuticals or radiochemicals used to produce such radiopharmaceuticals or radiographic exposure devices in quantities of 20 or more curies without first obtaining a certificate of handling from the Department.

(b) The Department, after consultation with the Superintendent of State Police, may issue to the applicant a certificate of handling for a period not exceeding 1 year subject to fulfillment of the following conditions of the applicant.

1. The applicant shall submit a written application to the Department containing the information required by N.J.A.C. 7:28-12.4(c) 1 to 9 except that where such information is unavailable at the time the application is made, the applicant shall submit his best judgement as to such information and report deviations in accordance with N.J.A.C. 7:28-12.6(b)(3).
2. The applicant shall submit a report to the Department which supplies the specific

information required by N.J.A.C. 7:28-12.4(c)3,4,5 for each shipment. Such reports shall be received by the Department not later than 30 days following each of the following periods or partial period during which the certificate of handling is in force: January 1 to March 31; April 1 to June 30; July 1 to September 30; October 1 to December 31.

3. The applicant shall request approval from the Department whenever a shipment deviates from the general conditions set forth in the applicants' annual certificate of handling.
4. When an applicant consistently or routinely applies to the Department for approval of deviations from the annual certificate of handling, the Department may require the applicant to reapply for new annual certificate of handling.
5. In the case of radiographic exposure devices, a statement shall be submitted that such devices and the radiation sources utilizing therein meet all the requirements of N.J.A.C. 7:28-17.1 et seq.

7:28-12.7 Application for certificate of handling for the storage of intransit radioactive material

(a) No person shall cause, suffer, allow, or permit any intransit storage of radioactive material unless measures are taken to insure that the material cannot be removed by other than authorized personnel, and to insure compliance with such provisions of N.J.A.C. 7:28-6.1 et seq., 7.1 et seq., and 8.1 et seq. as the Department may have imposed, on a case by case basis, as a condition of certification.

(b) Any person who holds, detains, or otherwise stores radioactive material while intransit, where the combined amounts of radioactive materials continually or periodically exceed the quantities specified in N.J.A.C. 7:28-12.3, shall apply for a certificate of handling for intransit storage.

(c) Any person seeking to obtain a certificate of handling for intransit storage shall submit to the Department the following information:

1. The type, maximum quantity, and maximum time period for storage of each radioactive material to be stored;
2. A description of the location and manner of storage;
3. Names, addresses and telephone numbers of the chiefs of local police and fire departments of the jurisdiction in which the storage facility is situated;
4. Names and phone numbers of individuals, with knowledge as to the type and quantities of materials in storage, who will be available on a 24-hr basis to assist in radiological assessment in the event of a public safety accident;
5. An affidavit of insurance which complies with the requirements of subsection(g) of this Section;
6. Any additional information required by the Department.

(d) The Department, upon receipt of the information specified in subsection (c) of this section, after consultation with the Superintendent of State Police, may issue to the applicant a certificate of handling for intransit storage upon finding that such material will be stored in a manner which does not jeopardize the public health or safety.

(e) Any person storing radioactive material while such material is in transit shall immediately notify the Department of any additions in type, or increases in quantities or length of time of storage.

(f) The certificate of handling for intransit storage shall be posted prominently in the storage facility.

(g) The applicant shall have adequate insurance coverage in order to indemnify all parties against injury, loss, or damage resulting from accidents.

Form DEQ-036
6/80

STATE OF NEW JERSEY
DEPARTMENT OF ENVIRONMENTAL PROTECTION
BUREAU OF RADIATION PROTECTION
380 Scotch Road, Trenton, N.J. 08628
Phone 609 - 292 - 5586

BRP USE ONLY
COH No. T ______
Received ______
COH Issued ______

APPLICATION FOR CERTIFICATE OF HANDLING

Transportation of Radioactive Material

(Not Irradiated Reactor Fuel)

— *Application must be made not less than 7 business days prior to shipment.* —

1. Name of Shipper ______
2. Name of Carrier ______
3. Name of Driver ______
4. Shipment Vehicle ______ (Year) ______ (Make) ______ (Color)

   State of Registration ______ Plate Number ______
5. Radioactive Material: Type ______ Form (liquid, encapsulation, etc.) ______

   Quantity ______ Curies
6. Date of Shipment ______ Time of Shipment ______ ☐ a.m. ☐ p.m.
7. (a) Point of Origin of Material: Street ______

   City ______

   State ______

   (b) Scheduled Route ______

   (c) Destination: Name of Consignee ______

   Address ______
8. Is this shipment to be stored during transit? Yes ______ No ______

   NOTE: If this shipment of radioactive material is to be stored during transit, "Application for Certificate of Handling for the Storage of Intransit Radioactive Material" must be completed.
9. Emergency Contact Person Supplied by Applicant for COH:

   Name ______ Telephone Number ______

I ______, heretofore known as the COH Holder, hereby swear that the information given above is correct to the best of my knowledge, and that this shipment complies with all rules and regulations applicable to it and that $______ of liability insurance is carried by the holder of the COH to compensate for injury, loss and damage due to a radiological emergency involving this shipment.

______ (Date) ______ (Signature)

* *Applicant to retain pink copy.*

7:28-12.8 Noncompliance with certification conditions

(a) Any person who deviates from the conditions of any certificate of handling issued by the Department, or who handles radioactive material in nonconformity with the required information submitted in applying for a certificate of handling, shall be considered to be transporting, storing, or otherwise handling radioactive material without such certificate.

(b) Any person who knowingly makes any false statement on any application, label, shipping document, record, report, or other document required to be submitted to the Department or maintained pursuant to these regulations shall, upon conviction, be guilty of a crime of the fourth degree.

Form DEQ-037
6/80

STATE OF NEW JERSEY
DEPARTMENT OF ENVIRONMENTAL PROTECTION
BUREAU OF RADIATION PROTECTION
380 Scotch Road, Trenton, N.J. 08628
Phone 609 - 292 - 5586

BRP USE ONLY
No. S ______
Received ______
COH Issued ______

APPLICATION FOR CERTIFICATE OF HANDLING

Intransit Storage of Radioactive Material

1. Address of Storage Site: ______ (Bldg.) ______ (Street) ______ (City)

2. Owner of Storage Site: ______ (Name) ______ (Telephone Number)

3. Type (s) and Maximum Quantity of Each Radioactive Material Stored:

TYPE	MAXIMUM QUANTITY	TYPE	MAXIMUM QUANTITY
______	______ Curies	______	______ Curies
______	______ Curies	______	______ Curies
______	______ Curies	______	______ Curies

4. Maximum Time of Storage ______

5. Description of Location, Manner and Security of Storage:

______

______

______

6. Names, Addresses and Telephone Numbers of Authorities in the Municipalities having Jurisdiction over Storage Site Property:

(a) Police Chief: Name ______
Address ______
Telephone Number ______

(b) Fire Chief: Name ______
Address ______
Telephone Number ______

7. Name and Telephone Number of Individual Available on a 24-hour Basis, Capable of Assisting in Radiological Assessment in the Event of a Public Safety Accident:

Name ______ Telephone Number ______

I ______, heretofore known as the COH Holder, hereby swear that the information given above is correct to the best of my knowledge, and that this storage of radioactive material complies with all rules and regulations applicable to it and that $______ ______ of liability insurance is carried by the holder of the COH to compensate for injury, loss and damage due to a radiological emergency. Any change in the information given in this application requires immediate notification of the Bureau of Radiation Protection.

______ (Date) ______ (Signature)

* *Applicant to retain pink copy.*

7:28-12.9 Fees

The Department may charge fees for any service performed pursuant to this subchapter in accordance with a fee schedule promulgated pursuant to N.J.S.A. 26:2D-1 et seq. if it determines that such is necessary for the efficient implementation of the provisions of this subchapter.

APPENDIX Q
VIRGINIA RAM TRANSPORT RULES

ANNEX "T"

Virginia Hazardous Radioactive Materials Transportation Act
(Title 44, Chapter 3.3, Section 44-146.30)

TRANSPORTATION OF HAZARDOUS RADIOACTIVE MATERIALS

Section 44.146.30

Office of Emergency Services to monitor within the Commonwealth the transportation of hazardous radioactive materials. The Coordinator of the Office of Emergency Services, by not later than January one, nineteen hundred eighty, pursuant to rules and regulations promulgated by the Board of Health, will monitor the transportation within the Commonwealth of those hazardous radioactive materials, as defined by the Board of Health, which may constitute a significant potential danger to the citizens of the Commonwealth in the event of accidental spillage or release. The rules and regulations promulgated by the Board shall not be in conflict with federal statutes, rules, or regulations. Other agencies and commissions of the Commonwealth shall cooperate with the Board of Health in the formulation of rules and regulations as herein provided.

If any part of this act or the application thereof to any person or circumstance is held invalid by a court of competent jurisdiction, such holding shall not affect the validity of the remainder of the provisions or applications of the act which can be given effect without the invalid provisions or application, and to this end the provisions of this act are severable.

SECTION 1.00 GENERAL PROVISIONS

1.01 Authority for Regulations

Plenary authority for promulgation of regulations to protect public health and safety from radiation hazards is contained in the Health Laws of Virginia, codified as Title 32.1, Section 227-238, Code of Virginia (1950), as amended. The Hazardous Radioactive Materials Transportation Act, which is codified as Chapter 3.3 of Title 44, Section 44-146.30 of the Code of Virginia (1950), as amended requires the Board of Health to promulgate regulations under which the Coordinator of the Office of Emergency and Energy Services will monitor the transportation of hazardous radioactive materials. Furthermore, the statute requires the Board of Health in its regulations to define hazardous radioactive materials which may constitute a significant potential danger to the citizens of the Commonwealth in the event of accidental spillage or release.

1.02 Conflicts with Federal Statutes or Regulations

It is the goal of the Board to eliminate conflicts between these regulations and Federal statutes or regulations. If (a) any provision of any federal statute or regulation relating to the subject matter of these regulations changes in such a way as to create a conflict with these regulations, and (b) if the Supreme Court of Virginia or the Fourth United States Circuit Court of Appeals determines that a conflict exists, the conflicting portion of these regulations shall be inoperative. Any person whose conduct is regulated by these regulations shall comply with the requirements of the applicable Federal regulations, as required by section 4.02 of these regulations.

1.03 Inoperability of Regulations on Judicial Finding of Conflict

If any provision of these regulations is found by the Supreme Court of Virginia or the Fourth United States Circuit Court of Appeals to conflict with any Federal statute or regulation, the conflicting provision of these regulations shall be inoperative.

1.04 Scope

Except as otherwise specifically provided, these regulations apply to all persons who transport or cause to be transported within the Commonwealth of Virginia hazardous radioactive materials as herein defined.

1.05 Administration of Regulations

These regulations are administered by the following:

- 1.05.01 State Board of Health — the Board of Health is the governing body of the State Department of Health.
- 1.05.02 State Health Commissioner — the State Health Commissioner is the chief executive officer of the State Department of Health. The Commissioner has the authority to act, within the scope of regulations promulgated by the Board, for the Board when it is not in session.
- 1.05.03 Radiation Advisory Council — the Radiation Advisory Council, established pursuant to Section 32.1-233 of the Code of Virginia (1950), as amended, makes recommendations to the Commissioner and the Board, furnishing such technical advice as may be required, on matters related to development, utilization, and regulation of sources of ionizing radiation.
- 1.05.04 Coordinator of the Office of Emergency and Energy Services — the Coordinator is the chief executive officer of the State Office of Emergency and Energy Services. The Coordinator is charged with the responsibility of monitoring the transportation of hazardous radioactive materials in accordance with these regulations.

1.06 Application of Regulations

These regulations have general application throughout the Commonwealth. No provisions of these regulations shall be construed to reduce or negate the responsibility of any person to comply with other State or federal statutes or regulations.*

1.07 Effective Date of Regulations

These regulations shall become effective on February 15, 1980.

1.08 Application of the Administrative Process Act

The provisions of the Virginia Administrative Process Act, codified as Chapter 1.1:1 of Title 9, Section 9-6.14:1 et seq, Code of Virginia, 1950, as amended, govern the adoption, amendment, modification, and revision of these regulations, and the conduct of all proceedings hereunder and appeals therefrom.

1.09 Severability

If any provision of these regulations or the application thereof is held to be invalid, such invalidity shall not affect other provisions or application of any other part of these regulations which can be given effect without the invalid provisions or application, and to this end the provisions of these regulations and the various applications thereof are declared to be severable.

* Applicable regulations of the U.S. Department of Transportation are contained in Title 49, Parts 170-179 of the Code of Federal Regulations (CFR). Applicable regulations of the U.S. Nuclear Regulatory Commission are found in Title 10, Parts 71 and 73, Code of Federal Regulations.

1.10 Emergency Regulations

The Board, pursuant to powers granted in Section 32.1-13, Code of Virginia, 1950, as amended, is authorized to promulgate emergency regulations. Any emergency regulations adopted under this section shall comply with the provisions of Section 9-6.14:6, Code of Virginia, 1950, as amended.

1.11 Enforcement

The following provisions of Chapter 1, Article 4 of Title 32.1 of the Code of Virginia, 1950, as amended, shall apply:

- 1.11(a) 32.1-25 Right of entry to inspect, etc: warrants — Upon presentation of appropriate credentials and upon consent of the owner or custodian, the Commissioner or his designee shall have the right to enter at any reasonable time onto any property to inspect, investigate, evaluate, conduct tests, or take samples for testing as he reasonably deems necessary in order to determine whether the provisions of these regulations, any order of the Board or Commissioner or conditions in a permit, license or certificate issued by the Board of Commissioner are being complied with. If the Commissioner or his designee is denied entry, he may apply to an appropriate circuit court for an inspection warrant authorizing such investigation, evaluation, inspection, testing or taking of samples for testing as provided in Chapter 24 of Title 19.2.
- 1.11(b) 32.126 Orders— The Board is authorized to issue orders to require any person to comply with the provisions of any law administered by it, the Commissioner or the Department or any regulations promulgated by the Board or to comply with any case decision as defined in 9-6.14:4 of the Board or Commissioner. Any such order shall be issued only after a hearing with at least 30 days notice to the affected person of the time, place, and purpose thereof. Such order shall become effective not less than 15 days after mailing a copy thereof by certified mail to the last known address of such person. The provisions of this section shall not affect the authority of the Board to issue separate orders and regulations to meet any emergency as provided in Section 32.1-13.
- 1.11(c) 32.1-27 Penalties, injunctions, civil penalties and charges for violations —

  A. Any person willfully violating or refusing, failing or neglecting to comply with any regulation or order of the Board or Commissioner or any provision of this title shall be guilty of a Class I misdemeanor unless a different penalty is specified.

  B. Any person violating or failing, neglecting, or refusing to obey any lawful regulation or order of the Board or Commissioner or any provision of this Title, may be compelled in a proceeding instituted in an appropriate court by the Board or Commissioner to obey such regulations, order or provision of this Title and to comply therewith by injunction, mandamus, or other appropriate remedy.

  C. Without limiting the remedies which may be obtained in subsection B, any person violating or failing, neglecting or refusing to obey any injunction, mandamus, or other remedy obtained pursuant to subsection B shall be subject, in the discretion of the court, to a civil penalty not to exceed $10,000 for each violation. Each day of violation shall constitute a separate offense.

  D. With the consent of any person who has violated or failed, neglected, or refused to obey any regulation or order of the Board or Commissioner or any provision of this title, the Board may provide, in an order issued by the Board against such person, for the payment of civil charges for past violations in specific sums not to exceed the limit specified in Subsection C. Such civil charges shall be instead of any appropriate civil penalty which could be imposed under subsection C of this section.

SECTION 2.00 DEFINITIONS

2.01 Nontechnical Definitions

- 2.01.01 *Board* means State Board of Health.
- 2.01.02 *Carrier* means any person who undertakes, whether directly or by a lease or any other arrangement, to transport property for compensation.
- 2.01.03 *Commissioner* means the State Health Commissioner.
- 2.01.04 *Coordinator* is the Chief Executive Officer of the State Office of Emergency and Energy Services.
- 2.01.05 *Monitor* means to keep track of the transport of hazardous radioactive materials within the Commonwealth pursuant to the provisions of these regulations.
- 2.01.06 *Person* means an individual, corporation, partnership, association, or any other legal entity.
- 2.01.07 *Shipper* means person who transfers possession of hazardous radioactive material to the carrier for transport through the Commonwealth.

2.02 Technical Definitions

As used in these regulations, these terms have the definitions set forth below:

- 2.02.01 *Curie* is a unit of activity equal to 37 billion disintegrations per second. A commonly used submultiple of the curie is the microcurie (μCi). 1 μCi – 0.000001 Ci = 37,000 dps. For the purpose of these regulations, 1 Ci of natural uranium means the sum of 37 billion dps from U-238 plus 37 billion dps from U-234 plus 1.7 billion dps from U-235; this is equivalent to 3000 kg, or 6615 lb of natural uranium. One curie of natural thorium means the sum of 37 billion dps from Th-232 plus 37 billion dps from Th-228; this is equivalent to 9000 kg or 19,850 lb of natural thorium.
- 2.02.02 *Hazardous radioactive materials* means quantities of radioactive materials exceeding Type B quantities as defined in these regulations and therefore subject to provisions of these regulations.
- 2.02.03 *Low specific activity material* means any of the following:

    - 2.02.03(a) Uranium or thorium ores and physical or chemical concentrates of those ores;
    - 2.02.03(b) Unirradiated natural or depleted uranium or unirradiated thorium;
    - 2.02.03(c) Tritium oxide in aqueous solutions provided the concentrations does not exceed 5.0 mCi/mℓ;
    - 2.02.03(d) Material in which the activity is essentially uniformly distributed and in which the estimated average concentration per gram of contents does not exceed:*

        - 2.02.03(d)(1) 0.0001 mCi of Group I radionuclides; or
        - 2.02.03(d)(2) 0.005 mCi of Group II radionuclides; or
        - 2.02.03(d)(3) 0.3 mCi of Group III or IV radionuclides.
        - 2.02.03(e) Objects of nonradioactive material externally contaminated with radioactive material, provided that the radioactive material is not readily dispersible and the surface contamination, when averaged over an area of 1 m^2, does not exceed 0.0001 mCi (220,000 disintegrations per minute)

* This includes, but is not limited to, materials of low radioactivity concentrations such as residues or solutions from chemical processing; wastes such as building rubble, metal, wood, and fabric scarp. glassware, paper, and cardboard; solid or liquid plant waste, sludges, and ashes.

per square centimeter of Group I radionuclides or 0.001 mCi (2,200,000 disintegrations per minute) per square centimeter of other radionuclides.

- 2.02.04 *Rem* is a measure of the dose of any ionizing radiation to body tissue in terms of its estimated biological effect relative to a dose received from an exposure to one roentgen (R) of X-rays. One millirem (mrem) = 0.001 rem. The relation of the rem to other dose units depends upon the biological effect under consideration and upon the condition of irradiation. For the purpose of these regulations, any of the following is considered to be equivalent to a dose of 1 rem:

1. An exposure to 1 R of X-, or gamma radiation;
2. A dose of 1 rad due to X-, gamma, or beta radiation;
3. A dose of 0.1 rad due to neutrons or high energy protons;*
4. A dose of 0.05 rad due to particles heavier than protons and with sufficient energy to reach the lens of the eye.

NEUTRON FLUX DOSE EQUIVALENTS

Neutron energy (MeV)	Number of neutrons/CM² equivalent to a dose of 1 rem (neutron/cm²)	Average flux to deliver 100 mrem in 40 hr (neutrons/ cm²/sec
Thermal	970 million	670
0.000001	720 million	500
0.005	820 million	570
0.02	400 million	280
0.1	120 million	80
0.5	43 million	30
1.0	26 million	18
2.5	29 million	20
5.0	26 million	18
7.5	24 million	17
10.0	24 million	17
10 to 30	14 million	10

- 2.02.05 *Special form* means any of the following physical forms of licensed material of any transport group:

  - 2.02.05(a) The material is in solid form having no dimension less than 0.5 mm; or at least one dimension greater than 5 mm; does not melt, sublime, or ignite in air at a temperature of 1000° F; will not shatter or crumble if subject to the percussion test described in 2.02.05(c) of this part; and is not dissolved or converted into dispersible form to the extent of more than 0.005% by weight by immersion for 1 week in water at 68° F or in air at 86° F; or
  - 2.02.05(b) The material is securely contained in a capsule having no dimension less than 0.5 mm or at least one dimension greater than 5 mm, which will retain its contents if subjected to the tests prescribed in 2.02.05(c) of this part; and which is constructed in materials which do not melt, sublime, or ignite in air at 1475° F, and do not dissolve or convert into dispersible form to the extent of

* If it is more convenient to measure the neutron flux, or equivalent, than to determine the neutron dose in rads, 1 rem of neutron radiation may, for purposes of these regulations, be assumed to be equivalent to 14 million neutrons per square centimeter incident upon the body; or, if there exists sufficient information to estimate with reasonable accuracy the approximate distribution in energy of the neutrons, the incident number of neutrons per square centimeter equivalent to one rem may be estimated from the following table:

more than 0.005% by weight by immersion for 1 week in water at 68° F or in air at 85° F.

- 2.02.05(c) Tests for special form radioactive material or containers:
    - 2.02.05(c)(1) Free drop — a free drop through a distance of 30 ft onto a flat essentially unyielding surface, striking that surface in such a position as to suffer maximum damage.
    - 2.02.05(c)(2) Percussion — impact of the flat circular end of a 1-in. diameter steel rod weighting 3 lb, dropped through a distance of 40 in. The capsule or material shall be placed on a sheet of lead, or hardness number 3.5 to 4.5 on the Vickers scale, and not more than 1 in. thick, supported by a smooth essentially unyielding surface.
    - 2.02.05(c)(3) Heating — heating in air to a temperature of 1475° F and remaining at that temperature for a period of 10 min.
    - 2.02.05(c)(4) Immersion — immersion for 24 hr in water at room temperature. The water shall be pH6 to pH8, with a maximum conductivity of 10 μmhos/cm^3.

- 2.02.06 *Transport group* means any one of seven groups into which radionuclides in normal form are classified, according to their toxicity and their relative potential hazard in transport, as found in Appendix A of these regulations. Any radionuclide not specifically listed in one of the groups in Appendix A shall be assigned to one of the groups in accordance with the following table:

	Radioactive half-life		
Radionuclide	**0 to 1000 days**	**1000 days to 1,000,000 years**	**Over 1,000,000 years**
Atomic Number 1—81	Group III	Group II	Group III
Atomic Number 82 and over	Group I	Group I	Group III

- 2.02.07 *Type A quantity* and *Type B quantity* means a quantity of radioactive material the aggregate radioactivity of which does not exceed that specified in the following table:

Transport groups	Type A quantity (in curies)	Type B quantity (in curies)
I	0.001	20
II	0.05	20
III	3	200
IV	20	200
V	20	5,000
VI and VII	1,000	50,000
Special form	20[a]	5,000

[a] Except that for californium - 252, the limit is 2 Ci.

Note: For mixed shipments (including radioactive components from more than one of the above groups), the provisions of Title 10, Part 71 of the Code of Federal Regulations shall be used to determined whether the shipment involves hazardous radioactive materials.

SECTION 3.00 REGISTRATION, REPORTS, NOTIFICATION, VARIANCES, AND EXEMPTIONS

3.01 Scope

This section provides for the registration of all persons who propose to transport or cause to be transported within the Commonwealth of Virginia hazardous radioactive materials as defined in section 2.00 of these regulations, and for certain reports and notifications to be filed.

3.02 Registration

Every person, shipper, or carrier, transporting or proposing to transport within the Commonwealth hazardous radioactive materials shall register this activity with the Department of Health within thirty (30) days following the effective date of these regulations or thereafter at least thirty (30) days prior to the transportation of such materials. Application for registration shall be completed on forms furnished by the Commissioner and shall contain all the information required by the forms and accompanying instructions. Upon receipt of a complete application form and any other information required by the Commissioner, the Commissioner shall issue a registration certificate. This certificate shall expire two (2) years from date issued. Registration information shall be provided by the Commissioner to the Coordinator.

3.03 Renewal of Registration

Application for renewal shall be made on forms provided by the Commissioner.

3.04 Reports

At least annually, the Coordinator of the Office of Emergency and Energy Services shall submit to the Commissioner, the Governor's Office and the General Assembly a report summarizing their activities carried out under the provisions of these regulations.

3.05 Notification

At least twenty four (24) hours prior to each shipment or series of shipments of hazardous radioactive materials by a registrant within the Commonwealth of Virginia, the registrant shall notify by telephone or in writing the Coordinator. As a part of the notification, the registrant shall give the number assigned his registration certificate, the date and time of each shipment, origin and destination, mode of transport, and any special circumstances applying to the shipment which were not described in the registration application. Any significant change of the notification data will be reported to the Coordinator also prior to shipment. The Coordinator shall disseminate the notification to local law enforcement agencies, emergency services coordinators, other designated local officials along the route as requested by county or municipal authorities, or as determined by the Coordinator to be necessary for effective implementation of these regulations. Joint notification by the shipper and carrier is permitted.

3.06 Exemptions

3.06.01 Low Specific Activity Material

The shipment or transportation of low specific activity materials is not subject to the requirements of these regulations. See section 2.02.03.

3.06.02 National Defense

The shipment or transportation of radioactive materials by the U.S. Government, for military or national defense, is not subject to the requirements of these regulations. Nothing herein shall be construed as requiring the disclosure of any defense information or restricted data as defined in the Atomic Energy Act of 1954 or the Energy Reorganization Act of 1974, as amended.

3.07 Authority for Variances

The Commissioner may grant on his own motion or by request, a variance from any part or all of these regulations. Such variances are to be granted only in situations involving national security or in circumstances where compliance with the regulations is not possible and when he determines that no adverse affect on the public health and safety will result.

3.08 Request for Variances

Any person or firm may make a request, in writing, or by telephone followed by written confirmation, for variance of any part of these regulations. Such requests shall fully and clearly describe the part of the regulations from which such a variance is sought, shall identify the substance(s) and quantity thereof to which such variance would apply, and shall set forth fully the reasons that such a variance should be made.

3.09 Variances Granted

The Commissioner shall cause to be maintained a listing of all variances granted. Such listing shall be available to the public. This information will be shared with the Coordinator.

SECTION 4.00 OTHER REQUIREMENTS

4.01 Routing

When selecting routes for the transportation of hazardous radioactive materials, congested metropolitan areas and hazardous environmental conditions shall be avoided wherever practicable. Interstate highway routing or frequently inspected railways shall be selected whenever possible.

4.02 Applicability of Federal Laws or Regulations

Every shipper or carrier of hazardous radioactive materials shall, as a requirement of these Virginia regulations, comply with all United States Department of Transportation, United States Nuclear Regulatory Commission, or other federal regulatory requirements imposed upon such shippers or carriers as a requirement of federal law or regulation.

4.03 Instructions and Procedures

No shipper shall deliver any hazardous radioactive material to a carrier for transport unless the shipper has established procedures for opening and closing packages in which hazardous radioactive material is transported. Such procedures shall provide for safety and assure that, prior to the delivery to a carrier for transport, each package is properly closed for transport and that any special instructions needed to open the package safetly are sent to or have been made available to the consignee. The shipper shall provide the carrier with written emergency instructions, which have been approved by the Coordinator.

4.04 Record-Keeping for Shippers

The shipper shall maintain complete files for inspection by the Commissioner. These files shall include:

- 4.04.01 Training programs offered — dates, times, who participated.
- 4.04.02 Escorts used — name, position, documentation of completion of required training.
- 4.04.03 Detailed shipping records — type of shipment, quantity, times, dates, routes, and destination.

- 4.04.04 Emergency instructions.
- 4.04.05 Detailed description of security measures used.

4.05 Records Available for Inspection

The shipper shall make any records required by Section 4.04 of these regulations immediately available for inspection by the Commissioner upon request.

SECTION 5.00 SPECIAL REQUIREMENTS FOR PHYSICAL PROTECTION OF EXTRAORDINARILY RADIOACTIVE MATERIALS

5.01 Advance Approval of Routes

Any person who transports or delivers to a carrier for transport quantities of hazardous radioactive materials having a total external radiation dose rate in excess of 100 rems/hr at a distance of 3 ft from any accessible surface without intervening shielding shall, in addition to the other requirements previously set forth in these regulations, use only routes approved by the Commissioner in advance of such shipment in the registration certificate or emergency routes prescribed by the Coordinator.

5.02 Filing of Federal Route Applications and Approvals with Commissioner

Any person required by federal law or regulation to obtain route approval from the Nuclear Regulatory Commission shall file copies of any applications to the NRC with the Commissioner at the same time that person files an application for route approval with the NRC. Any person receiving a route approval from the NRC shall forthwith file a copy of the route approval received from NRC with the Commissioner.

5.03 Certification

Any person who transports or delivers to a carrier for transport quantities of hazardous radioactive materials having a total external radiation dose rate in excess of 100 rems/hr at a distance of 3 ft from any accessible surface without intervening shielding shall:

- 5.03.01 Arrange to provide an armed escort for such shipments while in transit within the Commonwealth of Virginia.
- 5.03.02 Ensure that the shipment is scheduled where practicable without any intermediate stops except for refueling and obtaining provisions, and that at all stops at least one individual maintains surveillance of the transport vehicle.
- 5.03.03 Ensure that individuals other than law enforcement officials, serving as escorts have successfully completed a training program in accordance with Appendix B of these regulations.
- 5.03.04 Ensure that procedures for coping with threats and safeguards emergencies have been developed.
- 5.03.05 Certify the above information in writing to the Commissioner on Form HDF-121. Joint certification by shippers and carriers is permitted.

5.04 Shipments by Road

In addition to the provisions of section 5.02, for shipments by road, the shipper and carrier shall:

- 5.04.01 Ensure that each shipment is accompanied by (i) at least one driver and one escort in the transport vehicle, or (ii) at least one driver in the transport vehicle and two escorts in a separate vehicle.
- 5.04.02 Ensure that the transport or separate vehicle is equipped with a radio-telephone

or approved equal communications equipment and that calls are made at least every two (2) hours to a designated location to advise of the status of the shipment.

- 5.04.03 Ensure that the transport vehicle is equipped with features that permit immobilization of the cab or the cargo-carrying portion of the vehicle. This requirement of immobilization means the ability to render the vehicle incapable of moving under its own power through activation of a device located in the cab of the vehicle.
- 5.04.04 Certify the above information in writing to the Commissioner on Form HDF-121. Joint certification by shippers and carriers is permitted.

5.05 Shipments by Rail

In addition to the provisions of section 5.02, for shipments by rail, the shipper and carrier shall:

- 5.05.01 Ensure that each shipment is accompanied by at least one escort in the shipment car or in a separate car that will permit observation of the shipment car.
- 5.05.02 Ensure that two-way voice communication capability is available and that calls are made at least every two (2) hours to a designated location to advise of the status of the shipment.
- 5.05.03 Ensure that at least one escort maintains visual surveillance of the shipment car during periods when the train is stopped on sidings or in rail yards.
- 5.05.04 Certify the above information in writing to the Commissioner on Form HDF-121. Joint certification by shippers and carriers is permitted.

5.06 Shipments by Water

If any person shall transport hazardous radioactive material into Virginia waters for delivery to a land carrier for transportation within the Commonwealth or for storage prior to such land transportation, such transportation by vessel shall be exempt from the provisions of these regulations except that such person shall notify the Coordinator in advance of such shipment. Notification shall include a description of the radioactive material, the name of the port of entry, the name of the vessel delivering the hazardous radioactive material, the date and time of expected arrival in port and the name of the land carrier to which the shipment is to be delivered.

5.07 Implementation

For requirements contained in section 5.00, a period of sixty (60) days from the effective date of these regulations is allowed for the implementation of requirements that involve equipment modification or training. All requirements of section 5.00 apply only to persons who transport hazardous radioactive materials having a total external radiation dose rate in excess of 100 rems/hr at a distance of 3 ft from any accessible surface without intervening shielding.

APPENDIX A
TRANSPORT GROUPING OF RADIONUCLIDES

Element[a]	Radionuclide[b]	Group
Actinium (89)	AC-227	I
	AC-228	I
Americium (95)	AM-241	I
	AM-243	I
Antimony (51)	Sb-122	IV
	Sb-124	III
	Sb-125	III
Argon (18)	Ar-37	VI
	Ar-41	II
	Ar-41 (uncompressed)[c]	V
Arsenic (33)	As-73	IV
	As-74	IV
	As-76	IV
	As-77	IV
Astatine (85)	At-211	III
Barium (56)	Ba-131	IV
	Ba-133	II
	Ba-140	III
Berkelium (97)	Bk-249	I
Beryllium (4)	Be-7	IV
Bismuth (83)	Bi-206	IV
	Bi-207	III
	Bi-210	II
	Bi-212	III
Bromine (35)	Br-82	IV
Cadmium (48)	Cd-109	IV
	Cd-115 m[d]	III
	Cd-115	IV
Calcium (20)	Ca-45	IV
	Ca-47	IV
Californium (98)	Cf-249	I
	Cf-250	I
	Cf-252	I
Carbon (6)	C-14	IV
Cerium (58)	Ce-141	IV
	Ce-143	IV
	Ce-144	III
Cesium (55)	Cs-131	IV
	Cs-134 m[d]	III
	Cs-135	IV
	Cs-136	IV
	Cs-137	III
Chlorine (17)	Cl-36	III
	Cl-38	IV
Chromium (24)	Cr-51	IV
Cobalt (27)	Co-56	III
	Co-57	IV
	Co-58 m[d]	IV
	Co-58	IV
	Co-60	III
Copper (29)	Cu-64	IV
Curium (96)	Cm-242	I
	Cm-243	I
	Cm-244	I
	Cm-245	I
	Cm-246	I
Dysprosium (66)	Dy-154	III
	Dy-165	IV
	Dy-166	IV
Erbium (68)	Er-169	IV
	Er-171	IV
Europium (63)	Eu-150	III
	Eu-152 m[d]	IV
	Eu-152	III
	Eu-154	II
	Eu-155	IV
Fluorine (9)	F-18	IV
Gadolinium (64)	Gd-153	IV
	Gd-159	IV
Gallium (31)	Ga-67	III
	Ga-72	IV
Germanium (32)	Ge-71	IV
Gold (79)	Au-193	III
	Au-194	III
	Au-195	III
	Au-196	IV
	Au-198	IV
	Au-199	IV
Hafnium (72)	Hf-181	IV
Holmium (67)	Ho-166	IV
Hydrogen (1)	H-3 (see tritium)	
Indium (49)	In-113 m[d]	IV
	In-114 m[d]	III
	In-115 m[d]	IV
	In-115	IV
Iodine (53)	I-124	III
	I-125	III
	I-126	III
	I-129	III
	I-131	III
	I-132	IV
	I-133	III
	I-134	IV
	I-135	IV
Iridium (77)	Ir-190	IV
	Ir-192	III
	Ir-194	IV
Iron (26)	Fe-55	IV
	Fe-59	IV
Krypton (36)	Kr-85 m[d]	III
	Kr-85 m[d] (uncompressed)[c]	V
	Kr-85	III
	Kr-85 (uncompressed)[c]	VI
	Kr-87	II
	Kr-87 (uncompressed)[c]	V
Lanthanum (57)	La-140	IV
Lead (82)	Pb-203	IV
	Pb-210	II
	Pb-212	II
Lutecium (71)	Lu-172	III
	Lu-177	IV
Magnesium (12)	Mg-28	III

Element[a]	Radionuclide[b]	Group
Manganese (25)	Mn-52	IV
	Mn-54	IV
	Mn-56	IV
Mercury (80)	Hg-197 m[d]	IV
	Hg-197	IV
	Hg-203	IV
Mixed fission products M F P		II
Molybdenum (42)	Mo-99	IV
Neodymium (60)	Nd-147	IV
	Nd-149	IV
Neptunium (93)	Np-237	I
	Np-239	I
Nickel (28)	Ni-56	III
	Ni-59	IV
	Ni-63	IV
	Ni-65	IV
Niobium (41)	Nb-93 m[d]	IV
	Nb-95	IV
	Nb-97	IV
Osmium (76)	Os-185	IV
	Os-191 m[d]	IV
	Os-191	IV
	Os-193	IV
Palladium (46)	Pd-103	IV
	Pd-109	IV
Phosphorus (15)	P-32	IV
Platinum (78)	Pt-191	IV
	Pt-193	IV
	Pt-193 m[d]	IV
	Pt-197 m[d]	IV
	Pt-197	IV
Plutonium (94)	Pu-238 (F)[c]	I
	Pu-239 (F)[c]	I
	Pu-240	I
	Pu-241 (F)[c]	I
	Pu-242	I
Polonium (84)	Po-210	I
Potassium (19)	K-42	IV
	K-43	III
Praseodymium (59)	Pr-142	IV
	Pr-143	IV
Promethium (61)	Pm-147	IV
	Pm-149	IV
Protactinium (91)	Pa-230	I
	Pa-231	I
	Pa-233	II
Radium (88)	Ra-223	II
	Ra-224	II
	Ra-226	I
	Ra-228	I
Radon (86)	Rn-220	IV
	Rn-222	II
Rhenium (75)	Re-183	IV
	Re-186	IV
	RE-187	IV
	Re-188	IV
	Re-Natural	IV
Rhodium (45)	Rh-103 m[a]	IV
	Rh-105	IV
Rubidium (37)	Rb-86	IV
	Rb-87	IV
	Rb-Natural	IV
Ruthenium (44)	Ru-97	IV
	Ru-103	IV
	Ru-105	IV
	Ru-106	III
Samarium (62)	Sm-145	III
	Sm-147	III
	Sm-151	IV
	Sm-153	IV
Scandium (21)	Sc-46	III
	Sc-47	IV
	Sc-48	IV
Selenium (34)	Se-75	IV
Silicon (14)	Si-31	IV
Silver (47)	Ag-105	IV
	Ag-110 m[d]	III
	Ag-111	IV
Sodium (11)	Na-22	III
	Na-24	IV
Strontium (38)	Sr-85 m[d]	IV
	Sr-85	IV
	Sr-89	III
	Sr-90	II
	Sr-91	III
	Sr-92	IV
Sulfur (16)	S-35	IV
Tantalum (73)	Ta-182	III
Technetium (43)	Tc-96 m[d]	IV
	Tc-96	IV
	Tc-97 m[d]	IV
	Tc-97	IV
	Tc-99 m[d]	IV
	Tc-99	IV
Tellurium (52)	Te-125 m[d]	IV
	Te-127m[d]	IV
	Te-127	IV
	Te-129 m[d]	III
	Te-129	IV
	Te-131 m[d]	III
	Te-132	IV
Terbium (65)	Tb-160	III
Thallium (81)	Tl-200	IV
	Tl-201	IV
	Tl-202	IV
	Tl-204	III
Thorium (90)	Th-227	II
	Th-228	I
	Th-230	I
	Th-231	I
	Th-232	III
	Th-234	II
	Th-Natural	III
Thulium (69)	Tm-168	III
	Tm-170	III
	Tm-171	IV

Element[a]	Radionuclide[b]	Group
Tin (50)	Sn-113	IV
	Sn-117 m[d]	III
	Sn-121	III
	Sn-125	IV
Tritium (1)	H-3	IV
	H-3 (as a gas, as luminous paint, or absorbed on solid material)	VII
Tungsten (74)	W-181	IV
	W-185	IV
	W-187	IV
Uranium (92)	U-230	II
	U-232	I
	U-233 (F)[e]	II
	U-234	II
	U-235 (F)[e]	III
	U-236	II
	U-238	III
	U-Natural	III
	U-Enriched (F)[e]	III
	U-Depleted	III
Vanadium (23)	V-48	IV
	V-49	III
Xenon (54)	Xe-125	III
	Xe-131 m[d]	III
	Xe-131 m[d](uncompressed)[c]	V
	Xe-133	III
	Xe-133 (uncompressed)[c]	VI
Xenon (54)-Con.	Xe-135	II
	Xe-135 (uncompressed)[c]	V
Ytterbium (70)	Yb-175	IV
Yttrium (39)	Y-88	III
	Y-90	IV
	Y-91 m[d]	III
	Y-91	III
	Y-92	IV
	Y-93	IV
Zinc (30)	Zn-65	IV
	Zn-69 m[d]	IV
	Zn-69	IV
Zirconium (40)	Zr-93	IV
	Zr-95	III
	Zr-97	IV

[a] Atomic number shown in parentheses.
[b] Atomic weight shown after the radionuclide symbol.
[c] Uncompressed means a pressure not exceeding 1 atmosphere.
[d] m = Metastable state.
[e] (F) = Fissile material.

Appendix B
PHYSICAL PROTECTION OF CERTAIN HAZARDOUS RADIOACTIVE MATERIALS IN TRANSIT TRAINING PROGRAM SUBJECT SCHEDULE

Pursuant to the provisions of these regulations, each person who transports or delivers to a carrier for transport hazardous radioactive materials as herein defined, having a total external radiation dose rate in excess of 100 rems/hr at a distance of 3 ft from any accessible surface without intervening shielding, is required to assure that individuals other than law enforcement officers used as shipment escorts have completed a training program. The subjects that are to be included in this training program are as follows:

Security Enroute

Route planning and selection
Vehicle operation
Procedures at stops
Detours and use of alternate routes

Communications

Equipment operation
Status reporting
Contacts with law enforcement units
Procedures for reporting incidents
Communications discipline

Radiological Considerations

Description of the radioactive cargo
Function and characteristics of the shipping casks
Radiation hazards
Federal, State and local ordinances relative to the shipment of radioactive materials
Responsible agencies

Response to Contingencies

Accidents
Severe weather assistance
Vehicle breakdown
Communications problems
Radioactive "spills"
Use of special equipment (flares, emergency lighting, etc.)

Response to Threats

Reporting
Calling for assistance
Use of immobilization features
Hostage situations
Avoiding suspicious situations
Handling and use of firearms

APPENDIX R
FORMS

CERTIFICATION FOR TRANSPORTATION OF HAZARDOUS RADIOACTIVE MATERIALS

I hereby certify that, in accordance with regulations promulgated under Title 44, Code of Virginia, Chapter 3.3, Section 44-146.30, and under Sections 32.1-227 through 238 of the Code, the following conditions will be met with respect to the transportation of large quantities of hazardous radioactive materials as described in Section 5.01 of the regulations. Additionally, I certify that all conditions listed below will be met before any shipment subject to this certification is made.

1. Arrangements will be made to provide an armed escort for such shipments while in transit through the Commonwealth of Virginia.
2. All shipments will be scheduled where practicable without any intermediate stops except for refueling and obtaining provisions, and that at all stops at least one individual will maintain surveillance of the transport vehicle.
3. Individuals other than law enforcement officials serving as escorts will have successfully completed a training program in accordance with Appendix B of these regulations.
4. Procedures for coping with threats and safeguards emergencies will be developed.

I further certify that if any shipment, subject to this certification, is made by road, the following conditions will be met:

1. Each shipment will be accompanied by (i) at least one driver and one escort in the transport vehicle, or (ii) at least one driver in the transport vehicle and two escorts in a separate vehicle.
2. The transport or separate vehicle will be equipped with a radio-telephone or approved equal communications equipment and that calls will be made at least every 2 hr to a designated location to advise of the status of the shipment.
3. The transport vehicle will be equipped with features that permit immobilization of the cab or the cargo-carrying portion of the vehicle in such a manner as to render the vehicle incapable of moving under its own power.

I also certify that if any shipment, subject to this certification, is shipped by rail, the following conditions will be met:

1. Each shipment will be accompanied by at least one escort in the shipment car or in a separate car that will permit observation of the shipment car.
2. Two-way voice communication capability will be available and calls will be made at least every 2 hr to a designated location to advise of the status of the shipment.
3. At least one escort will maintain visual surveillance of the shipment car during periods when the train is stopped on sidings or in rail yards.

____
Signature

DATE:__________________________ ______________________________
Company

COMMONWEALTH OF VIRGINIA
NOTIFICATION GUIDELINES FOR SHIPMENTS OF HAZARDOUS RADIOACTIVE MATERIAL

The following is to be provided to the Office of Energy and Emergency Services (OEES) in writing or by phone, at least 24 hr prior to shipment.

(1a) Department of Health Registration

Number________________

(1b) Shipper: Name________________

Address________________

City________
State______
Zip________________

(1c) Carrier: Name________________

Address________________

City________
State______
Zip________________

(2a) Date of Notification:________________

(2b) Date of Shipment:________________

(3) Origin:________________

(4) Destination:________________

(5) Route to be used through the Commonwealth:________________

____

____

(6) Description of Radioactive Materials:

(6a) Type:________________

(6b) Quantity (in Curies):________________

(6c) Physical Form:________________

(7) Time of Shipment:

(7a) Entering Commonwealth:________________

(7b) Leaving Commonwealth:________________

(8) Vehicle Being Used:

(8a) License No(s):________________

(8b) Type & Description:________________

____

(9) Is Shipment to be escorted:________________

If so, by whom:________________

(10) Name & Title of Person Making Notification:

Name________________

Title________________

COMMONWEALTH OF VIRGINIA
APPLICATION FOR REGISTRATION TO TRANSPORT HAZARDOUS RADIOACTIVE MATERIALS

Instruction for Completion of HDF-123 on reverse side.

PLEASE TYPE OR PRINT:

Check one: _____Carrier or _____Shipper

1. Name______________________________
   Address______________________________
   City______________
   State______________________________
   Zip Code____________
2. Office Phone No.________________
3. Emergency Phone No.______________
4. Radiation Safety Officer (RSO)
   ____
5. Phone No. (RSO)________________
6. Emergency Phone No. (RSO)________
7. Estimated No. Shipments per year?
   ____
8. Mode of Transportation: _______Truck
   _______Rail _____Ship _______Air
   Other (Specify)________________
9. Type of Transport Vehicle:
   ____
10. Type of Escort Provided (See Instructions):
    ____
11. Proposed Routes:____
    ____
    ____
12. Estimated Mileage for Each Route______________________________
13. Travel Time for Each Route:______________________________
14. Names and Locations of Proposed Stops:______________________________
    ____
15. Type of Escort Provided:______________________________

Date of Application________________ Signature______________________

INSTRUCTIONS FOR COMPLETION OF HDF-123

1. Give legal name and mailing address of Company shipping or transporting material. If the carrier is an individual not employed by a company, give legal name and address of his office or home.
2. Give the office telephone number of the Company or individual listed in Item 1 which is routinely used in the conduct of business.
3. Give the telephone number of the company or individual listed in Item 1 which could be called in the event of an emergency involving the shipment.
4. Give the legal name of the person responsible for the owner's or shipper's radiation safety progam and who could be contacted *at any time* while the shipment is in transit.
5. Give the routine business telephone number of the person listed in Item 4.
6. Give the telephone number which will reach the individual listed in Item 4 *at any time* while the shipment is in transit.
7. Give approximate total number of shipments per year of the company or individual listed in item 1.
8. Check appropriate box showing how material is to be transported. If other, write specific means of transport.
9. Specify type of vehicle; e.g., detachable flatbed truck, railroad boxcar, etc.
10. Give the name or type of agency escorting shipment, e.g., Nuclear Company Security Force or Anytown Police Department.
11. List all usual and customary routes and alternate routes, including route numbers of (a) all roads, railroads and waterways to be traveled, (b) names of commercial carriers other than that listed in Item 1, (c) estimated mileage in Virginia for each route.
12. Give a numerical value for the *total mileage* in Virginia for each Route and alternate route proposed.
13. Give approximate travel time in Virginia for *each* route listed in Item 10.
14. Give names and locations of each proposed routine stop on *each* route. Include approximate time of each stop.
15. Give name of all agencies providing escort for material if applicable. Include copy of appropriate agreements and training programs.

NOTE:

1. Attach two (2) copies of all emergency instructions provided during a materials shipment, including specific instructions to drivers.
2. Forward the completed application to:

   Virginia State Health Department
   Bureau of Radiological Health
   James Madison Building — Room 910
   109 Governor Street
   Richmond, Virginia 23219

3. Fill in *all* blanks. Where an item is not applicable write N/A or "none" where appropriate.

APPENDIX S
N.Y.S. SUFFOLK CO. RAM
TRANSPORT RULES

ARTICLE 15 SUFFOLK COUNTY SANITARY CODE
ARTICLE 15 — RADIATION CONTROL

SECTION

ARTICLE 15

Section 1509 Notification of Transportation of Radioactive Materials

1. No person shall ship, transport, convey or receive radioactive materials in categories listed in Paragraph 2, unless said person, not less than 48 hr prior thereto shall notify the commissioner, in writing and by telephone, of the proposed shipment, transport, conveyance or receipt. It shall be the sole discretion of the commissioner, upon request, to accept any notice required herein within a period less than the 48-hr period.

Such notice shall set forth:

a. Date of shipment
b. Place of shipment
c. Name and address of shipper and official authorized to act for same
d. Category identification of the type and quantity of radioactive materials
e. Methods of transportation
f. Route of transportation
g. Date of destination
h. Place of destination
i. Name and address of person to receive such radioactive material and name of official authorized to act for same
j. Vehicle license number
k. Provisions for surveillance in the event that radioactive materials do not reach stated destination as scheduled
l. Procedures undertaken to minimize the limits of radiation and the possibility of contamination from said radioactive materials.

2. Notification is required of:

a. Any shipment of solid, liquid or gaseous radioactive materials equivalent to or exceeding the following amounts:*

- 20 Ci of Group I radionuclides
- 20 Ci of Group II radionuclides
- 200 Ci of Group III radionuclides
- 200 Ci of Group IV radionuclides
- 5000 Ci of Group V radionuclides
- 50,000 Ci of Group VI radionuclides
- 50,000 Ci of Group VII radionuclides

b. Spent nuclear fuel

c. Any quantity of radioactive materials of plutonium 238, 239, 241, uranium 233, 235, or any material containing these radioisotopes

d. Any shipment of radioactive wastes

e. Transportation of any package exceeding 10 mg of radium 226.

3. If the commissioner finds that any of the information included under Section 1509, No. 1 is unsatisfactory or the procedures are unsafe or are not in compliance with existing regulations, the commissioner may determine that a proposed shipment should not be made as scheduled. Notice of such determination shall be given to the shipper, transporter, receiver, and any others properly concerned whereupon the shipment will not be made until permission therefore has been given.

4. Any person transporting radioactive materials shall immediately notify the commissioner in the event of an accident, loss, theft, breakdown, or any other incident during transport that is not set forth in the notification required by Paragraph 1 herein above.

* From Title 49, Code of Federal Regulations, Section 173.390.

APPENDIX T
NUCLEAR ENERGY LIABILITY EXCLUSION ENDORSEMENT

Information regarding liability insurance aspects of shipping nuclear material can be found in ANSI N14 Guides (American National Standards Institute, 1430 Broadway, New York, N.Y. 10018.)

APPENDIX U
INSTRUCTIONS FOR REMOVING RAM FROM SHIPPING PACKAGE*

CAUTION: It is recommended that elution vial shields be used when eluting the generators, shielded syringes be used when preparing formulations, and appropriate vial shields be used for the formulations.

FIRST ELUTION

1. Remove generator system and accessories from carton.
2. Lift hinged cover exposing dispenser end. Remove protective cap from dispenser and attach a sterile needle — REMOVE PLASTIC NEEDLE COVER (Figure 2). Return cover to closed position.
3. Place an elution vial in the elution shield (Figure 1) and clean septum of elution vial with an antiseptic swab.
   Position elution shield on dispensing platform (Figure 3).
4. Rotate fluid path shut off valve full turns counter-clockwise until loose. Valve is located on left side of generator.
5. Slide elution shield to far left position (Figure 4). The dispensing needle will pierce the septum of the evacuated elution vial. The elution will begin immediately.
6. Step away to reduce your radiation exposure. Allow 3 to 5 min for complete elution. NOTE: If vacuum in elution vial is lost, i.e., no eluate present in vial, discard vial and use a new elution vial.
7. When elution is complete, slide elution shield to far right position. Remove elution shield, containing vial with Sodium Pertechnetate Tc99m eluate, from dispensing platform.
8. Replace dispensing needle with sterile needle with plastic cover in place. DO NOT REMOVE COVER FROM NEEDLE until next elution.
9. Affix the pressure-sensitive label to the dose vial shield. Sodium Pertechnetate Tc 99m is ready for use. Maintain adequate shielding of the radioactive preparation.

STORAGE

Store generator and eluate at room temperature (18 to 25°C).
Caution: Avoid Freezing.

Subsequent elutions

1. Lift hinged cover exposing dispenser needle. Remove plastic needle cover from dispensing needle and discard. Return cover to closed position.
2. Repeat steps 3, 5, 6, 7, 8, and 9.

20 mℓ elutions

To use the larger size elution vial, remove the spacer in the elution shield and replace with the spacer designed for 20 cc vials.

The radioactivity concentration of the final Sodium Pertechnetate Tc 99m preparation may be calculated by using the following formula:

$C = A/V$ where C is the radioactivity concentration of the Sodium pertechnetate Tc 99m preparation (millicuries/milliliter).

* Union Carbide Corporation brochure.

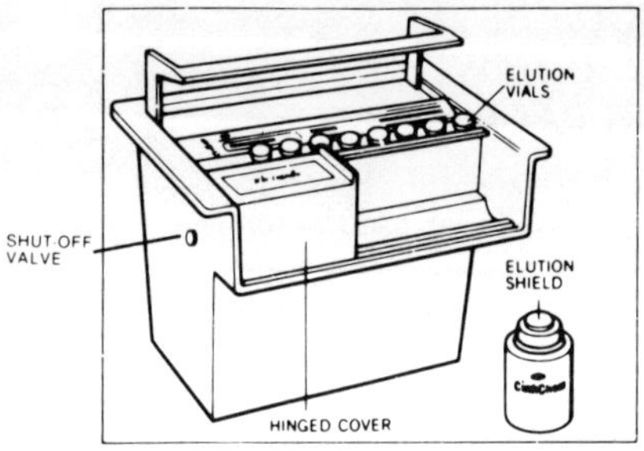

FIGURE 1

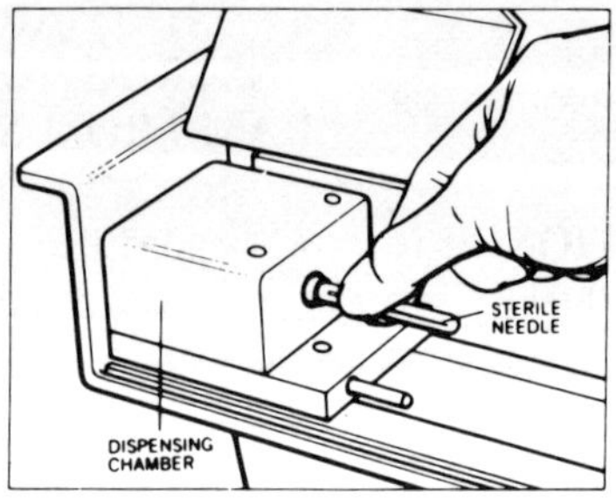

FIGURE 2

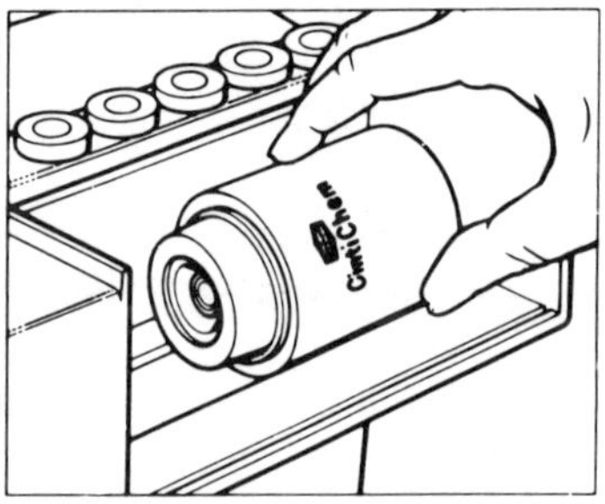

FIGURE 3

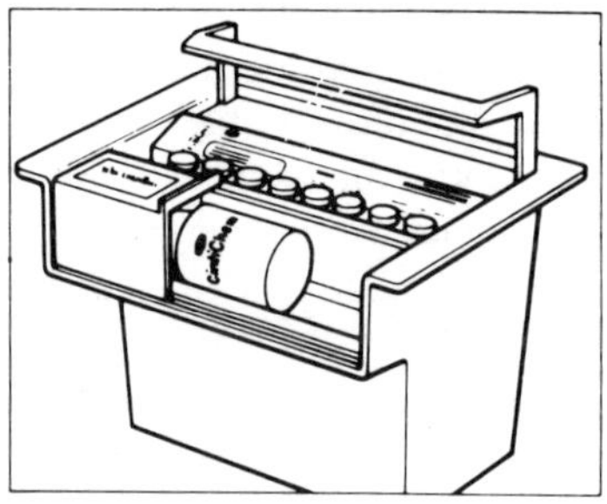

FIGURE 4

A is the Technetium Tc 99m activity added to the reaction vessel (millcuries), and
V is the total volume in the final mixture (milliliters).

Technetium Tc 99m assay procedure

1. Determine the equivalent Technetium Tc 99m value for a Cobalt Co 57 standard by multiplying the number of millicuries of the Cobalt Co 57 standard by the appropriate equivalent factor. This equivalent value of Cobalt Co 57 for the standard need only be decayed daily for use as a secondary standard.
2. Place the standard in the chamber and record μ amp reading.
3. Transfer the Technetium Tc 99m sample from the shield to the chamber. Record the μ amp reading.
4. Calculate activity:

$$\frac{\mu \text{ amps of Tc 99m}}{\mu \text{ amps of Co 57 std.}} \times \text{mCi Co 57 std.} = \text{mCi Tc 99m} ,$$

APPENDIX V
EXCERPTS FROM U.S. DOT ROUTING REQUIREMENTS

PART 171—GENERAL INFORMATION, REGULATIONS, AND DEFINITIONS

Preferred route or *Preferred highway* is a highway for shipment of large quantity radioactive materials so designated by a State routing agency, and any interstate System highway for which an alternate highway has not been designated by such State agency as provided by §177.825(b) of this subchapter.

State-designated route means a preferred route selected in accordance with U.S. DOT "Guidelines for Selecting Preferred Highway Routes for Large Quantity Shipments of Radioactive Materials" or an equivalent routing analysis which adequately considers overall risk to the public. Designation must have been preceded by substantive consultation with affected local jurisdictions and with any other affected states to ensure consideration of all impacts and continuity of designated routes.

"State routing agency" means an entity (including a common agency of more than one state such as one established by Interstate compact) which is authorized to use state legal process pursuant to §177.825 of this subchapter to impose routing requirements, enforceable by state agencies, on carriers of radioactive materials without regard to intrastate jurisdictional boundaries. This term also includes Indian tribal authorities which have police powers to regulate and enforce highway routing requirements within their lands.

PART 172—HAZARDOUS MATERIALS TABLE AND HAZARDOUS MATERIALS COMMUNICATIONS REGULATIONS

§172.507 Special placarding provisions: Highway

Each motor vehicle used to transport a package of large quantity radioactive materials (see §173.389(b) of this subchapter) must have the required RADIOACTIVE warning placard placed on a square background as described in §172.527.

§172.527 Background requirements for certain placards

(a) Except for size and color, the square background required by §172.510(a) for certain placards on rail cars, and §172.507 for placards on motor vehicles containing a package of large quantity radioactive materials, must be as follows:

PART 173—SHIPPERS — GENERAL REQUIREMENTS FOR SHIPMENTS AND PACKAGINGS

SUBPART B
PREPARATION OF HAZARDOUS MATERIALS FOR TRANSPORTATION

§173.22 Shipper's responsibility

(a) Unless otherwise provided in this part, before offering a hazardous material for shipment in a container the shipper shall determine that the container has been made, assembled with all parts or fittings in their proper place and properly secured, and marked in compliance with applicable specifications prescribed in Parts 178 and 179 of this subchapter or with specifications of the Department in effect at date of manufacture of container. In determining whether a specification container is manufactured in accordance with applicable specifications, the shipper may accept the manufacturer's certification or specification marking. (See §§178.0-2 and 179.1 of this subchapter.) For containers supplied by the carrier, the shipper may rely on the manufacturer's identification plate, specification marking, or on certification by the carrier. When a shipper performs a function covered by or having an effect on a specification requirement of Part 178 or Part 179, the shipper must perform that function in accordance with the specification.

(b) Prior to each shipment of fissile radioactive material, (see §173.389 of this subchapter), the shipper shall notify the consignee of the dates of shipment and expected arrival. The shipper shall also notify each consignee of any special loading/unloading instructions prior to his first shipment. For any shipment of irradiated reactor fuel, the shipper shall provide physical protection in compliance with a plan established under

(1) Requirements prescribed by the U.S. Nuclear Regulatory Commission, or
(2) Equivalent requirements approved by the Associate Director for Hazardous Materials Regulation, MTB.

(c) Within 90 days following acceptance by a carrier of any package containing a large quantity radioactive material (see §173.389(b)) for transportation by public highway, the shipper shall file the following information with the Associate Director for Hazardous Materials Regulation, MTB (this paragraph does not apply to packages shipped in compliance with physical security requirements of the U.S. Nuclear Regulatory Commission in 10 CFR Part 73):

(1) The route plan required under §177.825(c) of this subchapter (any supplement to the route plan prepared in accordance with §177.825(c) of this subchapter shall be filed within 90 days of receipt from the carrier):
(2) A statement identifying the name and address of the shipper, carrier, and consignee; and
(3) A copy of the shipping paper or the description of the radioactive material required by §§172.202 and 172.203 of this subchapter.

PART 177—CARRIAGE BY PUBLIC HIGHWAY

SUBPART A
GENERAL INFORMATION AND REGULATIONS

§177.810 Vehicular tunnels

(a) Except as regards radioactive materials, nothing contained in Parts 170 to 189 of this subchapter shall be so construed as to nullify or supersede regulations established and published under authority of state statue or municipal ordinance regarding the kind, character, or quantity of any hazardous material permitted by such regulations to be transported through any urban vehicular tunnel used for mass transportation. For radioactive materials, see §177.825 of this part.

§177.825 Routing and training requirements for radioactive materials

(a) The carrier shall ensure that any motor vehicle which contains a radioactive material for which placarding is required is operated on routes that minimize radiological risk. The carrier shall consider available information on accident rates, transit time, population density and activities, time of day, and day of week during which transportation will occur. In performance of this requirement the carrier shall tell the driver that the motor vehicle contains radioactive materials and shall indicate the general route to be taken. This requirement does not apply when

(1) There is only one practicable highway route available considering operating necessity and safety, or
(2) The motor vehicle is operated on a preferred highway under conditions described in paragraph (b) of this section.

(b) Unless otherwise permitted by this section, a carrier and any person who operates a motor vehicle containing a package of large quantity radioactive materials as defined in §173.389(b) of this subchapter shall ensure that the vehicle operates over preferred routes selected to reduce time in transit, except that an interstate system bypass or beltway around a city shall be used when available.

(1) A preferred route consists of

(i) An interstate system highway for which an alternative route is not designated by a state routing agency as provided in this section, and
(ii) A state-designated route selected by a state routing agency (see §171.8 of this subchapter) in accordance with the DOT "Guidelines for Selecting Preferred Highway Routes for Shipments of Large Quantity Radioactive Materials".

(2) When a deviation from a preferred route is necessary (including emergency deviation, to the extent time permits), routes shall be selected in accordance with paragraph(a) of this section. A motor vehicle may deviate from a preferred route under any of the following circumstances:

(i) Emergency conditions that would make continued use of the preferred route unsafe.
(ii) To make necessary rest, fuel, and vehicle repair stops.
(iii) To the extent necessary to pick up, deliver, or transfer a large quantity package of radioactive materials.

(c) A carrier (or his agent) who operates a motor vehicle which contains a package of large quantity radioactive material as defined in §173.389(b) of this subchapter shall prepare a written route plan and supply a copy before departure to the motor vehicle driver and a copy to the shipper (before departure for exclusive use shipments, or otherwise within 15 working days following departure). Any variation between the route plan and routes actually used, and the reason for it, shall be reported in an amendment to the route plan delivered to the shipper as soon as practicable but within 30 days following the deviation. The route plan shall contain

(1) A statement of the origin and destination points, a route selected in compliance with this section, all planned stops, and estimated departure and arrival times; and
(2) Telephone numbers which will access emergency assistance in each state to be entered.

(d) No person may transport a package of large quantity radioactive material, as defined in §173.389(b) of this subchapter, on a public highway unless

(1) The driver has received within the two preceding years, written training on

(i) Requirements in Parts 172, 173, and 177 of this subchapter pertaining to the radioactive materials transported;
(ii) The properties and hazards of the radioactive materials being tansported; and
(iii) Procedures to be followed in case of an accident or other emergency.

(2) The driver has in his immediate possession a certificate of training as evidence of training required by this section, and a copy is placed in this qualification file (see §391.51 of this title), showing

(i) The driver's name and operator's license number;
(ii) The dates training was provided;
(iii) The name and address of the person providing the training;
(iv) That the driver has been trained in the hazards and characteristics of large quantity radioactive materials; and
(v) A statement by the person providing the training that information on the certificate is accurate.

(3) The driver has in his immediate possession the route plan required by paragraph (c) of this section and operates the motor vehicle in accordance with the route plan.

(e) A person may transport irradiated reactor fuel only in compliance with a plan if required under §173.22(b) of this subchapter that will ensure the physical security of the material. Variation for security purposes from the requirements of this section is permitted so far as necessary to meet the requirements imposed under such a plan, or otherwise imposed by the U.S. Nuclear Regulatory Commission in 10 CFR Part 73.

In Part 177 Appendix A is added after §177.870 to read as follows:

APPENDIX A TO PART 177—RELATIONSHIP BETWEEN ROUTING REQUIREMENTS IN PART 177 WITH STATE AND LOCAL REQUIREMENTS

I. Purpose

This appendix is a statement of the Department of Transportation policy regarding the relationship of state and local rules with federal rules in Part 177 of this subchapter for routing motor carriers transporting radioactive materials. The purpose of this appendix is to advise a state or local government how it can exercise authority over motor carriers under its own laws in a manner that the Department of Transportation considers to be consistent with rules in Part 177 (see 49 U.S.C. 1811(a)). This appendix and Part 177 do not delegate federal authority to regulate motor carriers.

II. Definition

Routing rule means any action which effectively redirects or otherwise significantly restricts or delays the movement by public highway of motor vehicles containing hazardous materials, and which applies because of the hazardous nature of the cargo. Permits, fees, and similar requirements are included if they have such effects. Traffic controls are not included if they are not based on the nature of the cargo, such as truck routes based on vehicles weight or size, nor are emergency measures.

III. Large quantity radioactive materials

A. State routing rules

A state routing rule which applies to large quantity radioactive materials is inconsistent with Part 177 if

1. It prohibits transportation of large quantity radioactive by highway between any two points without providing an alternate route for the duration of the prohibition; or
2. It does not meet all of the following criteria:

(a) The rule is established by a state routing agency as defined in §171.8 of this subchapter:
(b) The rule is based on a comparative radiological risk assessment process at least as sensitive as that outlined in the ''DOT Guidelines'';
(c) The rule is based on evaluation of radiological risk wherever it may occur, and on a solicitation and substantive consideration of views from each affected jurisdiction, including local jurisdictions and other States; and
(d) The rule ensures reasonable continuity of routes between jurisdictions.

B. Local routing rules

A local routing rule that applies to large quantity radioactive materials is inconsistent with this Part if it prohibits or otherwise affects transportation on routes or at locations either

1. Authorized by Part 177, or
2. Authorized by a state routing agency in a manner consistent with Part 177.

IV. Quantities of radioactive materials required to be placarded

A State or local routing rule that applies to a radioactive material (other than a large quantity radioactive material), for which Part 177 requires placarding, is inconsistent with Part 177 unless it is identical to §177.825(a) of this part.

V. Radioactive materials for which placarding is not required

A state or local routing rule that applies to a radioactive material for which Part 172 does not require placarding is inconsistent with this part.

VI. Other related state and local rules

A State or local transportation rule is inconsistent with Part 177 if it

A. Conflicts with physical security requirements which the Nuclear Regulatory Commission has established in 10 CFR Part 73 or requirements approved by the Department of Transportation under §173.22(b) of this subchapter;

B. Requires additional or special personnel, equipment, or escort
C. Requires additional or different shipping paper entries, placards, or other hazard warning devices;
D. Requires filing route plans or other documents containing information that is specific to individual shipments;
E. Requires prenotification;
F. Requires accident or incident reporting other than as immediately necessary for emergency assistance; or
G. Unnecessarily delays a transportation. (49 U.S.C. 1803, 1804, 1808, 49 CFR 1.53 and App. A to Part 1)

Note — The Materials Transportation Bureau has determined that this document will not result in a major economic impact under the terms of Executive Order 12221 and DOT implementing procedures (44 FR 11034), nor require an environmental impact statement under the National Environmental Policy Act (49 U.S.C. 4321 et seq.). A regulatory evaluation and environmental assessment is available for review in the docket. Review of recordkeeping requirements under the Federal Reports Act is required by the Office of Management and Budget prior to the effective date of this document.

Issued in Washington, D.C. on January 13, 1981. L. D. Santman, Director, Materials Transportation Bureau.

APPENDIX W
U.S. NRC ADVANCED NOTIFICATION REQUIREMENTS

Date — Comment period expires March 9, 1981.

Addresses — Written comments should be submitted to the Secretary of the Commission, U.S. Nuclear Regulatory Commission, Washington, D.C. 20555, Attention: Docketing and Service Branch. Copies of comments on the proposed rule may be examined in the Commission's Public Document Room at 1717 H Street, N.W., Washington, D.C.

For further information contact — John P. Roberts, Office of Nuclear Material Safety and Safeguards, U.S. Nuclear Regulatory Commission, Washington, D.C. 20555 (Telephone 301-427-4205).

SUPPLEMENTARY INFORMATION

Background

Section 302(a) of Public Law 96-295 states:

> The Nuclear Regulatory Commission, within 90 days of enactment of this Act, shall promulgate regulations providing for timely notification to the Governor of any State prior to the transport of nuclear waste, including spent nuclear fuel, to, through, or across the boundaries of such State. Such notification requirement shall not apply to nuclear waste in such quantities and of such types as the Commission specifically determines do not pose a potentially significant hazard to the health and safety of the public.

Discussion of Proposed Rule

The Commission has examined the question of potential significant hazard to the health and safety of the public with respect to the transport of nuclear waste. The Commission and the Department of Transportation have established packaging standards for various quantities of radioactive material to provide for adequate safety of the public. There are two basic categories of packages, Type A and Type B. Type A packages must be designed to withstand the rigors of normal transport but are not designed to withstand transport accidents. Therefore, the quantities and types of radioactive material which may be transported in Type A packages are limited so that, if released in an accident, no significant hazard to public health and safety would result. Type B packages, on the other hand, must be designed to withstand both the normal conditions of transport and specified accident conditions. There are no quantity limits for radioactive material per se in Type B containers. Factors such as weight, volume, decay heat generation, and criticality control serve to place practical restirctions on the contents of Type B containers in demonstrating that the design meets regulatory requirements. Considering the types and quantities of materials shipped in Type A and Type B packages, it seems reasonable to conclude that quantities of radioactive waste required to be shipped in a Type A package do not pose a potentially significant hazard to the public health and safety. This is why the Type B packaging standards are more stringent than Type A standards. Although NUREG-0170, the Final Environmental Statement on the Transportation of Radioactive Material by Air and Other Modes (available from the Nuclear Regulatory Commission, Division of Technical Information and Document Control, Attention: Sales Manager, Washington, DC 20555) indicates that the potential risk is small, the Commission has determined that, in accordance with the intent of the Congress, the requirement for advance notification should be extended to those types and quantities of nuclear waste requiring specific packaging structural standards to withstand the effects of accidents, that is, Type B or large quantities of nuclear waste.

In NUREG-0170, it was estimated that about 389,000 packages of waste will be shipped in 1985. Most waste shipments will involve limited quantity or low specific activity packages which do not pose a potentially significant hazard to the health and safety of the public. Despite the exemption of these waste shipments from the advance notification requirement, it is expected that advance notifications for as many as 24,000 shipments may be required annually by 1985 under these proposed regulations.

Advance notification requirements for spent fuel shipments of 100 g or greater mass are being addressed by the Commission in a separate rulemaking action in 10 CFR Part 73 for safeguards purposes. A companion covering this action is published elsewhere in this issue of the *Federal Register*. Only quantities of spent fuel of less than 100 g mass requiring shipment in Type B packaging are covered in this proposed amendment to 10 CFR Part 71.

The proposed amendment to 10 CFR Part 71 will require licensees to supply the following information: the name, address, and telephone number of the shipper, carrier, and receiver of the shipment, a description of the material to be transported, point of origin, estimated period of departure, estimated periods of arrival at state boundaries, the destination of the shipment, the estimated period of arrival, and a point of contact for current shipment information. This information would be provided to the offices of the governors of states affected by mail postmarked at least 7 days, or delivered by messenger at least 4 days, in advance of the estimated period of departure. A potential new information requirement contained in a recent DOT proposed rulemaking may lessen the impact of this amendment since shippers are on notice that they may need to develop procedures for reporting to DOT and can arrange to extend this effort to include NRC. The DOT ''Highway Routing of Radioactive Materials; Proposed Rulemaking'' (45 FR 7140) would require that route plans for large quantity shipments be submitted to the DOT Materials Transportation Bureau (proposed 49 CFR 173.22(c). Some information would also be required for Type B quantity shipments (proposed 49 CFR 173.22(b)).

The proposed rule affects only NRC licensees, resulting, at the outset, in a situation where governors will not receive notification concerning a fraction of the total number of shipments, since some shipments of interest will be made by Agreement State licensees. This situation was anticipated, as noted in the additional views of several representative (opposed to the requirement of Section 301) appearing at page 37 of H. Rept. 96-194, Part 2 (June 29, 1979):

> Futher, the NRC currently licenses possession of radioactive materials in only 25 states. Under agreements between the NRC and the remaining states, those states would also have to implement regulations under this amendment.

NRC's Office of State Programs will work with the Agreement States to make regulations equivalent to the proposed rules a matter of compatibility.

Proposed Rule

Pursuant to the Atomic Energy Act of 1954, as amended, the Energy Reorganization Act of 1974, as amended, Section 301 of Public Law 96-295, and section 553 of Title 5 of the United States Code, notice is hereby given that adoption of the following amendments to 10 CFR Part 71 is contemplated.

1. In §71.4, immediately following paragraph (q) a new introductory phrase and new paragraphs (r) and (s) are added to read as follows:

§71.4 Definitions.

As used in this part:

(q)***

As used in §§71.5a to 71.5b of this part:

(r) ''Nuclear waste'' means (1) any quantity of source, byproduct, or special nuclear material required by this part to be in Type B packaging while transported to, through, or across state boundaries to a disposal site, or to a collection point for transport to a disposal site, and (2) any quantity of irradiated fuel required by this part to be in Type B packaging while transported to, through, or across state boundaries irrespective of destination provided that the quantity of irradiated fuel is less than 100 g mass.

(s) *State* means the several states of the union, the District of Columbia, the Commonwealth of Puerto Rico, the Virgin Islands, Guam, American Samoa, the Trust Territory of the Pacific Islands, and the Commonwealth of the Northern Mariana Islands.

2. Immediately following §71.5, a new centerhead and new §§71.5a-71.5b are added to read as follows:

Advance Notification to States of Transport of Nuclear Waste

§71.5a Transport of Nuclear Waste—Advance Notification Requirement

Prior to the transport of any nuclear waste outside of the confines of his plant or other place of use or storage, or delivery of any nuclear waste to a carrier for transport, each licensee shall comply with the procedures in §71.5b of this part for advance notification to the governor of a state for the transport of nuclear waste to, through, or across the boundary of the state.

§71.5b Advance Notification of Shipment of Nuclear Waste; Revision Notice; Cancellation Notice

(a) Where, when, and how advance notification must be sent.

The notification required by §71.5a must be in writing to the office of each appropriate governor and to the Director, Office of Nuclear Material Safety and Safeguards, U.S. Nuclear Regulatory Commission. A notification delivered by mail must be postmarked at least 7 days before the beginning of the estimated 7-day period of departure of the shipment. A notification delivered by messenger must reach the office of the governor at least 4 days before the beginning of the estimated seven day period of departure of the shipment.

(b) Information to be furnished in advance notification of shipment.

Each advance notification of shipment of nuclear waste must contain the following information:

(1) The name, address, and telephone number of the shipper, carrier, and receiver of the nuclear waste shipment.

(2) A description of the nuclear waste contained in the shipment as required by the regulations of the U.S. Department of Transportation in 49 CFR §§172.202 and 172.203(d).

(3) A plan which specifies

(i) The point of origin of the shipment and the estimated 7-day period of departure;

(ii) The estimated 7-day period of arrival of the shipment at state boundaries;

(iii) The destination of the shipment, and the estimated 7-day period of arrival; and

(iv) A point of contact with a telephone number for current shipment information.

(c) *Revision Notice.* A licensee who finds that schedule information previously furnished to a governor in accordance with §71.5b(b)(3) will not be met, shall notify a responsible individual in the office of the governor of the state and inform that individual of the extent of the delay relative to the schedule originally reported in writing under the provisions of §71.5b(b)(3). The licensee shall maintain a record of the name of the individual contacted for one year.

(d) *Cancellation notice*

(1) Each licensee described in paragraph (a) of this section who cancels a nuclear waste shipment for which advance notification has been sent shall send a cancellation notice to the governor of each state previously notified and to the Director, Office of Nuclear Material Safety and Safeguards, U.S. Nuclear Regulatory Commission.

(2) The notice is to state that it is a cancellation and is to identify the advance notification which is being canceled.

(Secs. 53, 57, 62, 63, 81, 161i and o, Pub. L. 83-703, 68 Stat. 930, 932, 933, 935, 948 (42 U.S.C. 2073, 2077, 2092, 2093, 2201(i) and (o)); Sec. 201 as amended, Pub. L. 93-438, 88 Stat. 1242, as amended by Publ. L. 94-79, 89 Stat. 413 (42 U.S.C.5841); Sec. 301, Pub. L. 96-295, 94 Stat. 780)

Dated at Washington, D.C. this 2nd day of December, 1980. For the U.S. Nuclear Regulatory Commission. Samuel J. Chilk, Secretary of the Commission.

10 CFR PART 73
ADVANCE NOTIFICATION TO GOVERNORS CONCERNING SHIPMENTS OF IRRADIATED REACTOR FUEL

Agency — Nuclear Regulatory Commission:

Action — Proposed rule.

Summary — The NRC is required by Federal statute to issue regulations which provide for the timely advance notification to the governor of any state prior to the transport of nuclear waste, including irradiated reactor fuel, within or through the state. This notification will provide governors advance information, not otherwise available to them, related to nuclear waste transportation in their states. To carry out the notification for irradiated reactor fuel the Commission proposes to amend its regulations in 10 CFR Part 73. The Commission is issuing a separate notice of proposed rulemaking elsewhere in this edition of the *Federal Register* with regard to the required notification for other kinds of nuclear waste.

Dates — Comments due on or before March 9, 1981.

Addresses — Written comments or suggestions for consideration in connection with the proposed amendments should be sent to the Secretary of the Commission, U.S. Nuclear Regulatory Commission, Washington, D.C. Attention: Docketing and Service Branch. Copies of comments received may be examined at the Commission's Public Document Room at 1717 H Street, NW, Washington, D.C. 20555.

For further information contact — L. J. Evans, Jr., Chief, Regulatory Improvement Branch, Division of Safeguards, Office of Nuclear Material Safety and Safeguards. (301) 427-4181.

SUPPLEMENTARY INFORMATION

Background

Section 301 of Pub. L. 96-295 requires the Nuclear Regulatory Commission to promulgate regulations for timely notification to the governor of any state, prior to the transport of nuclear waste, including spent nuclear fuel, to, through, or across the boundaries of the Due to information protection considerations, the notification requirements for spent fuel shipments will likely be different from the notification requirements for other forms of nuclear waste. Accordingly, the Commission proposes to amend 10 CFR Part 73 to implement notification for spent fuel shipments and 10 CFR Part 71 to implement notification for other forms of radioactive waste. The Part 71 proposed amendment is set forth elsewhere in this issue of the Federal Register.

Discussion of Proposed Rule

A. Synopsis of the proposed action

The proposed rule calls for the following:

1. The governor will be notified 4 days before entry of a shipment into a state.
2. The information to be supplied will be similar to that supplied for other shipments of radioactive waste, namely:

i. The shipment route,
ii. Estimated date and time of departure from point of origin,
iii. Estimated date and time of arrival at state boundary.
iv. Identification of shipper, carrier, and receiver, and
v. Description of the shipment as specified by the Department of Transportation in 49 CFR 172.202 and 172.203(d)

3. The governor will ensure that schedule information is appropriately protected from unauthorized disclosure; other information need not be protected.
4. The information protection measures are to be patterned after those for National Security Information — Confidential Level and in accordance with measures in the proposed 10 CFR 73.21, which is being issued separately.
5. The schedule information is to be automatically downgraded a short time after the shipment so that protection of the information need not be continued.
6. The licensee will renotify the office of the governor in the event of schedule changes in excess of 6 hr.

From the outset of its program for the protection of spent fuel shipments, the NRC has held that knowledge of the schedule of a shipment would be of significant value to an adversary planning to sabotage the shipment. Consistent with that longstanding policy, the proposed regulation provides for protection of schedule information pursuant to newly enacted §147 of the Atomic Energy Act (section 207, Public Law 96-295 94 Stat. 780). Accordingly, the Commission has determined that the unauthorized disclosure of the kinds of information required by §73.37(f)(3) could reasonably be expected to have a significant adverse effect on the health and safety of the public or the common defense and security by significantly increasing the likelihood of theft, diversion, or sabotage of irradiated nuclear reactor fuel.

The Commission's staff is preparing to make available to the public an atlas of spent fuel shipment routes that have been approved by the NRC. A copy will be provided to each governor. The atlas will be updated from time to time. Copies of this document, designated NUREG 0725, are or soon will be available from GPO Sales Program, Division of Technical Information and Document Control, U.S. Nuclear Regulatory Commission, Washington, D.C. 20555.

It is possible that some governors might prefer not to receive notifications. The staff proposes that no governor should be forced to receive and protect unwanted information. Accordingly, in response to a request from a governor, the staff will remove that governor's name from the list of governors to be notified.

B. Overview of proposed notification and information protection processes

Before any transport of spent fuel subject to the nondisclosure requirement of §147 is made, governors or their designees will be informed by the NRC of the applicable information protection provisions of a new proposed 10 CFR 73.21 now under consideration by the Commission. The Commission anticipates that §73.21 will be promulgated as a final rule concurrently with promulgation in final form of the amendments to §73.37 proposed herein. In the event that promulgation of §73.21 is delayed beyond the effective date of §73.37, the Commission will provide in §73.37 itself or by whatever other means are appropriate for protection of sensitive safeguards information as authorized by §147 of the Atomic Energy Act. It is anticipated that the interim protection will be substantially as provided by proposed §73.21. The significant provisions of proposed §73.21 and related law applicable to state employees would generally be as follows:

(1) State employees who receive, produce, or acquire schedule information are to protect it against unauthorized disclosure
(2) Only those persons authorized by the governor or his designee or otherwise authorized by §73.21 are to be allowed access to schedule information
(3) When not in use, written schedule information is to be stored in a security container within a building. A container such as a safe or bank safe deposit box is acceptable. Only authorized persons are to be allowed access to the content of the security container.
(4) Schedule information is not to be discussed by telephone except in an emergency or under extraordinary conditions. However, relative schedule information, such as the number of hours of delay resulting from a schedule change may be transmitted by telephone (or other means)
(5) Written schedule information may be destroyed by burning, pulping, or other positive method
(6) Written schedule information may be reproduced but only to the extent needed to carry out the state's official business.
(7) Newly enacted §147 of the Atomic Energy Act provides that a civil penalty can be assessed against a person who discloses schedule information without proper authorization or who fails to carry out the information protection requirements.

(The above requirements will be published in the *Federal Register* separately for public comment on their own merits. They are described here so that members of the public may comment more effectively on the proposed amendments to 10 CFR 73.37.)

Once the information protection arrangements are established within a state, a typical notification could be carried out as follows. Notification would be made to the governor shortly before the shipment is to be made. The notification would be by letter, with a "protected" enclosure. All information not protected under the provisions of §147 would be set forth in the body of the letter. The body of the letter would also contain a paragraph stating that the enclosure is protected from disclosure by law and that there is substantial civil penalty for unauthorized disclosure. The protected enclosure would be contained in a separate, sealed envelope appropriately identified. This practice would permit the basic letter to be opened by persons outside of the authorized chain of individuals who would need to know the protected information, without violation of §147 and implementing regulations. The letter with its unopened "protected" enclosure could then be passed on to those persons authorized to receive it.

A volume of protected information would likely accumulate in the absence of an information downgrading system. Downgrading of schedule information appears to be justified because the value of the information to an adversary declines after a shipment or series of shipments is completed. The NRC therefore proposes requirements that automatically downgrade schedule information 10 days after a one-of-a-kind shipment departs a state or 10 days after the last shipment of a series of related shipments departs the state. Downgraded schedule information need not be protected.

Proposed Rule

Pursuant to the Atomic Energy Act of 1954, as amended, the Energy Reorganization Act of 1974, as amended, and sections 552 and 553 of Title 5 of the United States Code, notice is hereby given that adoption of the following amendments to 10 CFR Part 73 is contemplated. Section 73.37 is amended by adding paragraphs (f) and (g) to read as follows:

§73.37 Requirements for physical protection of irradiated reactor fuel in transit

(f) Prior to the transport of spent fuel within or through a state a licensee subject to this section shall notify the governor. The licensee shall comply with the following criteria in regard to a notification:

(1) The notification must be in writing and sent to the office of each appropriate governor. A notification delivered by mail must be postmarked at least 7 days before transport of a shipment within or through the state. A notification delivered by messenger must reach the office of the governor at least 4 days before transport of a shipment within or through the state. A list of the mailing addresses of governors is available upon request from the Director, Office of State Programs, U.S. Nuclear Regulatory Commission, Washington, D.C. 20555.

(2) The notification must include the following information:

(i) A listing of the routes to be used within or through the state.
(ii) Identification of the shipper, the receiver, and the carrier(s).
(iii) A description of the shipment as specified by the Department of Transportation in 49 CFR 172.202 and 172.203(d).
(iv) A statement that the information described below in §73.37(f)(3) is required by NRC regulation to be protected in accordance with the requirements of §73.21.

(3) The licensee shall provide the following information on a separate enclosure to the written notification:

(i) The estimated date and time of departure from the point of origin of the shipment.
(ii) The estimated date and time of entry into the governor's state.
(iii) For the case of a single shipment whose schedule is not related to the schedule of any subsequent shipment, a statement that schedule information must be protected in accordance with the provisions of §73.21 until at least 10 days after the shipment has departed the state.
(iv) For the case of a shipment in a series of shipments whose schedules are related, a statement that schedule information must be protected in accordance with the provisions of §73.21 until 10 days after the last shipment in the series has departed the state and an estimate of the date on which the last shipment in the series will enter the state.

(4) A licensee shall notify a responsible individual in the office of the governor of any schedule change that differs by more than 6 hr from the schedule information previously furnished to a governor in accordance with §73.37(f)(3), and shall inform that individual of the number of hours of advance or delay relative to the written schedule information previously furnished.

(g) State officials, state employees, and other individuals, whether or not licensees of the Commission, who receive schedule information of the kind specified in §73.37(f)(3) shall protect that information against unauthorized disclosure as specified in §73.21.

(Secs. 53, 147, 161b, 161i, 161o, Pub. L. 83-703, 68 Stat. 930, 948, 949, sec. 201, Pub. L. 93-438, 88 Stat. 1242-1243, sec. 207 Pub. L. 96-295, 94 Stat. 780 (42 U.S.C. 2073, 2201, 5841))

Dated at Washington, D.C. this 2nd day of December, 1980. For the U.S. Nuclear Regulatory Commission. Samuel J. Chilk, Secretary of the Commission.

INDEX

A

D

E

F

G

H

I

J

K

L

M

N

O

P

Q

R

U

V

W

X

Y

Z